Netter's Clinical Anatomy

John T. Hansen, PhD
Associate Dean for Admissions
Professor of Neurobiology and Anatomy
University of Rochester School of
Medicine and Dentistry

David R. Lambert, MD
Associate Dean for Undergraduate Medical Education
Associate Professor of Medicine
University of Rochester School of
Medicine and Dentistry

Illustrations by Frank H. Netter, MD

Contributing Illustrators

John A. Craig, MD
Carlos A.G. Machado, MD
James A. Perkins, MS, MFA

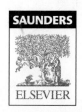

SAUNDERS

ELSEVIER

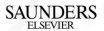

SAUNDERS
ELSEVIER

Published by Saunders, an imprint of Elsevier, Inc. Copyright © 2008 Elsevier Inc.
1600 John F. Kennedy Boulevard
Suite 1800
Philadelphia, PA 19103-2899

FIRST EDITION

ISBN-13: 978-1-929007-71-4
ISBN-10: 1-929007-71-X
Library of Congress Catalog No.: 2005920964

NOTICE

Medicine is an ever-changing field. Standard safety precautions must be followed,
but as new research and clinical experience broaden our knowledge, changes in
treatment and drug therapy may become necessary or appropriate. Readers
are advised to check the most current product information provided by the
manufacturer of each drug to be administered to verify the recommended dose,
the method and duration of administration, and contraindications. It is the
responsibility of the treating physician, relying on experience and knowledge of the
patient, to determine dosages and the best treatment for each individual patient.
Neither the Publisher nor the editor assume any liability for any injury and/or
damage to persons or property arising from this publication.

The Publisher

Printed in the U.S.A.

Tables on the following pages have been modified with permission from materials
contained in Hansen JT. *Essential Anatomy Dissection.* 2nd ed. Philadelphia, Pa.: Lippincott Williams & Wilkins; 2002: 531, 544, 557, 595, 608, 620, 622, 632.

10   9   8   7   6   5   4   3   2   1

We dedicate this book to our children,
Amy and Sean,
and
Remy, Siobhan, and Aurore;
and to our spouses,
Paula and Andrea.
Without their unconditional love and encouragement, little would
have been accomplished either professionally or personally.

About the Authors

John T. Hansen, PhD, is Professor and Associate Chair for Education in Neurobiology and Anatomy, Associate Dean for Admissions, and Director of Curriculum Development in the Offices of Medical Education at the University of Rochester School of Medicine and Dentistry. Dr. Hansen served as Chair of the Department of Neurobiology and Anatomy before becoming Associate Dean. Dr. Hansen is the recipient of numerous teaching awards from students at three different medical schools. In 1999, he was the recipient of The Alpha Omega Alpha Robert J. Glaser Distinguished Teacher Award given annually by the Association of American Medical Colleges to nationally recognized medical educators. Dr. Hansen's investigative career encompasses research of the peripheral chemoreceptor system, paraneurons, and neural plasticity and inflammation. He is coauthor of *Netter's Atlas of Human Physiology*, consulting editor of *Atlas of Human Anatomy*, third edition, author of *Essential Anatomy Dissector*, and consultant on the CD-ROM *Netter Presenter Human Anatomy Collection*.

David R. Lambert, MD, is Associate Professor of Medicine and Associate Dean for Undergraduate Medical Education at the University of Rochester School of Medicine and Dentistry. In addition, he is Chief of General Medicine in the Department of Medicine at the University of Rochester Medical Center. Dr. Lambert has received several teaching awards from medical students and was named the Lawrence Young Dean's Teaching Scholar at Rochester in 1999. In addition to practicing general internal medicine, his professional focus has been on medical student and resident education, serving as Medicine Clerkship Director and Associate Program Director for the Internal Medicine Residency at Strong Memorial Hospital. He was on the development team for *MKSAP for Students 2* published by the American College of Physicians and is an editor of *Diagnostic Strategies for Common Medical Problems*.

Preface

Human anatomy is the foundation upon which the education of our medical, dental, and allied health science students is built. However, today's biomedical science curriculum must cover an ever-increasing body of scientific knowledge, often in fewer hours, as competing disciplines and new technologies covet a greater portion of the limited curricular hours. Many of these same technologies, especially those in the diagnostic imaging fields, have made understanding the anatomy even more important and moved the discipline into the realm of clinical medicine. It is fair to say that competent clinicians and allied health professionals can no longer simply view their anatomical training in isolation from the clinical implications related to that anatomy.

In this context, we are proud to introduce *Netter's Clinical Anatomy*. Generations of students have used Dr. Frank H. Netter's elegant anatomical illustrations to learn anatomy, and this book combines his beautiful anatomical and embryological renderings with numerous clinical illustrations to help students bridge the gap between normal anatomy and its clinical implications.

This book provides succinct text, tables, and bulleted points, which offer students and practitioners a quick reference and review of the essential normal anatomy and the more commonly encountered clinical conditions seen in practice. These clinical correlations are drawn from a wide variety of fields including emergency medicine, radiology, orthopedics, and general surgery, but also include clinical anatomy related to the fields of cardiology, endocrinology, infectious diseases, neurology, oncology, reproductive biology, and urology.

An introductory chapter designed to orient students to the body's organ systems, clinical correlations pages cross-referenced with the normal anatomy pages, and end-of-chapter review questions help to reinforce student learning.

Our intent in creating *Netter's Clinical Anatomy* was to provide a concise and focused introduction to clinical anatomy, an essential review for students beginning their clinical clerkships or elective programs, and a reference book that clinicians will find useful for review and patient education.

We hope that you, the health science student-in-training or the practicing physician, will find *Netter's Clinical Anatomy* the link you've searched for to enhance your understanding of clinical anatomy.

Acknowledgments

Compiling the illustrations and researching and writing *Netter's Clinical Anatomy* has been both enjoyable and educational, confirming again the importance of lifelong learning in the health professions. No sooner was it completed then we had to begin the process of updating and reviewing our original material. Such is the nature of a dynamic field like medicine.

Netter's Clinical Anatomy is for our students, and we are indebted to all of them, who, like us, yearn for a better view to help us learn the relevant anatomy that informs the practice of medicine.

Thanks and appreciation to our colleagues and reviewers, who provided encouragement and constructive comments that clarified many aspects of the book. Especially, we wish to acknowledge Lawrence Rizzolo, PhD, Department of Surgery, Yale University School of Medicine, for review of the anatomy and John Mahoney, MD, Department of Emergency Medicine, University of Pittsburgh, for review of the clinical correlations. Our hope is that their professional dedication and love of clinical anatomy are embodied in the illustrations and pages of *Netter's Clinical Anatomy*. We would also like to express our gratitude to William J. Swartz, PhD, Marilyn L. Zimny Professor of Anatomy, Department of Cell Biology and Anatomy, LSU Health Sciences Center; Thomas R. Gest, PhD, Associate Professor, Director – Medical Gross Anatomy, Director – Anatomical Donations Program, Division of Anatomical Sciences, University of Michigan Medical School; and Kenneth H. Jones, PhD, Director, Division of Anatomy, The Ohio State University, for their efforts to ensure the accuracy of this text.

At Icon Learning Systems, it has been a distinct pleasure to work with dedicated, professional people who massaged, molded, and ultimately nourished our dream beyond our wildest imaginations. The published "dream" before you owes much to the efforts of Jennifer Surich, Managing Editor, and Marybeth Thiel, Editorial Assistant, who kept us organized, focused, and on time. Thanks and appreciation go to Colleen Quinn, Graphic Designer, Melanie Peirson Johnstone, Layout and Production, Mary Ellen Curry, Director of Manufacturing, Greg Otis, Editorial Director, and Joan Caldwell, Marketing Manager. We owe a big thank you to Judy Gandy, Developmental Editor, who, with patience and persistence, asked the right questions and taught us how to write the English language with clarity and conciseness.

Special thanks go to Jim Perkins, John A. Craig, MD, and Carlos A.G. Machado, MD, for their beautiful artistic renderings. Their work nicely complemented, updated, and supplemented the original Netter illustrations. Jonathan Dimes, Art Director, kept on top of all of the illustrative material, and his keen eye for perspective and design elements are a tribute to his own abilities as a medical illustrator. Without a doubt, Icon's medical illustration team is first-rate.

A very special thank you to Paul Kelly, Executive Editor, who kept our dream alive and continues to appreciate the importance of clarity and the visual image to teach. While Paul has never taught a medical student, thousands of health science students worldwide owe him a debt of gratitude for shepherding numerous Netter publications through the gauntlet, from vague idea to published reality.

Finally, we remain indebted to Frank H. Netter, MD, whose creative genius lives on in generations of biomedical professionals who have learned clinical anatomy from his rich collection of medical illustrations.

To all of these remarkable people, and others: thank you.

Contents

Table of Clinical Correlations

Table of Clinical Correlations

CHAPTER 4   LOWER LIMB

Table of Clinical Correlations

CHAPTER 5 THORAX

Table of Clinical Correlations

CHAPTER 6 **ABDOMEN**

Table of Clinical Correlations

CHAPTER 7   PELVIS AND PERINEUM

Table of Clinical Correlations

CHAPTER 8 **HEAD AND NECK**

Table of Clinical Correlations

Introduction

Introduction The study of anatomy requires a clinical vocabulary that defines position, movements, relationships, and planes of reference and describes the systems of the human body. This chapter introduces the essential terminology and the body's systems to prepare you for the clinical anatomy that follows.

Terminology: Anatomical Position

By convention, anatomical descriptions of the human body are based on a person in anatomical position:

- Standing erect, facing forward
- Arms hanging at the sides, palms facing forward
- Legs placed together, feet directed forward

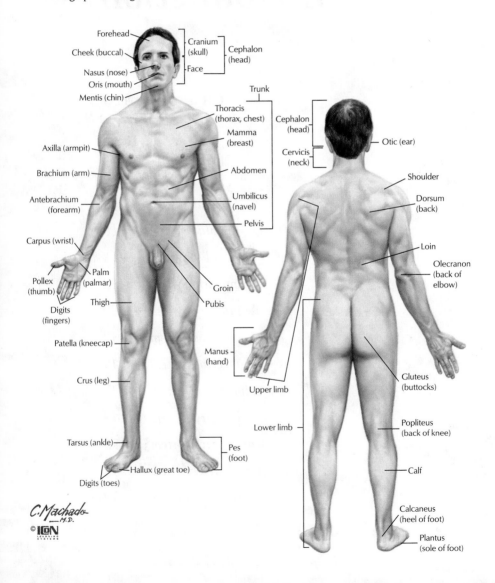

Forehead
Cheek (buccal)
Nasus (nose)
Oris (mouth)
Mentis (chin)
Cranium (skull)
Face
Cephalon (head)
Trunk
Thoracis (thorax, chest)
Mamma (breast)
Cephalon (head)
Cervicis (neck)
Otic (ear)
Axilla (armpit)
Brachium (arm)
Abdomen
Shoulder
Antebrachium (forearm)
Umbilicus (navel)
Dorsum (back)
Pelvis
Carpus (wrist)
Loin
Pollex (thumb)
Palm (palmar)
Groin
Olecranon (back of elbow)
Thigh
Pubis
Digits (fingers)
Patella (kneecap)
Manus (hand)
Gluteus (buttocks)
Crus (leg)
Upper limb
Popliteus (back of knee)
Lower limb
Tarsus (ankle)
Pes (foot)
Calf
Hallux (great toe)
Digits (toes)
Calcaneus (heel of foot)
Plantus (sole of foot)

C. Machado
—M.D.

© ICN

Terminology: Terms of Relationship and Body Planes

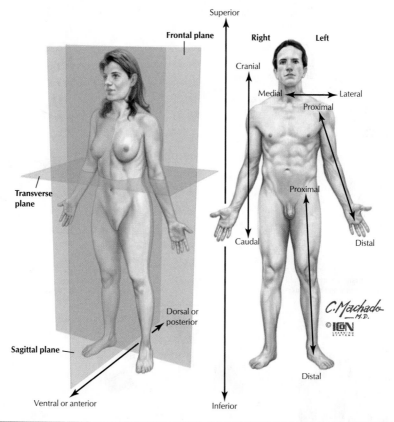

TERM	DESCRIPTION
Anterior (ventral)	Nearer the front
Posterior (dorsal)	Nearer the back
Superior (cranial)	Upward or nearer the head
Inferior (caudal)	Downward or nearer the feet
Medial	Toward the midline or median plane
Lateral	Farther from the midline or median plane
Proximal	Near a reference point
Distal	Away from a reference point
Superficial	Closer to the surface
Deep	Farther from the surface
Median plane	Divides body into equal right and left halves
Midsagittal plane	Median plane
Sagittal plane	Divides body into unequal right and left halves
Frontal (coronal) plane	Divides body into equal or unequal anterior and posterior parts
Transverse plane	Divides body into equal or unequal superior and inferior parts (cross sections)

Terminology: Terms of Movement

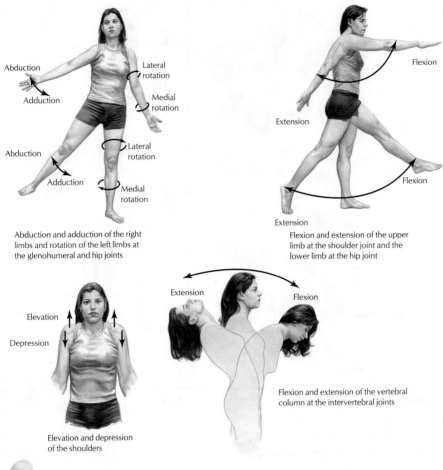

Abduction and adduction of the right limbs and rotation of the left limbs at the glenohumeral and hip joints

Flexion and extension of the upper limb at the shoulder joint and the lower limb at the hip joint

Elevation and depression of the shoulders

Flexion and extension of the vertebral column at the intervertebral joints

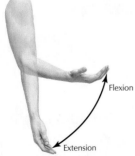

Flexion and extension of the forearm at the elbow joint

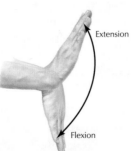

Flexion and extension of the hand at the wrist joint

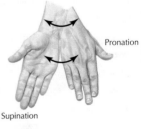

Pronation and supination of the forearm at the radioulnar joints

C. Machado M.D.

© ICN
LEARNING SYSTEMS

Terminology: Terms of Movement (continued)

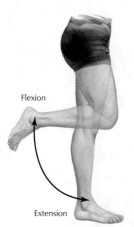

Flexion

Extension

Flexion and extension of the leg
at the knee joint

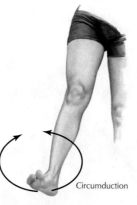

Circumduction

Circumduction (circular movement)
of the lower limb at the hip joint

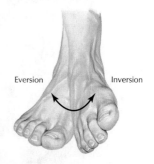

Eversion

Inversion

Inversion and eversion of the foot at
the subtalar and transverse tarsal joints

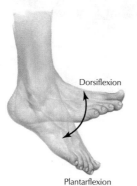

Dorsiflexion

Plantarflexion

Dorsiflexion and plantarflexion of
the foot at the ankle joint

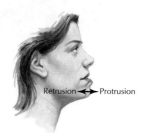

Retrusion ◄──► Protrusion

Protrusion and retrusion of the jaw
at the temporomandibular joints

C. Machado
—M.D.

© ICN

Skin

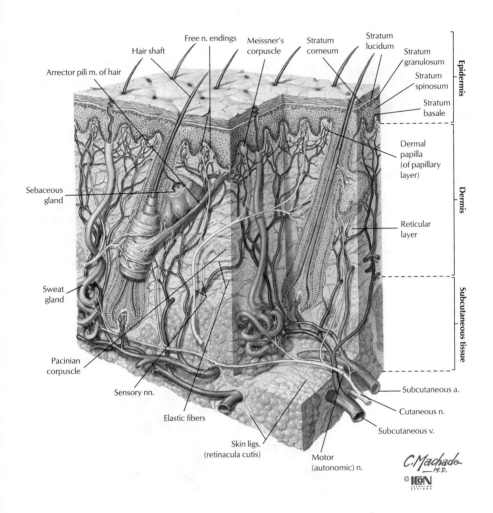

Arrector pili m. of hair — Hair shaft — Free n. endings — Meissner's corpuscle — Stratum corneum — Stratum lucidum — Stratum granulosum — Stratum spinosum — Stratum basale — Epidermis — Dermal papilla (of papillary layer) — Reticular layer — Dermis — Subcutaneous tissue — Sebaceous gland — Sweat gland — Pacinian corpuscle — Sensory nn. — Elastic fibers — Skin ligs. (retinacula cutis) — Motor (autonomic) n. — Subcutaneous a. — Cutaneous n. — Subcutaneous v.

C. Machado, M.D.

© ICON LEARNING SYSTEMS

The skin is the largest organ in the body and functions in protection (against mechanical abrasion and in immune responses); temperature regulation (via vasodilatation and vasoconstriction and by sweat glands); and sensations of touch (mechanoreceptors such as pacinian and Meissner's corpuscles), pain (nociceptors), and temperature (thermoreceptors). The skin consists of two layers: the epidermis, the outer protective layer composed of a specialized epithelium that varies in thickness depending on body region, and the dermis, the deeper layer of dense connective tissue that contains capillaries, specialized receptors and nerves, pigment and immune cells, sweat glands, hair follicles, sebaceous (oil) glands, and smooth muscle.

Clinical Correlation

Psoriasis
Anatomy on p. 6

Histopathologic features

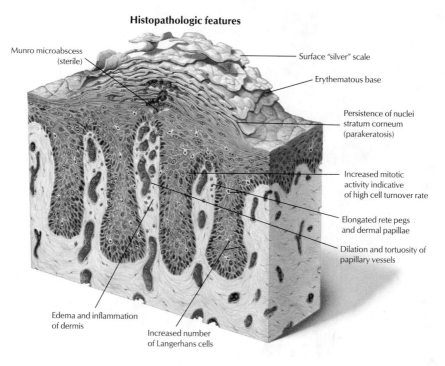

Munro microabscess (sterile)

Surface "silver" scale

Erythematous base

Persistence of nuclei stratum corneum (parakeratosis)

Increased mitotic activity indicative of high cell turnover rate

Elongated rete pegs and dermal papillae

Dilation and tortuosity of papillary vessels

Edema and inflammation of dermis

Increased number of Langerhans cells

Typical distribution

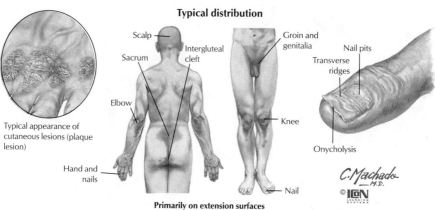

Typical appearance of cutaneous lesions (plaque lesion)

Scalp

Intergluteal cleft

Sacrum

Elbow

Hand and nails

Groin and genitalia

Nail pits

Transverse ridges

Knee

Onycholysis

Nail

Primarily on extension surfaces

C. Machado, M.D.

© IGN LEARNING SYSTEMS

Psoriasis, a chronic inflammatory skin disorder, affects women and men equally (approximately 1-3% of the population) and is characterized by defined red plaques, capped with a surface scale of desquamated epidermis. Although the pathogenesis of the disease is unknown, a genetic predisposition seems to be involved.

Clinical Correlation

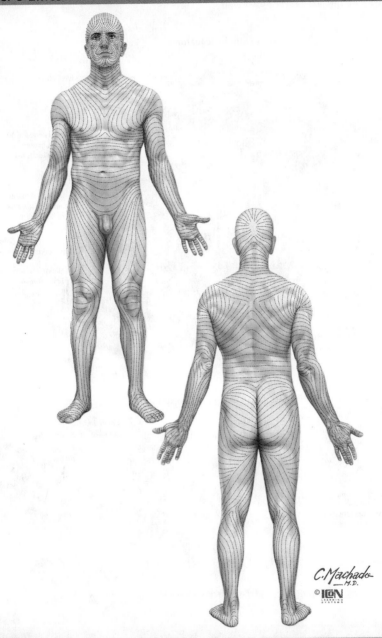

Collagen in the skin creates tension lines (Langer's lines) and, when possible, surgeons use these lines to make skin incisions. The resulting wounds have a tendency to gape less and usually leave a smaller scar after healing.

Skeletal System: Axial and Appendicular Skeleton

The skeleton is divided into two descriptive regions:
Axial skeleton: bones of the skull, vertebral column (spine), ribs, and sternum
Appendicular skeleton: bones of the limbs, including pectoral and pelvic girdles

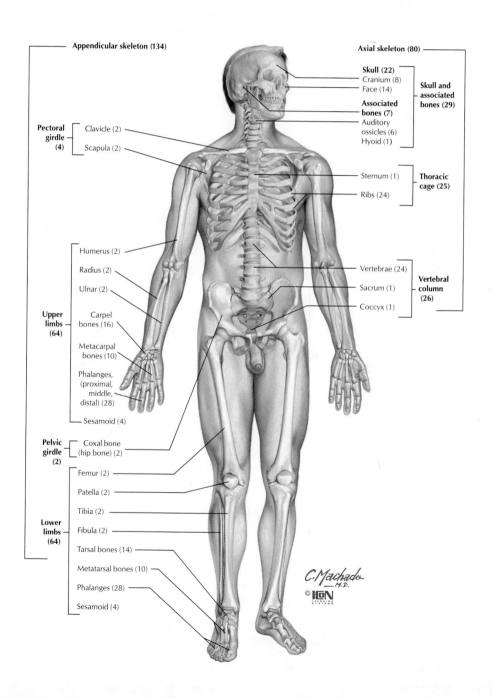

Appendicular skeleton (134)

Axial skeleton (80)

Skull (22)
Cranium (8)
Face (14)

Associated bones (7)
Auditory ossicles (6)
Hyoid (1)

Skull and associated bones (29)

Pectoral girdle (4)
Clavicle (2)
Scapula (2)

Sternum (1)
Ribs (24)

Thoracic cage (25)

Humerus (2)
Radius (2)
Ulnar (2)

Vertebrae (24)
Sacrum (1)
Coccyx (1)

Vertebral column (26)

Upper limbs (64)
Carpel bones (16)
Metacarpal bones (10)
Phalanges, (proximal, middle, distal) (28)
Sesamoid (4)

Pelvic girdle (2)
Coxal bone (hip bone) (2)

Lower limbs (64)
Femur (2)
Patella (2)
Tibia (2)
Fibula (2)
Tarsal bones (14)
Metatarsal bones (10)
Phalanges (28)
Sesamoid (4)

C. Machado
—M.D.
©ICON
LEARNING SYSTEMS

Skeletal System: Functions and Shapes of Bones

The skeletal system is composed of a living, dynamic, rigid connective tissue that forms the bones and cartilages of the human skeleton. Humans usually have approximately 214 bones (this number varies somewhat). Cartilage is attached to some bones, especially where flexibility is important, or covers the surfaces of some bones at points of articulation. Individual bones may be classified by their shape.

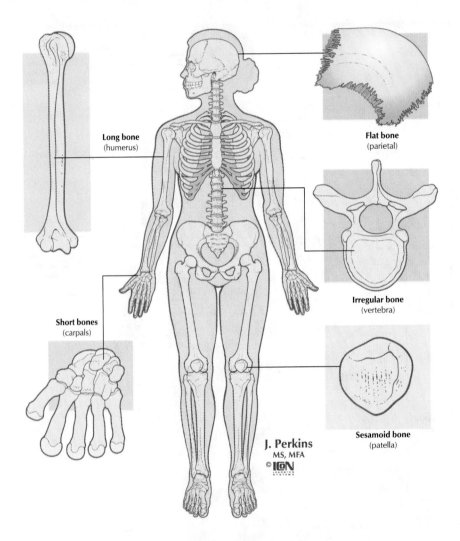

Long bone
(humerus)

Flat bone
(parietal)

Irregular bone
(vertebra)

Short bones
(carpals)

Sesamoid bone
(patella)

J. Perkins
MS, MFA
©ICN

Ninety-nine percent of the body's calcium is stored in bones. Many bones possess a central cavity that contains the bone marrow, a collection of hemopoietic (blood-forming) cells. Functions of the skeletal system and bones include

- Supporting the body
- Protecting vital tissues and organs
- Providing a mechanism for movement
- Storing calcium
- Providing a supply of blood cells

Skeletal System: Endochondral Bone Formation

Bones develop in one of two ways:

Intramembranous formation: Most flat bones develop in this way, by direct calcium deposition into a mesenchymal plate (precursor of the bone).

Endochondral formation: Most long bones develop by calcium deposition into a cartilaginous model of the bone that provides a scaffold for future bone.

The illustration shows growth and ossification of a long bone (humerus, midfrontal sections).

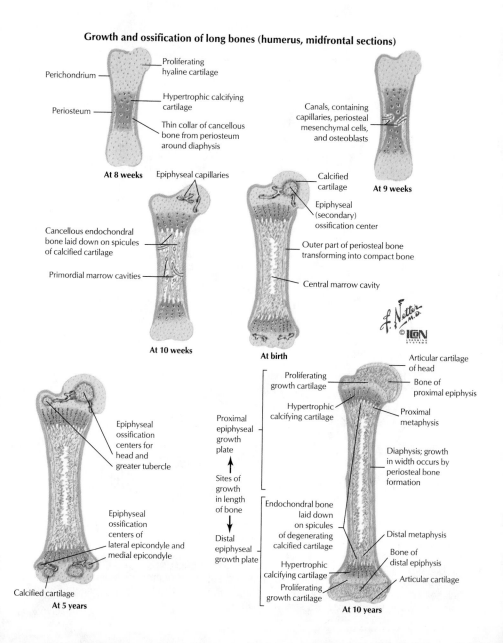

Growth and ossification of long bones (humerus, midfrontal sections)

Perichondrium — Proliferating hyaline cartilage

Periosteum — Hypertrophic calcifying cartilage

Thin collar of cancellous bone from periosteum around diaphysis

At 8 weeks   Epiphyseal capillaries

Canals, containing capillaries, periosteal mesenchymal cells, and osteoblasts

At 9 weeks

Cancellous endochondral bone laid down on spicules of calcified cartilage

Primordial marrow cavities

Calcified cartilage

Epiphyseal (secondary) ossification center

Outer part of periosteal bone transforming into compact bone

Central marrow cavity

At 10 weeks

At birth

Articular cartilage of head

Bone of proximal epiphysis

Proliferating growth cartilage

Hypertrophic calcifying cartilage

Proximal metaphysis

Proximal epiphyseal growth plate

Epiphyseal ossification centers for head and greater tubercle

Diaphysis; growth in width occurs by periosteal bone formation

Sites of growth in length of bone

Endochondral bone laid down on spicules of degenerating calcified cartilage

Distal metaphysis

Distal epiphyseal growth plate

Epiphyseal ossification centers of lateral epicondyle and medial epicondyle

Bone of distal epiphysis

Hypertrophic calcifying cartilage

Articular cartilage

Proliferating growth cartilage

Calcified cartilage

At 5 years

At 10 years

Clinical Correlation

Anatomy on pp. 9, 10

Fractures

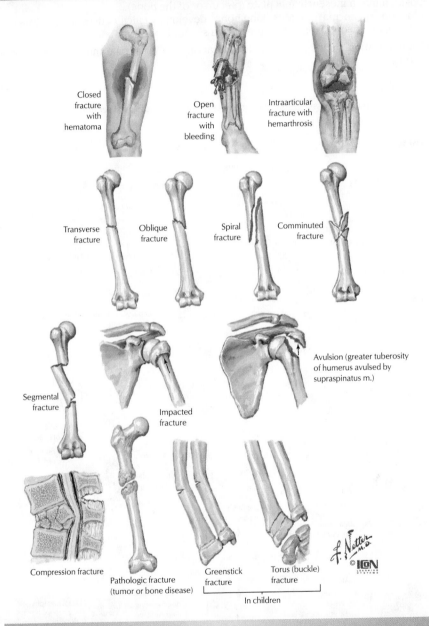

Closed fracture with hematoma

Open fracture with bleeding

Intraarticular fracture with hemarthrosis

Transverse fracture

Oblique fracture

Spiral fracture

Comminuted fracture

Segmental fracture

Impacted fracture

Avulsion (greater tuberosity of humerus avulsed by supraspinatus m.)

Compression fracture

Pathologic fracture (tumor or bone disease)

Greenstick fracture

Torus (buckle) fracture

In children

Fractures are classified as either closed (skin intact) or open (skin perforated). Whether fractures are compound or not is a separate distinction. One can have a closed compound fracture or an open simple fracture. The designations compound, simple, spiral, transverse, and so forth refer primarily to the bone.

Clinical Correlation

Bone Marrow Failure

Anatomy on pp. 11, 18

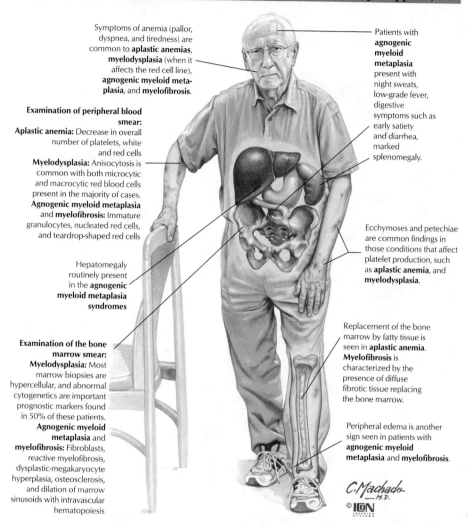

Symptoms of anemia (pallor, dyspnea, and tiredness) are common to **aplastic anemias**, **myelodysplasia** (when it affects the red cell line), **agnogenic myeloid metaplasia**, and **myelofibrosis**.

Patients with **agnogenic myeloid metaplasia** present with night sweats, low-grade fever, digestive symptoms such as early satiety and diarrhea, marked splenomegaly.

Examination of peripheral blood smear:
Aplastic anemia: Decrease in overall number of platelets, white and red cells
Myelodysplasia: Anisocytosis is common with both microcytic and macrocytic red blood cells present in the majority of cases.
Agnogenic myeloid metaplasia and **myelofibrosis:** Immature granulocytes, nucleated red cells, and teardrop-shaped red cells

Ecchymoses and petechiae are common findings in those conditions that affect platelet production, such as **aplastic anemia**, and **myelodysplasia**.

Hepatomegaly routinely present in the **agnogenic myeloid metaplasia syndromes**

Examination of the bone marrow smear:
Myelodysplasia: Most marrow biopsies are hypercellular, and abnormal cytogenetics are important prognostic markers found in 50% of these patients.
Agnogenic myeloid metaplasia and **myelofibrosis:** Fibroblasts, reactive myelofibrosis, dysplastic-megakaryocyte hyperplasia, osteosclerosis, and dilation of marrow sinusoids with intravascular hematopoiesis

Replacement of the bone marrow by fatty tissue is seen in **aplastic anemia**. **Myelofibrosis** is characterized by the presence of diffuse fibrotic tissue replacing the bone marrow.

Peripheral edema is another sign seen in patients with **agnogenic myeloid metaplasia** and **myelofibrosis**.

C. Machado, M.D.
© ICN

Bone marrow normally produces and stores a ready supply of blood cells for the circulatory system. Bone marrow failure is a condition that ultimately results in a decreased number of circulating blood cells and has many causes. On the basis of the histopathology of the bone marrow, this disease can be classified morphologically as

- **Aplastic anemia** (fatty bone marrow): decreased number of circulating platelets, white blood cells, and red blood cells
- **Myelodysplasia** (ineffective hematopoiesis): usually hypercellular bone marrow, but no cellular differentiation and maturation into mature blood cells
- **Agnogenic myeloid metaplasia and myelofibrosis** (fibrosis): bone marrow replaced by diffuse fibrotic tissue, with many immature cells present

Skeletal System: Types of Joints

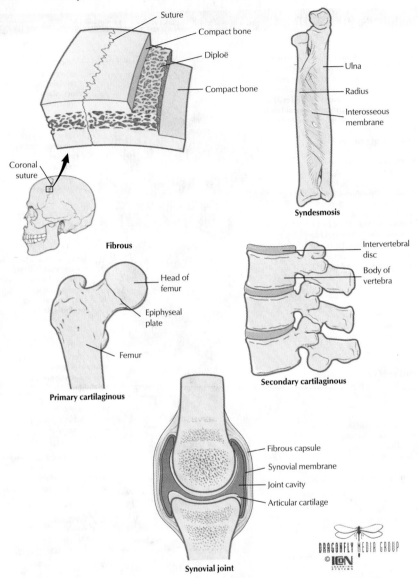

Adapted with permission from Moore K, Agur A. Essential Clinical Anatomy. 2nd ed. Philadelphia, Pa: Lippincott Williams & Wilkins; 2002.

Types of joints are

Fibrous (synarthroses): bones joined by fibrous connective tissue (sutures, syndesmoses, gomphoses)

Cartilaginous (amphiarthroses): bones joined by cartilage, or cartilage and fibrous tissue (primary [synchondrosis]; secondary [symphysis])

Synovial (diarthroses): bones joined by a joint cavity filled with synovial fluid and capsule with articular cartilage covering opposed surfaces (hinge, pivot, saddle, condyloid, plane, ball-and-socket)

Skeletal System: Types of Synovial Joints

Synovial joints generally allow considerable movement and are classified according to their shape and the type of movement that they permit (uniaxial, biaxial, or multiaxial movement):

Hinge (ginglymus): uniaxial joint for flexion and extension
Pivot (trachoid): uniaxial joint for rotation
Saddle: biaxial joint for flexion, extension, abduction, adduction, and circumduction
Condyloid (ellipsoid): biaxial joint for flexion, extension, abduction, adduction, and circumduction
Plane (gliding): joint for simple gliding movements
Ball-and-socket (spheroid): multiaxial joint for flexion, extension, abduction, adduction, medial and lateral rotation, and circumduction

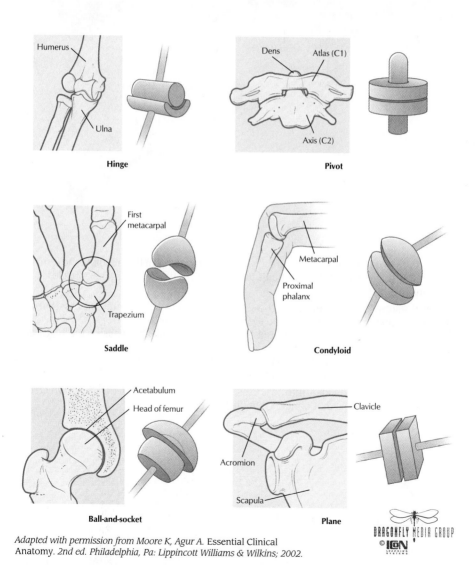

Adapted with permission from Moore K, Agur A. Essential Clinical Anatomy. *2nd ed. Philadelphia, Pa: Lippincott Williams & Wilkins; 2002.*

Muscular System: Structure of Skeletal Muscle

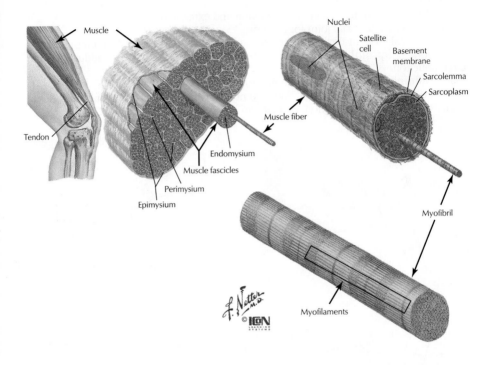

Muscle cells (fibers) produce contractions (shorten in length) that result in movements, changes in shape, or propulsion of fluids through hollow tissues or organs. Muscle is classified into three types:

Skeletal (simplistically referred to as voluntary muscle): striated fibers that are attached to bone and are responsible for movement of the skeleton
Cardiac (muscle of the heart): striated fibers that make up the walls of the heart and proximal portions of the great vessels
Smooth (simplistically referred to as involuntary muscle): unstriated fibers that line various organs, attach to hair follicles, and line blood vessels

Skeletal muscle is divided into fascicles (bundles) that consist of fibers, which are composed of myofibrils that contain myofilaments.

Muscular System: Skeletal Muscle Shapes

Skeletal muscle moves bones at their joints and possesses an origin (the muscle's fixed or proximal attachment) and an insertion (the muscle's moveable or distal attachment). Skeletal muscle appears striated under the microscope and can be classified on the basis of gross shape:

Flat: parallel fibers
Quadrate: four sides
Circular: sphincter
Fusiform: thick center and tapered ends
Pennate: feathered appearance

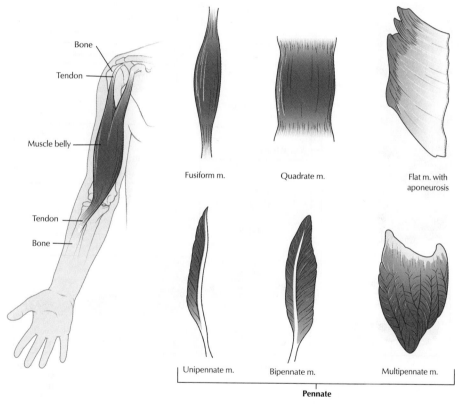

Bone

Tendon

Muscle belly

Tendon

Bone

Fusiform m.

Quadrate m.

Flat m. with aponeurosis

Unipennate m.

Bipennate m.

Multipennate m.

Pennate

Cardiovascular System: Composition of Blood

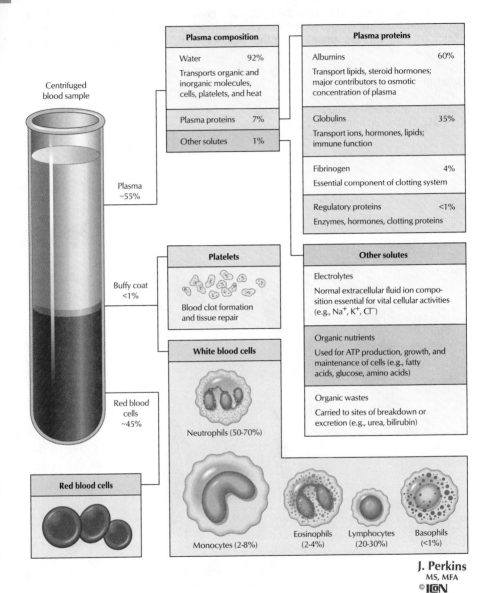

Centrifuged blood sample

Plasma ~55%

Buffy coat <1%

Red blood cells ~45%

Red blood cells

Plasma composition

Water	92%
Transports organic and inorganic molecules, cells, platelets, and heat	
Plasma proteins	7%
Other solutes	1%

Plasma proteins

Albumins	60%
Transport lipids, steroid hormones; major contributors to osmotic concentration of plasma	
Globulins	35%
Transport ions, hormones, lipids; immune function	
Fibrinogen	4%
Essential component of clotting system	
Regulatory proteins	<1%
Enzymes, hormones, clotting proteins	

Platelets

Blood clot formation and tissue repair

Other solutes

Electrolytes

Normal extracellular fluid ion composition essential for vital cellular activities (e.g., Na^+, K^+, Cl^-)

Organic nutrients

Used for ATP production, growth, and maintenance of cells (e.g., fatty acids, glucose, amino acids)

Organic wastes

Carried to sites of breakdown or excretion (e.g., urea, bilirubin)

White blood cells

Neutrophils (50-70%)

Monocytes (2-8%)

Eosinophils (2-4%)

Lymphocytes (20-30%)

Basophils (<1%)

J. Perkins
MS, MFA
© ION

Blood consists of formed elements: platelets, white and red blood cells, and plasma. Functions of the blood include
- Transport of dissolved gases, nutrients, metabolic waste products, and hormones to and from tissues
- Prevention of fluid loss via clotting mechanisms
- Immune defense activities
- Regulation of pH and electrolyte balance
- Thermoregulation (via vessel constriction and dilation)

Clinical Correlation

Leukemias

Anatomy on pp. 11, 18

Clinical presentation of leukemias

Acute myeloid leukemia (AML), acute lymphoblastic leukemia (ALL), chronic myelogenous leukemia (CML), and chronic lymphocytic leukemia (CLL)

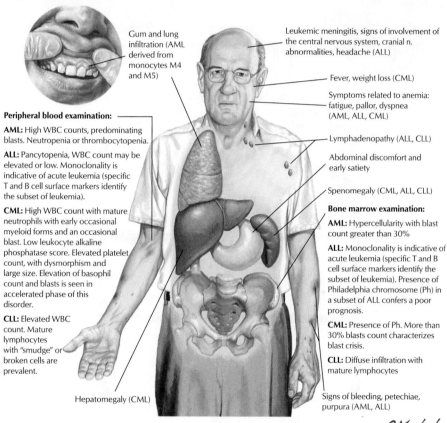

Gum and lung infiltration (AML derived from monocytes M4 and M5)

Leukemic meningitis, signs of involvement of the central nervous system, cranial n. abnormalities, headache (ALL)

Fever, weight loss (CML)

Symptoms related to anemia: fatigue, pallor, dyspnea (AML, ALL, CML)

Peripheral blood examination:

AML: High WBC counts, predominating blasts. Neutropenia or thrombocytopenia.

ALL: Pancytopenia, WBC count may be elevated or low. Monoclonality is indicative of acute leukemia (specific T and B cell surface markers identify the subset of leukemia).

CML: High WBC count with mature neutrophils with early occasional myeloid forms and an occasional blast. Low leukocyte alkaline phosphatase score. Elevated platelet count, with dysmorphism and large size. Elevation of basophil count and blasts is seen in accelerated phase of this disorder.

CLL: Elevated WBC count. Mature lymphocytes with "smudge" or broken cells are prevalent.

Lymphadenopathy (ALL, CLL)

Abdominal discomfort and early satiety

Spenomegaly (CML, ALL, CLL)

Bone marrow examination:

AML: Hypercellularity with blast count greater than 30%

ALL: Monoclonality is indicative of acute leukemia (specific T and B cell surface markers identify the subset of leukemia). Presence of Philadelphia chromosome (Ph) in a subset of ALL confers a poor prognosis.

CML: Presence of Ph. More than 30% blasts count characterizes blast crisis.

CLL: Diffuse infiltration with mature lymphocytes

Hepatomegaly (CML)

Signs of bleeding, petechiae, purpura (AML, ALL)

C.Machado
—M.D.

©ICN

The leukemias are a group of clinical disorders caused by neoplastic transformation of bone marrow stem cell progenitors that results in abnormal accumulation of white blood cells in bone marrow and often in circulating blood. Leukemias affect both children and adults, may arise from lymphoid or myeloid cells, and are termed acute when numerous immature or blast cells are present and chronic when these cells differentiate and mature.

Cardiovascular System: Organization

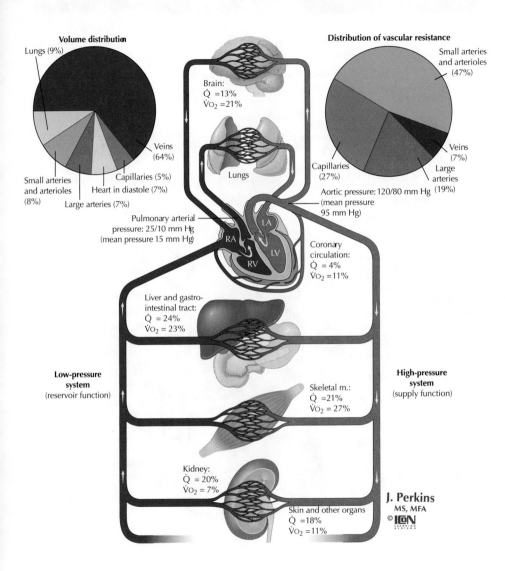

Volume distribution
Lungs (9%)
Veins (64%)
Small arteries and arterioles (8%)
Capillaries (5%)
Heart in diastole (7%)
Large arteries (7%)

Distribution of vascular resistance
Small arteries and arterioles (47%)
Veins (7%)
Capillaries (27%)
Large arteries (19%)
Aortic pressure: 120/80 mm Hg (mean pressure 95 mm Hg)

Brain:
$\dot{Q} = 13\%$
$\dot{V}O_2 = 21\%$

Lungs

Pulmonary arterial pressure: 25/10 mm Hg (mean pressure 15 mm Hg)

LA
RA
LV
RV

Coronary circulation:
$\dot{Q} = 4\%$
$\dot{V}O_2 = 11\%$

Liver and gastro-intestinal tract:
$\dot{Q} = 24\%$
$\dot{V}O_2 = 23\%$

Low-pressure system (reservoir function)

High-pressure system (supply function)

Skeletal m.:
$\dot{Q} = 21\%$
$\dot{V}O_2 = 27\%$

Kidney:
$\dot{Q} = 20\%$
$\dot{V}O_2 = 7\%$

Skin and other organs
$\dot{Q} = 18\%$
$\dot{V}O_2 = 11\%$

J. Perkins
MS, MFA
© ICN
LEARNING SYSTEMS

The cardiovascular system consists of the heart, which pumps blood into the pulmonary circulation for gas exchange and into the systemic circulation to supply body tissues, and the vessels carrying blood: arteries, arterioles, capillaries, and veins. At rest, cardiac output is approximately 5 L/min in both pulmonary and systemic circulations. The amount of blood flow per minute ($\dot{Q}$) (as percent cardiac output) and relative percent oxygen used per minute ($\dot{V}O_2$) in various organ systems are shown for the resting state. At any time point, most blood (64%) resides in the veins and is returned to the right side of the heart. Vascular resistance is mainly a function of the small muscular arteries and arterioles.

Clinical Correlation

Major Arteries and Pulse Points   *Anatomy on p. 20*

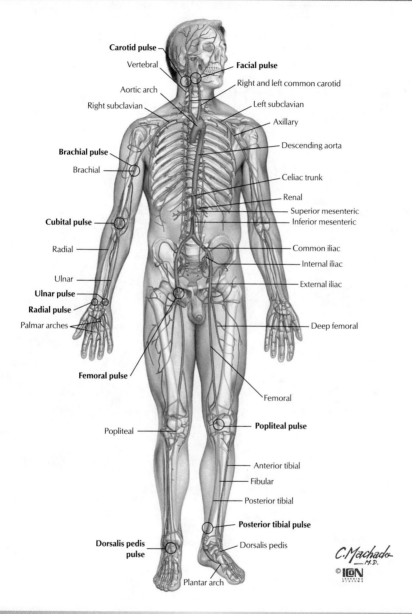

Carotid pulse
Vertebral
Aortic arch
Right subclavian
Brachial pulse
Brachial
Cubital pulse
Radial
Ulnar
Ulnar pulse
Radial pulse
Palmar arches
Femoral pulse
Popliteal
Dorsalis pedis pulse

Facial pulse
Right and left common carotid
Left subclavian
Axillary
Descending aorta
Celiac trunk
Renal
Superior mesenteric
Inferior mesenteric
Common iliac
Internal iliac
External iliac
Deep femoral
Femoral
Popliteal pulse
Anterior tibial
Fibular
Posterior tibial
Posterior tibial pulse
Dorsalis pedis
Plantar arch

C. Machado
M.D.

©ICN
LEARNING
SYSTEMS

At certain points along the pathway of the systemic arterial circulation, large and medium-sized arteries lie near the body's surface and can be used to take a pulse (via compressing an artery against a hard underlying structure, usually a bone). The most distal pulse (farthest from the heart) is usually that taken by using the dorsalis pedis artery on the dorsum of the foot or the posterior tibial artery medial to the ankle.

Clinical Correlation

Atherogenesis

Anatomy on pp. 18, 21, 25

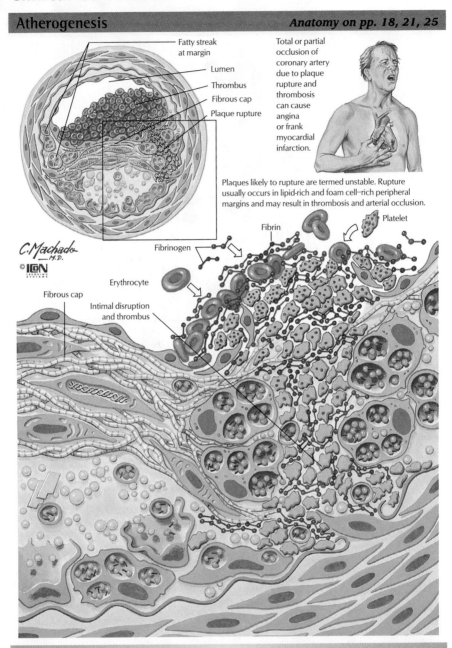

Fatty streak at margin

Lumen

Thrombus

Fibrous cap

Plaque rupture

Total or partial occlusion of coronary artery due to plaque rupture and thrombosis can cause angina or frank myocardial infarction.

Plaques likely to rupture are termed unstable. Rupture usually occurs in lipid-rich and foam cell-rich peripheral margins and may result in thrombosis and arterial occlusion.

Fibrin

Platelet

Fibrinogen

Erythrocyte

Fibrous cap

Intimal disruption and thrombus

C. Machado
M.D.

© ICN

Thickening and narrowing of the arterial wall and eventual deposition of lipid into the wall can lead to one form of atherosclerosis. The narrowed artery may not be able to meet metabolic needs of adjacent tissues, with the danger that they may become ischemic. Multiple factors, including focal inflammation of the arterial wall, may result in this condition. When development of plaque is such that it is likely to rupture and lead to thrombosis and arterial occlusion, the atherogenic process is termed unstable plaque formation, as illustrated.

Cardiovascular System: Major Veins

Veins are vessels that transport blood to the heart. Veins are capacitance vessels because they are easily distensible and can serve as reservoirs; they are often quite variable compared with arteries and usually occur as multiple vessels accompanying a single artery. Because veins carry blood at a low pressure and often against gravity, larger veins of the limbs and lower neck region have valves that aid venous return. Both the valves and the contractions of the adjacent skeletal muscles help to pump venous blood against gravity and toward the heart. In most of the body, veins occur as a superficial set in the subcutaneous tissue that connects to a deeper set, which often parallels arteries. During strenuous exercise, muscle contraction compresses thin-walled, low-pressure veins, which shunts venous blood to superficial veins. Blood then returns to the heart for recirculation. Types of veins include

Venules: collect blood from capillary beds
Veins: medium-sized to large vessels
Portal venous systems: veins that transport blood between two capillary beds, e.g., hepatic portal system

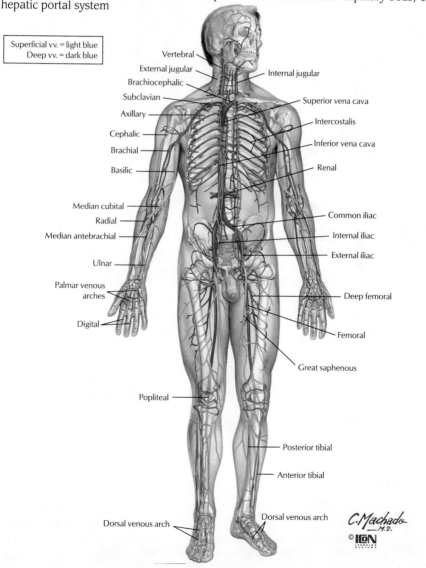

Superficial vv. = light blue
Deep vv. = dark blue

Vertebral
External jugular
Brachiocephalic
Subclavian
Axillary
Cephalic
Brachial
Basilic
Median cubital
Radial
Median antebrachial
Ulnar
Palmar venous arches
Digital
Popliteal
Dorsal venous arch

Internal jugular
Superior vena cava
Intercostalis
Inferior vena cava
Renal
Common iliac
Internal iliac
External iliac
Deep femoral
Femoral
Great saphenous
Posterior tibial
Anterior tibial
Dorsal venous arch

C. Machado
—M.D.
© ION
LEARNING SYSTEMS

Clinical Correlation

Varicose Veins

Anatomy on pp. 20, 23

Clinical features

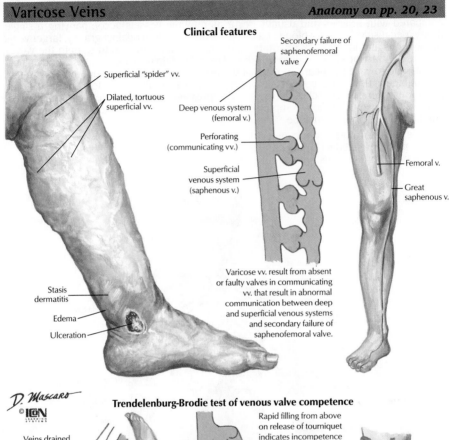

Secondary failure of saphenofemoral valve

Superficial "spider" vv.

Dilated, tortuous superficial vv.

Deep venous system (femoral v.)

Perforating (communicating vv.)

Superficial venous system (saphenous v.)

Femoral v.

Great saphenous v.

Stasis dermatitis

Edema

Ulceration

Varicose vv. result from absent or faulty valves in communicating vv. that result in abnormal communication between deep and superficial venous systems and secondary failure of saphenofemoral valve.

D. Mascaro
©ICN

Trendelenburg-Brodie test of venous valve competence

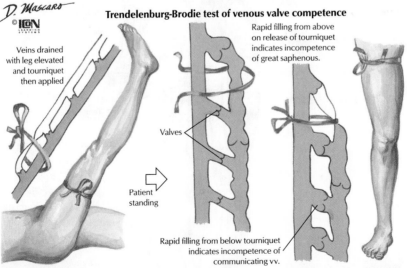

Rapid filling from above on release of tourniquet indicates incompetence of great saphenous.

Veins drained with leg elevated and tourniquet then applied

Valves

Patient standing

Rapid filling from below tourniquet indicates incompetence of communicating vv.

Walls of veins adjacent to the valves can become weakened and distended, thus compromising the ability of both the valve to work properly and the vein to facilitate return of blood toward the heart. Such veins are called varicose (enlarged and tortuous). This condition occurs most often in veins of the lower extremities.

Cardiovascular System: Heart

The heart is a hollow muscular organ that is divided into four chambers:

Right atrium: receives blood from the systemic circulation via superior and inferior venae cavae

Right ventricle: receives blood from the right atrium and pumps it into the pulmonary circulation via pulmonary arteries

Left atrium: receives blood from the lungs via pulmonary veins

Left ventricle: receives blood from the left atrium and pumps it into the systemic circulation via the aorta

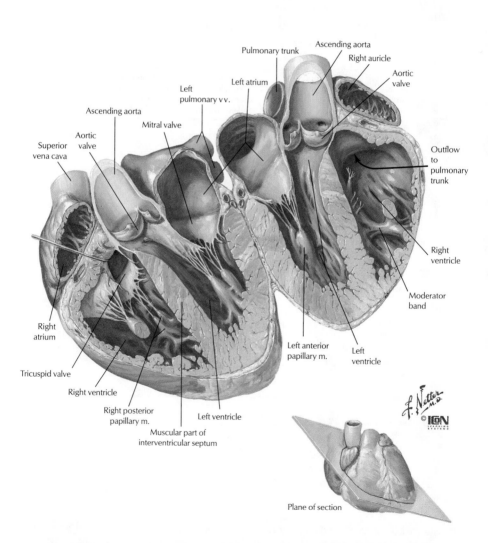

Clinical Correlation

Causes of Hypertension

Anatomy on pp. 20, 21, 25

Combined systolic and diastolic hypertension

Essential hypertension	Unknown etiology

Renal disorders

Parenchymal renal disease
- Glomerulonephritis
- Chronic pyelonephritis
- Diabetic nephropathy
- Interstitial nephritis
- Polycystic kidney
- Connective tissue disease
- Hydronephrosis

Renovascular disease
- Atherosclerotic, thrombotic, or embolic obstruction
- Fibromuscular hyperplasia
- Aneurysm or dissecting aneurysm

Adrenal disorders

Cortical
- Mineralocorticoid excess (primary or idiopathic hyperaldosteronism, DOC-excess syndromes)
- Cushing's or adrenogenital syndrome

Medullary—pheochromocytoma

Neurogenic disorders
- Increased intracranial pressure
- Brain tumors
- Encephalitis
- Cord transection
- Neuroblastoma

Hematologic disorders
- Polycythemia
- Erythropoietin

Parathyroid or thyroid disorders
- Hyperparathyroidism (also other causes of hypercalcemia)
- Myxedema

Coarctation of aorta
- Thoracic
- Abdominal (with or without renal a. involvement)

Toxemia of pregnancy

Preeclampsia   Eclampsia

Drug- or diet-induced

Oral contraceptives	Cocaine
Estrogens	Amphetamines
Licorice	Sympathomimetics
Cyclosporine	Monoamine oxidase inhibitors

Isolated systolic hypertension

Increased left ventricular stroke volume
- Aortic regurgitation
- Patent ductus arteriosus
- Hyperthyroidism
- Arteriovenous fistula

Decreased aortic distensibility
- Aortic arteriosclerosis
- Coarctation of aorta

F. Netter M.D.

©ICN

Hypertension (high blood pressure) is a major risk factor for atherogenesis, atherosclerotic cardiovascular disease, stroke, coronary artery disease, and renal failure. Hypertension can result from an unknown cause (idiopathic, or essential) or secondary causes. Associated morbidity and mortality are a significant public health concern.

Clinical Correlation

Hypertension in the Elderly

Anatomy on pp. 20, 21, 25

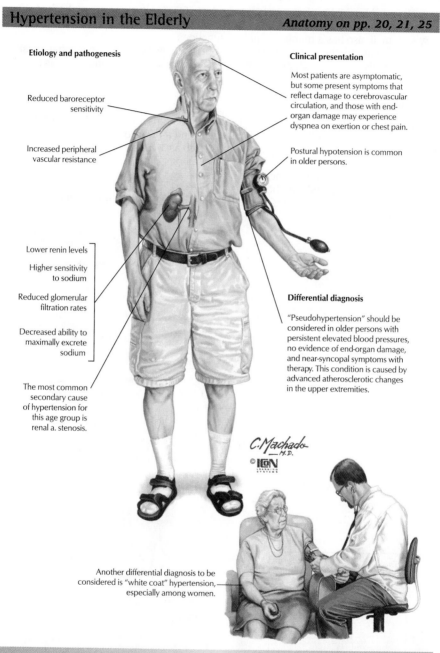

Etiology and pathogenesis

Reduced baroreceptor sensitivity

Increased peripheral vascular resistance

Lower renin levels

Higher sensitivity to sodium

Reduced glomerular filtration rates

Decreased ability to maximally excrete sodium

The most common secondary cause of hypertension for this age group is renal a. stenosis.

Clinical presentation

Most patients are asymptomatic, but some present symptoms that reflect damage to cerebrovascular circulation, and those with end-organ damage may experience dyspnea on exertion or chest pain.

Postural hypotension is common in older persons.

Differential diagnosis

"Pseudohypertension" should be considered in older persons with persistent elevated blood pressures, no evidence of end-organ damage, and near-syncopal symptoms with therapy. This condition is caused by advanced atherosclerotic changes in the upper extremities.

Another differential diagnosis to be considered is "white coat" hypertension, especially among women.

Hypertension has been defined as two or more readings of systolic blood pressure higher than 140 mm Hg or diastolic blood pressure higher than 90 mm Hg. One reading of over 210 mm Hg systolic or over 120 mm Hg diastolic also indicates hypertension. Each reading must be performed after the person has been sitting for 3 minutes. Approximately 50% of all people aged older than 60 years have hypertension.

Lymphatic System: Organization

Some consider the lymphatic system to be part of the circulatory system because of its extensive network of lymphatic vessels. However, although it complements the circulatory system, it also has a number of unique functions:

- Aids immunity (the ability to resist infection by activating defense mechanisms)
- Collects tissue fluids, solutes, hormones, and plasma proteins and conveys them to the bloodstream
- Absorbs fat from the small intestine

The lymphatic system includes

Lymph: a watery fluid that resembles plasma but contains fewer proteins and may contain fat, together with cells (mainly lymphocytes and a few red blood cells)

Lymphocytes: cellular components of lymph such as T cells, B cells, and natural killer (NK) cells

Lymph vessels: an extensive network of vessels and capillaries in peripheral tissues that transports lymph and lymphocytes

Lymphoid organs: lymph nodes, aggregates of lymphoid tissue, tonsils, thymus gland, spleen, and bone marrow

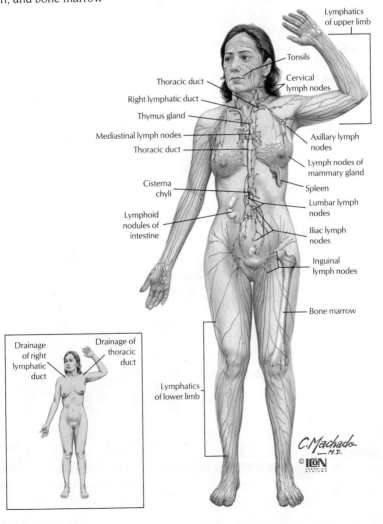

Lymphatics of upper limb

Tonsils

Thoracic duct

Cervical lymph nodes

Right lymphatic duct

Thymus gland

Mediastinal lymph nodes

Axillary lymph nodes

Thoracic duct

Lymph nodes of mammary gland

Cisterna chyli

Spleen

Lumbar lymph nodes

Lymphoid nodules of intestine

Iliac lymph nodes

Inguinal lymph nodes

Bone marrow

Drainage of right lymphatic duct

Drainage of thoracic duct

Lymphatics of lower limb

C. Machado
—M.D.

© ION
LEARNING SYSTEMS

Respiratory System: Organization

The respiratory system performs five basic functions:
- Filters and humidifies the air and moves air into and out of the lungs
- Provides a large surface area for gas exchange with blood
- Helps to regulate pH of body fluids
- Participates in vocalization
- Assists the olfactory system with detection of smells

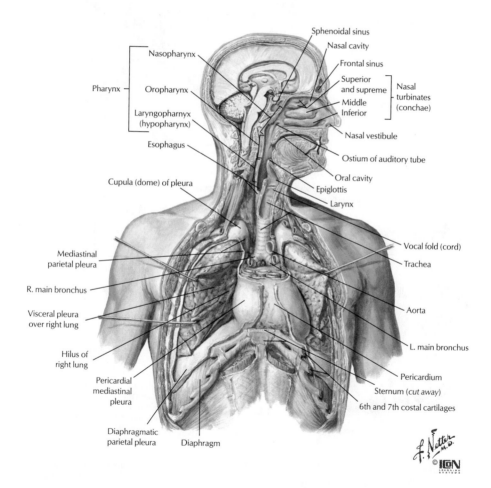

Clinical Correlation

Asthma: Pathophysiology   *Anatomy on p. 29*

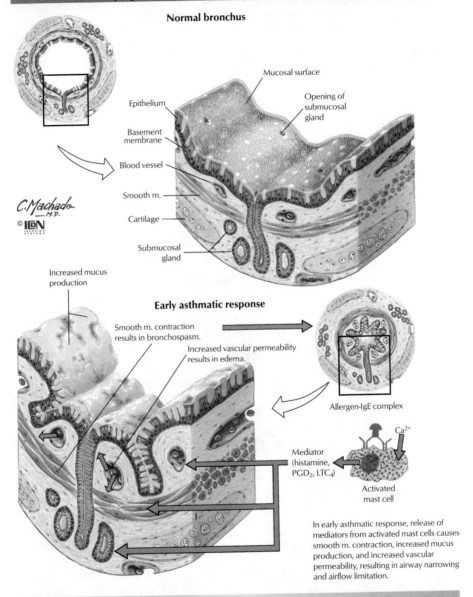

Normal bronchus

Mucosal surface

Epithelium

Opening of
submucosal
gland

Basement
membrane

Blood vessel

Smooth m.

Cartilage

Submucosal
gland

Increased mucus
production

Early asthmatic response

Smooth m. contraction
results in bronchospasm.

Increased vascular permeability
results in edema.

Allergen-IgE complex

Ca^{2+}

Mediator
(histamine,
PGD_2, LTC_4)

Activated
mast cell

In early asthmatic response, release of
mediators from activated mast cells causes
smooth m. contraction, increased mucus
production, and increased vascular
permeability, resulting in airway narrowing
and airflow limitation.

C.Machado
M.D.
© ION
LEARNING
SYSTEMS

Asthma can be intrinsic (has no defined environmental trigger) or extrinsic (has a
defined trigger). Asthma usually results from a hypersensitivity reaction to an allergen
(e.g., dust, pollen, molds), which leads to irritation of the respiratory passages and
smooth muscle contraction (narrowing of the passageways), swelling (edema) of the
epithelium lining the passageways, and increased production of mucus. Presenting
symptoms are often wheezing, shortness of breath, coughing, tachycardia, and feelings of chest tightness. Asthma is a pathologic inflammation of the airways and occurs
in both children and adults.

Clinical Correlation

Asthma: Late Pathophysiology
Anatomy on p. 29

Late asthmatic response

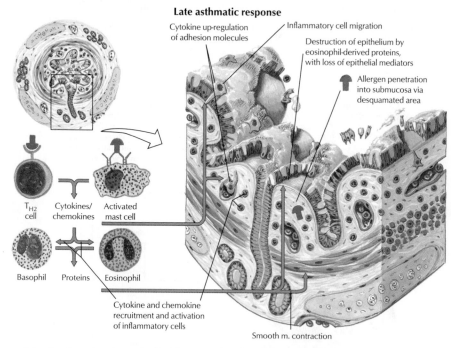

Cytokine up-regulation of adhesion molecules

Inflammatory cell migration

Destruction of epithelium by eosinophil-derived proteins, with loss of epithelial mediators

Allergen penetration into submucosa via desquamated area

T_{H2} cell

Cytokines/ chemokines

Activated mast cell

Basophil

Proteins

Eosinophil

Cytokine and chemokine recruitment and activation of inflammatory cells

Smooth m. contraction

Late asthmatic response characterized by inflammatory changes mediated by cytokines and chemokines, and epithelial destruction mediated by eosinophils and basophils

Chronic asthma

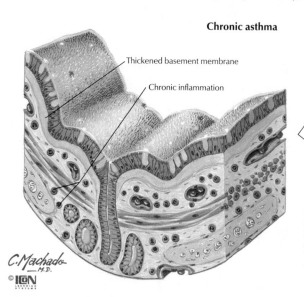

Thickened basement membrane

Chronic inflammation

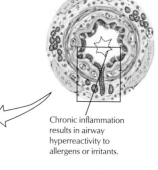

Chronic inflammation results in airway hyperreactivity to allergens or irritants.

Chronic asthma exhibits chronic low-grade inflammation, which extends beyond muscularis, where it is less susceptible to inhaled medications. Thickening of basement membrane occurs secondary to inflammation.

C. Machado
—M.D.

Nervous System: Organization

The nervous system integrates and regulates many body activities, sometimes at discrete locations (specific targets) and sometimes more globally. The nervous system usually acts quite rapidly and can also modulate effects of the endocrine and immune systems. The nervous system comprises two structural divisions:

Central nervous system (CNS): brain and spinal cord
Peripheral nervous system (PNS): somatic, autonomic, and enteric systems

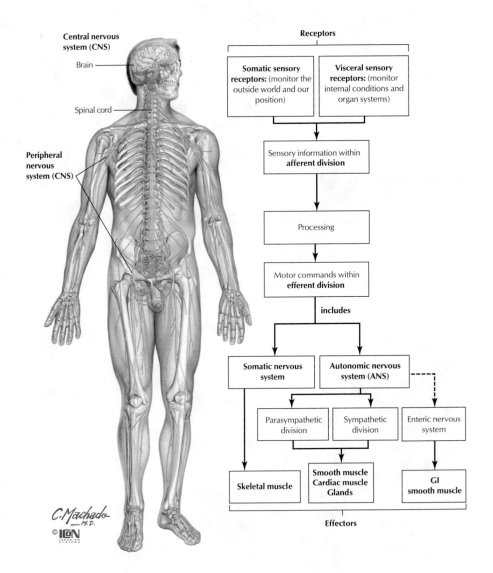

Central nervous system (CNS)

Brain

Spinal cord

Peripheral nervous system (CNS)

Receptors

Somatic sensory receptors: (monitor the outside world and our position)	Visceral sensory receptors: (monitor internal conditions and organ systems)

Sensory information within **afferent division**

Processing

Motor commands within **efferent division**

includes

Somatic nervous system	Autonomic nervous system (ANS)

Parasympathetic division	Sympathetic division	Enteric nervous system

Skeletal muscle	Smooth muscle Cardiac muscle Glands	GI smooth muscle

Effectors

C.Machado —M.D.
© ICN
LEARNING SYSTEMS

Nervous System: Neurons and Glial Cells

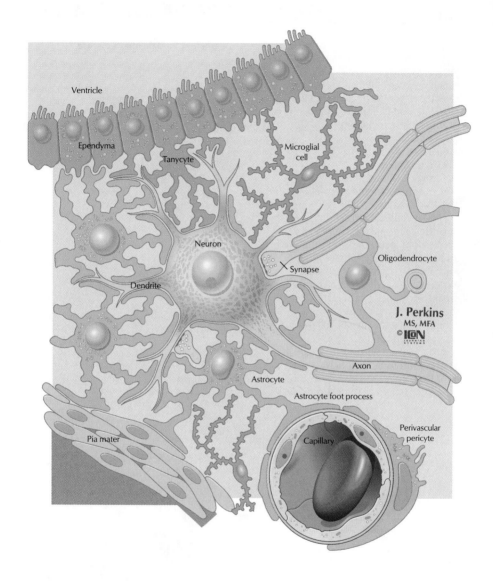

Neurons: nerve cells; may be multipolar, unipolar, or bipolar
Soma: cell body of a neuron; contains nucleus and organelles
Dendrites: cell processes of neurons that receive impulses
Axons: single processes of neurons that convey impulses away from soma
Synapses: contact points for communication
Astrocytes: glia that isolate CNS neurons and support their function
Oligodendrocytes: glia that myelinate CNS neuronal axons
Microglia: scavenger glia that participate in immune responses
Schwann cells: glia that myelinate neuronal processes in the PNS and provide trophic support

Clinical Correlation

Alzheimer's Disease
Anatomy on pp. 32, 33

Alzheimer's disease, characterized by progressive decline in social and cognitive skills, is the most common form of dementia (50-75%) and is linked to predisposing factors including

- Genetics
- Aging
- Female sex
- Previous head injury
- Presence of free radicals
- Toxic factors

The increased presence of neuritic plaques (accumulation of amyloid protein fragments) and neurofibrillary tangles (tau-microtubule complexes) is evidence of this disease. An increase in the loss of neurons in the hippocampus and posterior temporoparietal areas of the brain is often found. The disease is progressive, with both social and cognitive skills decreasing over time.

Pathology in Alzheimer's disease

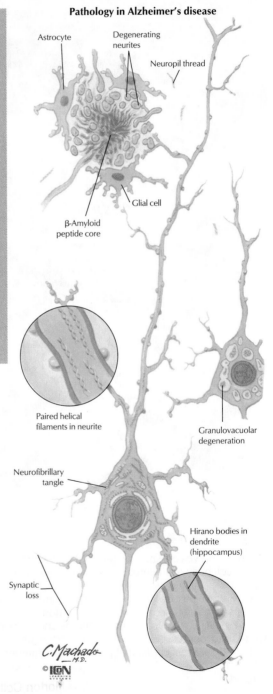

Astrocyte

Degenerating neurites

Neuropil thread

Glial cell

β-Amyloid peptide core

Paired helical filaments in neurite

Granulovacuolar degeneration

Neurofibrillary tangle

Hirano bodies in dendrite (hippocampus)

Synaptic loss

C. Machado M.D.

© ICN

Nervous System: Meninges

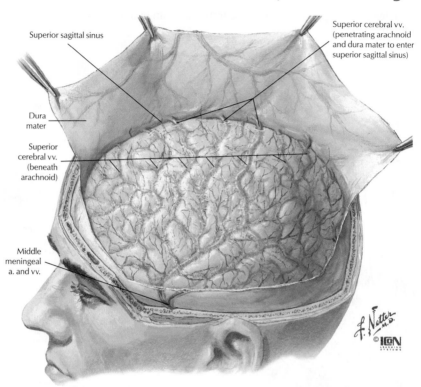

Superior sagittal sinus

Superior cerebral vv.
(penetrating arachnoid
and dura mater to enter
superior sagittal sinus)

Dura mater

Superior cerebral vv.
(beneath arachnoid)

Middle meningeal a. and vv.

The brain and spinal cord are surrounded by three membranous connective tissue layers called meninges:

Dura mater: the thick outermost layer

Arachnoid mater: a fine, weblike membrane beneath the dura mater

Pia mater: a delicate, transparent inner layer that intimately covers the brain and spinal cord

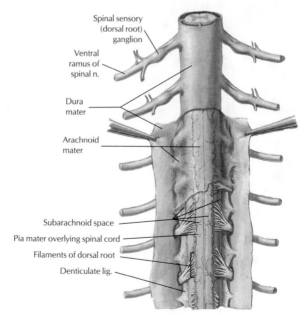

Spinal sensory (dorsal root) ganglion

Ventral ramus of spinal n.

Dura mater

Arachnoid mater

Subarachnoid space

Pia mater overlying spinal cord

Filaments of dorsal root

Denticulate lig.

Nervous System: Cranial Nerves

Twelve pairs of cranial nerves arise from the brain and pass through foramina in the cranium (skull).

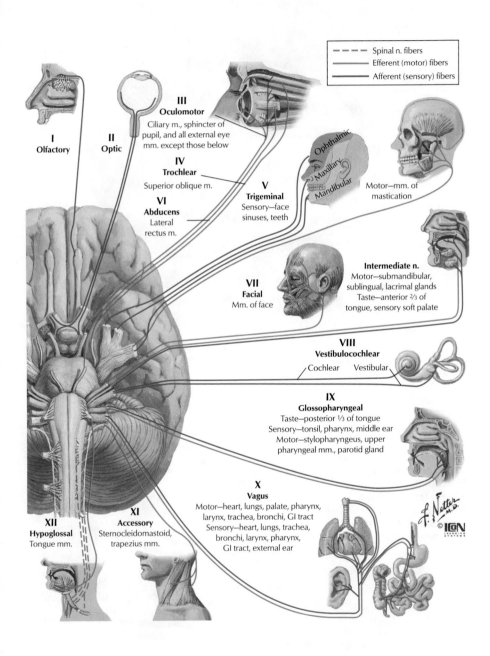

Spinal n. fibers
Efferent (motor) fibers
Afferent (sensory) fibers

I
Olfactory

II
Optic

III
Oculomotor
Ciliary m., sphincter of
pupil, and all external eye
mm. except those below

IV
Trochlear
Superior oblique m.

VI
Abducens
Lateral
rectus m.

V
Trigeminal
Sensory—face
sinuses, teeth

Ophthalmic
Maxillary
Mandibular

Motor—mm. of
mastication

VII
Facial
Mm. of face

Intermediate n.
Motor—submandibular,
sublingual, lacrimal glands
Taste—anterior ⅔ of
tongue, sensory soft palate

VIII
Vestibulocochlear
Cochlear   Vestibular

IX
Glossopharyngeal
Taste—posterior ⅓ of tongue
Sensory—tonsil, pharynx, middle ear
Motor—stylopharyngeus, upper
pharyngeal mm., parotid gland

X
Vagus
Motor—heart, lungs, palate, pharynx,
larynx, trachea, bronchi, GI tract
Sensory—heart, lungs, trachea,
bronchi, larynx, pharynx,
GI tract, external ear

XI
Accessory
Sternocleidomastoid,
trapezius mm.

XII
Hypoglossal
Tongue mm.

Nervous System: Spinal Nerves

Spinal cord and ventral rami in situ

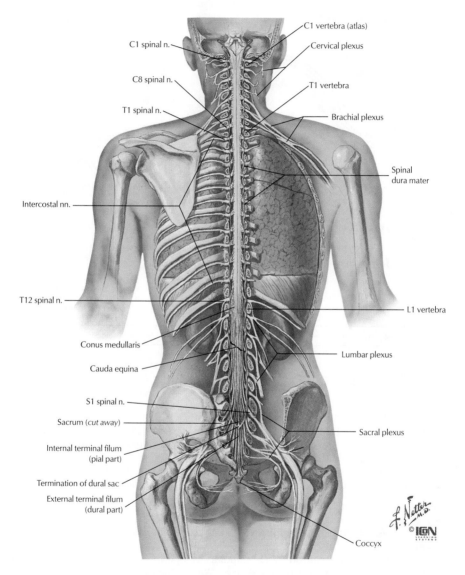

C1 vertebra (atlas)

C1 spinal n.

Cervical plexus

C8 spinal n.

T1 vertebra

T1 spinal n.

Brachial plexus

Spinal dura mater

Intercostal nn.

T12 spinal n.

L1 vertebra

Conus medullaris

Lumbar plexus

Cauda equina

S1 spinal n.

Sacrum (*cut away*)

Sacral plexus

Internal terminal filum (pial part)

Termination of dural sac

External terminal filum (dural part)

Coccyx

Features of spinal nerves are the following:
- They consist of 31 pairs (8 cervical, 12 thoracic, 5 lumbar, 5 sacral, 1 coccygeal).
- They are formed by ventral and dorsal roots.
- Motor nerve cell bodies reside in the spinal cord gray matter.
- Sensory nerve cell bodies reside in the spinal nerve dorsal root ganglia.
- Connections to the sympathetic trunk are via rami communicantes.
- Ventral rami of spinal nerves often converge to form plexuses (cervical, brachial, lumbar, sacral).

Nervous System: Elements of the PNS

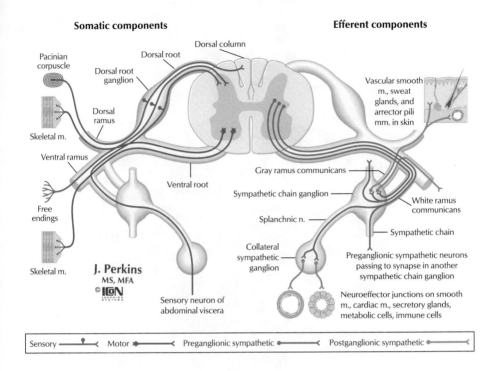

Somatic components

Pacinian corpuscle
Dorsal root
Dorsal root ganglion
Dorsal ramus
Skeletal m.
Ventral ramus
Free endings
Skeletal m.
Dorsal column
Dorsal root
Ventral root
Sensory neuron of abdominal viscera

Efferent components

Vascular smooth m., sweat glands, and arrector pili mm. in skin
Gray ramus communicans
Sympathetic chain ganglion
White ramus communicans
Splanchnic n.
Sympathetic chain
Collateral sympathetic ganglion
Preganglionic sympathetic neurons passing to synapse in another sympathetic chain ganglion
Neuroeffector junctions on smooth m., cardiac m., secretory glands, metabolic cells, immune cells

J. Perkins
MS, MFA
© ICON

Sensory   Motor   Preganglionic sympathetic   Postganglionic sympathetic

Functional components of the PNS include

Somatic nervous system: sensory and motor fibers to skin, skeletal muscle, and joints
Autonomic nervous system (ANS): sensory and motor fibers to all smooth muscle, cardiac muscle, and glands
Enteric nervous system: plexuses and ganglia of the gastrointestinal tract (GI) that regulate bowel secretion, absorption, and motility (originally said to be part of the ANS)

Features of the somatic division of the PNS include
- A one-neuron motor system
- A motor (efferent) neuron in the CNS and an axon that projects to a peripheral target, e.g., skeletal muscle
- A sensory (afferent) neuron (often unipolar) in a peripheral ganglion that conveys sensory impulses from the periphery, e.g., skin, to the CNS

Features of the ANS division of the PNS include
- A two-neuron motor system: the first neuron residing in the CNS and the second in a peripheral autonomic ganglion
- Axons termed preganglionic (those of the first motor neuron) and axons termed postganglionic (those of the second neuron)
- A system of two divisions: sympathetic and parasympathetic
- A single visceral sensory neuron (similar to the somatic system) that conveys sensory impulses (from viscera) to the CNS

Clinical Correlation

Myasthenia Gravis
Anatomy on pp. 32, 36-38

Pathophysiologic concepts

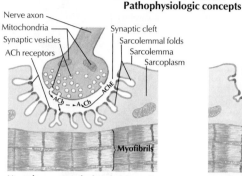

Nerve axon
Mitochondria
Synaptic vesicles
ACh receptors
Synaptic cleft
Sarcolemmal folds
Sarcolemma
Sarcoplasm
Myofibrils

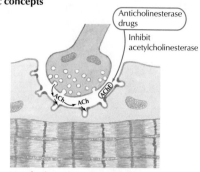

Anticholinesterase drugs
Inhibit acetylcholinesterase

Normal neuromuscular junction: Synaptic vesicles containing acetylcholine (ACh) form in n. terminal. In response to n. impulse, vesicles discharge ACh into synaptic cleft. ACh binds to receptor sites on m. sarcolemma to initiate m. contraction. Acetylcholinesterase (AChE) hydrolyzes ACh, thus limiting effect and duration of its action.

Myasthenia gravis: Marked reduction in number and length of subneural sarcolemmal folds indicates that underlying defect lies in neuromuscular junction. Anticholinesterase drugs increase effectiveness and duration of ACh action by slowing its destruction by AChE.

Clinical Manifestations

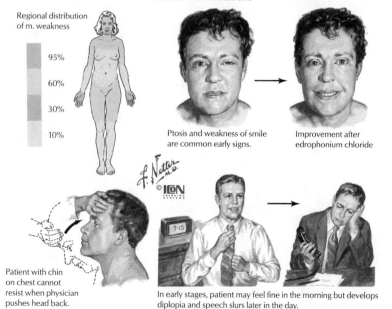

Regional distribution of m. weakness

95%
60%
30%
10%

Ptosis and weakness of smile are common early signs.

Improvement after edrophonium chloride

Patient with chin on chest cannot resist when physician pushes head back.

In early stages, patient may feel fine in the morning but develops diplopia and speech slurs later in the day.

Myasthenia gravis is a disease of the neuromuscular junction in which the postsynaptic membrane shows a reduction in folding and in the concentration of acetylcholine (ACh) receptors. It is usually an acquired immunologic disease, although a genetic component can exist. Patients present with muscle weakness, oculomotor abnormalities, ptosis, and diplopia; the disease is generally progressive. Muscle weakness fluctuates during the day, being less severe in the morning.

Nervous System: Effects of the Sympathetic Division of the ANS

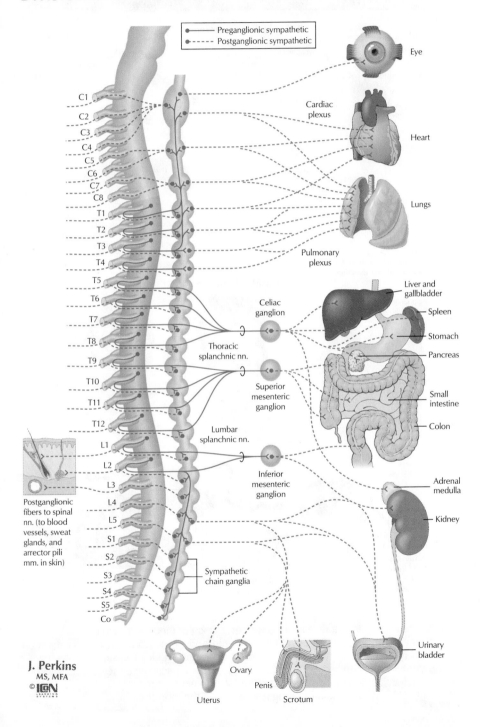

Preganglionic sympathetic
Postganglionic sympathetic

Eye

Cardiac plexus

Heart

Lungs

Pulmonary plexus

Liver and gallbladder
Spleen
Stomach
Pancreas

Celiac ganglion

Thoracic splanchnic nn.

Superior mesenteric ganglion

Small intestine

Colon

Lumbar splanchnic nn.

Inferior mesenteric ganglion

Adrenal medulla

Kidney

Postganglionic fibers to spinal nn. (to blood vessels, sweat glands, and arrector pili mm. in skin)

Sympathetic chain ganglia

C1
C2
C3
C4
C5
C6
C7
C8
T1
T2
T3
T4
T5
T6
T7
T8
T9
T10
T11
T12
L1
L2
L3
L4
L5
S1
S2
S3
S4
S5
Co

Urinary bladder

Ovary

Penis

Uterus

Scrotum

J. Perkins
MS, MFA
© ICN

Nervous System: Effects of the Sympathetic Division of the ANS (continued)

The sympathetic division acts globally to mobilize the body in "fright-fight-flight" situations.

STRUCTURE	EFFECTS
Eye	Dilates the pupil
Lacrimal glands	Reduces secretion slightly (vasoconstriction)
Skin	Causes goose bumps (arrector pili muscle contraction)
Sweat glands	Increases secretion
Peripheral vessels	Causes vasoconstriction
Heart	Increases heart rate and force of contraction
Coronary arteries	Assists in vasodilation
Lungs	Assists in bronchodilation and reduced secretion
Digestive tract	Decreases peristalsis, contracts internal anal sphincter muscle, causes vasoconstriction to shunt blood elsewhere
Liver	Causes glycogen breakdown, glucose synthesis and release
Salivary glands	Reduces and thickens secretion via vasoconstriction
Genital system	Causes ejaculation and orgasm, and remission of erection Constricts male internal urethral sphincter muscle
Urinary system	Decreases urine production via vasoconstriction Constricts male internal urethral sphincter muscle
Adrenal medulla	Increases secretion of epinephrine or norepinephrine

Nervous System: Effects of the Parasympathetic Division of the ANS

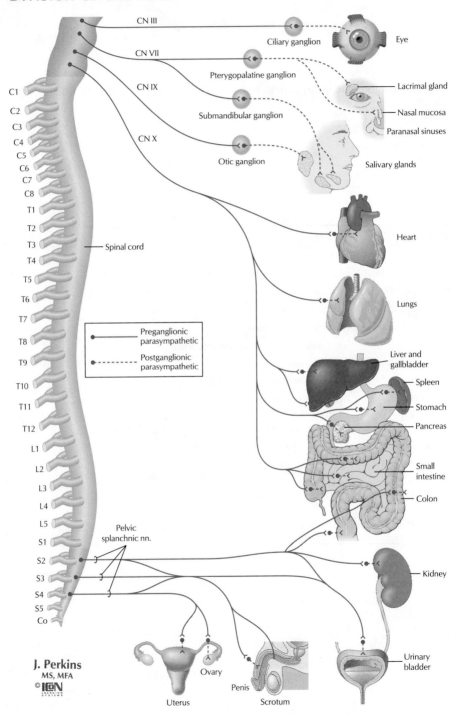

CN III
Ciliary ganglion
Eye
CN VII
Pterygopalatine ganglion
Lacrimal gland
CN IX
Nasal mucosa
Submandibular ganglion
Paranasal sinuses
CN X
Otic ganglion
Salivary glands

C1
C2
C3
C4
C5
C6
C7
C8
T1
T2
T3 — Spinal cord
T4
T5
T6
T7
T8
T9
T10
T11
T12
L1
L2
L3
L4
L5
S1
S2
S3
S4
S5
Co

Heart

Lungs

Preganglionic parasympathetic
Postganglionic parasympathetic

Liver and gallbladder
Spleen
Stomach
Pancreas
Small intestine
Colon

Pelvic splanchnic nn.

Kidney

Ovary
Uterus
Penis
Scrotum
Urinary bladder

J. Perkins
MS, MFA
©ICN
LEARNING SYSTEMS

Nervous System: Effects of the Parasympathetic Division of the ANS (continued)

The parasympathetic division usually acts focally and is primarily concerned with functions related to feeding or sexual arousal.

STRUCTURE	EFFECTS
Eye	Constricts pupil
Ciliary body	Constricts muscle for accommodation (near vision)
Lacrimal glands	Increases secretion
Heart	Decreases heart rate and force of contraction
Coronary arteries	Causes vasoconstriction with reduced metabolic demand
Lungs	Causes bronchoconstriction and increased secretion
Digestive tract	Increases peristalsis, increase secretion, inhibits internal anal sphincter for defecation
Liver	Aids glycogen synthesis and storage
Salivary glands	Increases secretion
Genital system	Promotes engorgement of erectile tissues
Urinary system	Contracts bladder (detrusor muscle) for urination, inhibits contraction of internal urethral sphincter, increases urine production

Nervous System: Enteric Nervous System

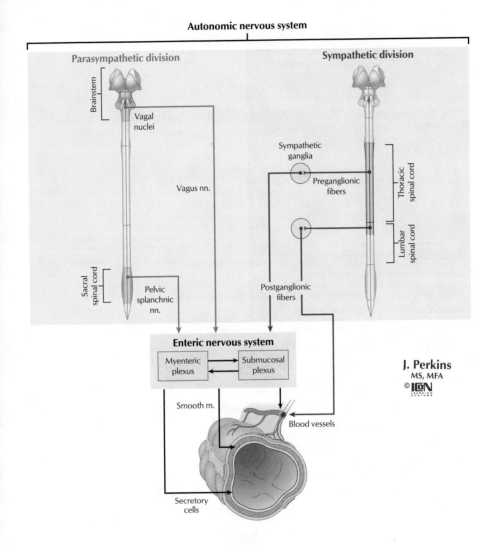

This system was formerly considered the third division of the ANS. The enteric (refers to the bowel) system consists of intrinsic ganglia and nerve plexuses in the walls of the GI tract. These ganglia and their neural networks include
• Myenteric (Auerbach's) plexuses
• Submucosal (Meissner's) plexuses
The enteric nervous system has links to sympathetic and parasympathetic divisions of the ANS for optimal regulation of bowel secretion, absorption, and motility. More than 20 transmitter substances have been identified in intrinsic neurons in the enteric system. Optimal GI functioning requires coordinated interactions of autonomic nerves, the enteric nervous system, and endocrine and paracrine secretions.

Endocrine System: Organization

The endocrine system performs a diverse array of regulatory functions in the body by interacting with target sites (cells and tissues), many a great distance away, via blood-borne molecules called hormones. The endocrine system interacts closely with the nervous and immune systems to facilitate communication, integration, and regulation. Endocrine glands and hormones share several additional features:

- Secretion is controlled via feedback mechanisms.
- Hormones bind target receptors on cell membranes or within cells.
- Hormone action may be slow to appear and may have long-lasting effects.
- Hormones are chemically diverse molecules.

In the illustration, only major hormones are given for each organ or system.

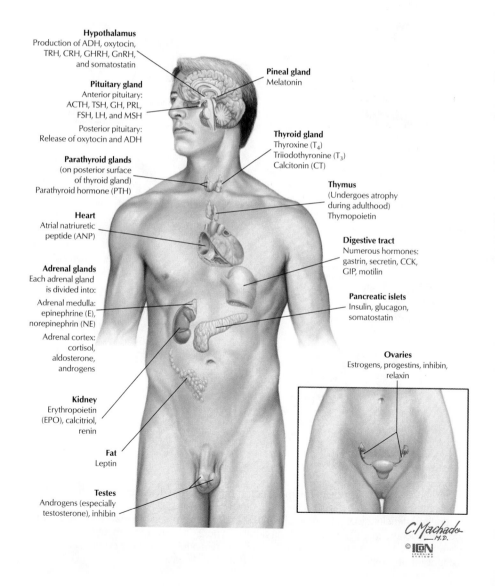

Hypothalamus
Production of ADH, oxytocin,
TRH, CRH, GHRH, GnRH,
and somatostatin

Pituitary gland
Anterior pituitary:
ACTH, TSH, GH, PRL,
FSH, LH, and MSH

Posterior pituitary:
Release of oxytocin and ADH

Parathyroid glands
(on posterior surface
of thyroid gland)
Parathyroid hormone (PTH)

Heart
Atrial natriuretic
peptide (ANP)

Adrenal glands
Each adrenal gland
is divided into:

Adrenal medulla:
epinephrine (E),
norepinephrin (NE)

Adrenal cortex:
cortisol,
aldosterone,
androgens

Kidney
Erythropoietin
(EPO), calcitriol,
renin

Fat
Leptin

Testes
Androgens (especially
testosterone), inhibin

Pineal gland
Melatonin

Thyroid gland
Thyroxine (T_4)
Triiodothyronine (T_3)
Calcitonin (CT)

Thymus
(Undergoes atrophy
during adulthood)
Thymopoietin

Digestive tract
Numerous hormones:
gastrin, secretin, CCK,
GIP, motilin

Pancreatic islets
Insulin, glucagon,
somatostatin

Ovaries
Estrogens, progestins, inhibin,
relaxin

C. Machado
_M.D.

©ICN
LEARNING
SYSTEMS

Clinical Correlation

Diabetes Mellitus and Its Vascular Consequences

Anatomy on pp. 20, 25, 45

Diabetic retinopathy

Diabetic retinopathy can be easily detected during a dialated eye examination and is the leading cause of blindness among adults in the United States. Visual loss can be prevented with early recognition and treatment of retinopathy.

Nonproliferative retinopathy (early stage)

- Microaneurysms
- Hemorrhages
- Cotton-wool spots
- Hard exudate
- Narrowed arterioles

Proliferative retinopathy (late stage)

Massive hemorrhage   Retinitis proliferans

Diabetic nephropathy

Histologic view of diabetic glomerulo-sclerosis

Diabetes mellitus is the leading cause of end-stage renal disease in the Western world.

Cerebrovascular disease

The high incidence of vascular complications among patients with diabetes is related not only to blood glucose elevations, but also to the frequent association of dyslipidemia, hypertension, a procoagulant state, and the tendency to form unstable plaques in the arterial wall.

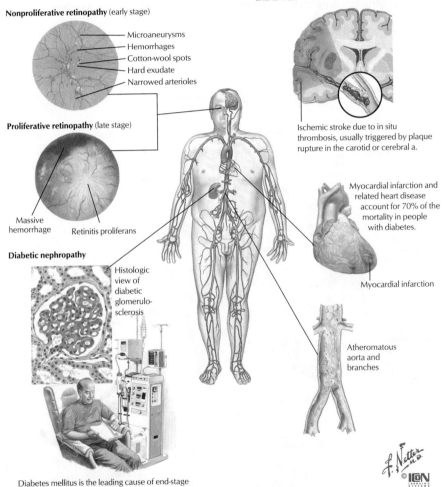

Ischemic stroke due to in situ thrombosis, usually triggered by plaque rupture in the carotid or cerebral a.

Myocardial infarction and related heart disease account for 70% of the mortality in people with diabetes.

Myocardial infarction

Atheromatous aorta and branches

Diabetes mellitus is one of the more common endocrine diseases; the lifetime risk of developing this disease is 30-50% in the developed world. Type 1 diabetes (insulin dependent: deficiency of pancreatic insulin secretion as a result of beta-cell destruction) usually occurs in children and young adults. Type 2 diabetes (non–insulin dependent: often caused by insulin resistance) is usually seen in adults. Vascular complications account for approximately 80% of all deaths from this disease.

Gastrointestinal System: Organization

The GI system includes the epithelium-lined tube from the mouth to the anus, plus structures such as the salivary glands, liver, gallbladder, and pancreas.

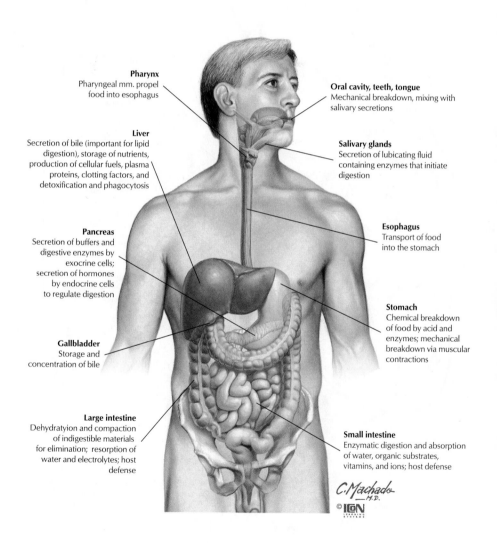

Pharynx
Pharyngeal mm. propel food into esophagus

Liver
Secretion of bile (important for lipid digestion), storage of nutrients, production of cellular fuels, plasma proteins, clotting factors, and detoxification and phagocytosis

Pancreas
Secretion of buffers and digestive enzymes by exocrine cells; secretion of hormones by endocrine cells to regulate digestion

Gallbladder
Storage and concentration of bile

Large intestine
Dehydratyion and compaction of indigestible materials for elimination; resorption of water and electrolytes; host defense

Oral cavity, teeth, tongue
Mechanical breakdown, mixing with salivary secretions

Salivary glands
Secretion of lubicating fluid containing enzymes that initiate digestion

Esophagus
Transport of food into the stomach

Stomach
Chemical breakdown of food by acid and enzymes; mechanical breakdown via muscular contractions

Small intestine
Enzymatic digestion and absorption of water, organic substrates, vitamins, and ions; host defense

C.Machado
—M.D.

©ICON

Clinical Correlation

Diarrhea *Anatomy on p. 47*

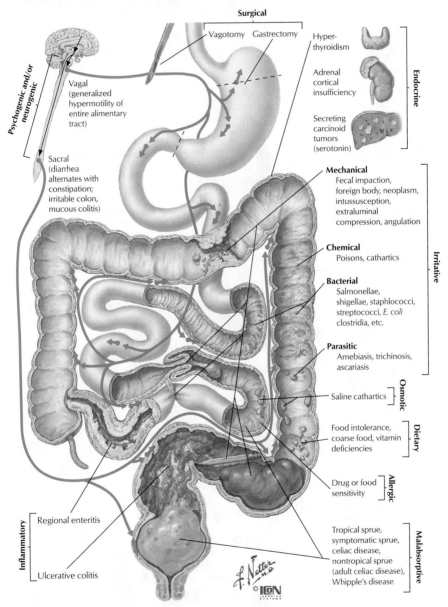

Surgical

Vagotomy   Gastrectomy

Hyper-thyroidism

Adrenal cortical insufficiency

Secreting carcinoid tumors (serotonin)

Endocrine

Psychogenic and/or neurogenic

Vagal (generalized hypermotility of entire alimentary tract)

Sacral (diarrhea alternates with constipation; irritable colon, mucous colitis)

Mechanical
Fecal impaction, foreign body, neoplasm, intussusception, extraluminal compression, angulation

Chemical
Poisons, cathartics

Bacterial
Salmonellae, shigellae, staphlococci, streptococci, E. coli clostridia, etc.

Parasitic
Amebiasis, trichinosis, ascariasis

Irritative

Saline cathartics — **Osmotic**

Food intolerance, coarse food, vitamin deficiencies — **Dietary**

Drug or food sensitivity — **Allergic**

Tropical sprue, symptomatic sprue, celiac disease, nontropical sprue (adult celiac disease), Whipple's disease — **Malabsorptive**

Inflammatory
Regional enteritis

Ulcerative colitis

Diarrhea, a common occurrence, is an increased stool output that may be caused by various neurogenic, surgical, endocrine, irritative, osmotic, dietary, allergic, malabsorptive, or inflammatory processes.

Urinary System: Organization

The kidneys lie in a retroperitoneal position (behind the peritoneum, outside the abdominal cavity), embedded in a cushion of fat, and just anterior to muscles of the posterior abdominal wall. The kidneys function to

- Filter plasma and begin the process of urine formation
- Reabsorb important electrolytes, organic molecules, vitamins, and water
- Excrete metabolic wastes, metabolites, and foreign chemicals, e.g., drugs
- Regulate fluid volume, composition, and pH
- Secrete hormones (regulate blood pressure, erythropoesis, and calcium metabolism)
- Convey urine to ureters, which conduct urine to the bladder for storage and then discharge via the urethra

Regional anatomy of kidney and ureter

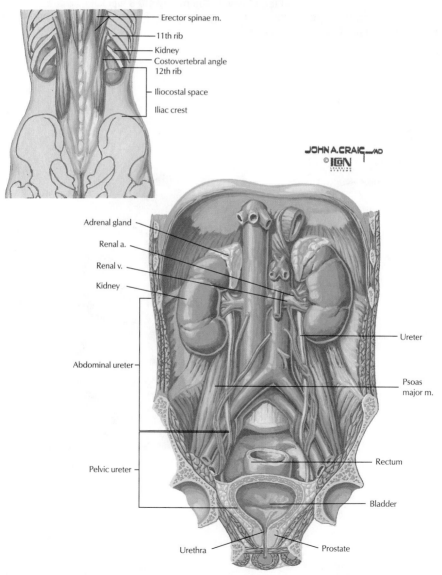

Erector spinae m.

11th rib

Kidney

Costovertebral angle

12th rib

Iliocostal space

Iliac crest

JOHN A.CRAIG—AD
© ICN

Adrenal gland

Renal a.

Renal v.

Kidney

Abdominal ureter

Pelvic ureter

Ureter

Psoas major m.

Rectum

Bladder

Urethra   Prostate

Reproductive System: Female Organs

Ovaries vary in size but are usually approximately the size of a large almond in pre-menopausal women and are suspended within the broad ligament (similar to a mesen-tery), which also supports the uterine tubes and uterus. Ovaries
- Produce female gametes called oocytes (ova, or eggs)
- Secrete sex hormones that support oogenesis and maintain pregnancy
- Secrete hormones that provide feedback to the pituitary gland

Female accessory organs include

Uterine tubes (fallopian tubes, or oviducts): open as fimbriated funnels into the pelvic cavity adjacent to the ovary (to capture ovulated oocytes) and convey the zygote (conceptus) to the uterus

Uterus: a pear-shaped, hollow muscular (smooth muscle) organ that protects and nour-ishes a developing embryo and fetus (development beyond 8 weeks)

Vagina: a musculoelastic distensible tube approximately 8-9 cm long that extends from the uterine cervix (neck) to the vestibule

Median (sagittal) section

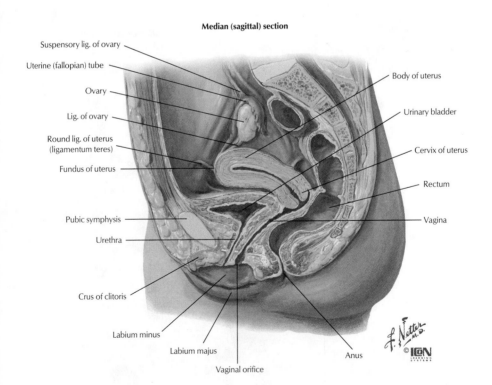

Suspensory lig. of ovary

Uterine (fallopian) tube

Ovary

Lig. of ovary

Round lig. of uterus (ligamentum teres)

Fundus of uterus

Pubic symphysis

Urethra

Crus of clitoris

Labium minus

Labium majus

Vaginal orifice

Body of uterus

Urinary bladder

Cervix of uterus

Rectum

Vagina

Anus

Reproductive System: Male Organs

The egg-shaped testes lie within the scrotum and are approximately the size of a chestnut. Male accessory organs include the

Epididymis: a structure on the posterior aspect of the testis that is a convoluted tubule folded on itself (stretched out, it is almost 23 feet long) where sperm mature

Ductus deferens (vas deferens): a muscular (smooth muscle) tube, approximately 40-45 cm long, that conveys sperm from the epididymis to the prostate gland (ejaculatory duct)

Seminal vesicles: tubular glands that lie posterior to the prostate, are approximately 15 cm long, produce seminal fluid, and join the vas deferens at the ejaculatory duct

Prostate gland: a walnut-sized gland that surrounds the urethra as it leaves the urinary bladder and produces prostatic fluid that is added to semen (sperm suspended in glandular secretions)

Urethra: a canal that passes through the prostate gland, enters the penis, and conveys semen for expulsion from the body

Paramedian (sagittal) dissection

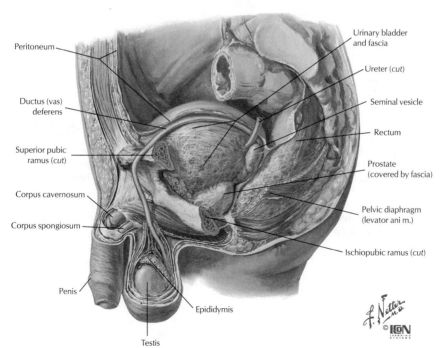

Embryology: Week 1, Fertilization and Implantation

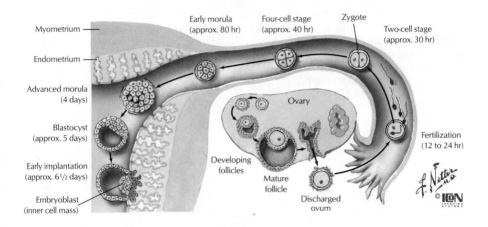

Fertilization normally occurs in the ampulla of the uterine tube (oviduct, fallopian tube) within 24 hours after ovulation. The fertilized ovum (the union of sperm and egg nuclei, with a diploid number of chromosomes) is termed a zygote. Subsequent cell division (cleavage) occurs at the 2-, 4-, 8-, and 16-cell stages, which results in formation of a ball of cells that travels down the uterine tube toward the uterine cavity. When the cell mass reaches day 3-4 of development, it resembles a mulberry and is called a morula (16-cell stage). As the morula enters the uterine cavity at approximately day 5, it develops a fluid-filled cyst in its interior and is then known as a blastocyst. At approximately day 5-6, implantation occurs as the blastocyst literally erodes or burrows its way into the uterine wall (endometrium).

Embryology: Week 2, Bilaminar Embryonic Disk

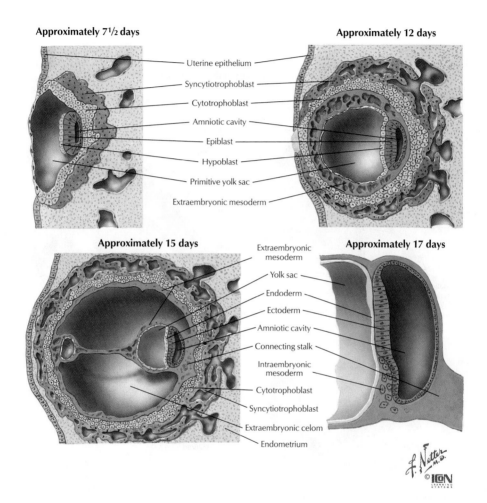

Approximately 7½ days

Approximately 12 days

- Uterine epithelium
- Syncytiotrophoblast
- Cytotrophoblast
- Amniotic cavity
- Epiblast
- Hypoblast
- Primitive yolk sac
- Extraembryonic mesoderm

Approximately 15 days

Approximately 17 days

- Extraembryonic mesoderm
- Yolk sac
- Endoderm
- Ectoderm
- Amniotic cavity
- Connecting stalk
- Intraembryonic mesoderm
- Cytotrophoblast
- Syncytiotrophoblast
- Extraembryonic celom
- Endometrium

As the blastocyst implants, it forms an inner cell mass (future embryo, embryoblast) and a larger fluid-filled cavity surrounded by an outer cell layer called the trophoblast. The trophoblast undergoes differentiation and complex cellular interactions with maternal tissues to initiate formation of uteroplacental circulation. Simultaneously, the inner cell mass develops into two cell types (bilaminar disk):

Epiblast: columnar cells on the dorsal surface of the embryoblast
Hypoblast: cuboidal cells on the ventral surface of the embryoblast

The epiblast forms a cavity on the dorsal side that gives rise to the amniotic cavity; the blastocyst cavity on the ventral side becomes the primitive yolk sac lined by simple squamous epithelium derived from the hypoblast. At approximately day 12, further hypoblast cell migration forms the true yolk sac, and the old blastocyst cavity becomes coated with extraembryonic mesoderm.

Embryology: Week 3, Gastrulation

Formation of intraembryonic mesoderm from the primitive streak and node (knot)

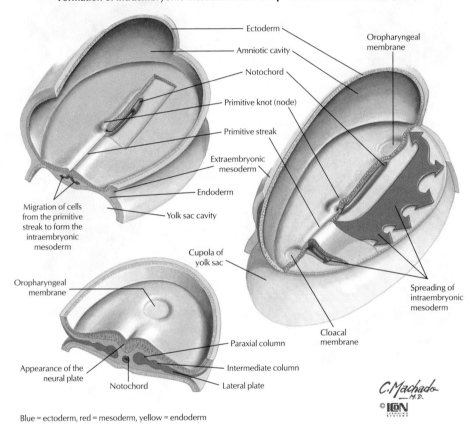

Blue = ectoderm, red = mesoderm, yellow = endoderm

Gastrulation (development of the trilaminar embryonic disk) begins with appearance of the primitive streak on the dorsal surface of the epiblast. This streak forms a groove demarcated at its cephalic (head) end by the primitive node. The node forms a midline cord of mesoderm that becomes the notochord. Migrating epiblast cells move toward the primitive streak, invaginate, and replace the underlying hypoblast cells to become the endoderm germ layer. Other invaginating epiblast cells develop between the endoderm and overlying epiblast and become the mesoderm. Finally, the surface epiblast cells form the ectoderm, the third germ layer. All body tissues are derived from one of these three embryonic germ layers.

Embryology: Ectodermal Derivatives

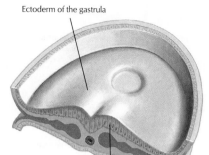

Ectoderm of the gastrula

Neural plate

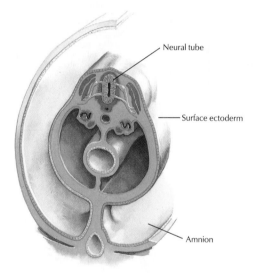

Neural tube

Surface ectoderm

Amnion

PRIMORDIA	DERIVATIVES OR FATE
Surface ectoderm	Epidermis of the skin Sweat, sebaceous, and mammary glands Nails and hair Tooth enamel Lacrimal glands Conjunctiva External auditory meatus
(Stomodeum and nasal placodes) (Otic placodes) (Lens placodes)	Oral and nasal epithelium Anterior pituitary Inner ear Lens of eye
Neural tube	Central nervous system Somatomotor neurons Branchiomotor neurons Presynaptic autonomic neurons Retina/optic nerves Posterior pituitary

Neural crest	Peripheral sensory neurons
	Postsynaptic autonomic
	    neurons
	All ganglia
	Adrenal medulla cells
	Melanocytes
	Bone, muscle, and connective
	    tissue in the head and
	    neck

Amnion	Protective bag (with chorion) around fetus

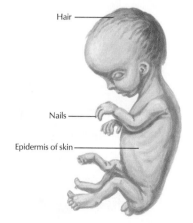

Hair

Nails

Epidermis of skin

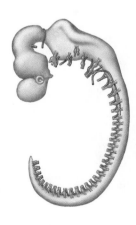

Central and
peripheral
nervous system

C. Machado
M.D.

© ICN
LEARNING
SYSTEMS

Embryology: Mesodermal Derivatives

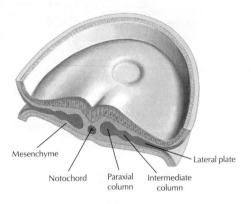

Mesenchyme

Notochord   Paraxial   Intermediate
             column   column

Lateral plate

PRIMORDIA	DERIVATIVES OR FATE
Notochord	Nucleus pulposus of an intervertebral disc Induces neurulation
Paraxial columns (somites)	Skeletal muscle Bone Connective tissue (e.g., dorsal dermis, meninges)
Intermediate mesoderm	Gonads Kidneys and ureters Uterus and uterine tubes Upper vagina Ductus deferens, epididymis, and related tubules Seminal vesicles and ejaculatory ducts
Lateral plate mesoderm	Dermis (ventral) Superficial fascia and related tissues (ventral) Bones and connective tissues of limbs Pleura and peritoneum GI tract connective tissue stroma
Cardiogenic mesoderm	Heart Pericardium

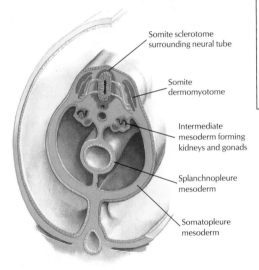

Somite sclerotome surrounding neural tube

Somite dermomyotome

Intermediate mesoderm forming kidneys and gonads

Splanchnopleure mesoderm

Somatopleure mesoderm

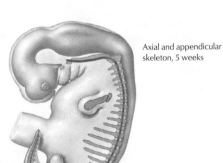

Axial and appendicular skeleton, 5 weeks

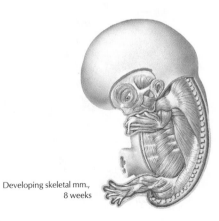

Developing skeletal mm., 8 weeks

Embryology: Endodermal Derivatives

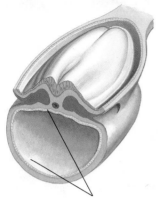

Endoderm of gastrula
and yolk sac

PRIMORDIA	EPITHELIAL DERIVATIVES OR FATE
Gut tube endoderm	GI tract (enterocytes) Mucosal glands of GI tract Parenchyma of GI organs (liver, pancreas) Airway lining (larynx, trachea, bronchial tree) Thyroid gland Tonsils
Cloaca (part of hindgut)	Rectum and anal canal Bladder, urethra, and related glands Vestibule Lower vagina
Pharyngeal pouches (part of foregut)	Auditory tube and middle ear epithelium Palatine tonsil crypts Thymus gland Parathyroid glands C cells of the thyroid gland
Yolk sac	Embryonic blood cell production (mesoderm) Pressed into umbilical cord, then disappears
Allantois (from yolk sac, then cloaca)	Embryonic blood cell production (mesoderm) Vestigial, fibrous urachus Umbilical cord part disappears

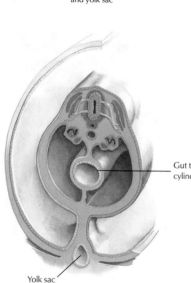

Gut tube of
cylindrical embryo

Yolk sac

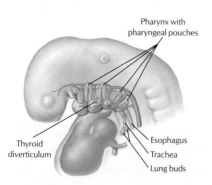

Pharynx with
pharyngeal pouches

Thyroid
diverticulum

Esophagus

Trachea

Lung buds

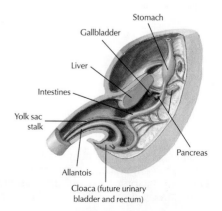

Stomach

Gallbladder

Liver

Intestines

Yolk sac
stalk

Allantois

Cloaca (future urinary
bladder and rectum)

Pancreas

Clinical Correlation

Developmental Defects
Anatomy on pp. 55-57

Malformation

Etiology
- Chromosomal
- Genetic
- Teratogenic
- Unknown

→ Morphogenic error →

Developed structure ↓ Primary structural defect

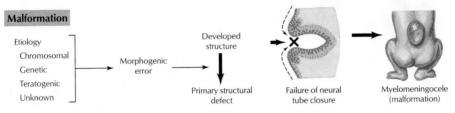

Failure of neural tube closure

Myelomeningocele (malformation)

Malformation. Primary structural defect resulting from error in tissue formation

Deformation

Etiology
- Extrinsic (fetal constraint)
- Intrinsic (fetal akinesia)

→ Abnormal force →

Normally developed structure ↓ Altered structure or position

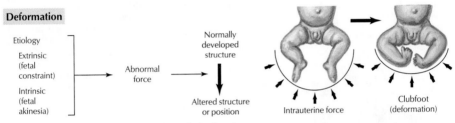

Intrauterine force

Clubfoot (deformation)

Deformation. Alteration in shape or position of normally developed structure

Disruption

Etiology
- Vascular
- Compressive
- Tearing

→ Vascular occlusion / Abnormal force →

Normally developed structure ↓ Tissue destruction

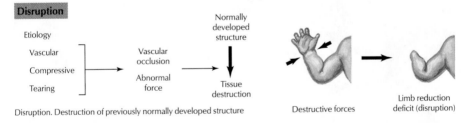

Destructive forces

Limb reduction deficit (disruption)

Disruption. Destruction of previously normally developed structure

JOHN A.CRAIG—AD
©ICN

In general, developmental defects may be classified as those occurring as a result of malformation, i.e., an error in tissue formation (usually caused by genetic or teratogenic factors); those occurring as a result of deformation of a normally developed structure by internal or external forces; and those resulting from a disruption of a normally developed structure.

Review Questions

Terminology

What is the anatomical position?	Descriptions and relationships based on a person standing erect, facing forward, with arms at the sides, palms facing forward, legs together, and feet directed forward.

Identify the following terms of relationship.
Closer to the surface:	Superficial
Closer to the midline:	Medial
Farther from a point of origin:	Distal
Closer to the head:	Superior (cranial)
Closer to the back:	Posterior (dorsal)

Identify the plane of section for each of the following descriptions.
Equal right and left halves:	Median plane
Anterior and posterior parts:	Coronal (frontal) section
Unequal right and left halves:	Sagittal or parasagittal section

Identify the movements described below.
A decrease in the joint angle:	Flexion
Move away from the body's midline:	Abduction
Movement superiorly:	Elevation
Rotation of palm so that it faces posteriorly in anatomical position:	Pronation
Turning the sole of the foot inward:	Inversion
Straightening the knee joint:	Extension
Bending the trunk forward:	Flexion (of the spine)

Skin

In which layer of the skin do pressure receptors and sweat glands reside?	Dermis.
What layer lies beneath the dermis?	Superficial fascia (hypodermis), which is subcutaneous tissue.
What are Langer's lines?	Tension lines in the skin created by orientation of collagen.

Skeletal System

What are the components of the axial skeleton?	Skull, vertebral column, ribs, and sternum.

Identify one bone for each descriptive shape listed below.
Irregular bone:	Vertebra
Long bone:	Humerus (radius, ulna,femur, tibia, fibula)
Largest sesamoid bone:	Patella (kneecap)

What kind of bone formation occurs when calcium is deposited into a cartilaginous model of that bone?	Endochondral bone formation.

Review Questions

In each description below, identify the type of fracture.

Intact skin over the fracture site: — Closed fracture

Fracture plane rotated along the long axis of the bone: — Spiral fracture

Fracture that results in many fragments: — Comminuted fracture

What type of joint is united by cartilage and possesses a cavity and capsule? — Synovial joint.

What are the two types of cartilaginous joints? — Primary (synchondroses) and secondary (symphyses).

For each synovial joint listed below, identify the type of joint it represents.

Hip joint: — Ball-and-socket (spheroid) joint
Base of the thumb: — Saddle joint
Elbow joint: — Hinge (ginglymus) joint

What does it mean when one says that a joint is biaxial? — The joint allows for movement in two directions, e.g., flexion and extension, and/or abduction and adduction.

What connection is there between the skeletal system and the cardiovascular system? — Besides the fact that vessels supply the bones, the bone marrow normally provides a ready supply of blood cells for the circulatory system.

Muscular System

What are the three different types of muscle? — Skeletal, cardiac, and smooth.

What term is used to describe the moveable distal site of a muscle's attachment? — Insertion (of the muscle).

Grossly, the fibers of the deltoid muscle appear feathered. What term is used to describe this appearance? — Pennate (multipennate).

Cardiovascular System

What two systemic veins return blood to the right atrium of the heart? — Superior and inferior venae cavae.

When the right ventricle contracts, where does the blood go? — Into the pulmonary trunk, then the right and left pulmonary arteries, and then the lungs.

Which vessels are resistance vessels and help to regulate blood pressure? — Arterioles.

Identify at least three places on the upper limb where one can detect a pulse. — At the wrist (radial artery), in the cubital fossa (brachial artery anterior to the elbow joint), and at the medial arm (brachial artery against the humerus).

Which vessels are capacitance vessels and can function as reservoirs? — Veins.

Review Questions

Which vessels possess valves?	Larger veins of the limbs and lower neck.
What clinical term is used to describe venous valve dysfunction, the resulting distention of the veins and possible compromised venous return to the heart?	Varicose veins.
Which heart chamber receives blood from the lungs?	Left atrium.
What arteries supply blood to the heart?	Right and left coronary arteries.
What is leukemia?	A group of clinical disorders caused by neoplastic transformation of the stem cells in the bone marrow that give rise to white blood cells.
What is the clinical term for the pain associated with myocardial ischemia?	Angina pectoris. Atherogenesis of the coronary arteries can compromise the blood supply to the myocardium and precipitate an ischemic episode that is felt as chest pain (angina).
What clinical term is used to describe irreparable damage to heart muscle after an ischemic episode?	Myocardial infarction.
What are varicose veins?	Distended veins (usually in a lower extremity) that result from absent or faulty valves in the communicating veins that link the superficial with the deep venous drainage.
Identify at least four different causes of hypertension.	Aortic arteriosclerosis, drugs, diet, endocrine disorders (renal, thyroid, parathyroid, adrenal), brain tumors.

Lymphatic System

Name four lymphoid organs.	Lymph nodes, thymus, spleen, tonsils, bone marrow.
What body regions are ultimately drained of lymph by the thoracic duct?	Left upper body quadrant, and both lower body quadrants.
Name three different groups of lymph nodes that could be palpated if they were enlarged because of infection.	Cervical (jugulodigastric), axillary, and inguinal.
What are the group of nodes surrounding the tracheal bifurcation and primary bronchi called?	Mediastinal nodes.

Respiratory System

The pharynx is divided into three regions. Name them.	Nasopharynx, oropharynx, and laryngopharynx (hypopharynx).
What are some common symptoms of asthma?	Wheezing, shortness of breath, coughing, tachycardia, and tightness in the chest.

Review Questions

Nervous System

What are the components of the CNS?	Brain and spinal cord.
What is the cell body of a neuron called?	Soma.
What types of neurons, based on classification by shape, are typically found in cranial nerve or spinal ganglia?	Unipolar (pseudounipolar) neurons.
What types of cells function as support cells to neurons in the CNS?	Neuroglia (astrocytes, oligodendrocytes, and microglia).
Functionally, what type of neuron conveys electrical impulses from the CNS to a peripheral target site?	Efferent (motor) neuron.
What is the most common form of dementia?	Alzheimer's disease.
Which meningeal layer intimately invests the spinal cord?	Pia mater.
Where is cerebrospinal fluid produced and how much is usually produced each day?	Choroid plexus; normally approximately 500 ml.
Where is cerebrospinal fluid usually found?	In brain ventricles and subarachnoid space.
What are the names of the 12 cranial nerves?	Use the mnemonic On (Olfactory) old (Optic) Olympus' (Oculomotor) towering (Trochlear) top (Trigeminal) a (Abducens) Finn (Facial) and (Auditory-Vestibulocochlear) German (Glossopharyngeal) viewed (Vagus) a (Accessory-Spinal Accessory) hop (Hypoglossal).
How are the 31 pairs of spinal nerves regionally distributed?	Eight cervical pairs, 12 thoracic pairs, 5 lumbar pairs, 5 sacral pairs, and 1 coccygeal pair.
Where are the cell bodies of all peripheral afferent (sensory) nerves located?	Dorsal root ganglia.
What type(s) of nerve fibers are found in spinal dorsal roots?	Afferent (sensory) fibers.
The ventral primary rami of many spinal nerves often converge and form a plexus. What are the major peripheral nerve plexuses?	Cervical plexus (neck), brachial plexus (upper limb), lumbar plexus (lower limb and abdominal region), and sacral plexus (lower limb, pelvis, and perineum).
What acquired immunologic disease is associated with a reduction in the presence of ACh receptors at the neuromuscular junction?	Myasthenia gravis.
What are the three functional components of the PNS?	Somatic nervous system, ANS, and enteric nervous system.

Review Questions

What are the two functional and anatomical divisions of the ANS?	Sympathetic (thoracolumbar) and parasympathetic (craniosacral) divisions.
What do neurons of the somatic nervous system innervate?	Skin and skeletal muscles (and the joints that the muscles act on).
What do neurons of the ANS innervate?	All smooth muscle (organs or viscera), cardiac muscle, bone marrow, and all glands.
Which cranial nerves give rise to preganglionic parasympathetic nerve axons?	Oculomotor (III), facial (VII), glossopharyngeal (IX), and vagus (X).
What component of the PNS provides an intrinsic network of nerves and ganglia in the GI tract?	Enteric nervous system.
What classical neurotransmitter is released at parasympathetic postganglionic synapses?	ACh.
What classical neurotransmitters are released at sympathetic pre-ganglionic synapses and post-ganglionic synapses?	ACh at all preganglionic synapses, and norepinephrine at all postganglionic synapses except those that end on sweat glands, where ACh is the neurotransmitter.
Which division of the ANS functions to mobilize the body in fight-or-flight situations?	Sympathetic division.

Endocrine System

For each hormone listed below, identify the endocrine gland or tissue that secretes it.	
FSH:	Anterior pituitary gland
T4:	Thyroid gland
Inhibin:	Ovary
GH:	Anterior pituitary gland
Cortisol:	Adrenal cortex
ANP:	Atria of the heart
Insulin:	Pancreas
Testosterone:	Testis
Renin:	Kidney
Melatonin:	Pineal
Oxytocin:	Hypothalamus
Prolactin:	Anterior pituitary
Besides the endocrine system, what systems play a key role in communication, integration, and regulation of bodily functions?	Nervous and immune systems.

Gastrointestinal System

What structures make up the small intestine?	Duodenum, jejunum, and ileum.
What nerves exert an influence on the function of the enteric nervous system?	Parasympathetic and sympathetic divisions of the ANS.

Review Questions

Identify three general causes of diarrhea.	Inflammatory (colitis), irritative (chemical, bacterial), and dietary (intolerance to foods, vitamin deficiencies).

Urinary System

Which two organs play a significant role in the regulation of the pH of body fluids?	Lungs and kidneys.

Reproductive System

As one looks into the abdomino-pelvic cavity, what visible structure partially supports the ovaries, uterine tubes, and uterus?	Broad ligament.
What is semen?	Sperm and secretions of the ducts, seminal vesicles, prostate gland, and bulbourethral glands.
How are sperm conveyed from the epididymis to the ejaculatory duct of the seminal vesicles?	Sperm travel in the ductus (vas) deferens.

Embryology Overview

What term is given to the union of the sperm and egg nuclei?	Fertilization, which results in a zygote.
When does the blastocyst begin implanting in the uterine wall?	Approximately the fifth or sixth day after fertilization.
The inner cell mass of the implanted blastocyst forms what two cell layers?	Epiblast and hypoblast.
What key event marks the third week of embryonic development?	Gastrulation.
Epiblast cells close to the primitive streak invaginate to form what two new cell layers?	The mesoderm and then the endoderm (by replacing the hypoblast cells). Surface epiblast cells then become the ectoderm.
For each tissue listed below, state whether it is derived from ectoderm, mesoderm, or endoderm:	
Notochord:	Mesoderm
Epidermis:	Ectoderm
Neurons:	Ectoderm
Lining of GI tract:	Endoderm
Nails and hair:	Ectoderm
Heart:	Mesoderm
Skeletal muscle:	Mesoderm
Dermis:	Mesoderm
Lining of airways:	Endoderm
Ganglia:	Ectoderm
Developmental defects may result from three general causes. Name them.	Abnormal development, abnormal forces on a normally developing tissue, and disruption or destruction of a normally developed structure.

2

Back

Introduction The back forms the axis (central line) of the human body and consists of the vertebral column, spinal cord, supporting muscles, and associated tissues (skin, connective tissues, vessels, and nerves). The hallmark of vertebrate anatomy is segmentation, which is particularly evident in the human back.

Surface Anatomy: Key Landmarks

Vertebra prominens: spinous process of C7
Scapula: spine, inferior angle, and medial border
Iliac crests: a horizontal line connecting the crests passes through the spinous process of L4 and the intervertebral disc of L4-5; a useful landmark for a lumbar puncture or epidural block
Posterior superior iliac spines: a line connecting these points passes through the spinous process of S2

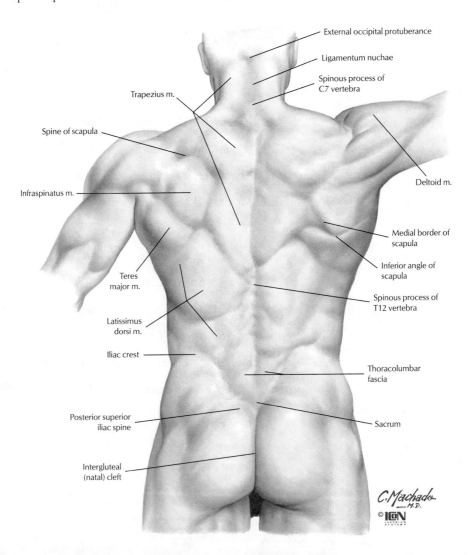

External occipital protuberance

Ligamentum nuchae

Spinous process of C7 vertebra

Trapezius m.

Spine of scapula

Deltoid m.

Infraspinatus m.

Medial border of scapula

Inferior angle of scapula

Teres major m.

Spinous process of T12 vertebra

Latissimus dorsi m.

Iliac crest

Thoracolumbar fascia

Posterior superior iliac spine

Sacrum

Intergluteal (natal) cleft

C.Machado
—M.D.

©IGN

Vertebral Column: The Spine

Vertebrae: 33 total: 7 cervical, 12 thoracic, 5 lumbar, 5 fused sacral, 4 coccygeal (last 3 fused)

Vertebral canal: formed by successive vertebral foramina of the articulated spine and containing the spinal cord

Primary curvatures: occur in the fetus (thoracic and sacral curvatures)

Secondary curvatures: occur when the infant supports its head (cervical lordosis) and assumes an upright posture (lumbar lordosis)

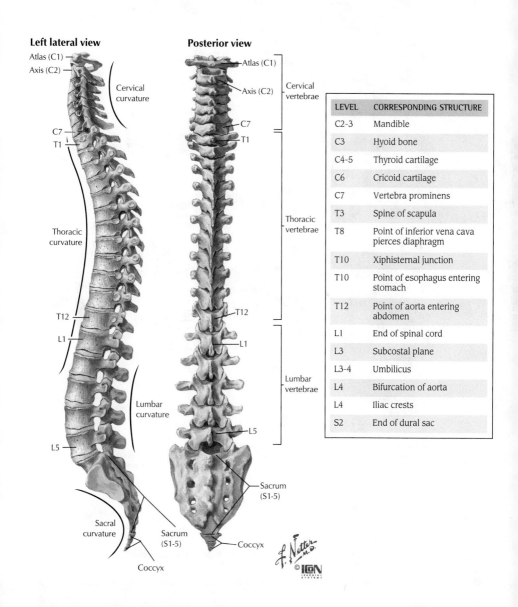

Left lateral view

Atlas (C1)
Axis (C2)
Cervical curvature
C7
T1
Thoracic curvature
T12
L1
Lumbar curvature
L5
Sacral curvature
Sacrum (S1-5)
Coccyx

Posterior view

Atlas (C1)
Axis (C2)
C7
T1
Cervical vertebrae
Thoracic vertebrae
T12
L1
Lumbar vertebrae
L5
Sacrum (S1-5)
Coccyx

LEVEL	CORRESPONDING STRUCTURE
C2-3	Mandible
C3	Hyoid bone
C4-5	Thyroid cartilage
C6	Cricoid cartilage
C7	Vertebra prominens
T3	Spine of scapula
T8	Point of inferior vena cava pierces diaphragm
T10	Xiphisternal junction
T10	Point of esophagus entering stomach
T12	Point of aorta entering abdomen
L1	End of spinal cord
L3	Subcostal plane
L3-4	Umbilicus
L4	Bifurcation of aorta
L4	Iliac crests
S2	End of dural sac

Clinical Correlation

Pathologic anatomy of scoliosis

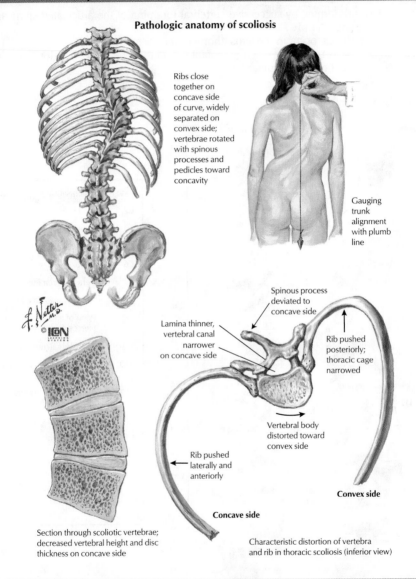

Ribs close together on concave side of curve, widely separated on convex side; vertebrae rotated with spinous processes and pedicles toward concavity

Gauging trunk alignment with plumb line

Spinous process deviated to concave side

Lamina thinner, vertebral canal narrower on concave side

Rib pushed posteriorly; thoracic cage narrowed

Vertebral body distorted toward convex side

Rib pushed laterally and anteriorly

Convex side

Concave side

Section through scoliotic vertebrae; decreased vertebral height and disc thickness on concave side

Characteristic distortion of vertebra and rib in thoracic scoliosis (inferior view)

DISORDER	DEFINITION	ETIOLOGY
Scoliosis (illustrated)	Accentuated lateral and rotational curve of thoracic or lumbar spine	Genetic, trauma, idiopathic; occurs in adolescent girls more than boys
Kyphosis	Hunchback, accentuated flexion of thoracic spine	Poor posture, osteoporosis
Lordosis	Swayback, accentuated extension of lumbar spine	Weakened trunk muscles, late pregnancy, obesity

Regional Vertebrae: Typical Vertebra

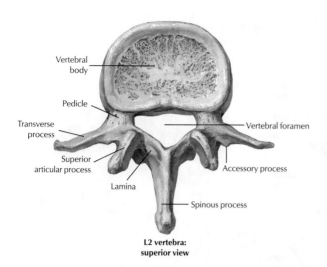

Vertebral body

Pedicle

Transverse process

Superior articular process

Lamina

Vertebral foramen

Accessory process

Spinous process

L2 vertebra: superior view

Vertebral body: weight-bearing portion that tends to increase in size as one descends the vertebral column
Vertebral arch: projection formed by paired pedicles and laminae
Transverse processes: lateral extensions from the union of the pedicle and lamina
Articular processes (facets): two superior and two inferior facets for articulation
Spinous process: projection that extends posteriorly from the union of two laminae
Vertebral notches: superior and inferior features that in articulated vertebrae form **intervertebral foramina** traversed by spinal nerve roots and associated vessels
Vertebral foramen: foramen formed from the vertebral arch and body
Transverse foramina: apertures that exist in transverse processes of cervical vertebrae and transmit vertebral vessels

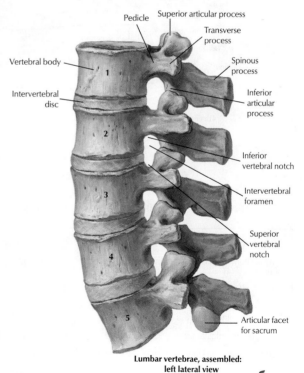

Pedicle

Superior articular process

Transverse process

Spinous process

Vertebral body

Intervertebral disc

Inferior articular process

Inferior vertebral notch

Intervertebral foramen

Superior vertebral notch

Articular facet for sacrum

Lumbar vertebrae, assembled: left lateral view

Regional Vertebrae: Cervical

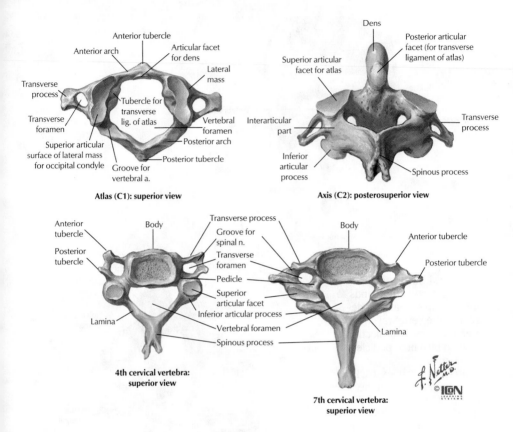

Atlas (C1): superior view

Anterior tubercle
Anterior arch
Articular facet for dens
Lateral mass
Transverse process
Tubercle for transverse lig. of atlas
Transverse foramen
Vertebral foramen
Posterior arch
Superior articular surface of lateral mass for occipital condyle
Posterior tubercle
Groove for vertebral a.

Axis (C2): posterosuperior view

Dens
Posterior articular facet (for transverse ligament of atlas)
Superior articular facet for atlas
Interarticular part
Transverse process
Inferior articular process
Spinous process

4th cervical vertebra: superior view

Anterior tubercle
Posterior tubercle
Body
Transverse process
Groove for spinal n.
Transverse foramen
Pedicle
Superior articular facet
Inferior articular process
Vertebral foramen
Spinous process
Lamina

7th cervical vertebra: superior view

Body
Anterior tubercle
Posterior tubercle
Lamina

The first two vertebrae (atlas and axis) are unique. C1 is the atlas and C2 is the axis.

ATLAS (C1)	OTHER CERVICAL VERTEBRAE (C3 TO C7)
Ringlike bone; superior facet articulates with occipital bone	Large triangular vertebral foramen
Two lateral masses with facets	Transverse foramen, through which vertebral artery passes
No body or spinous process	C3 to C5: short bifid spinous process
C1 rotates on articular facets of C2	C6 to C7: long spinous process
Vertebral artery runs in groove on posterior arch	C7 called vertebra prominens
	Narrow intervertebral foramina
	Nerve roots at risk of compression
AXIS (C2)	
Dens projects superiorly	
Strongest cervical vertebra	

Clinical Correlation

Cervical Vertebral Fractures   *Anatomy on pp. 67, 70*

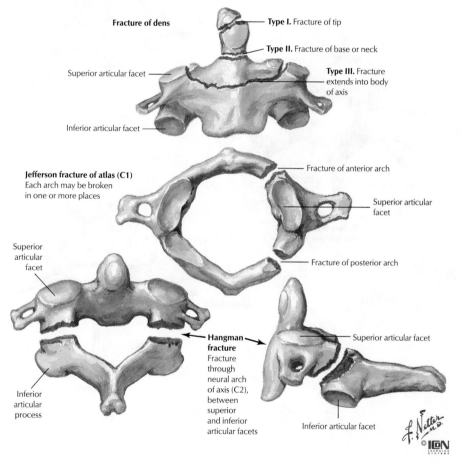

Fractures of cervical vertebrae

Fracture of dens

Type I. Fracture of tip

Type II. Fracture of base or neck

Superior articular facet

Type III. Fracture extends into body of axis

Inferior articular facet

Jefferson fracture of atlas (C1)
Each arch may be broken in one or more places

Fracture of anterior arch

Superior articular facet

Fracture of posterior arch

Superior articular facet

Superior articular facet

Hangman fracture
Fracture through neural arch of axis (C2), between superior and inferior articular facets

Inferior articular process

Inferior articular facet

Superior articular facet

Inferior articular facet

Fractures of the axis (C2) often involve the dens (odontoid process) and are classified as types I, II, and III. Type I is usually a stable fracture, type II is unstable, and type III (which extends into the body) usually reunites well when immobilized. The hangman fracture (pedicle fracture of C2) can be stabilized—if survived—with or without cord damage. A Jefferson fracture is a burst fracture of the atlas (C1), often caused by a blow to the top of the head.

Regional Vertebrae: Thoracic and Lumbar

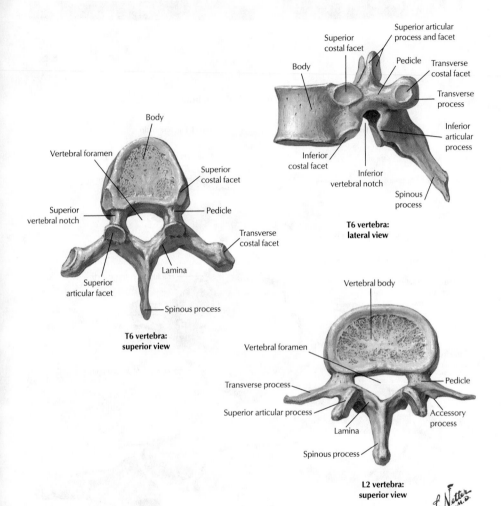

**T6 vertebra:
superior view**

**T6 vertebra:
lateral view**

**L2 vertebra:
superior view**

T1 TO T12	L1 TO L5
Heart-shaped body, with facets for rib articulation	Kidney-shaped body, massive for support
Small circular vertebral foramen	Midsized triangular vertebral foramen
Long transverse processes, which have facets for rib articulation in T1 to T10	Facets face medial or lateral direction, which permits good flexion and extension
Long spinous processes, which slope posteriorly and overlap next vertebra	Spinous process is short
	L5: largest vertebra

Regional Vertebrae: Sacrum and Coccyx

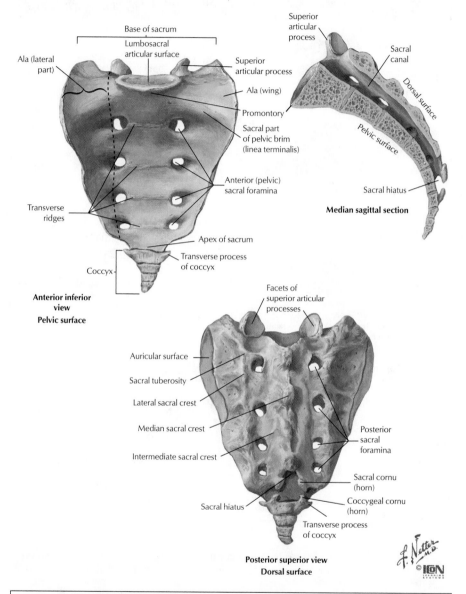

Base of sacrum
Lumbosacral articular surface
Ala (lateral part)
Superior articular process
Ala (wing)
Promontory
Sacral part of pelvic brim (linea terminalis)
Anterior (pelvic) sacral foramina
Transverse ridges
Apex of sacrum
Transverse process of coccyx
Coccyx

Anterior inferior view
Pelvic surface

Superior articular process
Sacral canal
Dorsal surface
Pelvic surface
Sacral hiatus

Median sagittal section

Facets of superior articular processes
Auricular surface
Sacral tuberosity
Lateral sacral crest
Median sacral crest
Intermediate sacral crest
Posterior sacral foramina
Sacral cornu (horn)
Coccygeal cornu (horn)
Sacral hiatus
Transverse process of coccyx

Posterior superior view
Dorsal surface

SACRUM	COCCYX
Large, wedge-shaped bone, which transmits body weight to pelvis	Co1 often not fused
Five fused vertebrae, with fusion complete by puberty	Co2 to Co4 fused
Four pairs of sacral foramina on dorsal and ventral (pelvic) side	No pedicles, laminae, spines
Sacral hiatus, the opening of sacral vertebral foramen	Remnant of our embryonic tail

Clinical Correlation

Osteoporosis

Anatomy on p. 67

Axial

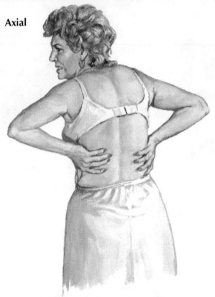

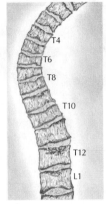

Multiple compression fractures of lower thoracic and upper lumbar vertebrae in patient with severe osteoporosis

Vertebral compression fractures cause continuous (acute) or intermittent (chronic) back pain from midthoracic to midlumbar region, occasionally to lower lumbar region.

Appendicular

Fractures caused by minimal trauma

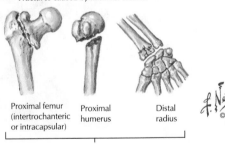

Proximal femur (intertrochanteric or intracapsular)   Proximal humerus   Distal radius

Most common types

   Osteoporosis (porous bone) is the most common bone disease and results from an imbalance in bone resorption and formation, which places bones at great risk for fracture.

CHARACTERISTIC	DESCRIPTION
Etiology	Postmenopausal women, genetics, vitamin D synthesis deficiency, idiopathic
Prevalence	Approximately 10 million Americans (8 million of them women), white
Risk factors	Family history, white female, increasing age, estrogen deficiency, vitamin D deficiency, low calcium intake, smoking, excessive alcohol use, inactive lifestyle
Complications	Vertebral compression fractures, fracture of proximal femur or humerus, ribs, and distal radius (Colles' fracture)

Clinical Correlation

Spondylolysis and Spondylolisthesis   *Anatomy on pp. 67, 69, 78*

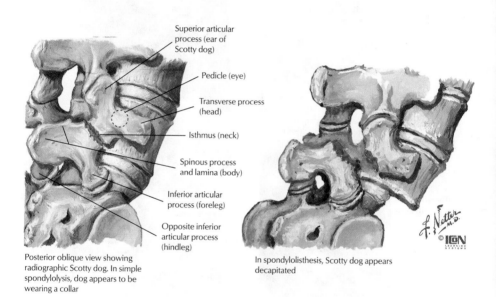

Superior articular
process (ear of
Scotty dog)

Pedicle (eye)

Transverse process
(head)

Isthmus (neck)

Spinous process
and lamina (body)

Inferior articular
process (foreleg)

Opposite inferior
articular process
(hindleg)

Posterior oblique view showing
radiographic Scotty dog. In simple
spondylolysis, dog appears to be
wearing a collar

In spondylolisthesis, Scotty dog appears
decapitated

Congenital and acquired conditions affect the spine. Spondylolysis is a congenital defect or an acquired stress fracture of the lamina that presents with no slippage of adjacent articulating vertebrae (most common at the L5-S1 site). Its radiographic appearance is a Scotty dog with a collar (highlighted in yellow, with the fracture site indicated as the red collar). However, a bilateral defect (a complete dislocation, or luxation), called spondylolisthesis, results in anterior displacement of the L5 body and transverse process while the posterior fragment (vertebral laminae and spinous process of L5) remains in proper alignment over the sacrum (S1). This defect has the radiographic appearance of a Scotty dog with a broken neck (highlighted in yellow, with the fracture in red). Pressure on spinal nerves often leads to low back and lower limb pain.

Clinical Correlation

Osteoarthritis
Anatomy on pp. 67, 69, 70, 101

Cervical spine involvement

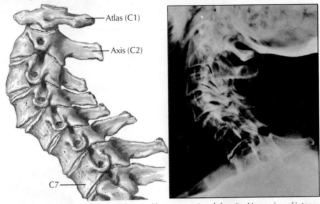

Atlas (C1)

Axis (C2)

C7

Extensive thinning of cervical discs and hyperextension deformity. Narrowing of intervertebral foramina. Lateral radiograph reveals similar changes.

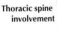

Thoracic spine involvement

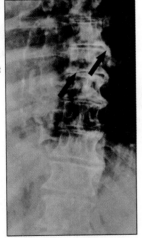

Lumbar spine involvement

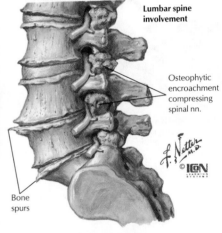

Osteophytic encroachment compressing spinal nn.

Bone spurs

Radiograph of thoracic spine shows narrowing of intervertebral spaces and spur formation (arrows).

Degeneration of lumbar intervertebral discs and hypertrophic changes at vertebral margins with spur formation. Osteophytic encroachment on intervertebral foramina compresses spinal nerves.

Osteoarthritis is the most common form of arthritis and often involves erosion of the articular cartilage of weight-bearing joints.

CHARACTERISTIC	DESCRIPTION
Etiology	Progressive erosion of cartilage in joints of spine, fingers, knee, and hip most commonly
Prevalence	20 million Americans, significant after age 65 years
Risk factors	Age, female sex, joint trauma, repetitive stress, obesity, genetic, race, previous inflammatory joint disease
Complications	In spine, involves intervertebral disc and facet joints, leading to hyperextension deformity and spinal nerve impingement

Joints and Ligaments of the Spine: Craniovertebral

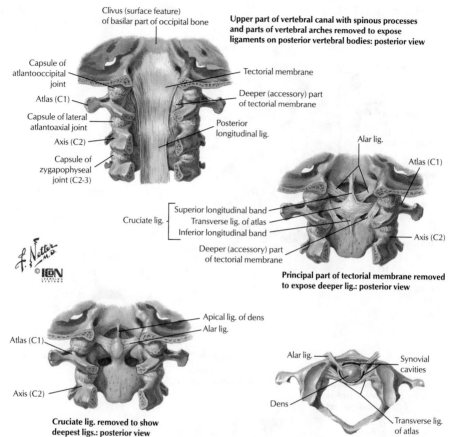

Clivus (surface feature) of basilar part of occipital bone

Upper part of vertebral canal with spinous processes and parts of vertebral arches removed to expose ligaments on posterior vertebral bodies: posterior view

Capsule of atlantooccipital joint

Atlas (C1)

Capsule of lateral atlantoaxial joint

Axis (C2)

Capsule of zygapophyseal joint (C2-3)

Tectorial membrane

Deeper (accessory) part of tectorial membrane

Posterior longitudinal lig.

Cruciate lig.
- Superior longitudinal band
- Transverse lig. of atlas
- Inferior longitudinal band

Deeper (accessory) part of tectorial membrane

Alar lig.

Atlas (C1)

Axis (C2)

Principal part of tectorial membrane removed to expose deeper lig.: posterior view

Atlas (C1)

Axis (C2)

Apical lig. of dens
Alar lig.

Cruciate lig. removed to show deepest ligs.: posterior view

Alar lig.

Synovial cavities

Dens

Transverse lig. of atlas

Median atlantoaxial joint: superior view

Craniovertebral joints include the atlantooccipital and atlantoaxial joints. Both are synovial joints that provide a relatively wide range of motion compared with other joints in the spine.

LIGAMENT	ATTACHMENT	COMMENT
Atlantooccipital (Biaxial Condyloid Synovial) Joint		
Articular capsule	Surrounds facets and occipital condyles	Allows flexion and extension
Anterior and posterior membranes	Anterior and posterior arches of C1 to foramen magnum	Limit movement of joint
Atlantoaxial (Uniaxial Synovial) Joint		
Tectorial membrane	Axis body to margin of foramen magnum	Is continuation of posterior longitudinal ligament
Apical	Dens to occipital bone	Is very small
Alar	Dens to occipital condyles	Limits rotation
Cruciate	Dens to lateral masses	Resembles a cross; allows rotation

Joints and Ligaments of the Spine: Vertebral Arches and Bodies

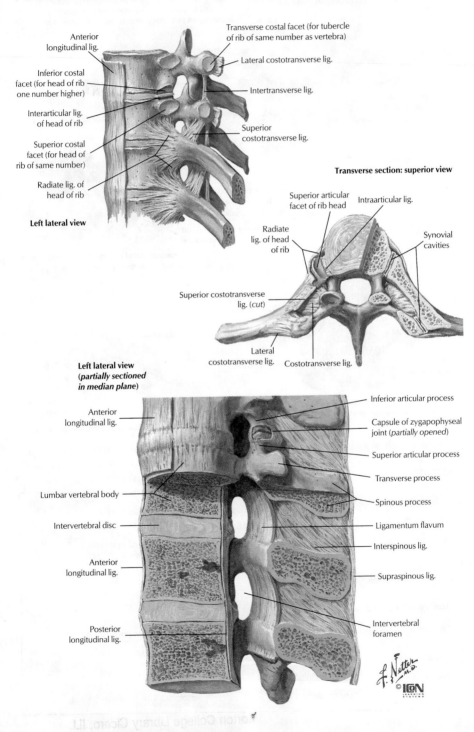

Anterior longitudinal lig.

Transverse costal facet (for tubercle of rib of same number as vertebra)

Lateral costotransverse lig.

Inferior costal facet (for head of rib one number higher)

Intertransverse lig.

Interarticular lig. of head of rib

Superior costotransverse lig.

Superior costal facet (for head of rib of same number)

Radiate lig. of head of rib

Left lateral view

Transverse section: superior view

Superior articular facet of rib head

Intraarticular lig.

Radiate lig. of head of rib

Synovial cavities

Superior costotransverse lig. (*cut*)

Lateral costotransverse lig.

Costotransverse lig.

Left lateral view
(***partially sectioned in median plane***)

Anterior longitudinal lig.

Inferior articular process

Capsule of zygapophyseal joint (*partially opened*)

Superior articular process

Transverse process

Lumbar vertebral body

Spinous process

Intervertebral disc

Ligamentum flavum

Anterior longitudinal lig.

Interspinous lig.

Supraspinous lig.

Posterior longitudinal lig.

Intervertebral foramen

Joints and Ligaments of the Spine: Vertebral Arches and Bodies (continued)

Joints of vertebral arches (which are plane synovial joints) between superior and inferior articular processes (facets) allow some gliding or sliding movement. Corresponding ligaments connect spinous processes, laminae, and bodies of adjacent vertebrae. Joints of vertebral bodies are secondary cartilaginous joints (symphyses) between adjacent vertebral bodies. These stable, weight-bearing joints also serve as shock absorbers. Intervertebral discs consist of an outer fibrocartilaginous anulus fibrosus and inner gelatinous nucleus pulposus (embryonic notochord remnant). Lumbar discs are thickest and upper thoracic spine discs are thinnest. Anterior and posterior longitudinal ligaments help to stabilize these joints.

LIGAMENT	ATTACHMENT	COMMENT
Zygapophyseal (Plane Synovial) Joints		
Articular capsule	Surrounds facets	Allows gliding motion C5-6 is most mobile L4-5 permits most flexion
Intervertebral (Secondary Cartilaginous [Symphyses]) Joints		
Anterior longitudinal (AL)	Anterior bodies and intervertebral discs	Is strong and prevents hyperextension
Posterior longitudinal (PL)	Posterior bodies and intervertebral discs	Is weaker than AL and prevents hyperflexion
Ligamenta flava	Connect adjacent laminae of vertebrae	Limit flexion and are more elastic
Interspinous	Connect spines	Are weak
Supraspinous	Connect spinous tips	Are stronger and limit flexion
Ligamentum nuchae	C7 to occipital bone	Is cervical extension of supraspinous ligament and is strong
Intertransverse	Connect transverse processes	Are weak ligaments
Intervertebral discs	Between adjacent bodies	Are secured by AL and PL ligaments

Clinical Correlation

Vertebral Dislocations and Fractures   *Anatomy on pp. 67, 69, 72, 78*

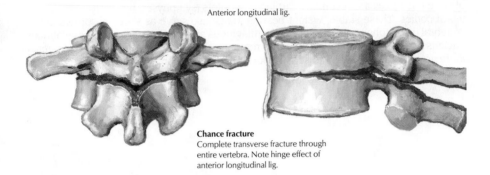

Anterior longitudinal lig.

Chance fracture
Complete transverse fracture through
entire vertebra. Note hinge effect of
anterior longitudinal lig.

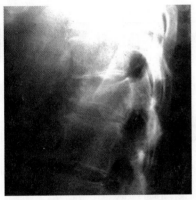

Lateral radiograph shows burst fracture of body of T12
with wedging, kyphosis, and retropulsion of fragments
into spinal canal.

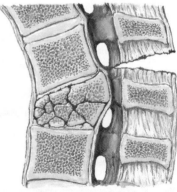

Sagittal view of fracture shown
in radiograph at left

A fracture through an entire vertebra, usually in the thoracolumbar spine, is a Chance
fracture, which used to be called a seat belt fracture because it occurred in vehicular
accidents when a lap belt but not a shoulder belt was worn (rare today). During rapid
deceleration, the spine flexes, with the lap belt as a pivot point; the fracture plane begins at the spinous process and travels through the vertebra. A fracture dislocation in
the thoracolumbar spine is unstable because both ligaments and bony structures are
involved, as are intervertebral discs. These ligaments include the following:

- Supraspinous
- Interspinous
- Ligamentum flavum
- Posterior longitudinal

Clinical Correlation

Ankylosing Spondylitis

Anatomy on pp. 78, 79

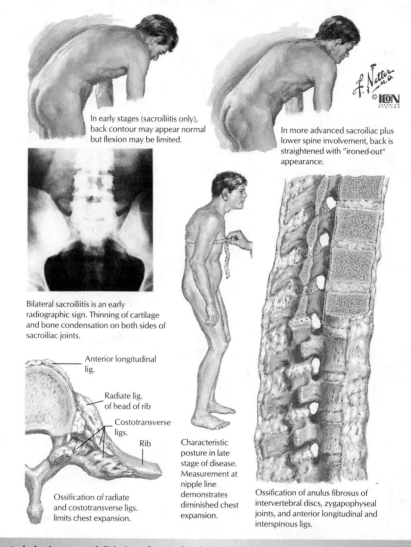

In early stages (sacroiliitis only), back contour may appear normal but flexion may be limited.

In more advanced sacroiliac plus lower spine involvement, back is straightened with "ironed-out" appearance.

Bilateral sacroiliitis is an early radiographic sign. Thinning of cartilage and bone condensation on both sides of sacroiliac joints.

Anterior longitudinal lig.

Radiate lig. of head of rib

Costotransverse ligs.

Rib

Ossification of radiate and costotransverse ligs. limits chest expansion.

Characteristic posture in late stage of disease. Measurement at nipple line demonstrates diminished chest expansion.

Ossification of anulus fibrosus of intervertebral discs, zygapophyseal joints, and anterior longitudinal and interspinous ligs.

Ankylosing spondylitis is a form of arthritis in which chronic inflammation affects the spine (spondylitis) and sacroiliac joint. Over time, vertebrae ossify and fuse (ankylosis), which causes a loss of spinal mobility.

CHARACTERISTIC	DESCRIPTION
Etiology	Genetic (90% of patients have HLA-B27 gene)
Prevalence	Three times more common in males, onset in second and third decades of life
Signs and symptoms	Inflammatory back pain, lower back stiffness, pain worse in morning, cardiac involvement, pain in other joints, iritis (uveitis)

Clinical Correlation

Low Back Pain

Anatomy on pp. 78, 79, 88, 92

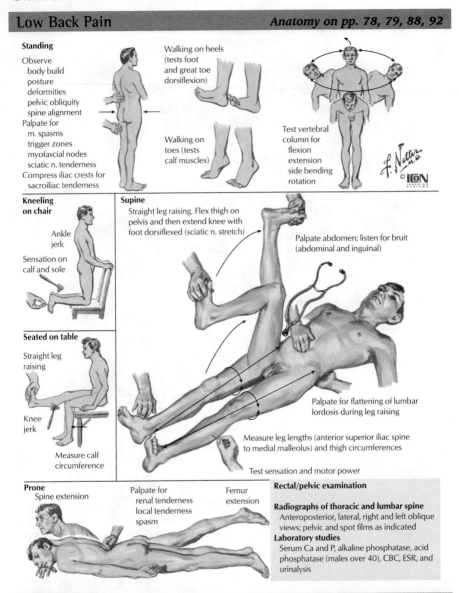

Standing

Observe
body build
posture
deformities
pelvic obliquity
spine alignment
Palpate for
m. spasms
trigger zones
myofascial nodes
sciatic n. tenderness
Compress iliac crests for
sacroiliac tenderness

Walking on heels
(tests foot
and great toe
dorsiflexion)

Walking on
toes (tests
calf muscles)

Test vertebral
column for
flexion
extension
side bending
rotation

Kneeling on chair

Ankle
jerk

Sensation on
calf and sole

Supine

Straight leg raising. Flex thigh on
pelvis and then extend knee with
foot dorsiflexed (sciatic n. stretch)

Palpate abdomen; listen for bruit
(abdominal and inguinal)

Palpate for flattening of lumbar
lordosis during leg raising

Seated on table

Straight leg
raising

Knee
jerk

Measure calf
circumference

Measure leg lengths (anterior superior iliac spine
to medial malleolus) and thigh circumferences

Test sensation and motor power

Prone
Spine extension

Palpate for
renal tenderness
local tenderness
spasm

Femur
extension

Rectal/pelvic examination

Radiographs of thoracic and lumbar spine
Anteroposterior, lateral, right and left oblique
views; pelvic and spot films as indicated
Laboratory studies
Serum Ca and P, alkaline phosphatase, acid
phosphatase (males over 40), CBC, ESR, and
urinalysis

Low back pain, the most common musculoskeletal disorder, can have various
causes. Those identified most often include

- Intervertebral disc rupture and herniation
- Nerve inflammation or compression
- Degenerative changes in vertebral facet joints
- Sacroiliac joint and ligament involvement
- Metabolic bone disease

- Psychosocial factors
- Abdominal aneurysm
- Metastatic cancer
- Myofascial disorders

Physical examination, although not always revealing a definite cause, may provide
clues to the level of spinal nerve involvement and relative sensitivity to pain.

Clinical Correlation

Process of Intervertebral Disc Herniation   *Anatomy on p. 78*

Intervertebral disc

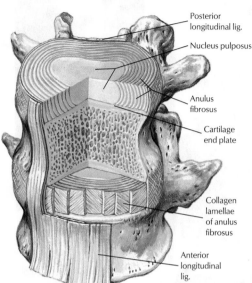

Posterior longitudinal lig.

Nucleus pulposus

Anulus fibrosus

Cartilage end plate

Collagen lamellae of anulus fibrosus

Anterior longitudinal lig.

Intervertebral disc composed of central nuclear zone
of collagen and hydrated proteoglycans surrounded
by concentric lamellae of collagen fibers

Pump mechanism of disc nutrition

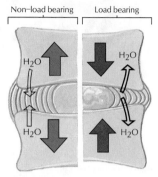

Non–load bearing   Load bearing

H_2O H_2O

H_2O H_2O

Movement-driven pump mechanism
alternately compresses and relaxes
pressure on disc, pumping water and
waste products out and water and
nutrients in.

*C. Machado
—M.D.*
© ICON
LEARNING SYSTEMS

Disc rupture and nuclear herniation

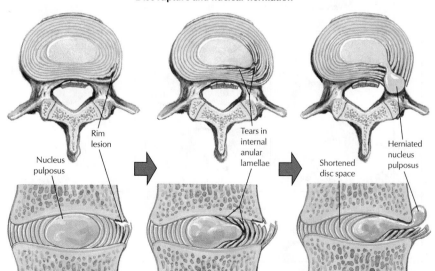

Rim lesion

Nucleus pulposus

Tears in internal anular lamellae

Shortened disc space

Herniated nucleus pulposus

Peripheral tear of anulus fibrosus and cartilage end plate (rim lesion) initiates sequence of events
that weaken and tear internal anular lamellae, allowing extrusion and herniation of nucleus pulposus.

Clinical Correlation

Herniation of a Cervical Disc   *Anatomy on pp. 78, 97, 101, 102, 104*

Cervical disc herniation: clinical manifestations

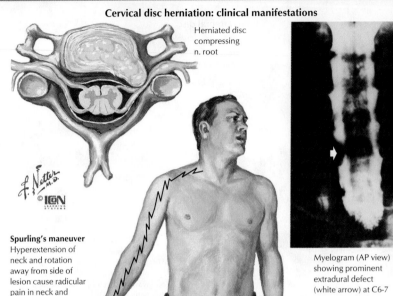

Herniated disc
compressing
n. root

Spurling's maneuver
Hyperextension of
neck and rotation
away from side of
lesion cause radicular
pain in neck and
down arm.

Myelogram (AP view)
showing prominent
extradural defect
(white arrow) at C6-7

Level	Motor signs (weakness)	Reflex signs	Sensory loss
C5	Deltoid	0	
C6	Biceps brachii	Biceps brachii — Weak or absent reflex	
C7	Triceps brachii	Triceps brachii — Weak or absent reflex	
C8	Interossei	Horner's syndrome	

Cervical disc herniation usually occurs in the absence of trauma and is often related to dehydration of the nucleus pulposus. Motor and sensory loss may occur, as indicated above.

Clinical Correlation

Inflammation and Lumbar Pain
Anatomy on pp. 78, 97, 100, 101, 104

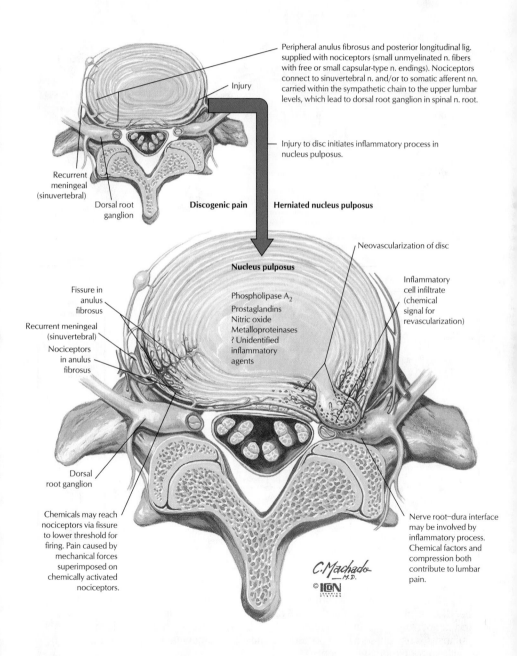

Peripheral anulus fibrosus and posterior longitudinal lig. supplied with nociceptors (small unmyelinated n. fibers with free or small capsular-type n. endings). Nociceptors connect to sinuvertebral n. and/or to somatic afferent nn. carried within the sympathetic chain to the upper lumbar levels, which lead to dorsal root ganglion in spinal n. root.

Injury

Recurrent meningeal (sinuvertebral)

Dorsal root ganglion

Injury to disc initiates inflammatory process in nucleus pulposus.

Discogenic pain   **Herniated nucleus pulposus**

Neovascularization of disc

Nucleus pulposus

Phospholipase A$_2$
Prostaglandins
Nitric oxide
Metalloproteinases
? Unidentified inflammatory agents

Inflammatory cell infiltrate (chemical signal for revascularization)

Fissure in anulus fibrosus

Recurrent meningeal (sinuvertebral)
Nociceptors in anulus fibrosus

Dorsal root ganglion

Chemicals may reach nociceptors via fissure to lower threshold for firing. Pain caused by mechanical forces superimposed on chemically activated nociceptors.

Nerve root–dura interface may be involved by inflammatory process. Chemical factors and compression both contribute to lumbar pain.

C. Machado
M.D.
© ICON
LEARNING SYSTEMS

Clinical Correlation

Herniation of a Lumbar Disc   *Anatomy on pp. 78, 97, 100, 101, 104*

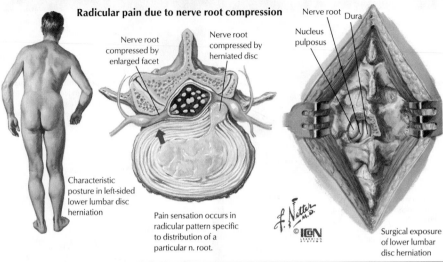

Radicular pain due to nerve root compression

Nerve root compressed by enlarged facet

Nerve root compressed by herniated disc

Nerve root

Dura

Nucleus pulposus

Characteristic posture in left-sided lower lumbar disc herniation

Pain sensation occurs in radicular pattern specific to distribution of a particular n. root.

Surgical exposure of lower lumbar disc herniation

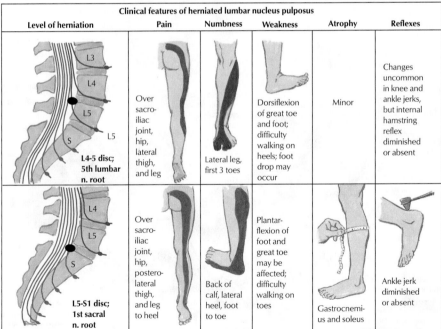

Clinical features of herniated lumbar nucleus pulposus					
Level of herniation	Pain	Numbness	Weakness	Atrophy	Reflexes
L4-5 disc; 5th lumbar n. root	Over sacro-iliac joint, hip, lateral thigh, and leg	Lateral leg, first 3 toes	Dorsiflexion of great toe and foot; difficulty walking on heels; foot drop may occur	Minor	Changes uncommon in knee and ankle jerks, but internal hamstring reflex diminished or absent
L5-S1 disc; 1st sacral n. root	Over sacro-iliac joint, hip, postero-lateral thigh, and leg to heel	Back of calf, lateral heel, foot to toe	Plantar-flexion of foot and great toe may be affected; difficulty walking on toes	Gastrocnemi-us and soleus	Ankle jerk diminished or absent

Lumbar disc disease is six times more common than cervical disc disease. Most lumbar disc herniations occur at the L4-5 or L5-S1 vertebral levels. The anterior aspects of the lumbar discs are under greater weight-bearing stress, so the herniating nucleus pulposus is usually squeezed posteriorly and often somewhat laterally, adjacent to the posterior longitudinal ligament.

Clinical Correlation

Back Pain Associated with Vertebral Facet Joints

Anatomy on pp. 78, 104

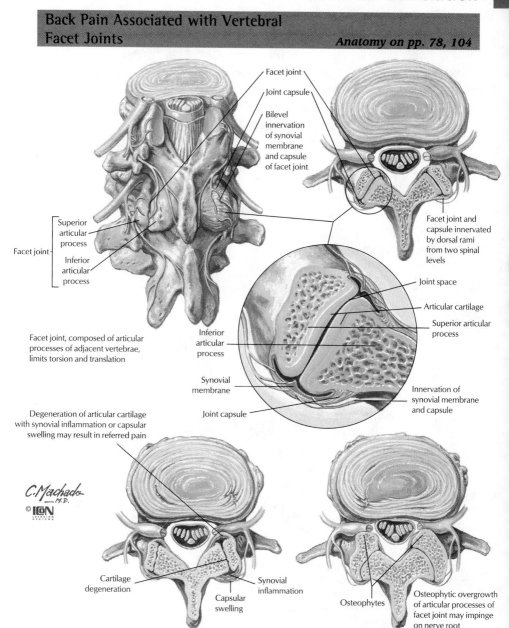

Facet joint

Joint capsule

Bilevel innervation of synovial membrane and capsule of facet joint

Facet joint and capsule innervated by dorsal rami from two spinal levels

Superior articular process

Facet joint

Inferior articular process

Joint space

Articular cartilage

Superior articular process

Inferior articular process

Facet joint, composed of articular processes of adjacent vertebrae, limits torsion and translation

Synovial membrane

Joint capsule

Innervation of synovial membrane and capsule

Degeneration of articular cartilage with synovial inflammation or capsular swelling may result in referred pain

C. Machado —M.D.

©ICON LEARNING SYSTEMS

Cartilage degeneration

Synovial inflammation

Capsular swelling

Osteophytes

Osteophytic overgrowth of articular processes of facet joint may impinge on nerve root

Although changes in vertebral facet joints are not the most common cause of back pain (approximately 15%), such alterations can lead to chronic pain. Articular surfaces of synovial facet joints are not directly innervated, but sensory nerve fibers supply synovial linings of the capsules surrounding the joints. Two examples of these conditions—degeneration of articular cartilage and osteophyte (bony outgrowth) overgrowth of facet articular processes—are illustrated.

Spine: Movements

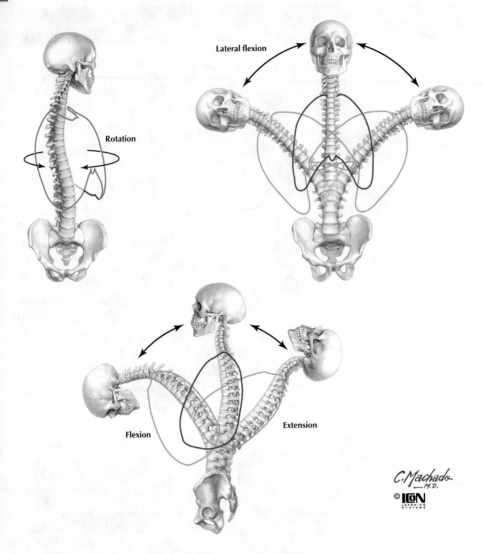

Movements of the spine are a function of the following features:
- Size and compressibility of intervertebral discs
- Tightness of joint capsules
- Orientation of articular facets
- Muscle and ligament function

The essential movements of the spine are flexion, extension, lateral flexion (lateral bending), and rotation. The greatest freedom of movement occurs in the cervical and lumbar spine, with the neck having the greatest range of motion. The atlantooccipital joint permits flexion and extension, as in nodding the head in acknowledgment. The atlantoaxial joint allows side-to-side movements (rotation), as in turning the head to indicate no. Alar ligaments limit side-to-side movement, so rotation of the atlantoaxial joint occurs with the skull and atlas rotating as a single unit, while the actual rotation occurs between the atlas and axis.

Clinical Correlation

Whiplash

Anatomy on pp. 77, 88

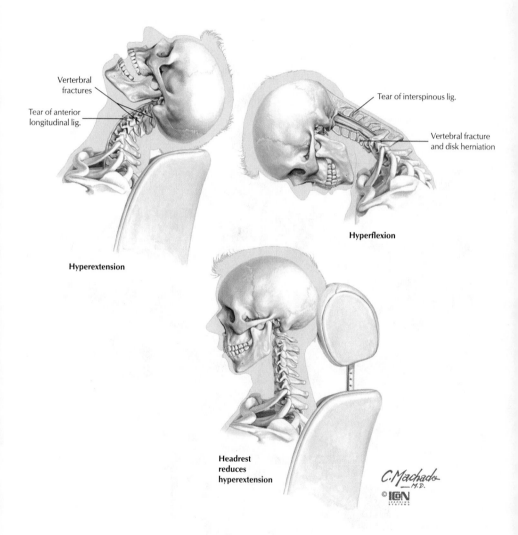

Verterbral fractures

Tear of anterior longitudinal lig.

Tear of interspinous lig.

Vertebral fracture and disk herniation

Hyperflexion

Hyperextension

Headrest reduces hyperextension

C. Machado —M.D.

© ICN
LEARNING
SYSTEMS

Whiplash is a nonmedical term for a cervical hyperextension injury, which is usually associated with a rear-end vehicular accident. The relaxed neck is thrown backward—is hyperextended—as the vehicle accelerates rapidly forward. Rapid recoil of the neck into extreme flexion occurs next. Properly adjusted headrests can significantly reduce the occurrence of hyperextension injury, which often results in stretched or torn cervical muscles and, in severe cases, ligament, bone, and nerve damage.

Back Muscles: Superficial and Intermediate Layers

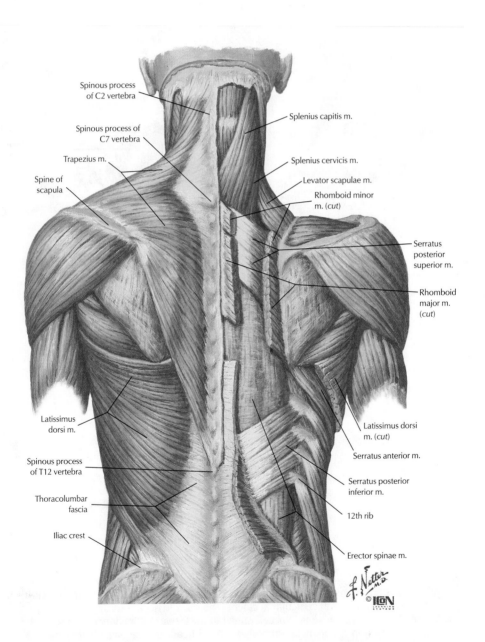

Spinous process of C2 vertebra

Spinous process of C7 vertebra

Trapezius m.

Spine of scapula

Latissimus dorsi m.

Spinous process of T12 vertebra

Thoracolumbar fascia

Iliac crest

Splenius capitis m.

Splenius cervicis m.

Levator scapulae m.

Rhomboid minor m. (cut)

Serratus posterior superior m.

Rhomboid major m. (cut)

Latissimus dorsi m. (cut)

Serratus anterior m.

Serratus posterior inferior m.

12th rib

Erector spinae m.

Back Muscles: Superficial and Intermediate Layers (continued)

Superficial muscles: muscles concerned with movements of upper limbs
Intermediate muscles: accessory muscles of respiration

This illustration shows superficial and intermediate muscles of the back. On the right side, the trapezius and latissimus dorsi muscles were removed to show the intermediate muscle layers. Deep muscles, not shown here, are postural muscles and muscles that move the spine (intrinsic or true back muscles).

MUSCLE	PROXIMAL ATTACHMENT (ORIGIN)	DISTAL ATTACHMENT (INSERTION)	INNERVATION	MAIN ACTIONS
Trapezius	Medial nuchal line, external occipital protuberance, nuchal ligament, and spinous processes of C7-T12	Lateral third of clavicle, acromion, and spine of scapula	Accessory nerve (cranial nerve XI) and C3-C4 (proprioception)	Elevates, retracts, and rotates scapula
Latissimus dorsi	Spinous processes of T7-T12, thoracolumbar fascia, iliac crest, and last three or four ribs	Humerus (intertubercular groove)	Thoracodorsal nerve (C6-C8)	Extends, adducts, and medially rotates humerus
Levator scapulae	Transverse processes of C1-C4	Medial border of scapula	C3-C4 and dorsal scapular (C5) nerve	Elevates scapula and tilts glenoid cavity inferiorly
Rhomboid minor and major	*Minor*: nuchal ligament and spinous processes of C7-T1 *Major*: spinous processes of T2-T5	Medial border of scapula	Dorsal scapular nerve (C4-C5)	Retract scapula, rotate it to depress glenoid cavity, and fix scapula to thoracic wall
Serratus posterior superior	Ligamentum nuchae and spinous processes of C7-T3	Superior border ribs 2-4	T1-T4	Elevates ribs
Serratus posterior inferior	Spinous processes of T11-L2	Inferior border ribs 9-12	T9-T12	Depresses ribs

Back Muscles: Deep Group (Superficial and Intermediate Layers)

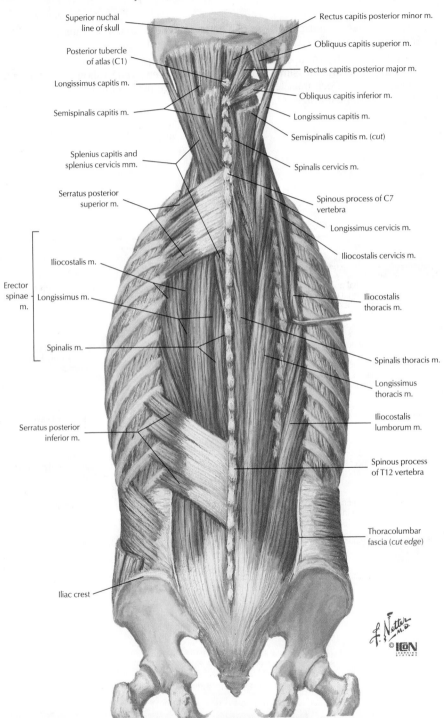

Superior nuchal line of skull

Posterior tubercle of atlas (C1)

Longissimus capitis m.

Semispinalis capitis m.

Splenius capitis and splenius cervicis mm.

Serratus posterior superior m.

Iliocostalis m.

Erector spinae m.

Longissimus m.

Spinalis m.

Serratus posterior inferior m.

Iliac crest

Rectus capitis posterior minor m.

Obliquus capitis superior m.

Rectus capitis posterior major m.

Obliquus capitis inferior m.

Longissimus capitis m.

Semispinalis capitis m. (cut)

Spinalis cervicis m.

Spinous process of C7 vertebra

Longissimus cervicis m.

Iliocostalis cervicis m.

Iliocostalis thoracis m.

Spinalis thoracis m.

Longissimus thoracis m.

Iliocostalis lumborum m.

Spinous process of T12 vertebra

Thoracolumbar fascia (cut edge)

Back Muscles: Deep Group (Superficial and Intermediate Layers) (continued)

Superficial muscles: splenius muscles that occupy the lateral and posterior neck
Intermediate muscles: erector spinae muscles that largely extend the spine
Deep: transversospinal muscles that fill spaces between transverse processes and spinous processes (see next page)

On the right side of the illustration, the dissection shows the intermediate muscle layer. All of these muscles are innervated by dorsal rami of spinal nerves.

MUSCLE	PROXIMAL ATTACHMENT (ORIGIN)	DISTAL ATTACHMENT (INSERTION)	INNERVATION*	MAIN ACTIONS
Superficial Layer				
Splenius capitis	Nuchal ligament and spinous process C7-T3	Mastoid process of temporal bone and lateral third of superior nuchal line	Middle cervical nerves	*Bilaterally*: extends head *Unilaterally*: laterally bends (flexes) and rotates face to same side
Splenius cervicis	Spinous process T3-T6	Transverse process (C1-C3)	Lower cervical nerves	*Bilaterally*: extends neck *Unilaterally*: laterally bends (flexes) and rotates neck toward same side
Intermediate Layer				
Erector spinae	Posterior sacrum, iliac crest, sacrospinous ligament, supraspinous ligament, and spinous processes of lower lumbar and sacral vertebrae	*Ilicostalis*: angles of lower ribs and cervical transverse processes *Longissimus*: between tubercles and angles of ribs, transverse processes of thoracic and cervical vertebrae, mastoid process *Spinalis*: spinous processes of upper thoracic and midcervical vertebrae	Respective spinal nerves of each region	Extend and laterally bend vertebral column and head

*Dorsal rami of spinal nerves.

Back Muscles: Deep Group (Deep Layer)

The transversospinal muscles (semispinalis, multifidus, and rotatores) are often referred to by clinicians as simply the paravertebral muscles because they form a solid mass of muscle tissue interposed between the transverse and spinous processes. On the right side, a deeper dissection shows underlying muscles of the transversospinal group.

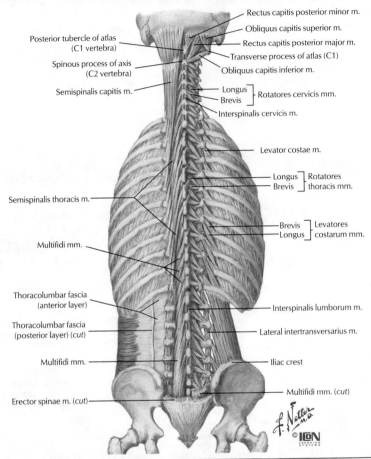

MUSCLE	PROXIMAL ATTACHMENT (ORIGIN)	DISTAL ATTACHMENT (INSERTION)	INNERVATION*	MAIN ACTIONS
Semispinalis	Transverse processes C4-T12	Spinous processes of cervical and thoracic regions	Respective spinal nerves of each region	Extends head, neck, and thorax and rotates them to opposite side
Multifidi	Sacrum, ilium, and transverse processes of T1-T12 and articular processes of C4-C7	Spinous processes of vertebrae above, spanning two to four segments	Respective spinal nerves of each region	Stabilizes spine during local movements
Rotatores	Transverse processes	Lamina and transverse process or spine above, spanning one or two segments	Respective spinal nerves of each region	Stabilize, extend, and rotate spine

*Dorsal rami of spinal nerves.

Back Muscles: Suboccipital Triangle and Muscles

Deep within the back of the neck, some transversospinal muscles that move the head and are attached to the skull, atlas, and axis form a triangle demarcated by the
- Rectus capitis posterior major muscle
- Obliquus capitis superior muscle (superior oblique muscle of head)
- Obliquus capitis inferior muscle (inferior oblique muscle of head)

Deep within this suboccipital triangle, the vertebral artery (a branch of the subclavian artery in the lower anterior neck) passes through the transverse foramen of the atlas and loops medially to enter the foramen magnum of the skull to supply the brainstem. The first three pairs of spinal nerves are also found in this region.

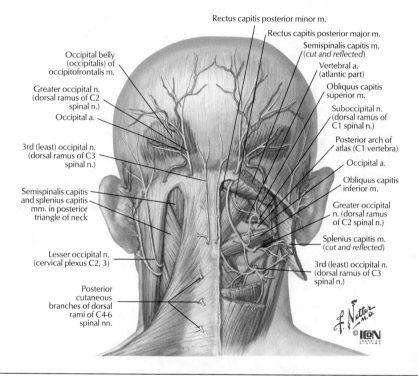

MUSCLE	PROXIMAL ATTACHMENT (ORIGIN)	DISTAL ATTACHMENT (INSERTION)	INNERVATION	MAIN ACTIONS
Rectus capitis posterior major	Spine of axis	Lateral inferior nuchal line	Suboccipital nerve (C1)	Extends head and rotates to same side
Rectus capitis posterior minor	Tubercle of posterior arch of atlas	Median inferior nuchal line	Suboccipital nerve (C1)	Extends head
Obliquus capitis superior	Atlas transverse process	Occipital bone	Suboccipital nerve (C1)	Extends head and bends it laterally
Obliquus capitis inferior	Spine of axis	Atlas transverse process	Suboccipital nerve (C1)	Rotates atlas to turn face to same side

Clinical Correlation

Myofascial Causes of Back Pain   *Anatomy on pp. 92, 99, 101, 104*

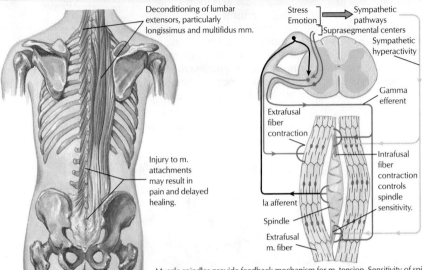

Deconditioning of lumbar extensors, particularly longissimus and multifidus mm.

Injury to m. attachments may result in pain and delayed healing.

Stress Emotion → Sympathetic pathways / Suprasegmental centers

Sympathetic hyperactivity

Gamma efferent

Extrafusal fiber contraction

Intrafusal fiber contraction controls spindle sensitivity.

Ia afferent

Spindle

Extrafusal m. fiber

Muscle spindles provide feedback mechanism for m. tension. Sensitivity of spindle modulated by gamma efferent system and by sympathetic innervaton of spindles. Sympathetic hyperactivity can result in painful spasm of spindles.

Deconditioning of extensor musculature

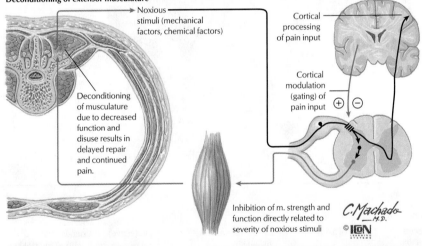

Noxious stimuli (mechanical factors, chemical factors)

Deconditioning of musculature due to decreased function and disuse results in delayed repair and continued pain.

Cortical processing of pain input

Cortical modulation (gating) of pain input ⊕ ⊖

Inhibition of m. strength and function directly related to severity of noxious stimuli

C.Machado—M.D.

© IGN LEARNING SYSTEMS

Myofascial pain syndrome is a common but poorly understood localized musculoskeletal pain (deep, aching or burning) associated with specific trigger points, usually over the erector spinae muscles that maintain posture (posterior neck and lower back regions).

CHARACTERISTIC	DESCRIPTION
Etiology	May follow trauma, poor posture or work ergonomics, stress
Prevalence	Women and men equally affected, usually aged 30-60 years
Pathophysiology	Noxious stimuli lead to deconditioning of extensor muscles, painful spasm of muscle spindles, and deep aching pain

Spinal Cord: Nerves

Thirty-one pairs of spinal nerves arise from the dorsal and ventral rootlets (filaments) of the cord and converge to form dorsal and ventral roots. These roots unite to form the spinal nerve pair (right and left spinal nerves for each spinal cord segment). Each spinal nerve then divides into a large ventral (primary) ramus and a smaller dorsal (primary) ramus.

Membranes removed: anterior view
(*greatly magnified*)

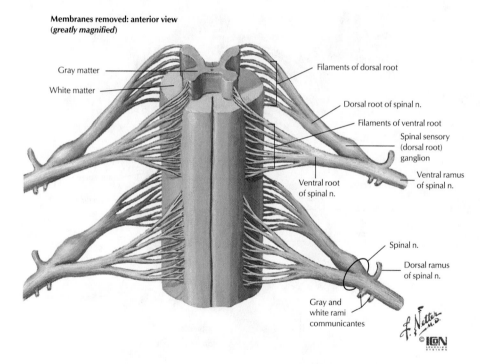

Gray matter

White matter

Filaments of dorsal root

Dorsal root of spinal n.

Filaments of ventral root

Spinal sensory
(dorsal root)
ganglion

Ventral ramus
of spinal n.

Ventral root
of spinal n.

Spinal n.

Dorsal ramus
of spinal n.

Gray and
white rami
communicantes

Spinal Cord: Cord and Nerves In Situ

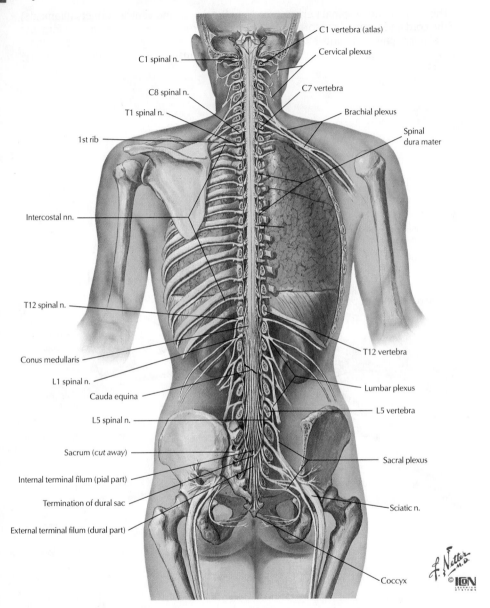

C1 vertebra (atlas)
Cervical plexus
C1 spinal n.
C8 spinal n.
C7 vertebra
T1 spinal n.
Brachial plexus
1st rib
Spinal dura mater
Intercostal nn.
T12 spinal n.
T12 vertebra
Conus medullaris
L1 spinal n.
Lumbar plexus
Cauda equina
L5 vertebra
L5 spinal n.
Sacrum (*cut away*)
Sacral plexus
Internal terminal filum (pial part)
Termination of dural sac
Sciatic n.
External terminal filum (dural part)
Coccyx

The 31 spinal segments and associated pairs of spinal nerves are regionally arranged as follows:
- 8 cervical pairs
- 12 thoracic pairs
- 5 lumbar pairs
- 5 sacral pairs
- 1 coccygeal pair

Key nerve plexuses include
- Cervical: C1-4
- Brachial: C5-T1
- Lumbar: L1-4
- Sacral: L4-S4

Spinal Cord: Somatic Nerve

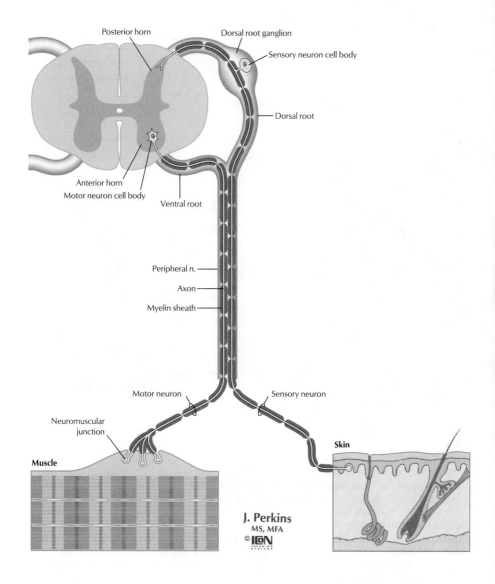

Posterior horn

Dorsal root ganglion

Sensory neuron cell body

Dorsal root

Anterior horn
Motor neuron cell body
Ventral root

Peripheral n.

Axon

Myelin sheath

Motor neuron

Sensory neuron

Neuromuscular
junction

Skin

Muscle

J. Perkins
MS, MFA
©IGN

Typical scheme for a peripheral nerve showing somatic motor and sensory components. Cell bodies of motor neurons reside in the anterior horn of the spinal cord; cell bodies of sensory neurons reside in the dorsal root ganglion. Autonomic fibers are not shown here.

Spinal Cord: Components of the Spinal Nerve (Thoracic)

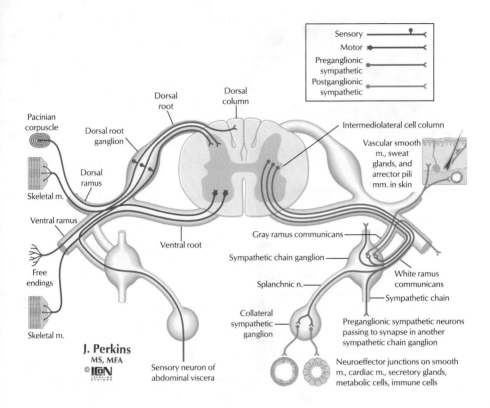

Sensory
Motor
Preganglionic sympathetic
Postganglionic sympathetic

Dorsal root
Dorsal column
Pacinian corpuscle
Dorsal root ganglion
Intermediolateral cell column
Vascular smooth m., sweat glands, and arrector pili mm. in skin
Dorsal ramus
Skeletal m.
Ventral ramus
Gray ramus communicans
Ventral root
Sympathetic chain ganglion
Free endings
White ramus communicans
Splanchnic n.
Sympathetic chain
Skeletal m.
Collateral sympathetic ganglion
Preganglionic sympathetic neurons passing to synapse in another sympathetic chain ganglion
J. Perkins
MS, MFA
©ICN
Sensory neuron of abdominal viscera
Neuroeffector junctions on smooth m., cardiac m., secretory glands, metabolic cells, immune cells

Regional spinal nerves convey sensory (afferent) nerve fibers from peripheral receptors into the spinal cord and motor (efferent) fibers from the cord to peripheral targets such as muscles. Dorsal roots contain sensory nerve fibers; ventral roots contain motor (somatic and sometimes autonomic) nerve fibers. Dorsal root (spinal) ganglia contain nerve cell bodies (neuronal soma) of sensory fibers (somatic and visceral); somatic motor axons arise from nerve cell bodies in the ventral (anterior) gray horns of the spinal cord. For simplicity, the left side of the cord shows only the somatic components of a spinal nerve, and the right side of the cord shows only the autonomic components. Each of the 31 pairs of spinal nerves contains three different types of nerve fibers:

- Somatic efferent fibers to skeletal muscle
- Postganglionic sympathetic efferent fibers to smooth muscle and glands
- Afferent fibers from skin, skeletal muscle and joints, or viscera

Also, each spinal nerve pair is connected to the sympathetic chain by a gray ramus communicans, and nerves arising from T1 to L2 spinal cord segments are connected to the sympathetic chain by white rami.

Spinal Cord: Relationship of Nerves to the Spine

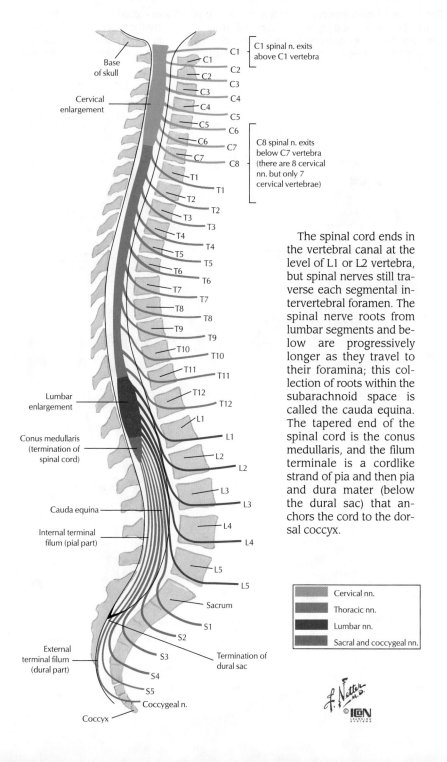

Base of skull

Cervical enlargement

C1 spinal n. exits above C1 vertebra

C8 spinal n. exits below C7 vertebra (there are 8 cervical nn. but only 7 cervical vertebrae)

Lumbar enlargement

Conus medullaris (termination of spinal cord)

Cauda equina

Internal terminal filum (pial part)

External terminal filum (dural part)

Coccyx

Termination of dural sac

The spinal cord ends in the vertebral canal at the level of L1 or L2 vertebra, but spinal nerves still traverse each segmental intervertebral foramen. The spinal nerve roots from lumbar segments and below are progressively longer as they travel to their foramina; this collection of roots within the subarachnoid space is called the cauda equina. The tapered end of the spinal cord is the conus medullaris, and the filum terminale is a cordlike strand of pia and then pia and dura mater (below the dural sac) that anchors the cord to the dorsal coccyx.

Cervical nn.

Thoracic nn.

Lumbar nn.

Sacral and coccygeal nn.

Spinal Cord: Dermatomes

The region of skin innervated by sensory nerve fibers associated with a single dorsal root and its dorsal root ganglion is called a dermatome. Dermatomes encircle the body in a segmental fashion corresponding to spinal cord segments. Knowledge of the dermatome pattern is useful in localizing specific spinal cord segments (intact or lesioned).

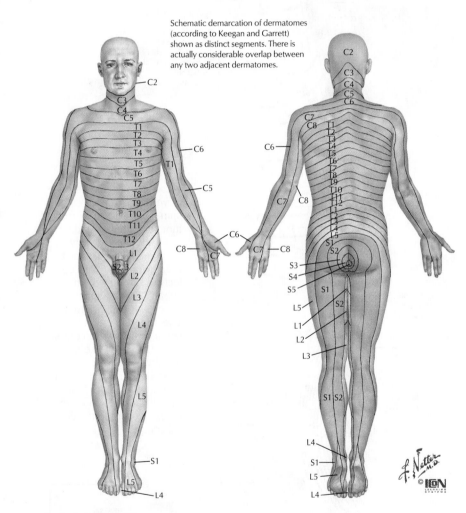

Schematic demarcation of dermatomes (according to Keegan and Garrett) shown as distinct segments. There is actually considerable overlap between any two adjacent dermatomes.

Levels of principal dermatomes

C5	Clavicles	T10	Level of umbilicus
C5, 6, 7	Lateral parts of upper limbs	T12, L1	Inguinal or groin regions
C8, T1	Medial sides of upper limbs	L1, 2, 3, 4	Anterior and inner surfaces of lower limbs
C6	Thumb	L4, 5, S1	Foot
C6, 7, 8	Hand	L4	Medial side of great toe
C8	Ring and little fingers	S1, 2, L5	Posterior and outer surfaces of lower limbs
T4	Level of nipples	S1	Lateral margin of foot and little toe
		S2, 3, 4	Perineum

Spinal Meninges

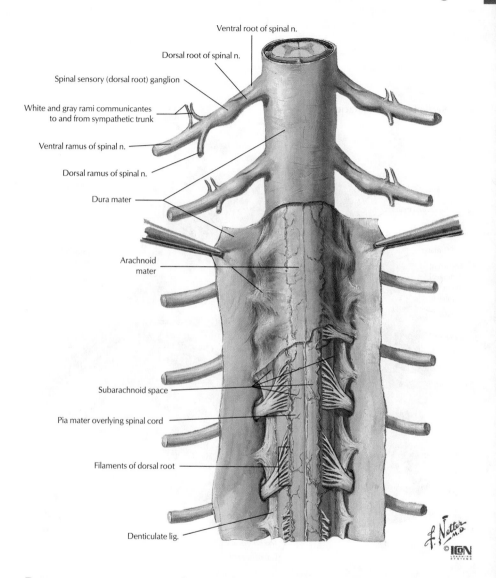

Ventral root of spinal n.

Dorsal root of spinal n.

Spinal sensory (dorsal root) ganglion

White and gray rami communicantes to and from sympathetic trunk

Ventral ramus of spinal n.

Dorsal ramus of spinal n.

Dura mater

Arachnoid mater

Subarachnoid space

Pia mater overlying spinal cord

Filaments of dorsal root

Denticulate lig.

Dura mater: thick outermost covering of the spinal cord and brain that forms a dural sac along the length of the spinal canal to the S2 level. The epidural (extradural) space lies between the vertebral canal walls and spinal dural sac and contains fat and vessels.

Arachnoid mater: very thin, avascular, impermeable membrane that lies just beneath the dura and lines the dural sac. Wispy threads of connective tissue extend from this layer to the underlying pia and span the subarachnoid space, which is filled with cerebrospinal fluid (CSF).

Pia mater: delicate membrane of thin connective tissue that envelops the cord. At the conus medullaris, it gives rise to the filum terminale. At cervical and thoracic cord levels, extensions of pia form approximately 21 pairs of triangular denticulate ("having small teeth") ligaments that help to anchor and stabilize the cord in the dural sac.

Spinal Meninges: Relationship to the Spinal Cord

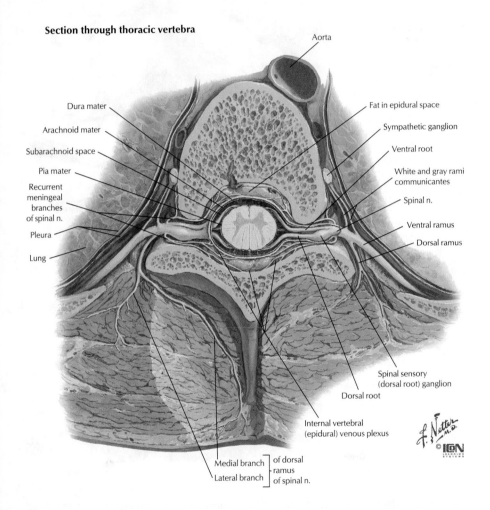

Section through thoracic vertebra

Aorta

Dura mater

Arachnoid mater

Subarachnoid space

Pia mater

Recurrent meningeal branches of spinal n.

Pleura

Lung

Fat in epidural space

Sympathetic ganglion

Ventral root

White and gray rami communicantes

Spinal n.

Ventral ramus

Dorsal ramus

Spinal sensory (dorsal root) ganglion

Dorsal root

Internal vertebral (epidural) venous plexus

Medial branch ⎤ of dorsal
Lateral branch ⎦ ramus of spinal n.

Cross section of the spine shows the thoracic spinal cord in the vertebral canal, meningeal layers, and spinal nerve roots traversing the intervertebral foramen. The epidural space (containing fat and veins) and the subarachnoid space (containing CSF) are easily seen. Components of the autonomic nervous system (rami communicantes and sympathetic ganglion) are shown in relationship to the ventral ramus.

Spinal Meninges: Cerebrospinal Fluid Circulation

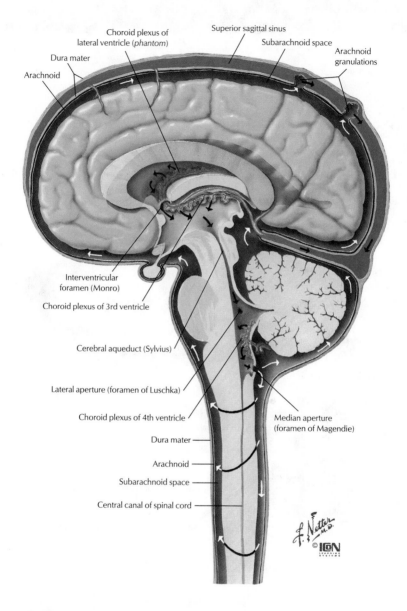

CSF circulates between the arachnoid mater and the pia mater, in the subarachnoid space surrounding the brain and spinal cord. The 500 ml CSF produced each day

- Supports and cushions the spinal cord
- Fulfills some functions normally provided by the lymphatic system
- Fills the 150-ml volume of the subarachnoid space
- Is produced by choroid plexuses in the brain's ventricles
- Is reabsorbed largely by arachnoid granulations and small central nervous system capillaries

Clinical Correlation

Lumbar Puncture and Epidural Anesthesia

Anatomy on pp. 66, 67, 101

Lumbar spinal puncture

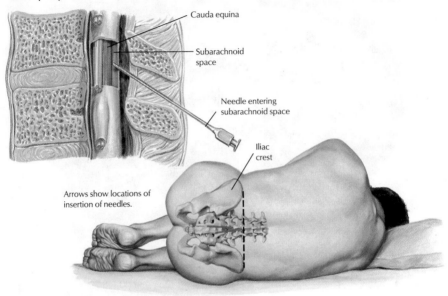

Cauda equina

Subarachnoid space

Needle entering subarachnoid space

Iliac crest

Arrows show locations of insertion of needles.

Epidural anesthesia

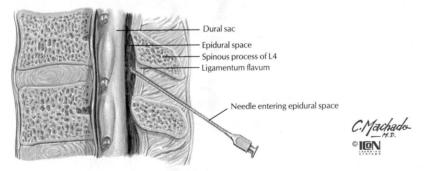

Dural sac

Epidural space

Spinous process of L4

Ligamentum flavum

Needle entering epidural space

CSF may be sampled clinically by performing a lumbar puncture. A spinal needle is inserted into the subarachnoid space of the lumbar cistern in the midline between either the L3 to L4 or L4 to L5 vertebral spinous processes. Because the spinal cord ends at approximately L1 or L2, the needle will not pierce or damage the cord. Administration of an anesthetic agent into the epidural space directly affects nerve roots of the cauda equina and is a common form of anesthesia used during childbirth. The agent infiltrates the epidural space and dural sac to reach the roots; it is usually administered at the same levels as those used for a lumbar puncture—L3-4 or L4-5.

Blood Supply to the Spine and Cord: Arteries of the Spine

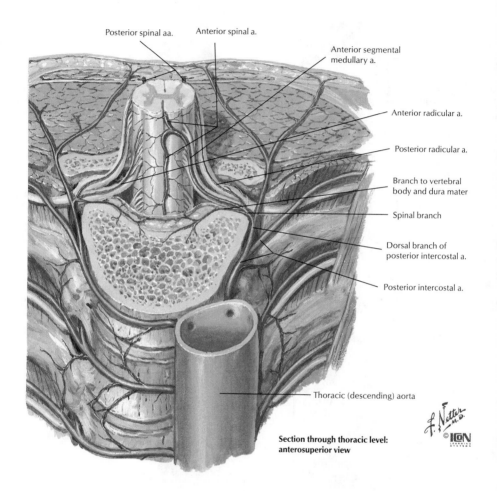

Posterior spinal aa.

Anterior spinal a.

Anterior segmental medullary a.

Anterior radicular a.

Posterior radicular a.

Branch to vertebral body and dura mater

Spinal branch

Dorsal branch of posterior intercostal a.

Posterior intercostal a.

Thoracic (descending) aorta

Section through thoracic level: anterosuperior view

The spine and spinal cord receive blood from spinal arteries derived from branches of larger arteries that serve each midline region of the body. The single anterior spinal artery and the two posterior spinal arteries ultimately arise from these larger parent arteries.
- Vertebral arteries arising from subclavian arteries in the neck
- Ascending cervical arteries arising from a branch of the subclavian arteries
- Posterior intercostal arteries arising from the thoracic aorta
- Lumbar arteries arising from the abdominal aorta
- Lateral sacral arteries arising from pelvic internal iliac arteries

The dorsal and ventral roots are supplied by segmental radicular (medullary) arteries. Also, longitudinal branches of radicular arteries course along the inside aspect of the vertebral canal and supply the vertebral column.

Blood Supply to the Spine and Cord: Arteries of the Cord

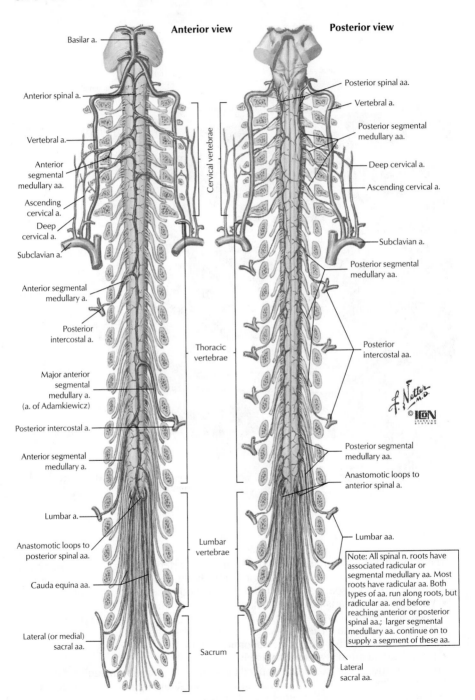

Anterior view

Basilar a.

Anterior spinal a.

Vertebral a.

Anterior segmental medullary aa.

Ascending cervical a.

Deep cervical a.

Subclavian a.

Anterior segmental medullary a.

Posterior intercostal a.

Major anterior segmental medullary a. (a. of Adamkiewicz)

Posterior intercostal a.

Anterior segmental medullary a.

Lumbar a.

Anastomotic loops to posterior spinal aa.

Cauda equina aa.

Lateral (or medial) sacral aa.

Cervical vertebrae

Thoracic vertebrae

Lumbar vertebrae

Sacrum

Posterior view

Posterior spinal aa.

Vertebral a.

Posterior segmental medullary aa.

Deep cervical a.

Ascending cervical a.

Subclavian a.

Posterior segmental medullary aa.

Posterior intercostal aa.

Posterior segmental medullary aa.

Anastomotic loops to anterior spinal a.

Lumbar aa.

Lateral sacral aa.

Note: All spinal n. roots have associated radicular or segmental medullary aa. Most roots have radicular aa. Both types of aa. run along roots, but radicular aa. end before reaching anterior or posterior spinal aa.; larger segmental medullary aa. continue on to supply a segment of these aa.

Blood Supply to the Spine and Cord: Venous Drainage

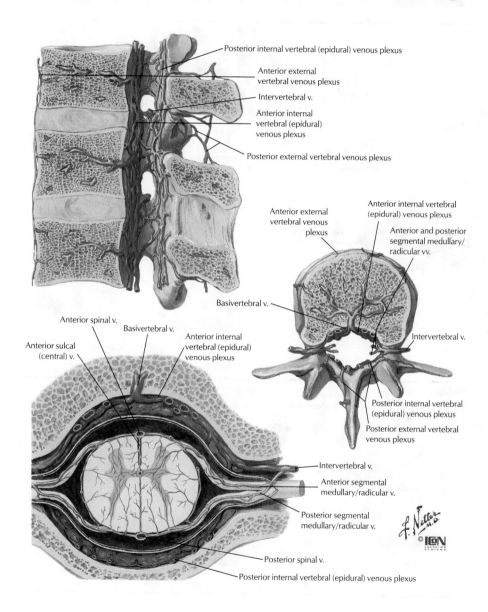

Posterior internal vertebral (epidural) venous plexus

Anterior external vertebral venous plexus

Intervertebral v.

Anterior internal vertebral (epidural) venous plexus

Posterior external vertebral venous plexus

Anterior external vertebral venous plexus

Anterior internal vertebral (epidural) venous plexus

Anterior and posterior segmental medullary/radicular vv.

Basivertebral v.

Intervertebral v.

Posterior internal vertebral (epidural) venous plexus

Posterior external vertebral venous plexus

Anterior spinal v.

Basivertebral v.

Anterior sulcal (central) v.

Anterior internal vertebral (epidural) venous plexus

Intervertebral v.

Anterior segmental medullary/radicular v.

Posterior segmental medullary/radicular v.

Posterior spinal v.

Posterior internal vertebral (epidural) venous plexus

Multiple anterior and posterior spinal veins run the length of the cord and drain into segmental (medullary) radicular veins. Radicular veins receive tributaries from internal vertebral veins that course within the vertebral canal (this internal venous plexus also anastomoses with external vertebral veins). Radicular veins then drain into segmental veins, with blood ultimately collecting in the superior vena cava, azygos venous system, and inferior vena cava.

Clinical Correlation

Acute Spinal Cord Syndromes   *Anatomy on pp. 78, 104, 107, 108*

Metastatic lesion

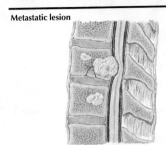

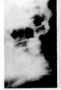

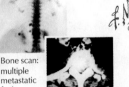

Bone lesions in spine (lateral view)

Myelogram evidencing CSF obstruction (AP view)

Bone scan: multiple metastatic foci

CT scan demonstrating destruction of vertebral body

Infarction

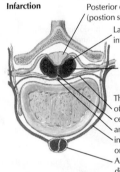

Posterior columns intact (postion sense intact)

Lateral corticospinal tract infarcted (motor funtion lost)

Spinothalamic tract infarcted (pain and temperature sensation lost)

Thrombosis of artery of Adamkiewicz, central (sulcal) artery, anterior spinal artery, intercostal artery or to:

Aortic obstruction by dissecting aneurysm or clamping during heart surgery

Sensory dissociation

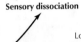

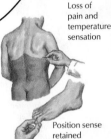

Loss of pain and temperature sensation

Position sense retained

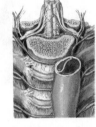

Dissecting aortic aneurysm obstructing artery of Adamkiewicz by blocking intercostal artery

Epidural abscess

Pus

Sources of infection

Hematogenous

    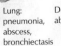

Skin: furuncle, carbuncle

Urinary tract: renal, perirenal, or prostatic abscess; pyelonephritis

Lung: pneumonia, abscess, bronchiectasis

Dental: abscess

Throat: pharyngitis, tonsillitis, abscess

Direct

  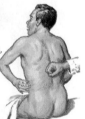

Psoas abscess

Dermal sinus

Decubitus ulcer, direct or hematogenous

Pain on percussion of spine. Local warmth may be noted.

Acute spinal cord syndromes present with neurologic deficits that are associated with the spinal cord level affected. Predisposing causes often include one of the following:
- Metastatic lesions from a primary source (lung, breast, prostate, kidney, thyroid)
- Infarction of a spinal artery (infarct of the anterior spinal artery is illustrated)
- Epidural abscess, usually from a predisposing infection

Embryology: Somite Formation and Differentiation

Differentiation of somites into myotomes, sclerotomes, and dermatomes
Cross section of human embryos

At 19 days

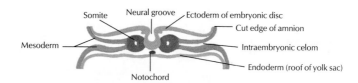

At 22 days

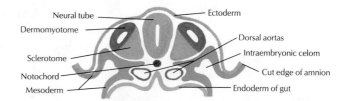

At 27 days

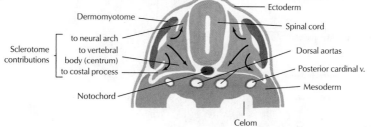

At 30 days

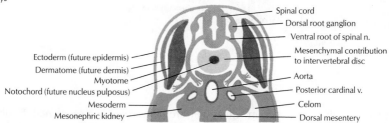

Somites (mesoderm) divide into dermomyotomes and medially placed sclerotomes.
Dermomyotomes divide into dermatomes (dermis of the skin) and myotomes.
Myotomes differentiate into segmental masses of muscle.
Sclerotomes and the notochord form the vertebral column.

Embryology: Segmentation

Segmental distribution of myotomes in fetus of 6 weeks

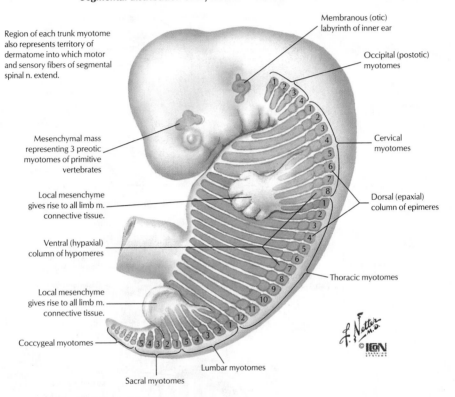

Region of each trunk myotome also represents territory of dermatome into which motor and sensory fibers of segmental spinal n. extend.

Membranous (otic) labyrinth of inner ear

Occipital (postotic) myotomes

Mesenchymal mass representing 3 preotic myotomes of primitive vertebrates

Cervical myotomes

Local mesenchyme gives rise to all limb m. connective tissue.

Dorsal (epaxial) column of epimeres

Ventral (hypaxial) column of hypomeres

Local mesenchyme gives rise to all limb m. connective tissue.

Thoracic myotomes

Coccygeal myotomes

Lumbar myotomes

Sacral myotomes

Myotomes, like somites from which they are derived, have a segmental distribution. Each segment is innervated by a pair of spinal nerves originating from a spinal cord segment. The small dorsal portion of the myotome becomes the epimere; the larger ventral segment becomes the hypomere. Adjacent myotome segments often merge so that an individual skeletal muscle derived from those myotomes may be innervated by more than one spinal segment.

Embryology: Epimeres and Hypomeres

Somatic development

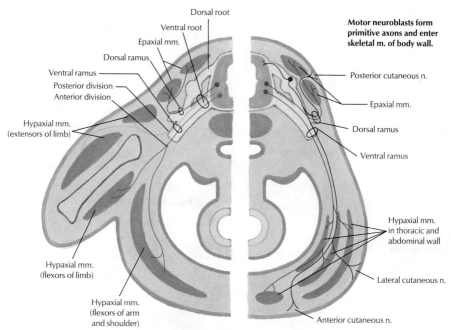

Motor neuroblasts form
primitive axons and enter
skeletal m. of body wall.

Dorsal root
Ventral root
Epaxial mm.
Dorsal ramus
Ventral ramus
Posterior division
Anterior division
Hypaxial mm.
(extensors of limb)
Posterior cutaneous n.
Epaxial mm.
Dorsal ramus
Ventral ramus
Hypaxial mm.
in thoracic and
abdominal wall
Hypaxial mm.
(flexors of limb)
Lateral cutaneous n.
Hypaxial mm.
(flexors of arm
and shoulder)
Anterior cutaneous n.

Somatic nervous system innervates somatopleure (body wall).

JOHN A. CRAIG—AD
©ICN

Epimeres (epaxial): form true or "intrinsic" back muscles (e.g., erector spinae) that are innervated by a dorsal ramus of the spinal nerve
Hypomeres (hypaxial): form the remainder of the trunk and limb musculature and are innervated by a ventral ramus of the spinal nerve

Right side shows embryo body wall and left side shows body wall with upper limb bud attached.

Embryology: Ossification of the Vertebral Column

Fate of body, costal process, and neural arch components of vertebral column, with sites and time of appearance of ossification centers

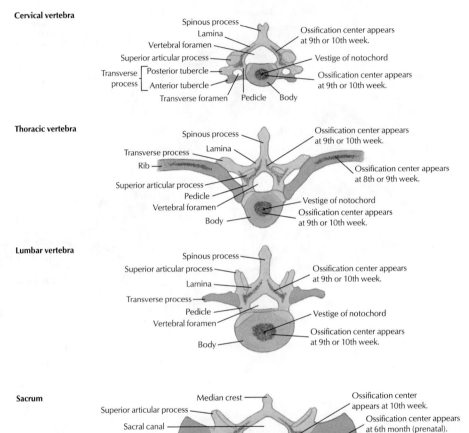

Each vertebra first appears as a cartilaginous model that then ossifies (endochondral bone formation), beginning in an ossification center. Ossification centers include

- Body (forms vertebral body)
- Costal process (forms ribs or, in vertebra without ribs, part of the transverse process)
- Neural arch (pedicle, lamina, and spinous process)

Embryology: Neurulation

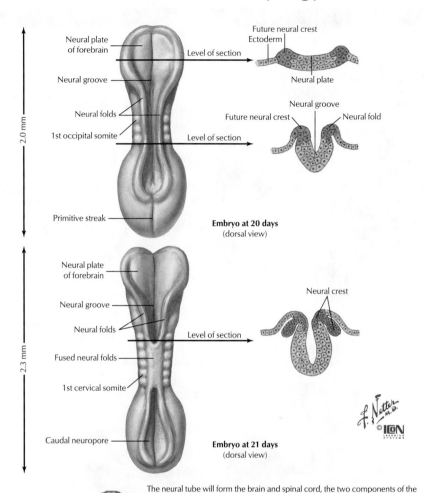

Future neural crest
Ectoderm

Level of section

Neural plate

Neural plate
of forebrain

Neural groove

Neural groove

Neural folds

Future neural crest

Neural fold

1st occipital somite

Level of section

Primitive streak

Embryo at 20 days
(dorsal view)

2.0 mm

Neural crest

Neural plate
of forebrain

Neural groove

Neural folds

Level of section

Fused neural folds

1st cervical somite

Caudal neuropore

Embryo at 21 days
(dorsal view)

2.3 mm

The neural tube will form the brain and spinal cord, the two components of the central nervous system (CNS). The neural crest will give rise to all of the neurons whose cell bodies are located outside the CNS in the peripheral nervous system (PNS) of nerves, ganglia, and plexuses.

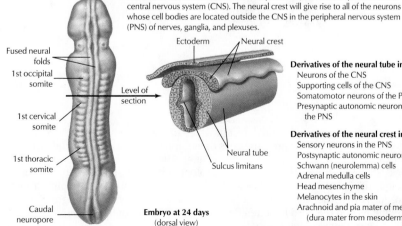

Fused neural
folds

1st occipital
somite

Level of
section

Ectoderm   Neural crest

1st cervical
somite

1st thoracic
somite

Neural tube

Sulcus limitans

Caudal
neuropore

Embryo at 24 days
(dorsal view)

2.6 mm

Derivatives of the neural tube include
Neurons of the CNS
Supporting cells of the CNS
Somatomotor neurons of the PNS
Presynaptic autonomic neurons of
the PNS

Derivatives of the neural crest include
Sensory neurons in the PNS
Postsynaptic autonomic neurons
Schwann (neurolemma) cells
Adrenal medulla cells
Head mesenchyme
Melanocytes in the skin
Arachnoid and pia mater of meninges
(dura mater from mesoderm)

Clinical Correlation

Neural Tube Defects

Anatomy on pp. 111, 114, 115

Spina bifida occulta

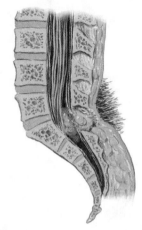

Dermal sinus

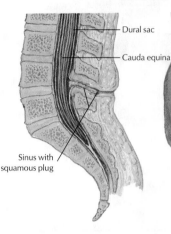

- Dural sac
- Cauda equina

Sinus with squamous plug

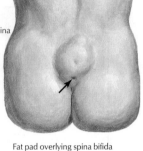

Fat pad overlying spina bifida occulta. Tuft of hair or only skin dimple may be present, or there may be no external manifestation. Dermal sinus also present in this case (arrow).

Types of spina bifida cystica with protrusion of spinal contents

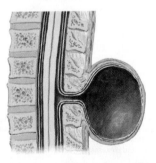

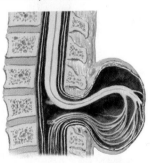

Meningocele

Meningomyelocele

Spina bifida is a congenital defect in which the neural tube remains too close to the surface such that the sclerotome cells do not migrate over the tube and form the neural arch of the vertebra (spina bifida occulta). This defect occurs most often at the L5 or S1 level and may present with neurologic findings. Spina bifida, one of several neural tube defects, is linked to low folic acid ingestion during the first trimester of pregnancy. If the meninges and CSF protrude as a cyst (meningocele) or if the meninges and the cord itself reside in the cyst (meningomyelocele), significant neurologic problems often develop.

Embryology: Development of the Spinal Cord

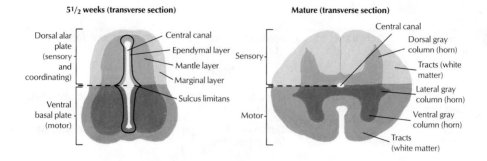

5¹/₂ weeks (transverse section)

Dorsal alar plate (sensory and coordinating)

Central canal
Ependymal layer
Mantle layer
Marginal layer
Sulcus limitans

Ventral basal plate (motor)

Mature (transverse section)

Central canal
Dorsal gray column (horn)
Tracts (white matter)
Lateral gray column (horn)
Ventral gray column (horn)
Tracts (white matter)

Sensory

Motor

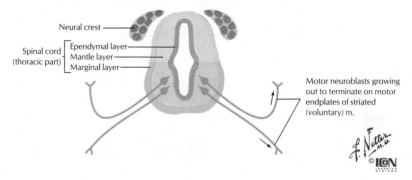

Differentiation and growth of neurons at 26 days

Neural crest

Spinal cord (thoracic part)
Ependymal layer
Mantle layer
Marginal layer

Motor neuroblasts growing out to terminate on motor endplates of striated (voluntary) m.

The neuroepithelium (cells of the neural tube) develop into three zones:

Ependymal: inner layer lining the central canal of the spinal cord
Mantle: intermediate layer that develops into the gray mater of the cord
Marginal: outer layer that becomes the white mater of the cord

A dorsal alar plate forms sensory derivatives of the cord, and the ventral basal plate gives rise to somatic and autonomic motor neurons whose axons leave the spinal cord.

Review Questions

As one views the back from cranial to caudal down the median furrow, which vertebral spine usually is the first to be seen?	Vertebra prominens (C7).
An imaginary horizontal line drawn posteriorly, connecting the iliac crests, will pass through what vertebral level?	Spinous process of L4 (and the intervertebral disc of L4-5).
Why is the line connecting the iliac crests clinically important?	It is a useful landmark for a lumbar puncture or an epidural block.
What does the dermatome portion of the dermomyotome become?	Dermis of the skin (epidermis comes from the surface ectoderm).
How many vertebrae do humans have, and what is their regional distribution?	Thirty-three vertebrae (7 cervical, 12 thoracic, 5 lumbar, 5 fused sacral, and 4 coccygeal).
What are the primary curvatures of the spine?	Thoracic and sacral.

What are the lay terms for the following accentuated curvatures?
    Lordosis:
    Kyphosis:
    Scoliosis:
	
	Swayback
	Hunchback
	Curved back

What two features of a typical vertebra form the vertebral arch?	Paired pedicles and laminae.
Two laminae fuse to form what vertebral feature?	Spinous process.
What portion of the embryonic somite gives rise to the cartilaginous precursor of the axial skeleton?	Sclerotome.
What other mesodermal structure contributes to the formation of the spine?	Notochord.
What is another name for the C1 vertebra?	Atlas.
What are the craniovertebral joints?	Synovial joints between the atlas and occipital bone (atlantooccipital joint) and between the atlas and axis (atlantoaxial joint).
What is a Jefferson fracture of the cervical spine and how might it be caused?	It is a burst fracture of the atlas, often from a blow to the top of the head.
Most herniated intervertebral discs occur at which vertebral levels?	L4-5 or L5-S1.

Review Questions

What embryonic structure gives rise to the nucleus pulposus of the intervertebral disc?	Notochord.
A herniated disc at the L4-5 level that impinges on a spinal nerve root will most likely involve components of which spinal nerve?	L5.
Which portions of the articulated spine possess the greatest range of movement?	Cervical and lumbar regions.
In a fracture dislocation injury to the thoracolumbar spine, what ligaments are often torn or stretched?	Supraspinous, interspinous, ligamentum flavum, and posterior longitudinal, and the intervertebral disc.
Which vertebral joint allows for turning the head side to side to indicate "no"?	Atlantoaxial.
What ligament(s) prevent(s) excessive rotation of the head?	Alar.
What is the extension of the supraspinous ligament in the cervical region called?	Ligamentum nuchae.
Which vertebral ligament connects adjacent laminae?	Ligamentum flavum.
Identify four characteristics or signs of ankylosing spondylitis.	Inflammatory back pain, stiffness, onset in teens or early 20s, more common in males, complications with other joints, HLA-B27 histocompatibility antigen present.
Why is low back pain caused by muscle strain so common?	The "postural" muscles of the back must counteract the fact that the body's center of gravity lies anterior to the spine. The greatest stress is on the lower back muscles because the lumbar vertebrae support most of the weight.
How may the back muscles be grouped functionally?	Into three groups: superficial (upper limb muscles), intermediate (muscles of respiration), and deep (postural muscles).
Which of the back muscles are innervated by dorsal primary rami of spinal nerves?	Deep intrinsic back muscles.
Back muscles innervated by dorsal primary rami are derived from what portion of a typical embryonic myotome?	Epimere.
Which group of the deep intrinsic back muscles fills the spaces between the spinous process and the transverse processes of the vertebrae?	Transversospinal (paravertebral) muscles.

Review Questions

Which neck muscles take origin from the ligamentum nuchae?	Splenius capitis and splenius cervicis (the cervicis also arises from the spinous processes of the C6 to C7 vertebrae).
What are the three major groups of erector spinae muscles?	Iliocostalis, longissimus, and spinalis.
What deep transversospinal muscles form the suboccipital triangle?	Rectus capitis posterior major, obliquus capitis superior, and obliquus capitis inferior.
What is the innervation of the suboccipital muscles?	Suboccipital nerve (dorsal ramus of C1).
What important artery passes through the transverse foramina of C1-C6 and appears in the suboccipital triangle?	Vertebral artery, a branch of the subclavian in the neck.
How are 31 pairs of spinal nerves distributed regionally?	Eight cervical pairs, 12 thoracic, 5 lumbar, 5 sacral, and 1 coccygeal pair.
What ectodermal derivative gives rise to the central nervous system (brain and spinal cord)?	Neural tube.
What is the collection of ventral and dorsal roots of the lumbar, sacral, and coccygeal cord levels called?	Cauda equina.
What anchors the spinal cord at its distal end to the coccyx?	Filum terminale.
Which meningeal layer lies between the other two and is avascular?	Arachnoid matter.
What pial extensions stabilize the spinal cord laterally and minimize side-to-side movements?	Denticulate ligaments.
Where is CSF found?	In the brain ventricles and subarachnoid space of the brain and spinal cord.
In what space does one find the cauda equina and filum terminale?	Subarachnoid space.
What is a common neural tube defect that leads to incomplete development of the vertebral arch?	Spina bifida.
What arteries run the length of the spinal cord, and where are they situated?	A single anterior and two posterior spinal arteries run the length of the spinal cord.

Review Questions

The venous drainage of the spine and spinal cord ultimately drains into which veins?	Superior vena cava, azygos venous system, and inferior vena cava.
What three layers are derived from the neuroepithelial cells of the developing neural tube?	Ependymal, mantle, and marginal zones.
What layer of the neuroepithelium develops into the gray matter of the spinal cord?	Mantle zone.
What is the term for the region of skin innervated by cutaneous fibers from a single spinal cord segment?	Dermatome.
What is the location of the nerve cell bodies of the sensory fibers that convey pain from over the nipples? From over the umbilicus?	Nipple: Dorsal root ganglia of T4. Umbilicus: Dorsal root ganglia of T10.
What is the dermatome overlying most of the back of the head?	C2 (derived from sensory fibers in the greater occipital nerve).

Upper Limb

Introduction The upper limb, which includes the arm, forearm, and hand, is continuous with the lower neck and is suspended from the trunk at the shoulder. Clinically, it is convenient to divide the limb into its functional muscle compartments and to assess the nerve(s) innervating each compartment's muscles. The upper limb is ideally suited for a wide range of motion and for manipulating our surrounding environment.

Surface Anatomy: Key Landmarks

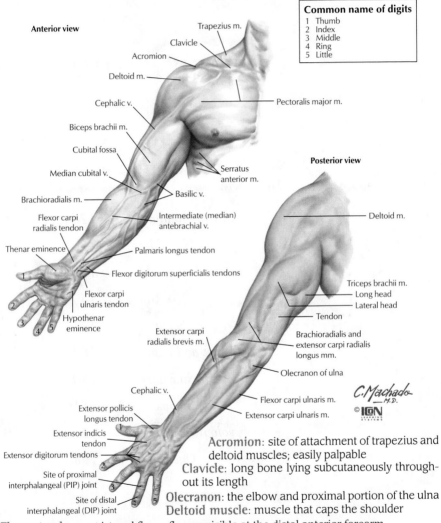

Anterior view

Trapezius m.

Clavicle

Acromion

Deltoid m.

Cephalic v.

Biceps brachii m.

Cubital fossa

Median cubital v.

Brachioradialis m.

Flexor carpi radialis tendon

Thenar eminence

Flexor carpi ulnaris tendon

Hypothenar eminence

Pectoralis major m.

Serratus anterior m.

Basilic v.

Intermediate (median) antebrachial v.

Palmaris longus tendon

Flexor digitorum superficialis tendons

Posterior view

Deltoid m.

Triceps brachii m.
Long head
Lateral head

Tendon

Brachioradialis and extensor carpi radialis longus mm.

Extensor carpi radialis brevis m.

Olecranon of ulna

Cephalic v.

Extensor pollicis longus tendon

Extensor indicis tendon

Extensor digitorum tendons

Site of proximal interphalangeal (PIP) joint

Site of distal interphalangeal (DIP) joint

Flexor carpi ulnaris m.

Extensor carpi ulnaris m.

Common name of digits
1 Thumb
2 Index
3 Middle
4 Ring
5 Little

Acromion: site of attachment of trapezius and deltoid muscles; easily palpable

Clavicle: long bone lying subcutaneously throughout its length

Olecranon: the elbow and proximal portion of the ulna

Deltoid muscle: muscle that caps the shoulder

Flexor tendons: wrist and finger flexors visible at the distal anterior forearm

Extensor tendons: wrist and finger extensors visible on the dorsum of the hand

Thenar eminence: cone of muscles at the base of the thumb

Hypothenar eminence: cone of muscles at the base of the little finger

Dorsal venous network: vessels seen on the dorsum of the hand

Cephalic vein: subcutaneous vein draining the lateral forearm and arm into the axillary vein

Basilic vein: vein draining the medial forearm and distal arm into the axillary vein

Median cubital vein: vein lying in the cubital fossa; commonly used for venipuncture

Surface Anatomy: Superficial Veins and Nerves

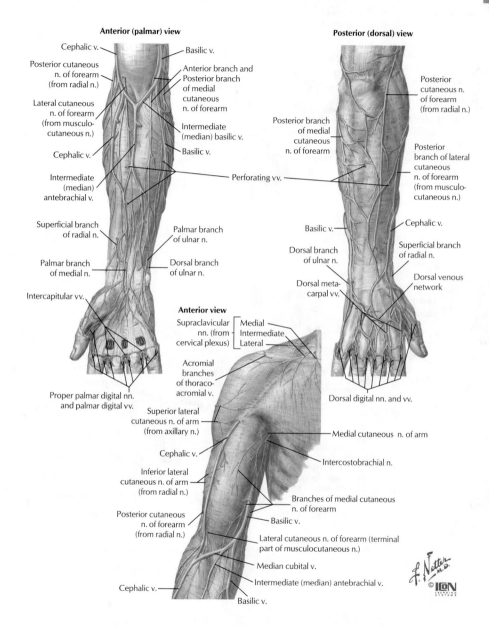

Anterior (palmar) view

Cephalic v.

Posterior cutaneous n. of forearm (from radial n.)

Lateral cutaneous n. of forearm (from musculo-cutaneous n.)

Cephalic v.

Intermediate (median) antebrachial v.

Superficial branch of radial n.

Palmar branch of medial n.

Intercapitular vv.

Basilic v.

Anterior branch and Posterior branch of medial cutaneous n. of forearm

Intermediate (median) basilic v.

Basilic v.

Perforating vv.

Palmar branch of ulnar n.

Dorsal branch of ulnar n.

Proper palmar digital nn. and palmar digital vv.

Posterior (dorsal) view

Posterior cutaneous n. of forearm (from radial n.)

Posterior branch of medial cutaneous n. of forearm

Posterior branch of lateral cutaneous n. of forearm (from musculo-cutaneous n.)

Cephalic v.

Basilic v.

Dorsal branch of ulnar n.

Dorsal meta-carpal vv.

Superficial branch of radial n.

Dorsal venous network

Dorsal digital nn. and vv.

Anterior view

Supraclavicular nn. (from cervical plexus)   Medial   Intermediate   Lateral

Acromial branches of thoraco-acromial v.

Superior lateral cutaneous n. of arm (from axillary n.)

Cephalic v.

Inferior lateral cutaneous n. of arm (from radial n.)

Posterior cutaneous n. of forearm (from radial n.)

Cephalic v.

Medial cutaneous n. of arm

Intercostobrachial n.

Branches of medial cutaneous n. of forearm

Basilic v.

Lateral cutaneous n. of forearm (terminal part of musculocutaneous n.)

Median cubital v.

Intermediate (median) antebrachial v.

Basilic v.

f. Netter M.D.

© ICON LEARNING SYSTEMS

Superficial veins drain blood toward the heart and communicate with deep veins that parallel arteries of the upper limb. When vigorous muscle contraction compresses the deep veins, some of the venous blood is shunted into superficial veins and thereby returned to the heart (the veins become more prominent when the limb is being exercised, e.g., when lifting weights). These veins have valves to assist in venous return. Corresponding cutaneous nerves are terminal sensory branches of the major nerves arising from the brachial plexus (C5-T1 spinal levels).

Shoulder: Bones (Pectoral Girdle)

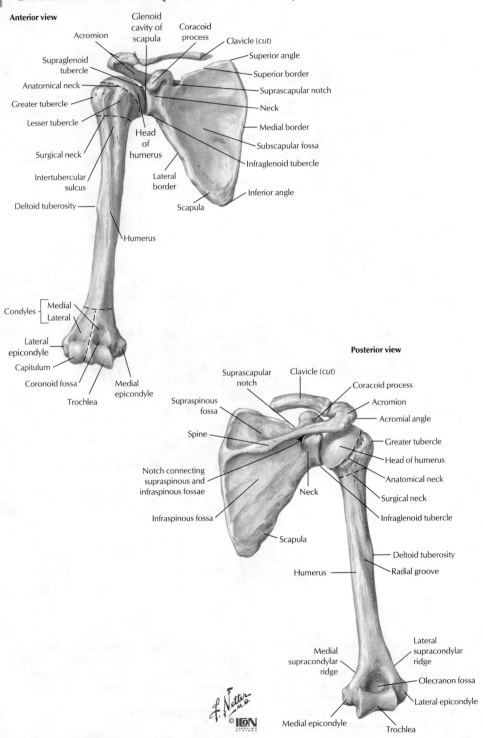

Anterior view

Acromion
Supraglenoid tubercle
Anatomical neck
Greater tubercle
Lesser tubercle
Surgical neck
Intertubercular sulcus
Deltoid tuberosity
Humerus

Glenoid cavity of scapula
Coracoid process
Head of humerus
Lateral border
Scapula

Clavicle (*cut*)
Superior angle
Superior border
Suprascapular notch
Neck
Medial border
Subscapular fossa
Infraglenoid tubercle
Inferior angle

Condyles { Medial Lateral
Lateral epicondyle
Capitulum
Coronoid fossa
Trochlea
Medial epicondyle

Posterior view

Suprascapular notch
Supraspinous fossa
Spine
Notch connecting supraspinous and infraspinous fossae
Infraspinous fossa

Clavicle (*cut*)
Coracoid process
Acromion
Acromial angle
Greater tubercle
Head of humerus
Anatomical neck
Surgical neck
Infraglenoid tubercle

Neck
Scapula
Humerus

Deltoid tuberosity
Radial groove

Medial supracondylar ridge
Lateral supracondylar ridge
Olecranon fossa
Lateral epicondyle
Medial epicondyle
Trochlea

Shoulder: Bones (Pectoral Girdle) (continued)

Right clavicle

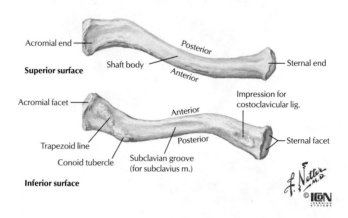

The scapula provides a large surface area for muscle attachment. Seventeen different muscles attach here; many are concerned with movements of the upper limb.

CLAVICLE	SCAPULA	HUMERUS
Cylindrical bone with slight S-shaped curve	Flat triangular bone	Long bone
Middle third: narrowest portion	Shallow glenoid cavity	Proximal head: articulates with glenoid cavity of scapula
First bone to ossify but last to fuse	Attachment locations for 17 muscles	Distal medial and lateral condyles: articulate at elbow with ulna and radius
Formed by intramembranous ossification	Fractures relatively uncommon	Surgical neck a common fracture site, which endangers axillary nerve
Most commonly fractured bone		
Acts as strut to keep limb away from trunk		

Shoulder: Joints and Ligaments

Anterior view

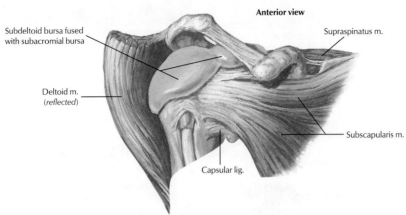

Subdeltoid bursa fused with subacromial bursa

Supraspinatus m.

Deltoid m. (*reflected*)

Subscapularis m.

Capsular lig.

Joint opened: lateral view

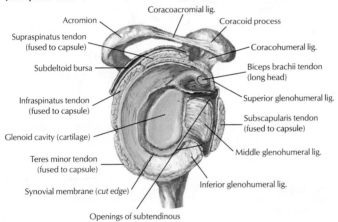

Coracoacromial lig.

Acromion

Coracoid process

Supraspinatus tendon (fused to capsule)

Coracohumeral lig.

Subdeltoid bursa

Biceps brachii tendon (long head)

Infraspinatus tendon (fused to capsule)

Superior glenohumeral lig.

Subscapularis tendon (fused to capsule)

Glenoid cavity (cartilage)

Middle glenohumeral lig.

Teres minor tendon (fused to capsule)

Synovial membrane (*cut edge*)

Inferior glenohumeral lig.

Openings of subtendinous bursa of subscapularis

Coronal section through joint

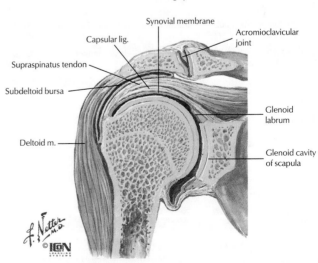

Synovial membrane

Capsular lig.

Acromioclavicular joint

Supraspinatus tendon

Subdeltoid bursa

Glenoid labrum

Deltoid m.

Glenoid cavity of scapula

Shoulder: Joints and Ligaments (continued)

Anterior view

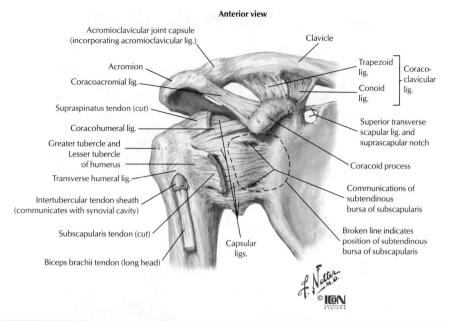

LIGAMENT OR BURSA	ATTACHMENT	COMMENT
Acromioclavicular (Synovial Plane) Joint		
Capsule and articular disc	Surrounds joint	Allows gliding movement as arm is raised and scapula rotates
Acromioclavicular	Acromion to clavicle	
Coracoclavicular (conoid and trapezoid ligaments)	Clavicle to coracoid process	Reinforces the joint
Glenohumeral (Multiaxial Synovial Ball-and-Socket) Joint		
Capsule	Surrounds joint	Permits flexion, extension, abduction, adduction, circumduction; most frequently dislocated joint
Coracohumeral	Coracoid process to greater tubercle of humerus	
Glenohumeral	Supraglenoid tubercle to lesser tubercle of humerus	Composed of superior, middle, and inferior thickenings
Transverse humeral	Spans greater and lesser tubercles of humerus	Holds long head of biceps tendon in intertubercular groove
Glenoid labrum	Margin of glenoid cavity of scapula	Is fibrocartilaginous ligament that deepens glenoid cavity
Bursae		
Subacromial		Between coracoacromial arch and suprascapular muscle
Subdeltoid		Between deltoid muscle and capsule
Subscapular		Between subscapularis tendon and scapular neck

Clinical Correlation

Tendonitis and Bursitis   *Anatomy on pp. 128, 129*

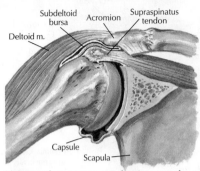

Subdeltoid bursa   Acromion   Supraspinatus tendon
Deltoid m.

Capsule
Scapula

Abduction of arm causes repeated impingement of greater tubercle of humerus on acromion, leading to degeneration and inflammation of supraspinatus tendon, secondary inflammation of bursa, and pain on abduction of arm. Calcific deposit in degenerated tendon produces elevation that further aggravates inflammation and pain.

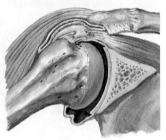

Calcific deposit may rupture spontaneously beneath floor of bursa, with relief of pain and inflammation.

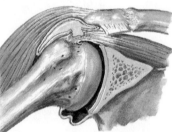

Deposit may rupture spontaneously into bursa and be resorbed, relieving pain and acute inflammation.

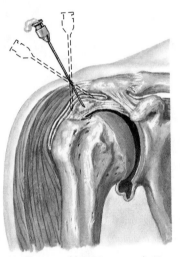

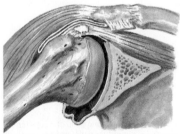

Chronic tendonitis and bursitis with calcific deposit in tendon and minimal inflammation. Chronic deposits do not rupture spontaneously but may be resorbed.

Needle rupture of deposit in acute tendonitis promptly relieves acute symptoms. After administration of local anesthetic, needle introduced at point of greatest tenderness. Several probings may be necessary to reach deposit. Toothpastelike deposit may ooze from needle. Irrigation of bursa with saline solution using two needles often done to remove more calcific material. Corticosteroid may be injected for additional relief.

Movement at the shoulder joint (or almost any joint) can lead to inflammation of the tendons surrounding that joint and secondary inflammation of the bursa that cushions the joint from overlying muscle or tendon. A painful joint can result, possibly even with calcification within the degenerated tendon. The supraspinatus muscle tendon is especially vulnerable because it can become pinched by the greater tubercle of the humerus, the acromion, and the coracoacromial ligament.

Clinical Correlation

Fractures of lateral third of clavicle

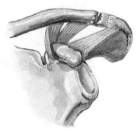

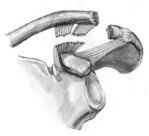

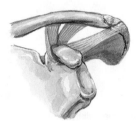

Type I. Fracture with no disruption of ligaments and therefore no displacement. Treated with simple sling for few weeks.

Type II. Fracture with tear of coracoclavicular ligament and upward displacement of medial fragment. Requires open repair; if pin used, must be bent to prevent migration.

Type III. Fracture through acromioclavicular joint; no displacement. Often missed and may later cause painful osteoarthritis requiring resection arthroplasty.

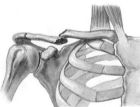

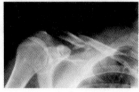

Fracture of middle third of clavicle (most common) Medial fragment displaced upward by pull of sterno-cleidomastoid muscle; lateral fragment displaced downward by weight of shoulder. Fractures occur most often in children.

Anteroposterior radiograph. Fracture of middle third of clavicle

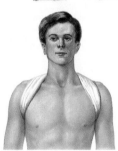

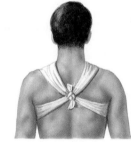

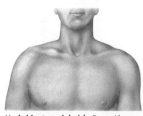

Healed fracture of clavicle. Even with proper treatment, small lump may remain.

Fracture of middle third of clavicle best treated with snug figure-of-8 bandage or clavicle harness for 3 weeks or until pain subsides. Bandage or harness must be tightened occasionally because it loosens with wear.

Fracture of the clavicle is quite common, especially in children. The fracture usually results from a fall on an outstretched hand or direct trauma to the shoulder. Fractures of the medial third of the clavicle are rare, but those of the middle third are common. In a complete fracture, the proximal bone fragment is pulled superiorly by the sternocleidomastoid muscle while the distal fragment is pulled inferiorly by the shoulder. Fractures of the lateral third can involve coracoclavicular ligament tears.

Clinical Correlation

Shoulder Dislocation   *Anatomy on pp. 128, 129, 142*

Anterior Dislocation of Glenohumeral Joint

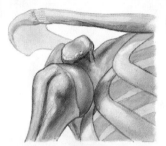

Subcoracoid dislocation (most common)

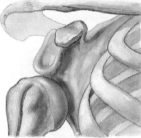

Subglenoid dislocation

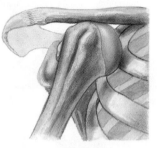

Subclavicular dislocation (uncommon). Very rarely, humeral head penetrates between ribs, producing intrathoracic dislocation.

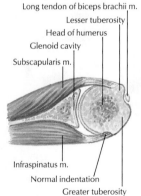

Subcoracoid dislocation. Anteroposterior radiograph

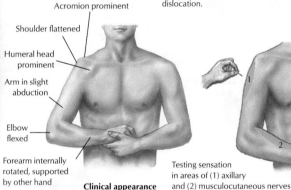

Acromion prominent

Shoulder flattened

Humeral head prominent

Arm in slight abduction

Elbow flexed

Forearm internally rotated, supported by other hand

Clinical appearance

Testing sensation in areas of (1) axillary and (2) musculocutaneous nerves

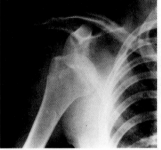

Long tendon of biceps brachii m.
Lesser tuberosity
Head of humerus
Glenoid cavity
Subscapularis m.

Infraspinatus m.
Normal indentation
Greater tuberosity

Section through normal glenohumeral joint

Almost 95% of shoulder (glenohumeral joint) dislocations occur in an anterior direction. Abduction, extension, and lateral (external) rotation of the arm at the shoulder (e.g., the throwing motion) place stress on the capsule and anterior elements of the rotator cuff (subscapularis tendon). Types of anterior dislocations are
- Subcoracoid (most common)
- Subglenoid
- Subclavicular (rare)

The axillary (most often) and musculocutaneous nerves may be injured during such dislocations.

Shoulder: Muscles

MUSCLE	PROXIMAL ATTACHMENT (ORIGIN)	DISTAL ATTACHMENT (INSERTION)	INNERVATION	MAIN ACTIONS
Trapezius	Medial third of superior nuchal line; external occipital protuberance, ligamentum nuchae, and spinous processes of C7-T12	Lateral third of clavicle, acromion, and spine of scapula	Spinal root of accessory nerve (cranial nerve XI) and cervical nerves (C3 and C4)	Elevates, retracts, and rotates scapula; superior fibers elevate, middle fibers retract, and inferior fibers depress scapula
Latissimus dorsi	Spinous processes of T7-T12, thoracolumbar fascia, iliac crest, and inferior three or four ribs	Intertubercular groove of humerus	Thoracodorsal nerve	Extends, adducts, and medially rotates humerus at shoulder
Levator scapulae	Transverse processes of C1-C4	Superior part of medial border of scapula	Dorsal scapular and cervical (C3 and C4) nerves	Elevates scapula and tilts its glenoid cavity inferiorly by rotating scapula
Rhomboid minor and major	*Minor*: ligamentum nuchae and spinous processes of C7 and T1 *Major*: spinous processes of T2-T5	Medial border of scapula from level of spine to inferior angle	Dorsal scapular nerve	Retracts scapula and rotates it to depress glenoid cavity; fixes scapula to thoracic wall
Deltoid	Lateral third of clavicle, acromion, and spine of scapula	Deltoid tuberosity of humerus	Axillary nerve	*Anterior part*: flexes and medially rotates arm at shoulder *Middle part*: abducts arm at shoulder *Posterior part*: extends and laterally rotates arm at shoulder
Supraspinatus (rotator cuff muscle)	Supraspinous fossa of scapula	Superior facet on greater tubercle of humerus	Suprascapular nerve	Helps deltoid abduct arm at shoulder and acts with rotator cuff muscles
Infraspinatus (rotator cuff muscle)	Infraspinous fossa of scapula	Middle facet on greater tubercle of humerus	Suprascapular nerve	Laterally rotates arm at shoulder; helps to hold head in glenoid cavity
Teres minor (rotator cuff muscle)	Lateral border of scapula	Inferior facet on greater tubercle	Axillary nerve	Laterally rotates arm at shoulder; helps to hold head in glenoid cavity
Teres major	Dorsal surface of inferior angle of scapula	Medial lip of intertubercular groove of humerus	Lower subscapular nerve	Adducts arm and medially rotates shoulder
Subscapularis (rotator cuff muscle)	Subscapular fossa of scapula	Lesser tubercle of humerus	Upper and lower subscapular nerves	Medially rotates arm at shoulder and adducts it; helps to hold humeral head in glenoid cavity

Shoulder: Muscles (continued)

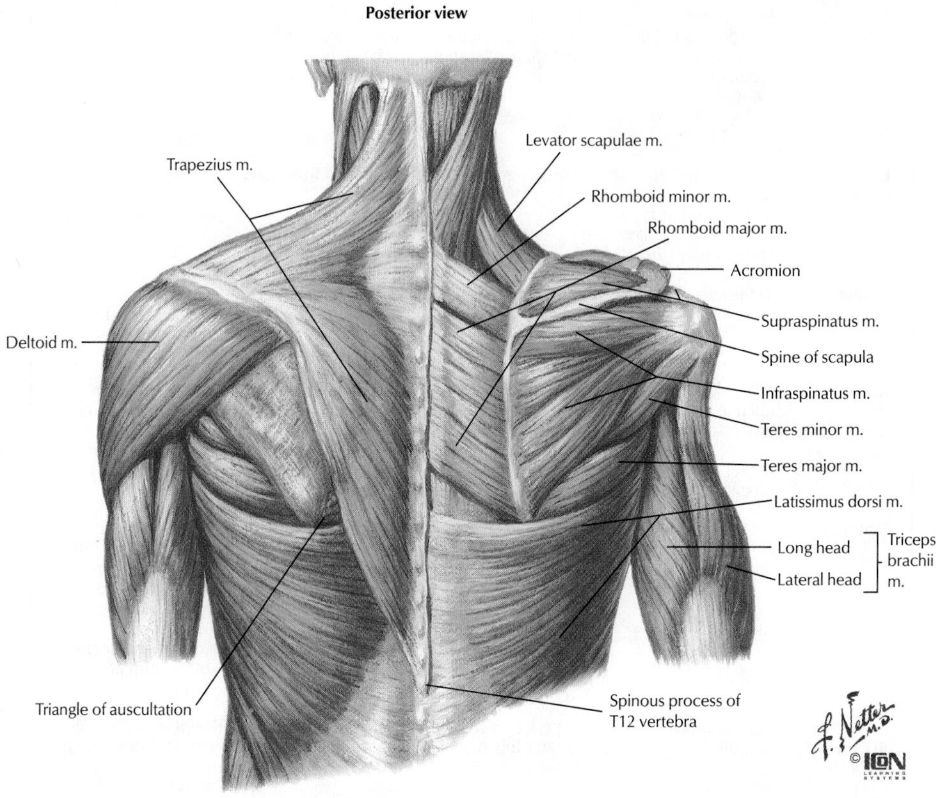

Posterior view

Trapezius m.

Levator scapulae m.

Rhomboid minor m.

Rhomboid major m.

Acromion

Deltoid m.

Supraspinatus m.

Spine of scapula

Infraspinatus m.

Teres minor m.

Teres major m.

Latissimus dorsi m.

Long head — Triceps brachii m.

Lateral head

Triangle of auscultation

Spinous process of T12 vertebra

Shoulder: Muscles (continued)

Anterior view

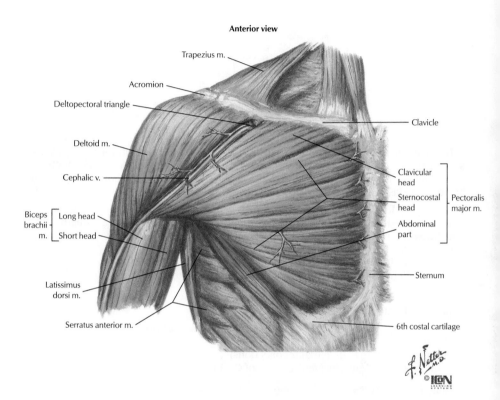

MUSCLE	PROXIMAL ATTACHMENT (ORIGIN)	DISTAL ATTACHMENT (INSERTION)	INNERVATION	MAIN ACTIONS
Pectoralis major	Medial half of clavicle; sternum; superior six costal cartilages; aponeurosis of external abdominal oblique	Intertubercular groove of humerus	Lateral and medial pectoral nerves	Flexes, adducts, and medially rotates arm at shoulder
Pectoralis minor	Third to fifth ribs	Coracoid process of scapula	Medial pectoral nerve	Depresses scapula and stabilizes it
Serratus anterior	Upper eight ribs	Medial border of scapula	Long thoracic nerve	Rotates scapula upward and pulls it anterior toward thoracic wall
Subclavius	Junction of first rib and costal cartilage	Inferior surface of clavicle	Nerve to subclavius	Depresses clavicle

Axilla: Boundaries

The axilla (armpit) is a pyramid-shaped area that contains important neurovascular structures that pass through the shoulder region. These neurovascular elements are enclosed in a fascial sleeve called the axillary sheath, which is a direct continuation of the prevertebral fascia of the neck. The axilla has six boundaries:

Base: axillary fascia and skin of armpit
Apex: bounded by first rib, clavicle, and superior part of the scapula; passageway for structures entering or leaving shoulder and arm
Anterior wall: pectoralis major and minor muscles
Posterior wall: subscapularis, teres major, and latissimus dorsi muscles
Medial wall: upper rib cage, intercostal and serratus anterior muscles
Lateral wall: humerus (intertubercular groove)

Important structures in the axilla include the

Axillary artery (divided into three parts for descriptive purposes)
Axillary vein
Axillary lymph nodes (five major collections)
Brachial plexus of nerves (ventral rami of C5-T1)

Axillary fasciae are the

Pectoral fascia: invests pectoralis major muscle; attaches to sternum and clavicle
Clavipectoral fascia: invests subclavius and pectoralis minor muscles
Axillary fascia: forms base of axilla
Axillary sheath: invests axillary neurovascular structures

Axilla: Boundaries (continued)

Anterior view

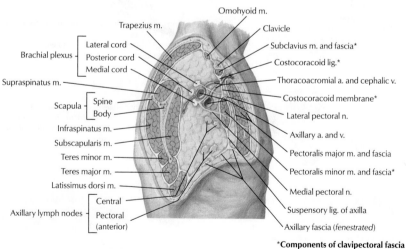

Thoracoacromial a.

Coracoid process

Cephalic v.

Deltoid m.

Pectoralis major m. (*cut*)

Biceps brachii m.
Short head
Long head

Brachial fascia
(*cut edge*)

Clavicle

Fascia investing subclavius m.*

Costocoracoid membrane*

Fascia investing pectoralis minor m.*

Pectoralis major m. and pectoral fascia
(superficial and deep layers)

Suspensory lig. of axilla*

Serratus anterior fascia

Axillary fascia (anterior part)

Oblique parasagittal section of axilla

Omohyoid m.

Trapezius m.

Brachial plexus
Lateral cord
Posterior cord
Medial cord

Supraspinatus m.

Scapula
Spine
Body

Infraspinatus m.

Subscapularis m.

Teres minor m.

Teres major m.

Latissimus dorsi m.

Axillary lymph nodes
Central
Pectoral
(anterior)

Clavicle

Subclavius m. and fascia*

Costocoracoid lig.*

Thoracoacromial a. and cephalic v.

Costocoracoid membrane*

Lateral pectoral n.

Axillary a. and v.

Pectoralis major m. and fascia

Pectoralis minor m. and fascia*

Medial pectoral n.

Suspensory lig. of axilla

Axillary fascia (*fenestrated*)

*Components of clavipectoral fascia

Clinical Correlation

Rotator Cuff Injury Anatomy on pp. 133, 134, 136, 137

Extensive rupture of left cuff. To bring about abduction, deltoid muscle contracts strongly but only pulls humerus upward toward acromion while scapula rotates and shoulder girdle is elevated. 45° abduction is thus possible.

Test for partial tear of cuff is inability to maintain 90° abduction against mild resistance.

Communication between shoulder joint and subdeltoid bursa on arthrogram is pathognomonic of cuff tear.

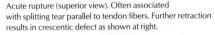

Subscapularis m.

Supraspinatus m.

Humerus

Biceps brachii tendon

Infraspinatus m.

Thickened, edematous biceps brachii tendon

Acute rupture (superior view). Often associated with splitting tear parallel to tendon fibers. Further retraction results in crescentic defect as shown at right.

Retracted tear, commonly found in surgery. Broken line indicates extent of debridement of degenerated tendon for repair.

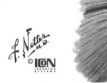

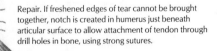

Repair. If freshened edges of tear cannot be brought together, notch is created in humerus just beneath articular surface to allow attachment of tendon through drill holes in bone, using strong sutures.

The tendons of insertion of the rotator cuff muscles form a musculotendinous cuff about the shoulder joint on its anterior, superior, and posterior aspects. The muscles of the rotator cuff group are the

- Subscapularis
- Supraspinatus
- Infraspinatus
- Teres minor

Repeated abduction and flexion (e.g., a throwing motion) cause wear and tear on the tendons as they rub on the acromion and coracoacromial ligament, which may lead to cuff tears or rupture. The tendon of the supraspinatus is the most vulnerable to injury.

Clinical Correlation

Lipoma

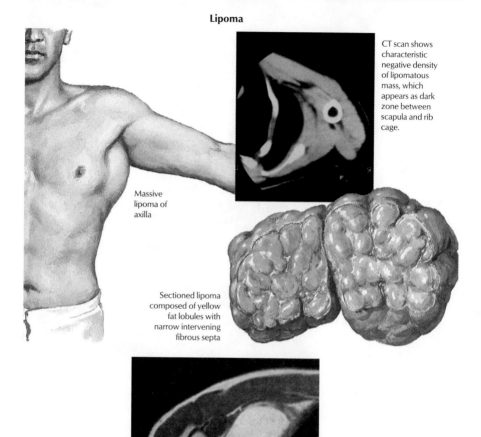

CT scan shows characteristic negative density of lipomatous mass, which appears as dark zone between scapula and rib cage.

Massive lipoma of axilla

Sectioned lipoma composed of yellow fat lobules with narrow intervening fibrous septa

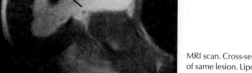

MRI scan. Cross-sectional view of same lesion. Lipoma wraps around adjacent humerus (*arrow*)

   Benign soft tissue tumors occur much more often than do malignant tumors. In adults, the most common type is the lipoma. A lipoma is composed of mature fat; is usually large and soft, asymptomatic, and more common than all other soft tissue tumors combined; and presents as a solitary mass. Most lipomas are found on the
   • Back
   • Shoulders
   • Axilla
   • Abdomen
   • Proximal region of the limbs

Axilla: Branches of the Axillary Artery

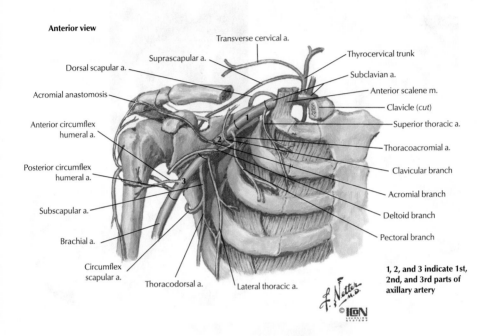

Anterior view

Transverse cervical a.

Suprascapular a.

Dorsal scapular a.

Acromial anastomosis

Anterior circumflex humeral a.

Posterior circumflex humeral a.

Subscapular a.

Brachial a.

Circumflex scapular a.

Thoracodorsal a.

Lateral thoracic a.

Thyrocervical trunk

Subclavian a.

Anterior scalene m.

Clavicle (*cut*)

Superior thoracic a.

Thoracoacromial a.

Clavicular branch

Acromial branch

Deltoid branch

Pectoral branch

1, 2, and 3 indicate 1st, 2nd, and 3rd parts of axillary artery

The axillary artery begins at the first rib and is divided into three descriptive parts by the pectoralis minor muscle. It continues as the brachial artery distally at the inferior border of the teres major muscle.

PART OF AXILLARY ARTERY	BRANCH	COURSE AND STRUCTURES SUPPLIED
1	Superior thoracic	Supplies first two intercostal spaces
2	Thoracoacromial	Has clavicular, pectoral, deltoid, and acromial branches
	Lateral thoracic	Runs with long thoracic nerve and supplies muscles that it traverses
3	Subscapular	Divides into thoracodorsal and circumflex scapular branches
	Anterior humeral circumflex	Passes around surgical neck of humerus
	Posterior humeral circumflex	Runs with axillary nerve through the quadrangular space to anastomose with anterior circumflex branch

Axilla: Scapular Anastomosis

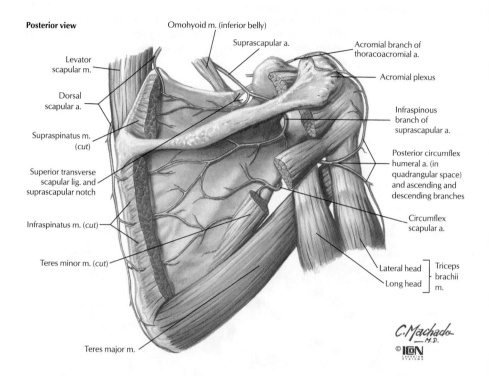

Posterior view

Omohyoid m. (inferior belly)

Suprascapular a.

Acromial branch of thoracoacromial a.

Acromial plexus

Levator scapular m.

Dorsal scapular a.

Infraspinous branch of suprascapular a.

Supraspinatus m. (cut)

Posterior circumflex humeral a. (in quadrangular space) and ascending and descending branches

Superior transverse scapular lig. and suprascapular notch

Circumflex scapular a.

Infraspinatus m. (cut)

Teres minor m. (cut)

Lateral head ⎤ Triceps
Long head ⎦ brachii m.

Teres major m.

C. Machado
—M.D.

©ICN
LEARNING
SYSTEMS

Like most joints, the shoulder joint has a rich vascular anastomosis. This anastomosis not only supplies the 17 muscles attaching to the scapula and some other shoulder muscles but also provides collateral circulation to the upper limb should the proximal part of the axillary artery become occluded (proximal to the subscapular branch). Important component arteries of this anastomosis include the

- Dorsal scapular (transverse cervical) branch of the subclavian (thyrocervical artery)
- Suprascapular from the subclavian (thyrocervical artery)
- Subscapular and its circumflex scapular and thoracodorsal branches

Axilla: Brachial Plexus and Axillary Artery

The axillary artery, axillary vein (lies medial to the artery), and cords of the brachial plexus are all bound in the axillary sheath. In this illustration, the sheath and some parts of the axillary vein have been removed and several muscles have been reflected to better visualize arrangement of the plexus as it invests the axillary artery. Key nerves and branches of the axillary artery also are shown supplying muscles.

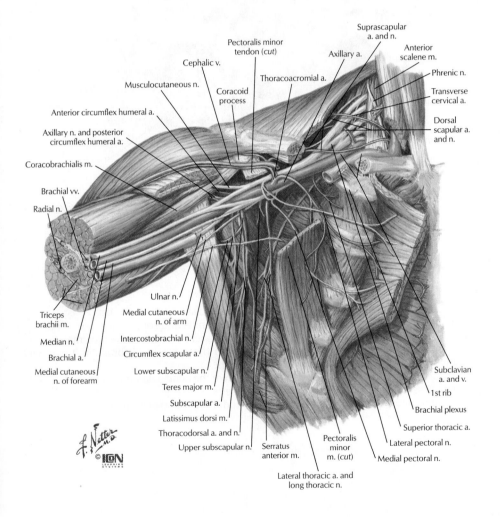

Pectoralis minor tendon (cut)
Suprascapular a. and n.
Axillary a.
Anterior scalene m.
Cephalic v.
Phrenic n.
Thoracoacromial a.
Musculocutaneous n.
Coracoid process
Transverse cervical a.
Anterior circumflex humeral a.
Dorsal scapular a. and n.
Axillary n. and posterior circumflex humeral a.
Coracobrachialis m.
Brachial vv.
Radial n.
Ulnar n.
Triceps brachii m.
Medial cutaneous n. of arm
Median n.
Intercostobrachial n.
Brachial a.
Circumflex scapular a.
Medial cutaneous n. of forearm
Lower subscapular n.
Subclavian a. and v.
Teres major m.
1st rib
Subscapular a.
Brachial plexus
Latissimus dorsi m.
Superior thoracic a.
Thoracodorsal a. and n.
Lateral pectoral n.
Upper subscapular n.
Serratus anterior m.
Pectoralis minor m. (cut)
Medial pectoral n.
Lateral thoracic a. and long thoracic n.

Axilla: Brachial Plexus

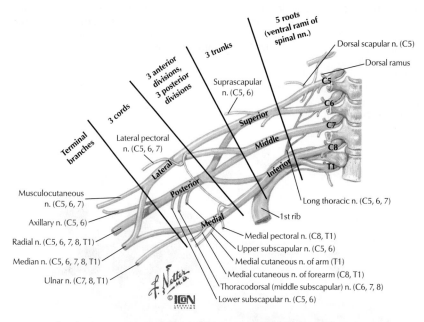

Nerves that innervate most of the shoulder muscles and all of the muscles of the upper limb arise from the brachial plexus. The plexus arises from ventral rami of spinal nerves C5 to T1. The plexus is descriptively divided into five roots (ventral rami), three trunks, six divisions (three anterior, three posterior), three cords (named for their relationship to the axillary artery), and five large terminal branches. Important motor branches of the brachial plexus are indicated in the table.

ARISE FROM	NERVE	MUSCLES INNERVATED
Roots	Dorsal scapular	Levator scapulae and rhomboids
	Long thoracic	Serratus anterior
Upper trunk	Suprascapular	Supraspinatus and infraspinatus
	Subclavius	Subclavius
Lateral cord	Lateral pectoral	Pectoralis major
	Musculocutaneous	Anterior compartment muscles of arm
Medial cord	Medial pectoral	Pectoralis minor and major
	Ulnar	Some forearm and most hand muscles
Medial and lateral cords	Median	Most forearm and some hand muscles
Posterior cord	Upper subscapular	Subscapularis
	Thoracodorsal	Latissimus dorsi
	Lower subscapular	Subscapularis and teres major
	Axillary	Deltoid and teres minor
	Radial	Posterior compartment muscles of the arm and forearm

Axilla: Lymph Nodes

The axillary lymph nodes lie in the fatty connective tissue of the axilla and are major collection nodes for lymph draining from the upper limb and portions of the chest wall, especially the breast (approximately 75% of lymphatic drainage from the breast passes through these nodes). The nodes are divided into five groups:

- Central nodes
- Lateral (brachial) nodes
- Posterior (subscapular) nodes
- Anterior (pectoral) nodes
- Apical (subclavian) nodes

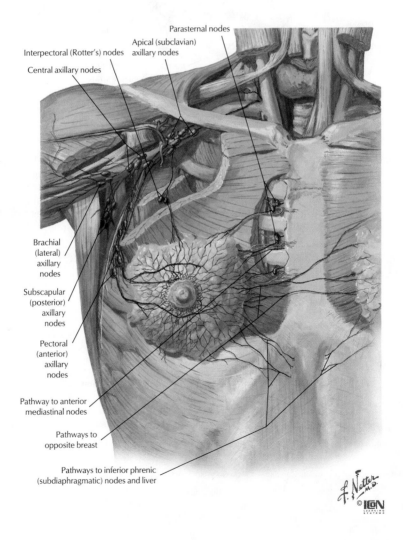

Parasternal nodes

Apical (subclavian)
Interpectoral (Rotter's) nodes   axillary nodes

Central axillary nodes

Brachial
(lateral)
axillary
nodes

Subscapular
(posterior)
axillary
nodes

Pectoral
(anterior)
axillary
nodes

Pathway to anterior
mediastinal nodes

Pathways to
opposite breast

Pathways to inferior phrenic
(subdiaphragmatic) nodes and liver

Arm: Anterior Compartment Muscles and Nerves

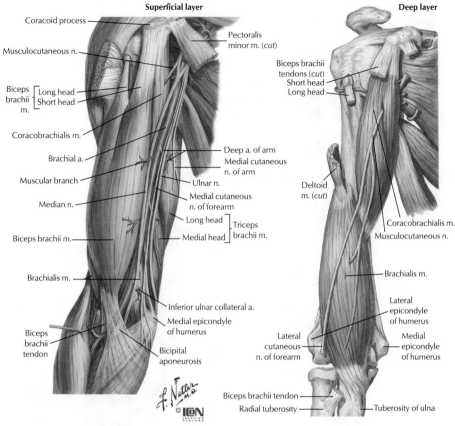

The arm is divided into an anterior (flexor) compartment and a posterior (extensor) compartment by an intramuscular septum. Muscles of the anterior compartment

- Are innervated by the musculocutaneous nerve
- Are supplied with blood from the brachial artery
- Are primarily flexors of the forearm at the elbow
- Are secondarily flexors of the arm at the shoulder (biceps and coracobrachialis)
- Can supinate the flexed forearm (biceps only)

MUSCLE	PROXIMAL ATTACHMENT (ORIGIN)	DISTAL ATTACHMENT (INSERTION)	INNERVATION	MAIN ACTIONS
Biceps brachii	*Short head:* apex of coracoid process of scapula *Long head:* supraglenoid tubercle of scapula	Tuberosity of radius and fascia of forearm via bicipital aponeurosis	Musculocutaneous nerve	Supinates flexed forearm; flexes forearm at elbow
Brachialis	Distal half of anterior humerus	Coronoid process and tuberosity of ulna	Musculocutaneous nerve	Flexes forearm at elbow in all positions
Coraco-brachialis	Tip of coracoid process of scapula	Middle third of medial surface of humerus	Musculocutaneous nerve	Helps to flex and adduct arm at shoulder

Arm: Posterior Compartment Muscles and Nerves

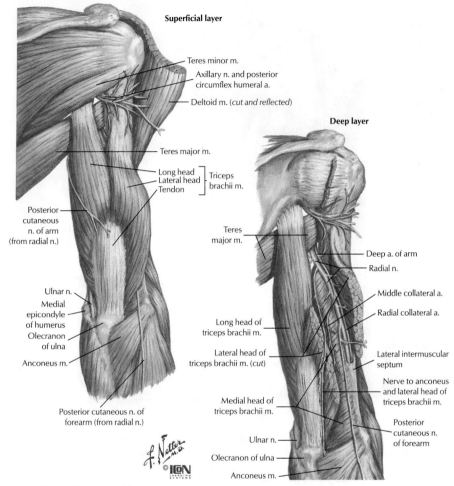

Superficial layer

Teres minor m.

Axillary n. and posterior circumflex humeral a.

Deltoid m. (*cut and reflected*)

Deep layer

Teres major m.

Long head
Lateral head } Triceps
Tendon   } brachii m.

Posterior cutaneous n. of arm (from radial n.)

Teres major m.

Deep a. of arm

Radial n.

Ulnar n.

Medial epicondyle of humerus

Olecranon of ulna

Anconeus m.

Long head of triceps brachii m.

Lateral head of triceps brachii m. (*cut*)

Middle collateral a.

Radial collateral a.

Lateral intermuscular septum

Nerve to anconeus and lateral head of triceps brachii m.

Posterior cutaneous n. of forearm (from radial n.)

Medial head of triceps brachii m.

Posterior cutaneous n. of forearm

Ulnar n.

Olecranon of ulna

Anconeus m.

Muscles of the posterior compartment
- Are innervated by the radial nerve
- Are supplied with blood from the deep artery of the arm (profunda brachii)
- Are largely extensors of the forearm at the elbow

MUSCLE	PROXIMAL ATTACHMENT (ORIGIN)	DISTAL ATTACHMENT (INSERTION)	INNERVATION	MAIN ACTIONS
Triceps brachii	*Long head*: infraglenoid tubercle of scapula *Lateral head*: posterior surface of humerus *Medial head*: posterior surface of humerus, inferior to radial groove	Proximal end of olecranon of ulna and fascia of forearm	Radial nerve	Extends forearm at elbow; is chief extensor of elbow; steadies head of abducted humerus (long head)
Anconeus	Lateral epicondyle of humerus	Lateral surface of olecranon and superior part of posterior surface of ulna	Radial nerve	Assists triceps in extending elbow; abducts ulna during pronation

Arm: Brachial Artery and Anastomoses

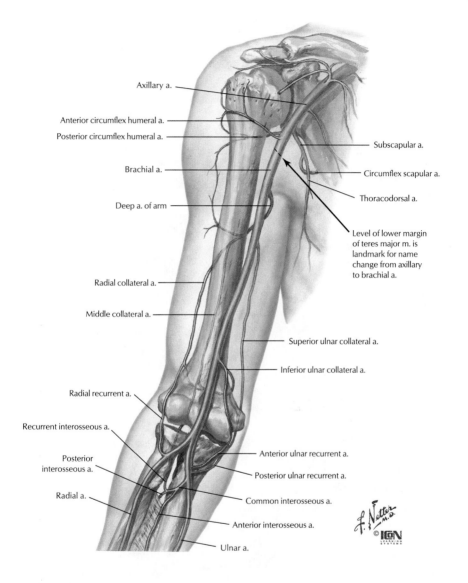

Axillary a.

Anterior circumflex humeral a.

Posterior circumflex humeral a.

Brachial a.

Deep a. of arm

Radial collateral a.

Middle collateral a.

Radial recurrent a.

Recurrent interosseous a.

Posterior interosseous a.

Radial a.

Subscapular a.

Circumflex scapular a.

Thoracodorsal a.

Level of lower margin of teres major m. is landmark for name change from axillary to brachial a.

Superior ulnar collateral a.

Inferior ulnar collateral a.

Anterior ulnar recurrent a.

Posterior ulnar recurrent a.

Common interosseous a.

Anterior interosseous a.

Ulnar a.

ARTERY	COURSE
Brachial	Begins at inferior border of teres major and ends at its bifurcation in cubital fossa
Deep artery of arm	Runs with radial nerve around humeral shaft
Superior ulnar collateral	Runs with ulnar nerve
Inferior ulnar collateral	Passes anterior to medial epicondyle of humerus
Radial	Is smaller lateral branch of brachial artery
Ulnar	Is larger medial branch of brachial artery

Arm: Serial Cross Sections

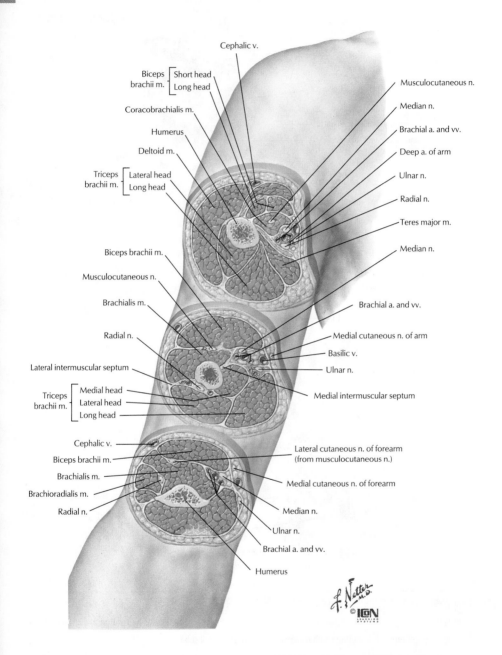

Cephalic v.

Biceps [Short head
brachii m. [Long head

Coracobrachialis m.

Humerus

Deltoid m.

Triceps [Lateral head
brachii m. [Long head

Biceps brachii m.

Musculocutaneous n.

Brachialis m.

Radial n.

Lateral intermuscular septum

Triceps [Medial head
brachii m. [Lateral head
[Long head

Cephalic v.

Biceps brachii m.

Brachialis m.

Brachioradialis m.

Radial n.

Musculocutaneous n.

Median n.

Brachial a. and vv.

Deep a. of arm

Ulnar n.

Radial n.

Teres major m.

Median n.

Brachial a. and vv.

Medial cutaneous n. of arm

Basilic v.

Ulnar n.

Medial intermuscular septum

Lateral cutaneous n. of forearm
(from musculocutaneous n.)

Medial cutaneous n. of forearm

Median n.

Ulnar n.

Brachial a. and vv.

Humerus

Cross sections clearly show anterior and posterior compartments and their respective flexor and extensor muscles. Note the nerve of each compartment and the medially situated neurovascular bundle containing the brachial artery, median nerve, and ulnar nerve. These last two nerves do not innervate arm muscles but simply pass through the arm to reach the forearm and hand.

Clinical Correlation

Rupture of the Biceps Brachii Muscle

Anatomy on p. 145

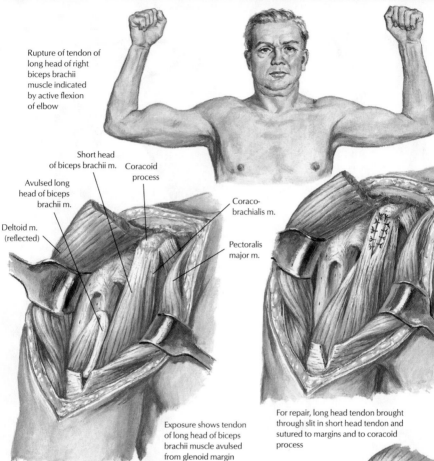

Rupture of tendon of long head of right biceps brachii muscle indicated by active flexion of elbow

Short head of biceps brachii m.

Coracoid process

Avulsed long head of biceps brachii m.

Coraco-brachialis m.

Deltoid m. (reflected)

Pectoralis major m.

Exposure shows tendon of long head of biceps brachii muscle avulsed from glenoid margin of scapula.

For repair, long head tendon brought through slit in short head tendon and sutured to margins and to coracoid process

Rupture of the biceps brachii may occur at the tendon or, rarely, the muscle belly. This tendon has the highest rate of spontaneous rupture of any tendon in the body. Rupture is seen most often in patients aged older than 40 years, in association with rotator cuff injuries (as the tendon begins to undergo degenerative changes), and with repetitive lifting (weight lifters). Rupture of the long head tendon is most common and may occur at the
- Shoulder joint
- Intertubercular (bicipital) groove of humerus
- Musculotendinous junction

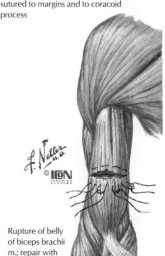

Rupture of belly of biceps brachii m.; repair with mattress sutures

Clinical Correlation

Fractures of the Humerus
Anatomy on pp. 126, 129, 134

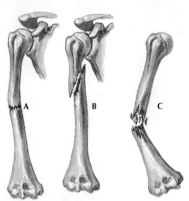

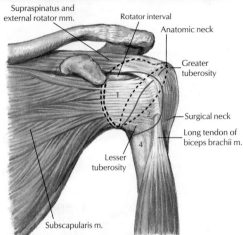

A. Transverse fracture of midshaft
B. Oblique (spiral) fracture
C. Comminuted fracture with marked angulation

Supraspinatus and external rotator mm.
Rotator interval
Anatomic neck
Greater tuberosity
Surgical neck
Long tendon of biceps brachii m.
Lesser tuberosity
Subscapularis m.

Neer four-part classification of fractures of proximal humerus.
1. Articular fragment (humeral head). 2. Lesser tuberosity. 3. Greater tuberosity. 4. Shaft. If no fragments displaced, fracture considered stable (most common) and treated with minimal external immobilization and early range-of-motion exercise.

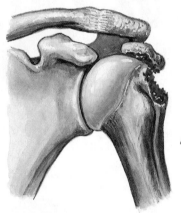

Displaced fracture of greater tuberosity surgically repaired using wires through small drill holes and suturing cuff tears. Small fragment may be excised and supraspinatus tendon reattached

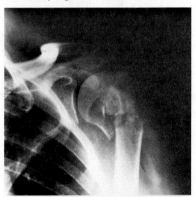

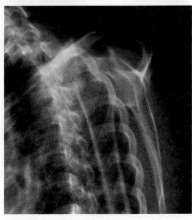

Fractures of the humerus may occur proximally (common in older persons) as a result of a fall on an outstretched hand; along the midshaft, usually from direct trauma; and distally (uncommon in adults). Proximal fractures occur mainly at four sites:
- Humeral head (articular fragment)
- Lesser tuberosity
- Greater tuberosity
- Proximal shaft

Midshaft fractures usually heal well but may involve entrapment of the radial nerve as it spirals around the shaft to reach the arm's posterior compartment (triceps muscle).

Forearm: Bones

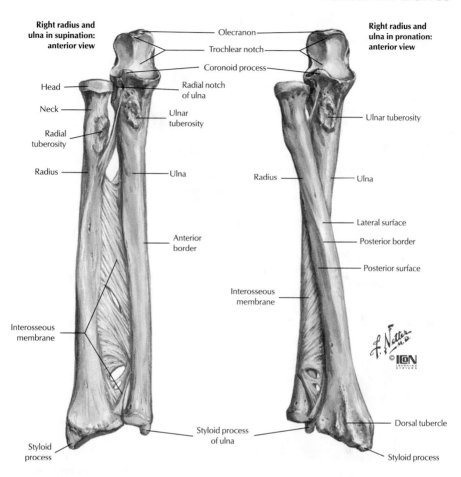

Right radius and ulna in supination: anterior view

Right radius and ulna in pronation: anterior view

Olecranon
Trochlear notch
Coronoid process
Head
Neck
Radial tuberosity
Radial notch of ulna
Ulnar tuberosity
Radius
Ulna
Anterior border
Interosseous membrane
Styloid process
Interosseous membrane
Ulnar tuberosity
Radius
Ulna
Lateral surface
Posterior border
Posterior surface
Interosseous membrane
Dorsal tubercle
Styloid process of ulna
Styloid process

FEATURE	DESCRIPTION
Radius	
Long bone	Is shorter than ulna
Proximal head	Articulates with capitulum of humerus and radial notch of ulna
Distal styloid process	Articulates with scaphoid, lunate, and triquetrum carpal bones
Ulna	
Long bone	Is longer than radius
Proximal olecranon	Is attachment point of triceps tendon
Proximal trochlear notch	Articulates with trochlea of humerus
Radial notch	Articulates with head of radius
Distal head	Articulates with disc at distal radioulnar joint

The radioulnar fibrous (syndesmosis) joint unites both bones via an interosseous membrane, which also divides the forearm into anterior and posterior compartments.

Forearm: Elbow Joint and Ligaments

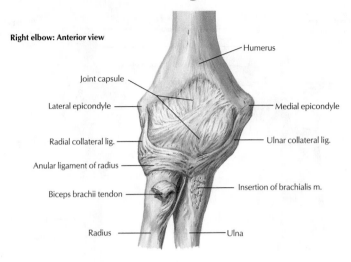

Right elbow: Anterior view

Humerus

Joint capsule

Lateral epicondyle

Medial epicondyle

Radial collateral lig.

Ulnar collateral lig.

Anular ligament of radius

Biceps brachii tendon

Insertion of brachialis m.

Radius

Ulna

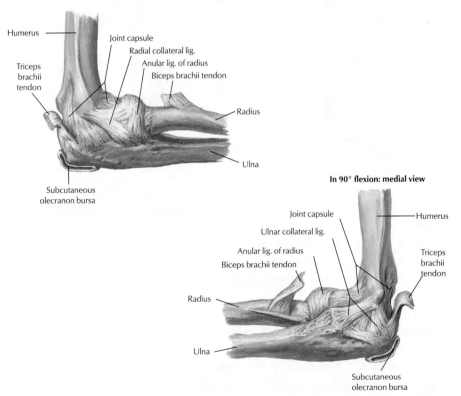

In 90° flexion: lateral view

Humerus

Joint capsule

Radial collateral lig.

Anular lig. of radius

Biceps brachii tendon

Triceps brachii tendon

Radius

Ulna

Subcutaneous olecranon bursa

In 90° flexion: medial view

Joint capsule

Humerus

Ulnar collateral lig.

Anular lig. of radius

Triceps brachii tendon

Biceps brachii tendon

Radius

Ulna

Subcutaneous olecranon bursa

Forearm: Elbow Joint and Ligaments (continued)

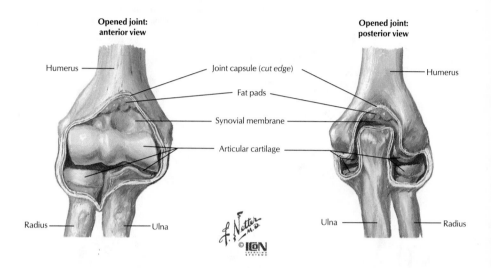

Opened joint: anterior view

Humerus — Joint capsule (*cut edge*) — Fat pads — Synovial membrane — Articular cartilage

Radius — Ulna

Opened joint: posterior view

Humerus

Ulna — Radius

The elbow joint is composed of the humeroulnar and humeroradial joints for flexion and extension and the proximal radioulnar joint for pronation and supination.

LIGAMENT	ATTACHMENT	COMMENT
Humeroulnar (Uniaxial Synovial Hinge [Ginglymus]) Joint		
Capsule	Surrounds joint	Provides flexion and extension
Ulnar (medial) collateral	Medial epicondyle of humerus to coronoid process and olecranon of ulna	Is triangular ligament with anterior, posterior, and oblique bands
Humeroradial Joint		
Capsule	Surrounds joint	Capitulum of humerus to head of radius
Radial (lateral) collateral	Lateral epicondyle of humerus to radial notch of ulna and anular ligament	Is weaker than ulnar collateral ligament but provides posterolateral stability
Proximal Radioulnar (Uniaxial Synovial Pivot) Joint		
Anular ligament	Surrounds radial head and radial notch of ulna	Keeps radial head in radial notch; allows pronation and supination

Clinical Correlation

Elbow Dislocation
Anatomy on pp. 151-153

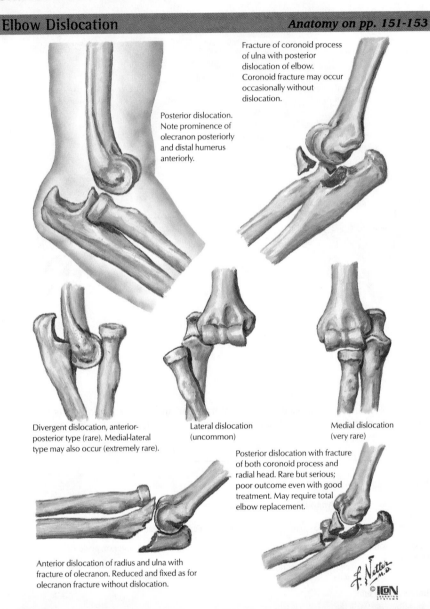

Posterior dislocation. Note prominence of olecranon posteriorly and distal humerus anteriorly.

Fracture of coronoid process of ulna with posterior dislocation of elbow. Coronoid fracture may occur occasionally without dislocation.

Divergent dislocation, anterior-posterior type (rare). Medial-lateral type may also occur (extremely rare).

Lateral dislocation (uncommon)

Medial dislocation (very rare)

Posterior dislocation with fracture of both coronoid process and radial head. Rare but serious; poor outcome even with good treatment. May require total elbow replacement.

Anterior dislocation of radius and ulna with fracture of olecranon. Reduced and fixed as for olecranon fracture without dislocation.

Elbow dislocations are third in frequency after shoulder and finger dislocations. Dislocation often results from a fall on an outstretched hand and includes the following types:
- Posterior (most common)
- Lateral (uncommon)
- Anterior (rare; may lacerate brachial artery)
- Medial (quite rare)

Dislocations may be accompanied by fractures of the humeral medial epicondyle, olecranon (ulna), radial head, or coronoid process of the ulna, and injury to the ulnar (most common) or median nerves.

Forearm: Anterior Compartment Superficial Muscles and Nerves

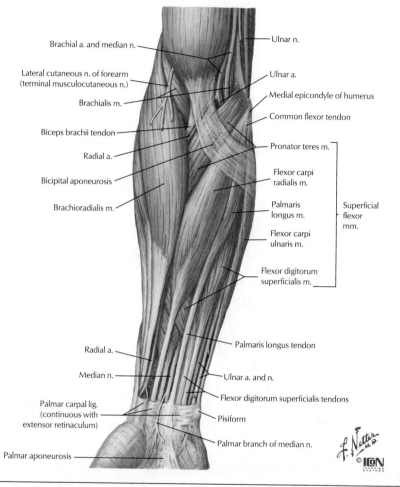

Brachial a. and median n.

Lateral cutaneous n. of forearm (terminal musculocutaneous n.)

Brachialis m.

Biceps brachii tendon

Radial a.

Bicipital aponeurosis

Brachioradialis m.

Radial a.

Median n.

Palmar carpal lig. (continuous with extensor retinaculum)

Palmar aponeurosis

Ulnar n.

Ulnar a.

Medial epicondyle of humerus

Common flexor tendon

Pronator teres m.

Flexor carpi radialis m.

Palmaris longus m.

Flexor carpi ulnaris m.

Flexor digitorum superficialis m.

Superficial flexor mm.

Palmaris longus tendon

Ulnar a. and n.

Flexor digitorum superficialis tendons

Pisiform

Palmar branch of median n.

MUSCLE	PROXIMAL ATTACHMENT (ORIGIN)	DISTAL ATTACHMENT (INSERTION)	INNERVATION	MAIN ACTIONS
Pronator teres	Medial epicondyle of humerus and coronoid process of ulna	Middle of lateral surface of radius	Median nerve	Pronates forearm and flexes elbow
Flexor carpi radialis	Medial epicondyle of humerus	Base of second metacarpal bone	Median nerve	Flexes hand at wrist and abducts it
Palmaris longus	Medial epicondyle of humerus	Distal half of flexor retinaculum and palmar aponeurosis	Median nerve	Flexes hand at wrist and tightens palmar aponeurosis
Flexor carpi ulnaris	*Humeral head*: medial epicondyle of humerus *Ulnar head*: olecranon and posterior border of ulna	Pisiform bone, hook of hamate bone, and fifth metacarpal bone	Ulnar nerve	Flexes hand at wrist and adducts it

Forearm: Anterior Compartment Deep Muscles and Nerves

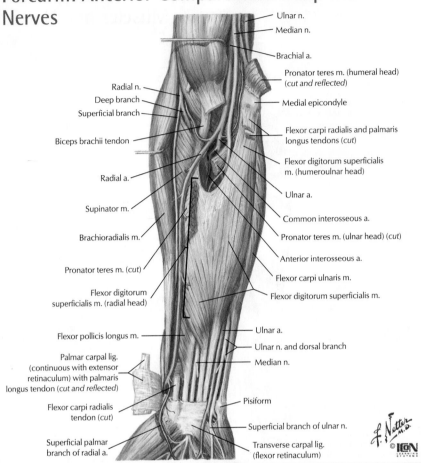

Ulnar n.
Median n.
Brachial a.
Pronator teres m. (humeral head) (cut and reflected)
Radial n.
Deep branch
Superficial branch
Medial epicondyle
Flexor carpi radialis and palmaris longus tendons (cut)
Biceps brachii tendon
Flexor digitorum superficialis m. (humeroulnar head)
Radial a.
Ulnar a.
Supinator m.
Common interosseous a.
Brachioradialis m.
Pronator teres m. (ulnar head) (cut)
Anterior interosseous a.
Pronator teres m. (cut)
Flexor carpi ulnaris m.
Flexor digitorum superficialis m. (radial head)
Flexor digitorum superficialis m.
Flexor pollicis longus m.
Ulnar a.
Ulnar n. and dorsal branch
Palmar carpal lig. (continuous with extensor retinaculum) with palmaris longus tendon (cut and reflected)
Median n.
Flexor carpi radialis tendon (cut)
Pisiform
Superficial branch of ulnar n.
Superficial palmar branch of radial a.
Transverse carpal lig. (flexor retinaculum)

MUSCLE	PROXIMAL ATTACHMENT (ORIGIN)	DISTAL ATTACHMENT (INSERTION)	INNERVATION	MAIN ACTIONS
Flexor digitorum superficialis	*Humeroulnar head*: medial epicondyle of humerus, ulnar collateral ligament, and coronoid process of ulna *Radial head*: superior half of anterior radius	Bodies of middle phalanges of medial four digits	Median nerve	Flexes middle phalanges of medial four digits; also weakly flexes proximal phalanges, forearm, and wrist
Flexor digitorum profundus	Proximal three fourths of medial and anterior surfaces of ulna and interosseous membrane	Bases of distal phalanges of medial four digits	*Medial part*: ulnar nerve *Lateral part*: median nerve	Flexes distal phalanges of medial four digits; assists with flexion of wrist
Flexor pollicis longus	Anterior surface of radius and adjacent interosseous membrane	Base of distal phalanx of thumb	Median nerve (anterior interosseous)	Flexes phalanges of first digit (thumb)
Pronator quadratus	Distal fourth of anterior surface of ulna	Distal fourth of anterior surface of radius	Median nerve (anterior interosseous)	Pronates forearm

Forearm: Posterior Compartment Superficial Muscles and Nerves

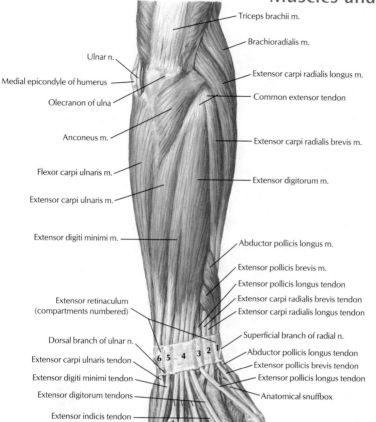

Triceps brachii m.

Brachioradialis m.

Ulnar n.

Medial epicondyle of humerus

Olecranon of ulna

Extensor carpi radialis longus m.

Common extensor tendon

Anconeus m.

Extensor carpi radialis brevis m.

Flexor carpi ulnaris m.

Extensor digitorum m.

Extensor carpi ulnaris m.

Extensor digiti minimi m.

Abductor pollicis longus m.

Extensor pollicis brevis m.

Extensor pollicis longus tendon

Extensor carpi radialis brevis tendon

Extensor retinaculum (compartments numbered)

Extensor carpi radialis longus tendon

Superficial branch of radial n.

Dorsal branch of ulnar n.

Abductor pollicis longus tendon

Extensor carpi ulnaris tendon

6 5 4 3 2 1

Extensor pollicis brevis tendon

Extensor digiti minimi tendon

Extensor pollicis longus tendon

Extensor digitorum tendons

Anatomical snuffbox

Extensor indicis tendon

MUSCLE	PROXIMAL ATTACHMENT (ORIGIN)	DISTAL ATTACHMENT (INSERTION)	INNERVATION	MAIN ACTIONS
Brachio-radialis	Proximal two thirds of lateral supracondylar ridge of humerus	Lateral surface of distal end of radius	Radial nerve	Flexes forearm at elbow
Extensor carpi radialis longus	Lateral supracondylar ridge of humerus	Base of second metacarpal bone	Radial nerve	Extends and abducts hand at wrist
Extensor carpi radialis brevis	Lateral epicondyle of humerus	Base of third metacarpal bone	Radial nerve (deep branch)	Extends and abducts hand at wrist
Extensor digitorum	Lateral epicondyle of humerus	Extensor expansions of medial four digits	Radial nerve (posterior interosseous)	Extends medial four digits at metacarpophalangeal joints; extends hand at wrist joint
Extensor digiti minimi	Lateral epicondyle of humerus	Extensor expansion of fifth digit	Radial nerve (posterior interosseous)	Extends fifth digit at metacarpophalangeal and interphalangeal joints
Extensor carpi ulnaris	Lateral epicondyle of humerus and posterior border of ulna	Base of fifth metacarpal bone	Radial nerve (posterior interosseous)	Extends and adducts hand at wrist

Forearm: Posterior Compartment Deep Muscles and Nerves

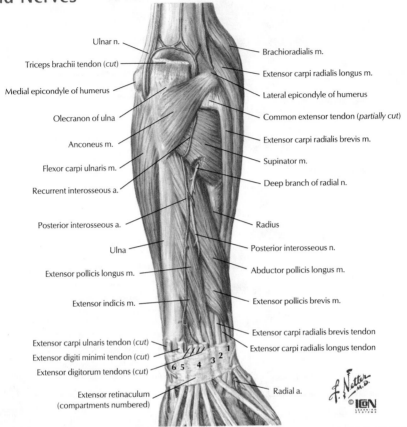

Ulnar n.

Triceps brachii tendon (*cut*)

Medial epicondyle of humerus

Olecranon of ulna

Anconeus m.

Flexor carpi ulnaris m.

Recurrent interosseous a.

Posterior interosseous a.

Ulna

Extensor pollicis longus m.

Extensor indicis m.

Extensor carpi ulnaris tendon (*cut*)

Extensor digiti minimi tendon (*cut*)

Extensor digitorum tendons (*cut*)

Extensor retinaculum (compartments numbered)

Brachioradialis m.

Extensor carpi radialis longus m.

Lateral epicondyle of humerus

Common extensor tendon (*partially cut*)

Extensor carpi radialis brevis m.

Supinator m.

Deep branch of radial n.

Radius

Posterior interosseous n.

Abductor pollicis longus m.

Extensor pollicis brevis m.

Extensor carpi radialis brevis tendon

Extensor carpi radialis longus tendon

6 5 4 3 2 1

Radial a.

MUSCLE	PROXIMAL ATTACHMENT (ORIGIN)	DISTAL ATTACHMENT (INSERTION)	INNERVATION	MAIN ACTIONS
Supinator	Lateral epicondyle of humerus; radial collateral, and anular ligaments; supinator fossa; and crest of ulna	Lateral, posterior, and anterior surfaces of proximal third of radius	Radial nerve (deep branch)	Supinates forearm, i.e., rotates radius to turn palm anteriorly
Abductor pollicis longus	Posterior surfaces of ulna, radius, and interosseous membrane	Base of first metacarpal bone	Radial nerve (posterior interosseous)	Abducts thumb and extends it at carpometacarpal joint
Extensor pollicis brevis	Posterior surfaces of radius and interosseous membrane	Base of proximal phalanx of thumb	Radial nerve (posterior interosseous)	Extends proximal phalanx of thumb at carpometacarpal joint
Extensor pollicis longus	Posterior surface of middle third of ulna and interosseous membrane	Base of distal phalanx of thumb	Radial nerve (posterior interosseous)	Extends distal phalanx of thumb at metacarpophalangeal and interphalangeal joints
Extensor indicis	Posterior surface of ulna and interosseous membrane	Extensor expansion of second digit	Radial nerve (posterior interosseous)	Extends second digit and helps to extend hand at wrist

Forearm: Arteries

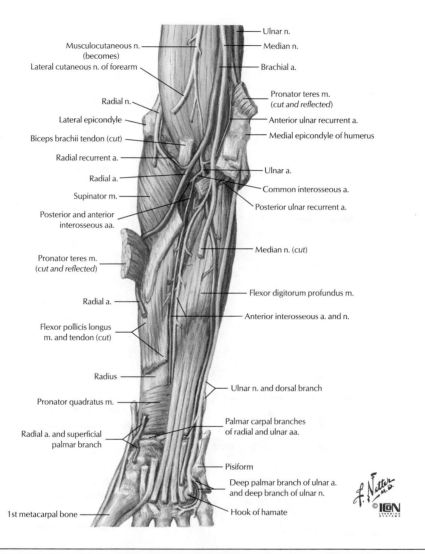

Musculocutaneous n.
(becomes)
Lateral cutaneous n. of forearm

Radial n.

Lateral epicondyle

Biceps brachii tendon (cut)

Radial recurrent a.

Radial a.

Supinator m.

Posterior and anterior
interosseous aa.

Pronator teres m.
(cut and reflected)

Radial a.

Flexor pollicis longus
m. and tendon (cut)

Radius

Pronator quadratus m.

Radial a. and superficial
palmar branch

1st metacarpal bone

Ulnar n.

Median n.

Brachial a.

Pronator teres m.
(cut and reflected)

Anterior ulnar recurrent a.

Medial epicondyle of humerus

Ulnar a.

Common interosseous a.

Posterior ulnar recurrent a.

Median n. (cut)

Flexor digitorum profundus m.

Anterior interosseous a. and n.

Ulnar n. and dorsal branch

Palmar carpal branches
of radial and ulnar aa.

Pisiform

Deep palmar branch of ulnar a.
and deep branch of ulnar n.

Hook of hamate

ARTERY	COURSE
Radial	Arises from brachial artery in cubital fossa
Radial recurrent branch	Anastomoses with radial collateral artery in arm
Palmar carpal branch	Anastomoses with carpal branch of ulnar artery
Ulnar	Arises from brachial artery in cubital fossa
Anterior ulnar recurrent	Anastomoses with inferior ulnar collateral in arm
Posterior ulnar recurrent	Anastomoses with superior ulnar collateral in arm
Common interosseous	Gives rise to anterior and posterior interosseous arteries
Palmar carpal branch	Anastomoses with carpal branch of radial artery

Forearm: Serial Cross Sections

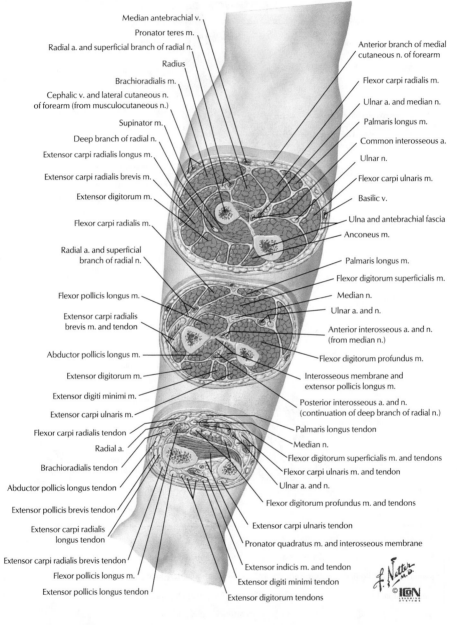

Median antebrachial v.
Pronator teres m.
Radial a. and superficial branch of radial n.
Radius
Brachioradialis m.
Cephalic v. and lateral cutaneous n. of forearm (from musculocutaneous n.)
Supinator m.
Deep branch of radial n.
Extensor carpi radialis longus m.
Extensor carpi radialis brevis m.
Extensor digitorum m.
Flexor carpi radialis m.
Radial a. and superficial branch of radial n.
Flexor pollicis longus m.
Extensor carpi radialis brevis m. and tendon
Abductor pollicis longus m.
Extensor digitorum m.
Extensor digiti minimi m.
Extensor carpi ulnaris m.
Flexor carpi radialis tendon
Radial a.
Brachioradialis tendon
Abductor pollicis longus tendon
Extensor pollicis brevis tendon
Extensor carpi radialis longus tendon
Extensor carpi radialis brevis tendon
Flexor pollicis longus m.
Extensor pollicis longus tendon

Anterior branch of medial cutaneous n. of forearm
Flexor carpi radialis m.
Ulnar a. and median n.
Palmaris longus m.
Common interosseous a.
Ulnar n.
Flexor carpi ulnaris m.
Basilic v.
Ulna and antebrachial fascia
Anconeus m.
Palmaris longus m.
Flexor digitorum superficialis m.
Median n.
Ulnar a. and n.
Anterior interosseous a. and n. (from median n.)
Flexor digitorum profundus m.
Interosseous membrane and extensor pollicis longus m.
Posterior interosseous a. and n. (continuation of deep branch of radial n.)
Palmaris longus tendon
Median n.
Flexor digitorum superficialis m. and tendons
Flexor carpi ulnaris m. and tendon
Ulnar a. and n.
Flexor digitorum profundus m. and tendons
Extensor carpi ulnaris tendon
Pronator quadratus m. and interosseous membrane
Extensor indicis m. and tendon
Extensor digiti minimi tendon
Extensor digitorum tendons

The interosseous membrane divides the forearm into anterior (flexors and pronators) and posterior (extensor and supinator) compartments. The median nerve innervates all but the flexor carpi ulnaris and ulnar half of flexor digitorum profundus muscles in the anterior compartment (ulnar nerve innervates these); the radial nerve innervates all posterior compartment muscles. Deep veins run with radial and ulnar arteries and communicate with superficial (subcutaneous) veins.

Clinical Correlation

Fracture of the Radial Head and Neck   *Anatomy on pp. 151-153*

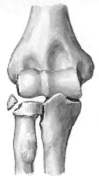 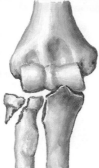 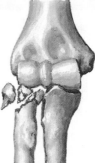 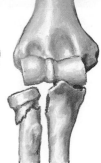

Small chip fracture of radial head

Large fracture of radial head with displacement

Comminuted fracture of radial head

Fracture of radial neck, tilted and impacted

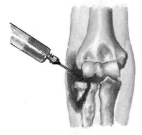 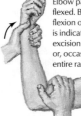

Elbow passively flexed. Blocked flexion or crepitus is indication for excision of fragments or, occasionally, entire radial head.

Hematoma aspirated, and 20-30 ml of xylocaine injected to permit painless testing of joint mobility

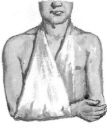

Small fractures without limitation of flexion heal well after aspiration with only sling support.

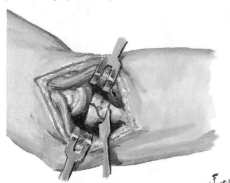 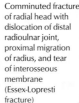 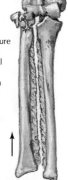

Comminuted fracture of radial head with dislocation of distal radioulnar joint, proximal migration of radius, and tear of interosseous membrane (Essex-Lopresti fracture)

Excision of fragment or entire radial head via posterolateral incision. Radial head may be replaced with Swanson silicone implant in selected patients.

Fractures to the proximal radius often involve either the head or the neck of the radius and can result from a fall on an outstretched hand (indirect trauma) or a direct blow to the elbow. Fracture of the radial head is more common in adults; fracture of the neck is more common in children.

Clinical Correlation

Biomechanics of Forearm Radial Fractures
Anatomy on pp. 151, 157, 158

Tuberosity of radius useful indicator of degree of pronation or supination of radius
A. In full supination, tuberosity directed toward ulna
B. In about 40° supination, tuberosity primarily posterior
C. In neutral position, tuberosity directly posterior
D. In full pronation, tuberosity directed laterally

A   B   C   D

Biceps brachii m.

Supinator m.

Pronator teres m.

Pronator quadratus m.

In fractures of radius above insertion of pronator teres muscle, proximal fragment flexed and supinated by biceps brachii and supinator muscles. Distal fragment pronated by pronator teres and pronator quadratus muscles.

In fractures of middle or distal radius that are distal to insertion of pronator teres muscle, supinator and pronator teres muscles keep proximal fragment in neutral position. Distal fragment pronated by pronator quadratus muscle.

Ulna

Radius

Interosseous membrane

Neutral   Pronation   Supination

Normally, radius bows laterally, and interosseous space is wide enough to allow rotation of radius on ulna. Space widest when forearm is in neutral rotation, narrower in pronation and in supination. (Lateral views to better demonstrate changes in space widths.)

Malunion may diminish or reverse radial bow, which impinges on ulna, impairing ability of radius to rotate over ulna.

The ulna is a straight bone with a stable articulation (elbow), but the radius is not uniform in size, proximal to distal. Natural lateral bowing of the radius is essential for optimal pronation and supination. When the radius is fractured, the muscles attaching to the bone deform this alignment. Careful reduction of the fracture should attempt to replicate normal anatomy to maximize pronation and supination, as well as to maintain integrity of the interosseous membrane.

Clinical Correlation

Fracture of the Ulnar Shaft
Anatomy on pp. 151, 152, 158

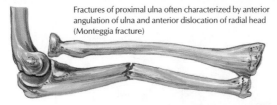

Fractures of proximal ulna often characterized by anterior angulation of ulna and anterior dislocation of radial head (Monteggia fracture)

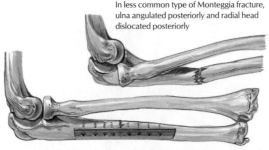

In less common type of Monteggia fracture, ulna angulated posteriorly and radial head dislocated posteriorly

Fracture treated with open reduction and internal fixation using compression plate and screws. Dislocation of radial head reduced. Postoperative immobilization in long arm cast or functional splint for 6-8 weeks. Early exercise of fingers and shoulder encouraged.

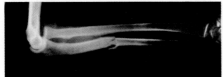

Preoperative radiograph shows anterior Monteggia fracture

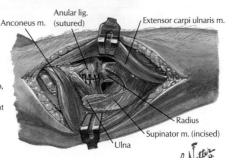

If dislocation of radial head does not reduce easily or joint remains unstable after reduction, open reduction and repair of anular ligament needed.

Anular lig. (sutured)
Anconeus m.
Extensor carpi ulnaris m.
Radius
Supinator m. (incised)
Ulna

Usually, a direct blow to or forced pronation of the forearm is the most common cause of a fracture of the shaft of the ulna. Fracture of the ulna with dislocation of the proximal radioulnar joint is termed a Monteggia fracture. The radial head usually dislocates anteriorly, but posterior, medial, or lateral dislocation also may occur. Such dislocations may put the posterior interosseous nerve (branch of the radial nerve) at risk.

Wrist and Hand: Bones

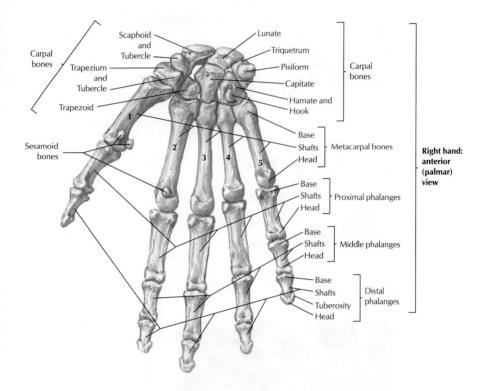

FEATURE	CHARACTERISTICS
Proximal Row of Carpals	
Scaphoid (boat shaped) Lunate (moon or crescent shaped) Triquetrum (triangular) Pisiform (pea shaped)	Lies beneath anatomical snuffbox Is most commonly fractured carpal All three bones (scaphoid, lunate, triquetrum) articulate with distal radius
Distal Row of Carpals	
Trapezium (four sided) Trapezoid Capitate (round bone) Hamate (hooked bone)	Distal row articulates with proximal row of carpals and with metacarpals
Metacarpals	
Numbered 1-5 (thumb to little finger) Two sesamoid bones	Possess a base, shaft, and head Are triangular in cross section Fifth metacarpal most commonly fractured Are associated with head of first metacarpal
Phalanges	
Three for each digit except thumb	Possess a base, shaft, and head Termed proximal, middle, and distal Distal phalanx of middle finger commonly fractured

Clinical Correlation

Fracture of the Scaphoid   *Anatomy on pp. 164, 166, 167, 170*

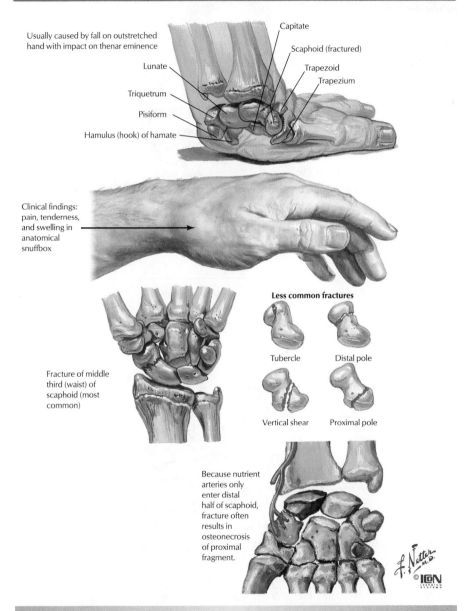

Usually caused by fall on outstretched hand with impact on thenar eminence

Capitate

Scaphoid (fractured)

Lunate

Trapezoid
Trapezium

Triquetrum

Pisiform

Hamulus (hook) of hamate

Clinical findings: pain, tenderness, and swelling in anatomical snuffbox

Less common fractures

Tubercle   Distal pole

Vertical shear   Proximal pole

Fracture of middle third (waist) of scaphoid (most common)

Because nutrient arteries only enter distal half of scaphoid, fracture often results in osteonecrosis of proximal fragment.

The scaphoid (navicular) bone is the most frequently fractured carpal and may be injured by falling on an extended wrist. Fracture of the middle third (waist) of the bone is most common. Pain and swelling in the anatomical snuffbox often occur; optimal healing depends on an adequate blood supply (from the palmar carpal branch of the radial artery). Loss of the blood supply can lead to nonunion or avascular osteonecrosis.

Wrist and Hand: Wrist Joint and Ligaments

Posterior (dorsal) view

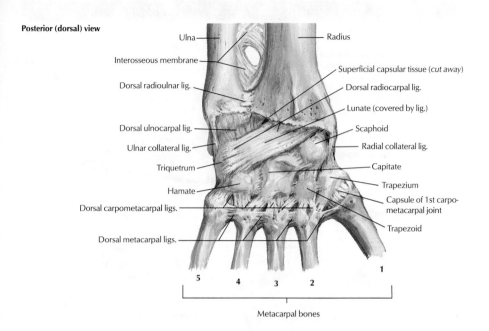

Ulna

Radius

Interosseous membrane

Superficial capsular tissue (*cut away*)

Dorsal radioulnar lig.

Dorsal radiocarpal lig.

Lunate (covered by lig.)

Dorsal ulnocarpal lig.

Scaphoid

Ulnar collateral lig.

Radial collateral lig.

Triquetrum

Capitate

Hamate

Trapezium

Dorsal carpometacarpal ligs.

Capsule of 1st carpo-
metacarpal joint

Dorsal metacarpal ligs.

Trapezoid

5   4   3   2

1

Metacarpal bones

Coronal section: dorsal view

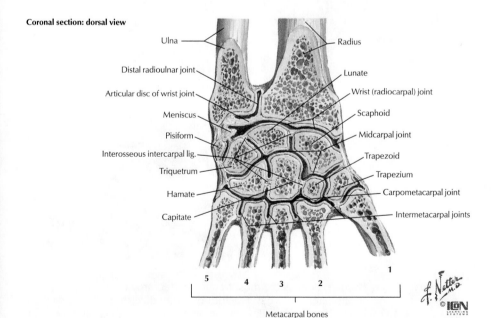

Ulna

Radius

Distal radioulnar joint

Lunate

Articular disc of wrist joint

Wrist (radiocarpal) joint

Meniscus

Scaphoid

Pisiform

Midcarpal joint

Interosseous intercarpal lig.

Trapezoid

Triquetrum

Trapezium

Hamate

Carpometacarpal joint

Capitate

Intermetacarpal joints

5   4   3   2

1

Metacarpal bones

Wrist and Hand: Wrist Joint and Ligaments (continued)

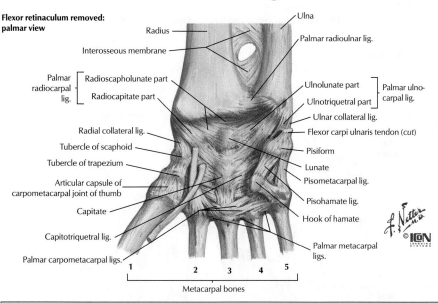

Flexor retinaculum removed: palmar view

Radius

Interosseous membrane

Palmar radiocarpal lig. — Radioscapholunate part / Radiocapitate part

Radial collateral lig.

Tubercle of scaphoid

Tubercle of trapezium

Articular capsule of carpometacarpal joint of thumb

Capitate

Capitotriquetral lig.

Palmar carpometacarpal ligs.

1   2   3   4   5

Metacarpal bones

Ulna

Palmar radioulnar lig.

Ulnolunate part / Ulnotriquetral part — Palmar ulno-carpal lig.

Ulnar collateral lig.

Flexor carpi ulnaris tendon (cut)

Pisiform

Lunate

Pisometacarpal lig.

Pisohamate lig.

Hook of hamate

Palmar metacarpal ligs.

LIGAMENT	ATTACHMENT	COMMENT
Radiocarpal (Biaxial Synovial Ellipsoid) Joint		
Capsule and disc	Surrounds joint; radius to scaphoid, lunate, and triquetrum	Provides little support; allows flexion, extension, abduction, adduction, circumduction
Palmar (volar) radiocarpal ligaments	Radius to scaphoid, lunate, and triquetrum	Are strong and stabilizing
Dorsal radiocarpal	Radius to scaphoid, lunate, and triquetrum	Is weaker ligament
Radial collateral	Radius to scaphoid and triquetrum	Stabilizes proximal row of carpals
Distal Radioulnar (Uniaxial Synovial Pivot) Joint		
Capsule	Surrounds joint; ulnar head to ulnar notch of radius	Is thin superiorly; allows pronation, supination
Palmar and dorsal radioulnar	Extends transversely between the two bones	Articular disc binds bones together
Intercarpal (Synovial Plane) Joints		
Proximal row of carpals	Adjacent carpals	Permits gliding and sliding movements
Distal row of carpals	Adjacent carpals	Are united by anterior, posterior, and interosseous ligaments
Midcarpal (Synovial Plane) Joints		
Palmar (volar) intercarpal	Proximal and distal rows of carpals	Is location for one third of wrist extension and two thirds of flexion; permits gliding and sliding movements
Carpal collaterals	Scaphoid, lunate, and triquetrum to capitate and hamate	Stabilize distal row (ellipsoid synovial joint)

Wrist and Hand: Finger Joints and Ligaments

Metacarpophalangeal and interphalangeal ligaments

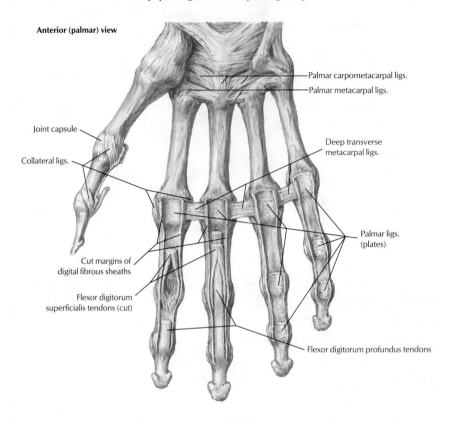

Anterior (palmar) view

Palmar carpometacarpal ligs.

Palmar metacarpal ligs.

Joint capsule

Deep transverse metacarpal ligs.

Collateral ligs.

Palmar ligs. (plates)

Cut margins of digital fibrous sheaths

Flexor digitorum superficialis tendons (*cut*)

Flexor digitorum profundus tendons

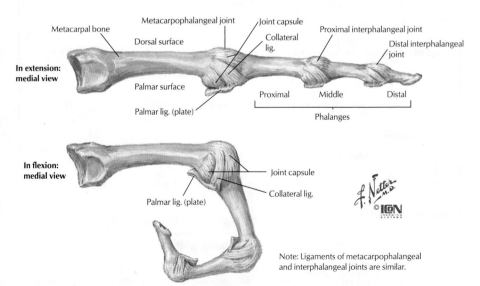

Metacarpophalangeal joint

Joint capsule

Proximal interphalangeal joint

Metacarpal bone

Dorsal surface

Collateral lig.

Distal interphalangeal joint

In extension: medial view

Palmar surface

Proximal   Middle   Distal

Palmar lig. (plate)

Phalanges

In flexion: medial view

Joint capsule

Collateral lig.

Palmar lig. (plate)

Note: Ligaments of metacarpophalangeal and interphalangeal joints are similar.

Wrist and Hand: Finger Joints and Ligaments (continued)

LIGAMENT	ATTACHMENT	COMMENT
Carpometacarpal (CMC) (Plane Synovial) Joints (except Thumb)		
Capsule	Carpals to metacarpals of digits 2-5	Surrounds joints; allows some gliding movement
Palmar and dorsal CMC	Carpals to metacarpals of digits 2-5	Dorsal ligament strongest
Interosseous CMC	Carpals to metacarpals of digits 2-5	
Thumb (Biaxial Saddle) Joint		
Same ligaments as CMC	Trapezium to first metacarpal	Allow flexion, extension, abduction, adduction, circumduction Is common site for arthritis
Metacarpophalangeal (Biaxial Condyloid Synovial) Joint		
Capsule	Metacarpal to proximal phalanx	Surrounds joint; allows flexion, extension, abduction, adduction, circumduction
Radial and ulnar collaterals	Metacarpal to proximal phalanx	Are tight in flexion and loose in extension
Palmar (volar) plate	Metacarpal to proximal phalanx	If broken digit, cast in flexion or ligament will shorten
Interphalangeal (Uniaxial Synovial Hinge) Joints		
Capsule	Adjacent phalanges	Surrounds joints; allow flexion and extension
Two collaterals	Adjacent phalanges	Are oriented obliquely
Palmar (volar) plate	Adjacent phalanges	Prevents hyperextension

Wrist and Hand: Intrinsic Hand Muscles

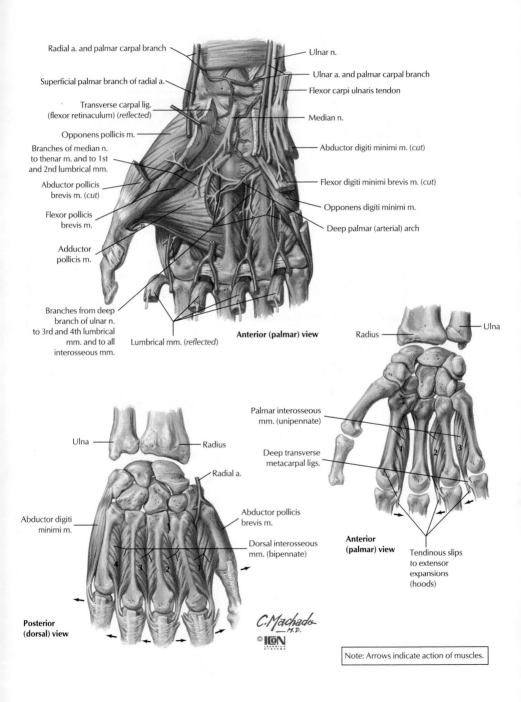

Radial a. and palmar carpal branch

Ulnar n.

Superficial palmar branch of radial a.

Ulnar a. and palmar carpal branch

Flexor carpi ulnaris tendon

Transverse carpal lig.
(flexor retinaculum) (reflected)

Median n.

Opponens pollicis m.

Branches of median n.
to thenar m. and to 1st
and 2nd lumbrical mm.

Abductor digiti minimi m. (cut)

Abductor pollicis
brevis m. (cut)

Flexor digiti minimi brevis m. (cut)

Opponens digiti minimi m.

Flexor pollicis
brevis m.

Deep palmar (arterial) arch

Adductor
pollicis m.

Branches from deep
branch of ulnar n.
to 3rd and 4th lumbrical
mm. and to all
interosseous mm.

Lumbrical mm. (reflected)

Anterior (palmar) view

Radius

Ulna

Palmar interosseous
mm. (unipennate)

Ulna

Radius

Deep transverse
metacarpal ligs.

Radial a.

Abductor digiti
minimi m.

Abductor pollicis
brevis m.

**Anterior
(palmar) view**

Dorsal interosseous
mm. (bipennate)

Tendinous slips
to extensor
expansions
(hoods)

**Posterior
(dorsal) view**

C. Machado
—M.D.
©ICN
LEARNING
SYSTEMS

Note: Arrows indicate action of muscles.

Wrist and Hand: Intrinsic Hand Muscles (continued)

MUSCLE	PROXIMAL ATTACHMENT (ORIGIN)	DISTAL ATTACHMENT (INSERTION)	INNERVATION	MAIN ACTIONS
Abductor pollicis brevis	Flexor retinaculum and tubercles of scaphoid and trapezium	Lateral side of base of proximal phalanx of thumb	Median nerve (recurrent branch)	Abducts thumb
Flexor pollicis brevis	Flexor retinaculum and tubercle of trapezium	Lateral side of base of proximal phalanx of thumb	Median nerve (recurrent branch)	Flexes proximal phalanx of thumb
Opponens pollicis	Flexor retinaculum and tubercle of trapezium	Lateral side of first metacarpal bone	Median nerve (recurrent branch)	Opposes thumb toward center of palm and rotates it medially
Adductor pollicis	*Oblique head*: bases of second and third metacarpals and capitate *Transverse head*: anterior surface of body of third metacarpal bone	Medial side of base of proximal phalanx of thumb	Ulnar nerve (deep branch)	Adducts thumb toward middle digit
Abductor digiti minimi	Pisiform and tendon of flexor carpi ulnaris	Medial side of base of proximal phalanx of fifth digit	Ulnar nerve (deep branch)	Abducts fifth digit
Flexor digiti minimi brevis	Hook of hamate and flexor retinaculum	Medial side of base of proximal phalanx of fifth digit	Ulnar nerve (deep branch)	Flexes proximal phalanx of fifth digit
Opponens digiti minimi	Hook of hamate and flexor retinaculum	Palmar surface of fifth metacarpal bone	Ulnar nerve (deep branch)	Draws fifth metacarpal bone anteriorly and rotates it, bringing fifth digit into opposition with thumb
Lumbricals 1 and 2	Lateral two tendons of flexor digitorum profundus	Lateral sides of extensor expansions of second to fifth digits	Median nerve	Flex digits at metacarpophalangeal joints and extend interphalangeal joints
Lumbricals 3 and 4	Medial three tendons of flexor digitorum profundus	Lateral sides of extensor expansions of second to fifth digits	Ulnar nerve (deep branch)	Flex digits at metacarpophalangeal joints and extend interphalangeal joints
Dorsal interossei	Adjacent sides of two metacarpal bones	Extensor expansions and bases of proximal phalanges of second to fourth digits	Ulnar nerve (deep branch)	Abduct digits; flex digits at metacarpo-phalangeal joint and extend interphalangeal joints
Palmar interossei	Palmar surfaces of second, fourth, and fifth metacarpal bones	Extensor expansions of digits and bases of proximal phalanges of second, fourth, and fifth digits	Ulnar nerve (deep branch)	Adduct digits; flex digits at metacarpophalangeal joint and extend interphalangeal joints

Wrist and Hand: Tendon Sheaths

Long flexor tendons (flexor digitorum superficialis and profundus) course on the palmar side of the digits, with the superficialis tendon splitting to allow the profundus tendon to pass to the distal phalanx. On the dorsum of the digits, the extensor expansion (hood) provides for insertion of the long extensor tendons and lumbrical and interosseous muscles. Lumbricals and interossei flex the metacarpophalangeal joint and extend the proximal and distal interphalangeal joints.

Flexor and extensor tendons in fingers

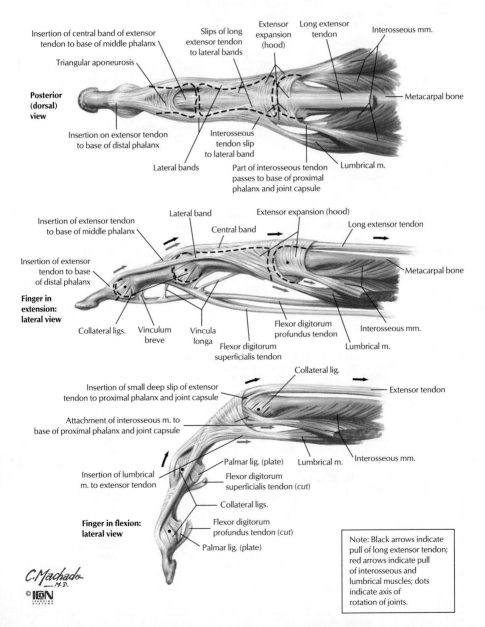

Insertion of central band of extensor tendon to base of middle phalanx

Slips of long extensor tendon to lateral bands

Extensor expansion (hood)

Long extensor tendon

Interosseous mm.

Triangular aponeurosis

Posterior (dorsal) view

Metacarpal bone

Insertion on extensor tendon to base of distal phalanx

Interosseous tendon slip to lateral band

Lateral bands

Part of interosseous tendon passes to base of proximal phalanx and joint capsule

Lumbrical m.

Insertion of extensor tendon to base of middle phalanx

Lateral band

Central band

Extensor expansion (hood)

Long extensor tendon

Insertion of extensor tendon to base of distal phalanx

Metacarpal bone

Finger in extension: lateral view

Collateral ligs.

Vinculum breve

Vincula longa

Flexor digitorum profundus tendon

Interosseous mm.

Flexor digitorum superficialis tendon

Lumbrical m.

Collateral lig.

Insertion of small deep slip of extensor tendon to proximal phalanx and joint capsule

Extensor tendon

Attachment of interosseous m. to base of proximal phalanx and joint capsule

Palmar lig. (plate)

Lumbrical m.

Interosseous mm.

Insertion of lumbrical m. to extensor tendon

Flexor digitorum superficialis tendon (cut)

Collateral ligs.

Finger in flexion: lateral view

Flexor digitorum profundus tendon (cut)

Palmar lig. (plate)

Note: Black arrows indicate pull of long extensor tendon; red arrows indicate pull of interosseous and lumbrical muscles; dots indicate axis of rotation of joints.

C. Machado
—M.D.

© ICN

Clinical Correlation

Colles' (Distal Radial) Fracture   *Anatomy on pp. 151, 166, 167*

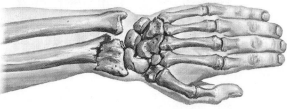

Most commonly results from fall on outstretched dorsiflexed hand

Immediate prehospital care: limb splinted, wrist elevated above level of heart on pillows or folded garment, ice pack applied

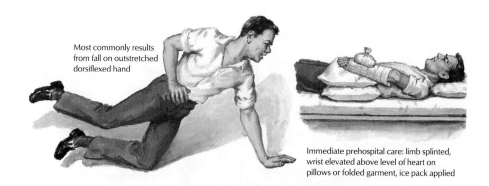

Lateral view of Colles' fracture demonstrates characteristic dinner fork deformity with dorsal and proximal displacement of distal fragment. Note dorsal instead of normal volar slope of articular surface of distal radius.

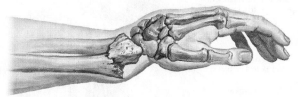

Dorsal view shows radial deviation of hand with ulnar prominence of styloid process of ulna and decrease of reverse of normal radial slope of articular surface of distal radius.

Fractures of the distal radius are common (approximately 80% of forearm fractures) in all age groups and often result from a fall on an outstretched hand. Colles' fracture is an extension-compression fracture of the distal radius that produces a typical dinner fork deformity.

Wrist and Hand: Vessels and Nerves

Palmar views: Superficial

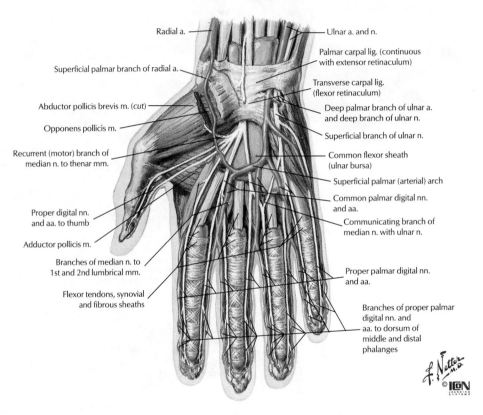

Radial a.

Superficial palmar branch of radial a.

Abductor pollicis brevis m. (*cut*)

Opponens pollicis m.

Recurrent (motor) branch of median n. to thenar mm.

Proper digital nn. and aa. to thumb

Adductor pollicis m.

Branches of median n. to 1st and 2nd lumbrical mm.

Flexor tendons, synovial and fibrous sheaths

Ulnar a. and n.

Palmar carpal lig. (continuous with extensor retinaculum)

Transverse carpal lig. (flexor retinaculum)

Deep palmar branch of ulnar a. and deep branch of ulnar n.

Superficial branch of ulnar n.

Common flexor sheath (ulnar bursa)

Superficial palmar (arterial) arch

Common palmar digital nn. and aa.

Communicating branch of median n. with ulnar n.

Proper palmar digital nn. and aa.

Branches of proper palmar digital nn. and aa. to dorsum of middle and distal phalanges

Wrist and Hand: Vessels and Nerves

Palmar view: Deep

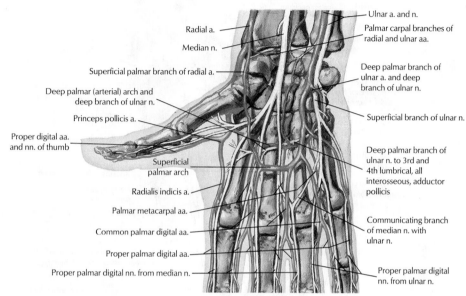

Radial a.

Median n.

Superficial palmar branch of radial a.

Deep palmar (arterial) arch and deep branch of ulnar n.

Princeps pollicis a.

Proper digital aa. and nn. of thumb

Superficial palmar arch

Radialis indicis a.

Palmar metacarpal aa.

Common palmar digital aa.

Proper palmar digital aa.

Proper palmar digital nn. from median n.

Ulnar a. and n.

Palmar carpal branches of radial and ulnar aa.

Deep palmar branch of ulnar a. and deep branch of ulnar n.

Superficial branch of ulnar n.

Deep palmar branch of ulnar n. to 3rd and 4th lumbrical, all interosseous, adductor pollicis

Communicating branch of median n. with ulnar n.

Proper palmar digital nn. from ulnar n.

ARTERY	COURSE
Radial	
Superficial palmar branch	Forms superficial palmar arch with ulnar artery
Princeps pollicis	Passes under flexor pollicis longus tendon and divides into two proper digital arteries to thumb
Radialis indicis	Passes to index finger on its lateral side
Deep palmar arch	Is formed by terminal part of radial artery
Ulnar	
Deep palmar branch	Forms deep palmar arch with radial artery
Superficial palmar arch	Is formed by termination of ulnar artery; gives rise to three common digital arteries, each of which gives rise to two proper digital arteries

Wrist and Hand: Palmar Spaces

Bursae, spaces and tendon sheaths of hand

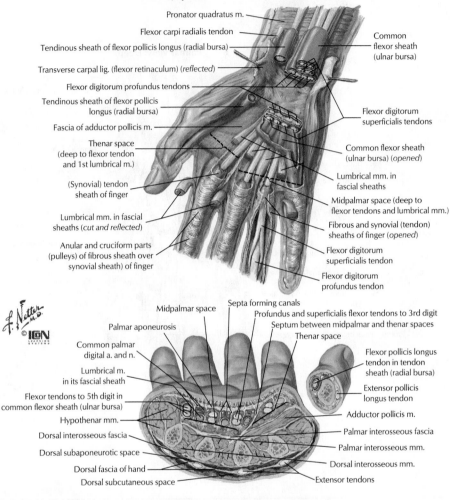

Pronator quadratus m.
Flexor carpi radialis tendon
Tendinous sheath of flexor pollicis longus (radial bursa)
Transverse carpal lig. (flexor retinaculum) (reflected)
Flexor digitorum profundus tendons
Tendinous sheath of flexor pollicis longus (radial bursa)
Fascia of adductor pollicis m.
Thenar space (deep to flexor tendon and 1st lumbrical m.)
(Synovial) tendon sheath of finger
Lumbrical mm. in fascial sheaths (cut and reflected)
Anular and cruciform parts (pulleys) of fibrous sheath over synovial sheath) of finger

Common flexor sheath (ulnar bursa)
Flexor digitorum superficialis tendons
Common flexor sheath (ulnar bursa) (opened)
Lumbrical mm. in fascial sheaths
Midpalmar space (deep to flexor tendons and lumbrical mm.)
Fibrous and synovial (tendon) sheaths of finger (opened)
Flexor digitorum superficialis tendon
Flexor digitorum profundus tendon

Midpalmar space
Palmar aponeurosis
Common palmar digital a. and n.
Lumbrical m. in its fascial sheath
Flexor tendons to 5th digit in common flexor sheath (ulnar bursa)
Hypothenar mm.
Dorsal interosseous fascia
Dorsal subaponeurotic space
Dorsal fascia of hand
Dorsal subcutaneous space

Septa forming canals
Profundus and superficialis flexor tendons to 3rd digit
Septum between midpalmar and thenar spaces
Thenar space
Flexor pollicis longus tendon in tendon sheath (radial bursa)
Extensor pollicis longus tendon
Adductor pollicis m.
Palmar interosseous fascia
Palmar interosseous mm.
Dorsal interosseous mm.
Extensor tendons

SPACE	COMMENT
Carpal tunnel	Osseofascial tunnel composed of carpal bones (carpal arch) and overlying flexor retinaculum; contains median nerve and nine tendons
Thenar eminence	Muscle compartment at base of thumb
Thenar space	Potential space just above adductor pollicis muscle
Hypothenar eminence	Muscle compartment at base of little finger
Central compartment	Compartment containing long flexor tendons and lumbrical muscles
Midpalmar space	Potential space deep to central compartment
Adductor compartment	Compartment containing adductor pollicis muscle
Synovial sheaths	Osseofibrous sheaths (tunnels) lined with synovium to facilitate sliding movements

Clinical Correlation

Finger Injuries
Anatomy on pp. 168, 172

Mallet finger

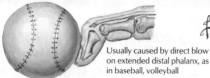

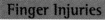

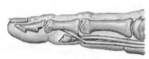

Usually caused by direct blow on extended distal phalanx, as in baseball, volleyball

Degrees of mallet finger injury. **A.** Extensor tendon stretched but not completely severed; mild finger drop and weak extensor ability retained. **B.** Tendon torn from its insertion. **C.** Bone fragment avulsed with tendon. In **B** and **C** there is 40-45° flexion deformity and loss of active extension.

Avulsion of flexor digitorum profundus tendon

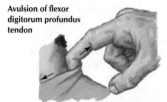

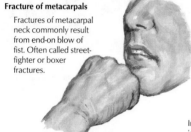

Flexor digitorum profundus tendon may be torn directly from distal phalanx or may avulse small or large bone fragment. Tendon usually retracts to about level of proximal interphalangeal joint, where it is stopped at its passage through flexor digitorum superficialis tendon; occasionally, it retracts into palm.

Caused by violent traction on flexed distal phalanx, as in catching on jersey of running football player

Fracture of metacarpals

Fractures of metacarpal neck commonly result from end-on blow of fist. Often called street-fighter or boxer fractures.

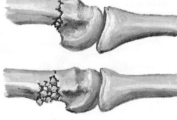

In fractures of metacarpal neck, volar cortex often comminuted, resulting in marked instability after reduction, which often necessitates pinning

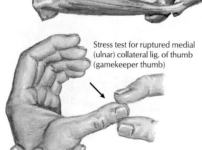

Transverse fractures of metacarpal shaft usually angulated dorsally by pull of interosseous mm.

Stress test for ruptured medial (ulnar) collateral lig. of thumb (gamekeeper thumb)

Thumb injury other than fracture

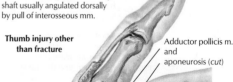

Adductor pollicis m. and aponeurosis (*cut*)

Torn medial collateral lig.

Ruptured medial collateral lig. of metacarpophalangeal joint of thumb

Various traumatic finger injuries may occur, causing fractures, disruption of flexor and extensor tendons, and torn ligaments. Each element must be carefully examined for normal function, including muscle groups, capillary refill, and two-point sensory discrimination.

Clinical Correlation

Proximal Interphalangeal Joint Dislocations

Anatomy on pp. 168, 172

Dorsal dislocation (most common)
Usually reducible by closed means, immobilized with palmar splint for 3 weeks, then active range-of-motion exercises begun

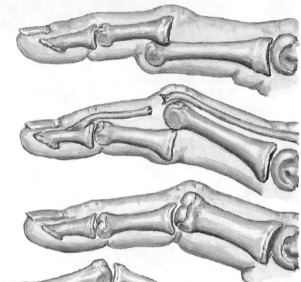

Palmar dislocation (uncommon)
Causes boutonnière deformity. Central slip of extensor tendon often torn, requiring open fixation, followed by dorsal splinting to allow passive and active exercises of distal interphalangeal joint.

Rotational dislocation (rare)
Note middle and distal phalanges seen in true lateral radiograph, proximal phalanx in oblique view. After reduction, treated as for dorsal dislocation.

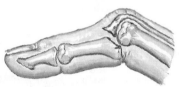

Dorsal dislocation of proximal interphalangeal joint with disruption of volar plate and collateral ligament may result in swan-neck deformity and compensatory flexion deformity of distal interphalangeal joint.

Volar dislocation of middle phalanx with avulsion of central slip of extensor tendon, with or without bone fragment. Failure to recognize and properly treat this condition results in boutonnière deformity and severely restricted function.

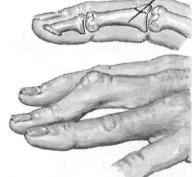

DEFECT	COMMENT
Coach's finger	Dorsal dislocation of the joint
Boutonnière deformity	Dislocation or avulsion fracture of middle phalanx, with failure to treat causing deformity and chronic pain
Rotational	Rare dislocation
Swan-neck deformity	Dorsal dislocation with disruption of palmar (volar) and collateral ligaments

Clinical Correlation

Rheumatoid Arthritis   *Anatomy on pp. 166-168, 172*

Early and moderate hand involvement in rheumatoid arthritis

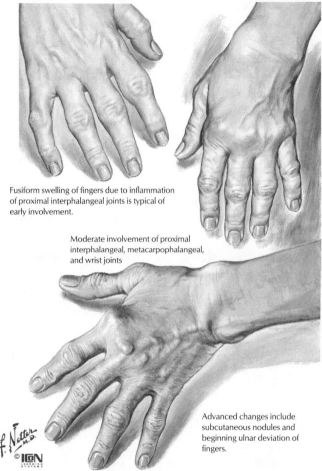

Fusiform swelling of fingers due to inflammation of proximal interphalangeal joints is typical of early involvement.

Moderate involvement of proximal interphalangeal, metacarpophalangeal, and wrist joints

Advanced changes include subcutaneous nodules and beginning ulnar deviation of fingers.

Rheumatoid arthritis, a multifactorial disease with a clear genetic component, affects approximately 1% of the population worldwide and is more common in women than men. The clinical presentation includes
- Onset usually between 40 and 50 years of age
- Morning stiffness
- Warm joints and joint swelling
- Arthritis in three or more joints
- More common in small joints of wrist and hand than in large joints
- Symmetric disease
- Rheumatoid nodules
- Serum IgM rheumatoid factor
- Vasculitis

Muscle Summary: Actions of Major Muscles

The following list summarizes actions of major muscles on joints of the upper limb. The list is not exhaustive and highlights only major muscles responsible for each movement (the separate muscle tables provide more detail).

SCAPULA

Elevate: levator scapulae, trapezius

Depress: pectoralis minor

Protrude: serratus anterior

Depress glenoid: rhomboids

Elevate glenoid: serratus anterior, trapezius

Retract: rhomboids, trapezius

SHOULDER

Flex: pectoralis major, coracobrachialis

Extend: latissimus dorsi

Abduct: deltoid, supraspinatus

Adduct: pectoralis major, latissimus dorsi

Rotate medially: subscapularis, teres major, pectoralis major, latissimus dorsi

Rotate laterally: infraspinatus, teres minor

ELBOW

Flex: brachialis, biceps

Extend: triceps, anconeus

RADIOULNAR

Pronate: pronators (teres and quadratus)

Supinate: supinator, biceps brachii

WRIST

Flex: flexor carpi radialis, ulnaris

Extend: all extensor carpi muscles

Abduct: flexor/extensor carpi radialis muscles

Adduct: flexor and extensor carpi ulnaris

Circumduct: combination of all movements

METACARPOPHALANGEAL

Flex: interossei and lumbricals

Extend: extensor digitorum

Abduct: dorsal interossei

Adduct: palmar interossei

Circumduct: combination of all movements

INTERPHALANGEAL-PROXIMAL

Flex: flexor digitorum superficialis

Extend: interossei and lumbricals

INTERPHALANGEAL-DISTAL

Flex: flexor digitorum profundus

Extend: interossei and lumbricals

Clinical Correlation

Nerve Summary: Shoulder Region Neuropathy

Anatomy on pp. 134, 141, 146

Suprascapular nerve

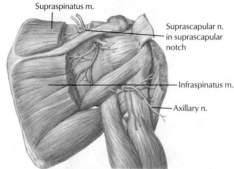

Suprapsinatus m.

Suprascapular n. in suprascapular notch

Infraspinatus m.

Axillary n.

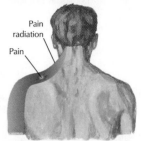

Pain radiation

Pain

Compression of suprascapular nerve may cause lateral shoulder pain and atrophy of supraspinatus and intraspinatus muscles

Musculocutaneous nerve

Musculocutaneous nerve compression within coracobrachialis muscle causes hypesthesia in lateral forearm and weakness of elbow flexion

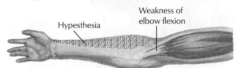

Hypesthesia

Weakness of elbow flexion

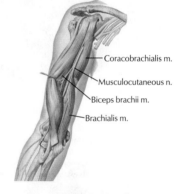

Coracobrachialis m.

Musculocutaneous n.

Biceps brachii m.

Brachialis m.

Long thoracic nerve

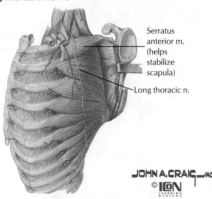

Serratus anterior m. (helps stabilize scapula)

Long thoracic n.

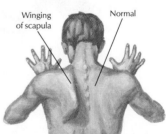

Winging of scapula

Normal

JOHN A. CRAIG—AD
©ICN
LEARNING SYSTEMS

INVOLVED NERVE	CONDITION
Suprascapular	Posterolateral shoulder pain, which may radiate to arm and neck; weakness in shoulder rotation
Musculocutaneous	Coracobrachialis compression and weakened flexion at the elbow, with hypesthesia of lateral forearm
Long thoracic	Injury at level of neck caused by stretching during lateral flexion of neck to opposite side; winged scapula
Axillary	Rare condition (quadrilateral space syndrome) (not shown in illustration)

Nerve Summary: Normal Radial Nerve Distribution in the Arm

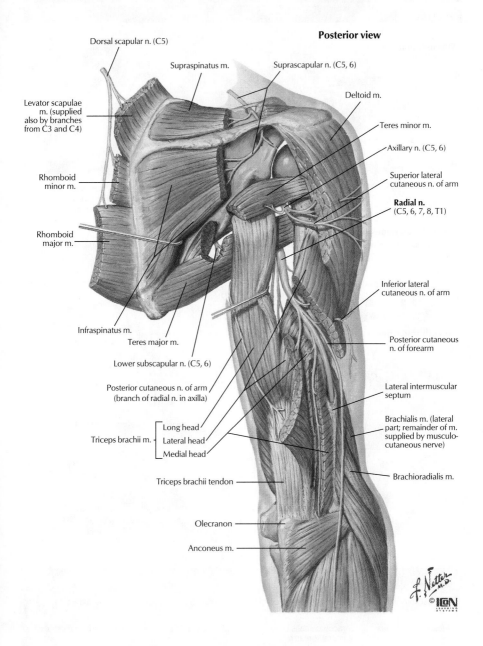

Posterior view

Dorsal scapular n. (C5)

Supraspinatus m.

Suprascapular n. (C5, 6)

Deltoid m.

Levator scapulae m. (supplied also by branches from C3 and C4)

Teres minor m.

Axillary n. (C5, 6)

Rhomboid minor m.

Superior lateral cutaneous n. of arm

Radial n. (C5, 6, 7, 8, T1)

Rhomboid major m.

Inferior lateral cutaneous n. of arm

Infraspinatus m.

Teres major m.

Posterior cutaneous n. of forearm

Lower subscapular n. (C5, 6)

Posterior cutaneous n. of arm (branch of radial n. in axilla)

Lateral intermuscular septum

Brachialis m. (lateral part; remainder of m. supplied by musculo-cutaneous nerve)

Triceps brachii m. ⎡ Long head
              ⎢ Lateral head
              ⎣ Medial head

Triceps brachii tendon

Brachioradialis m.

Olecranon

Anconeus m.

The radial nerve innervates muscles that extend the forearm at the elbow (posterior compartment muscles) and the skin of the posterior arm, via the inferior lateral and posterior cutaneous nerves of the arm.

Nerve Summary: Normal Radial Nerve Distribution in the Forearm

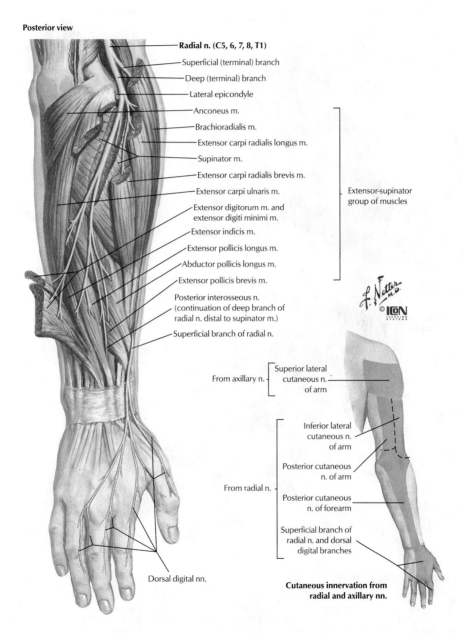

Posterior view

- Radial n. (C5, 6, 7, 8, T1)
- Superficial (terminal) branch
- Deep (terminal) branch
- Lateral epicondyle
- Anconeus m.
- Brachioradialis m.
- Extensor carpi radialis longus m.
- Supinator m.
- Extensor carpi radialis brevis m.
- Extensor carpi ulnaris m.
- Extensor digitorum m. and extensor digiti minimi m.
- Extensor indicis m.
- Extensor pollicis longus m.
- Abductor pollicis longus m.
- Extensor pollicis brevis m.
- Posterior interosseous n. (continuation of deep branch of radial n. distal to supinator m.)
- Superficial branch of radial n.

Extensor-supinator group of muscles

From axillary n. — Superior lateral cutaneous n. of arm

From radial n. —
- Inferior lateral cutaneous n. of arm
- Posterior cutaneous n. of arm
- Posterior cutaneous n. of forearm
- Superficial branch of radial n. and dorsal digital branches

Dorsal digital nn.

Cutaneous innervation from radial and axillary nn.

The radial nerve innervates extensor muscles of the wrist and fingers and the supinator (posterior compartment muscles). It also conveys cutaneous sensory information from the posterior forearm and the radial side of the dorsum of the hand. Pure radial nerve sensation is tested on the skin overlying the first dorsal interosseous muscle.

Clinical Correlation

Radial Nerve Compression

Anatomy on pp. 182, 183

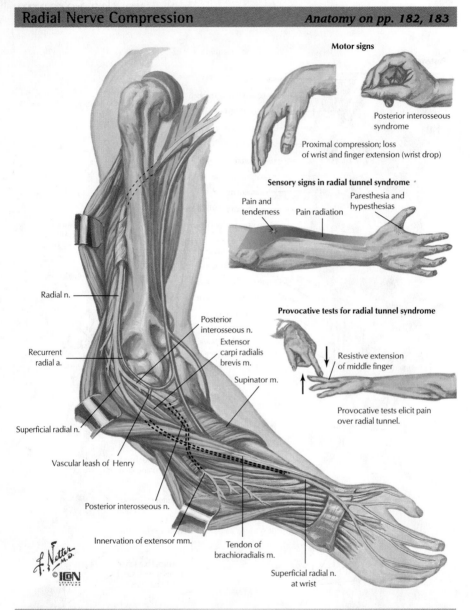

Motor signs

Posterior interosseous
syndrome

Proximal compression; loss
of wrist and finger extension (wrist drop)

Sensory signs in radial tunnel syndrome

Pain and
tenderness

Pain radiation

Paresthesia and
hypesthesias

Radial n.

Recurrent
radial a.

Posterior
interosseous n.

Extensor
carpi radialis
brevis m.

Supinator m.

Provocative tests for radial tunnel syndrome

Resistive extension
of middle finger

Provocative tests elicit pain
over radial tunnel.

Superficial radial n.

Vascular leash of Henry

Posterior interosseous n.

Innervation of extensor mm.

Tendon of
brachioradialis m.

Superficial radial n.
at wrist

COMPRESSION SITE	ETIOLOGY AND EFFECTS
Proximal	Humeral fracture, tourniquet injury, or chronic direct compression (Saturday night paralysis); weakened elbow, wrist, and finger extension, and supination
Elbow	Repetitive forearm rotation or fracture; posterior compartment neuropathies and radial tunnel syndrome
Wrist	Trauma, tight handcuffs, cast, or watchband; paresthesias in dorsolateral aspect of hand

Nerve Summary: Normal Median Nerve Distribution

The median nerve innervates all but the flexor carpi ulnaris and ulnar half of the flexor digitorum profundus muscles of the anterior compartment of the forearm (wrist and finger flexors, and forearm pronators). Pure median nerve sensation is tested on the skin overlying the palmar aspect of the tip of the index finger.

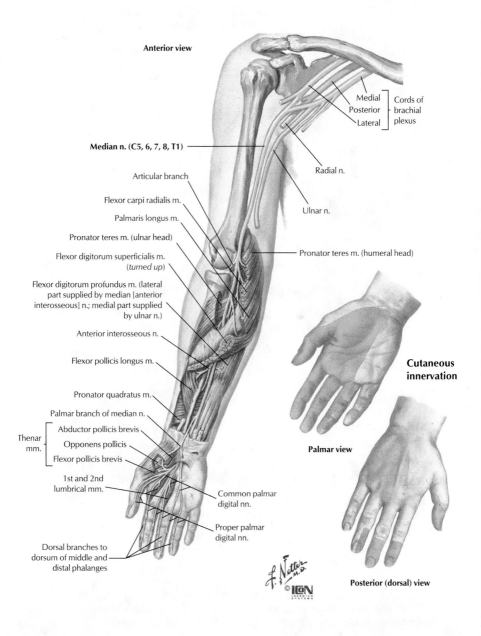

Anterior view

Medial ⎤
Posterior ⎬ Cords of brachial plexus
Lateral ⎦

Median n. (C5, 6, 7, 8, T1)

Radial n.

Articular branch

Flexor carpi radialis m.

Palmaris longus m.

Ulnar n.

Pronator teres m. (ulnar head)

Flexor digitorum superficialis m. (turned up)

Pronator teres m. (humeral head)

Flexor digitorum profundus m. (lateral part supplied by median [anterior interosseous] n.; medial part supplied by ulnar n.)

Anterior interosseous n.

Flexor pollicis longus m.

Cutaneous innervation

Pronator quadratus m.

Palmar branch of median n.

Abductor pollicis brevis

Thenar mm. ⎱ Opponens pollicis

Flexor pollicis brevis

Palmar view

1st and 2nd lumbrical mm.

Common palmar digital nn.

Proper palmar digital nn.

Dorsal branches to dorsum of middle and distal phalanges

Posterior (dorsal) view

Clinical Correlation

Proximal Median Nerve Compression Anatomy on p. 185

Median n.

Hypesthesia and activity-induced paresthesias

Pronator syndrome

Pain location

Provocative maneuvers

Flexion of middle finger against resistance

Compression by flexor digitorum superficialis m.

Compression by pronator teres m.

Pronation against resistance

Supra-condylar process

Lig. of Struthers

Medial epicondyle

Bicipital aponeurosis

Pronator teres m.
Humeral head
Ulnar head

Anterior interosseous n.

Compression by bicipital aponeurosis

Flexion of wrist against resistance

JOHN A. CRAIG—AD
© ICON

Flexor digitorum superficialis m. and arch

Flexor pollicis longus m.

Anterior interosseous syndrome

Normal

Abnormal

Hand posture in anterior interosseous syndrome due to paresis of flexor digitorum profundis and flexor pollicis longus mm.

Compression at the elbow is the second most common site of median nerve entrapment, after the wrist. Repetitive forearm pronation and finger flexion, especially against resistance, can cause muscle hypertrophy and entrap the nerve.

Clinical Correlation

Median Nerve and Carpal Tunnel Syndrome

Anatomy on pp. 174, 175, 185

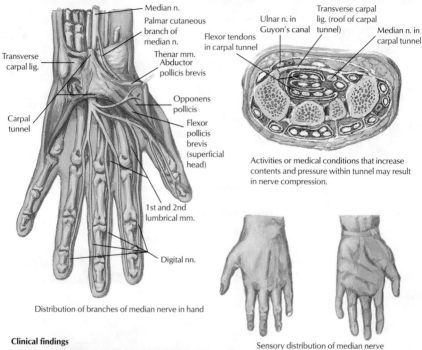

Median n.
Palmar cutaneous branch of median n.
Flexor tendons in carpal tunnel
Transverse carpal lig.
Thenar mm. Abductor pollicis brevis
Transverse carpal lig.
Opponens pollicis
Carpal tunnel
Flexor pollicis brevis (superficial head)
1st and 2nd lumbrical mm.
Digital nn.

Distribution of branches of median nerve in hand

Ulnar n. in Guyon's canal
Transverse carpal lig. (roof of carpal tunnel)
Median n. in carpal tunnel

Activities or medical conditions that increase contents and pressure within tunnel may result in nerve compression.

Sensory distribution of median nerve

Clinical findings

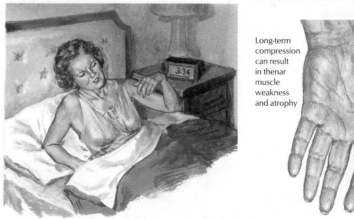

Long-term compression can result in thenar muscle weakness and atrophy

Thenar atrophy

Patient awakened by tingling, pain, or both in sensory distribution of median nerve

Median nerve compression in the carpal tunnel, the most common compression neuropathy, is often linked to occupational repetitive movements related to wrist flexion and extension, holding the wrist in an awkward position, or strong gripping of objects. Long-term compression commonly leads to thenar atrophy and weakness of the thumb and index fingers.

Clinical Correlation

Carpal Tunnel Syndrome: Testing and Management

Anatomy on pp. 174, 185

Provocative maneuvers

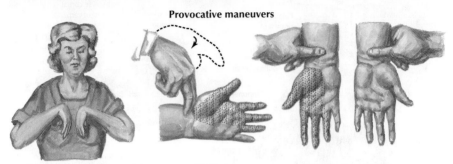

Phalen's test (wrist flexion)

Tinel's sign

Digital compression test

Provocative tests elicit paresthesias in hand.

Nonsurgical management

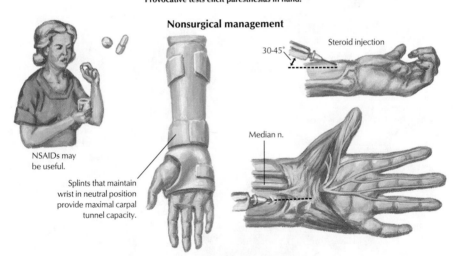

NSAIDs may be useful.

Splints that maintain wrist in neutral position provide maximal carpal tunnel capacity.

30-45°

Steroid injection

Median n.

Surgical decompression of carpal tunnel

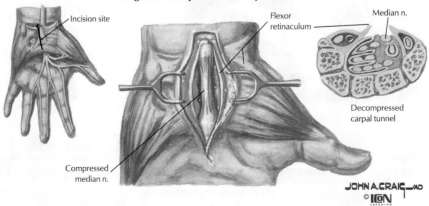

Incision site

Compressed median n.

Flexor retinaculum

Median n.

Decompressed carpal tunnel

JOHN A. CRAIG—AD
©ICN
LEARNING SYSTEMS

Nerve Summary: Normal Ulnar Nerve Distribution

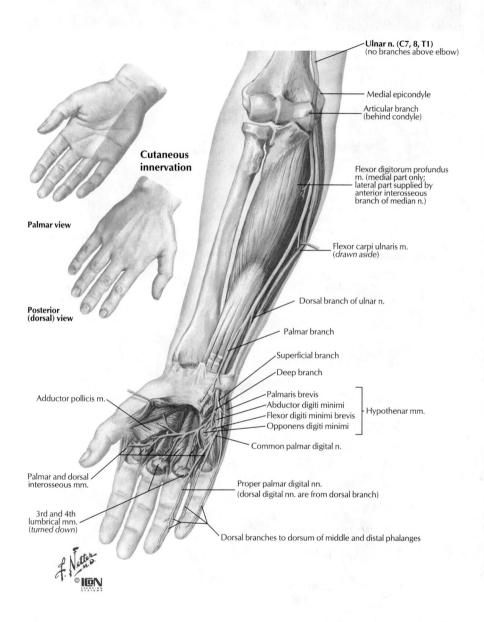

Ulnar n. (C7, 8, T1)
(no branches above elbow)

Medial epicondyle

Articular branch
(behind condyle)

Cutaneous
innervation

Flexor digitorum profundus
m. (medial part only;
lateral part supplied by
anterior interosseous
branch of median n.)

Palmar view

Flexor carpi ulnaris m.
(*drawn aside*)

Posterior
(dorsal) view

Dorsal branch of ulnar n.

Palmar branch

Superficial branch

Deep branch

Adductor pollicis m.

Palmaris brevis
Abductor digiti minimi
Flexor digiti minimi brevis   Hypothenar mm.
Opponens digiti minimi

Common palmar digital n.

Palmar and dorsal
interosseous mm.

Proper palmar digital nn.
(dorsal digital nn. are from dorsal branch)

3rd and 4th
lumbrical mm.
(*turned down*)

Dorsal branches to dorsum of middle and distal phalanges

The ulnar nerve innervates the flexor carpi ulnaris muscle and the ulnar half of the flexor digitorum profundus muscle in the anterior forearm and most of the intrinsic hand muscles (hypothenar muscles, two lumbricals, adductor pollicis, and all interossei). Pure ulnar nerve sensation is tested on the skin overlying the palmar aspect of the tip of the little finger.

Clinical Correlation

Ulnar Nerve Compression: Cubital Tunnel

Anatomy on pp. 158, 159, 189

Compression of ulnar nerve

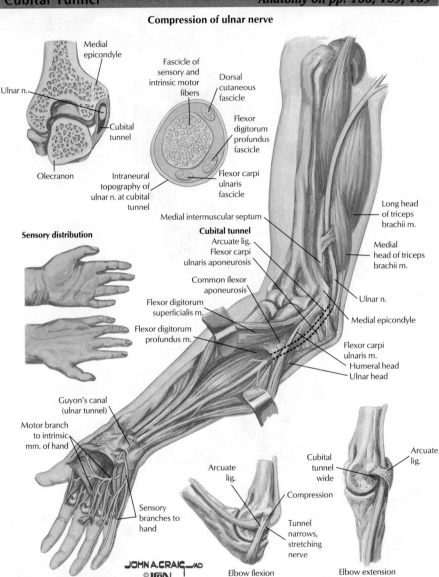

Medial epicondyle

Ulnar n.

Cubital tunnel

Olecranon

Intraneural topography of ulnar n. at cubital tunnel

Fascicle of sensory and intrinsic motor fibers

Dorsal cutaneous fascicle

Flexor digitorum profundus fascicle

Flexor carpi ulnaris fascicle

Sensory distribution

Medial intermuscular septum

Cubital tunnel
Arcuate lig.
Flexor carpi ulnaris aponeurosis

Common flexor aponeurosis

Flexor digitorum superficialis m.

Flexor digitorum profundus m.

Long head of triceps brachii m.

Medial head of triceps brachii m.

Ulnar n.

Medial epicondyle

Flexor carpi ulnaris m.
Humeral head
Ulnar head

Guyon's canal (ulnar tunnel)

Motor branch to intrinsic mm. of hand

Sensory branches to hand

Arcuate lig.

Cubital tunnel wide

Arcuate lig.

Compression

Tunnel narrows, stretching nerve

Elbow flexion

Elbow extension

JOHN A.CRAIG—AD

Cubital tunnel syndrome results from compression of the ulnar nerve as it passes beneath the ulnar collateral ligament and between the two heads of the flexor carpi ulnaris muscle. This syndrome is the second most common compression neuropathy after carpal tunnel syndrome. The tunnel space is significantly reduced with elbow flexion, which compresses and stretches the ulnar nerve. The nerve also may be injured by direct trauma to the subcutaneous portion as it passes around the medial epicondyle.

Clinical Correlation

Ulnar Tunnel Syndrome

Anatomy on pp. 171, 189

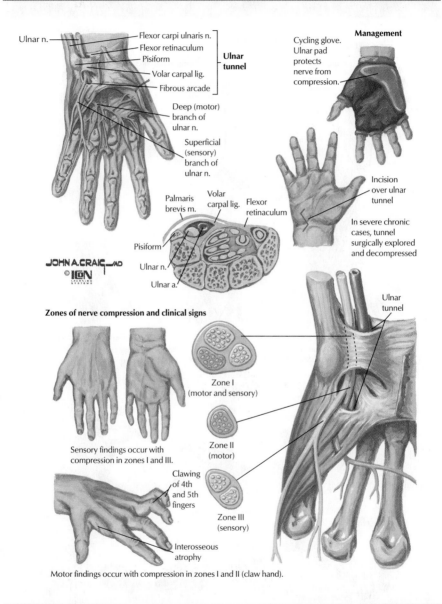

Ulnar n.

Flexor carpi ulnaris n.
Flexor retinaculum
Pisiform
Volar carpal lig.
Fibrous arcade

Ulnar tunnel

Deep (motor) branch of ulnar n.

Superficial (sensory) branch of ulnar n.

Palmaris brevis m.
Volar carpal lig.
Flexor retinaculum

Pisiform
Ulnar n.
Ulnar a.

JOHN A. CRAIG—AD
© ICON LEARNING SYSTEMS

Management

Cycling glove. Ulnar pad protects nerve from compression.

Incision over ulnar tunnel

In severe chronic cases, tunnel surgically explored and decompressed

Ulnar tunnel

Zones of nerve compression and clinical signs

Zone I (motor and sensory)

Zone II (motor)

Zone III (sensory)

Ulnar tunnel

Sensory findings occur with compression in zones I and III.

Clawing of 4th and 5th fingers

Interosseous atrophy

Motor findings occur with compression in zones I and II (claw hand).

The ulnar tunnel exists at the wrist where the ulnar nerve and artery pass deep to the palmaris brevis muscle and palmar (volar) carpal ligament, just lateral to the pisiform bone. Within the tunnel, the nerve divides into superficial sensory and deep motor branches. Injury may result from trauma, ulnar artery thrombosis, fractures (hook of the hamate), dislocations (ulnar head, pisiform), arthritis, or repetitive movements. Claw hand may be present with motor injury.

Clinical Correlation

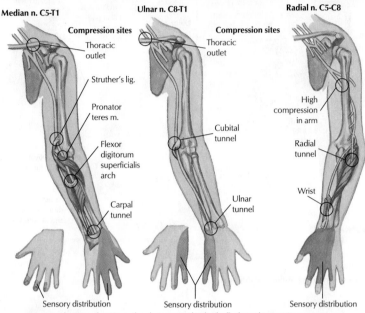

Median n. C5-T1

Compression sites

Thoracic outlet

Struther's lig.

Pronator teres m.

Flexor digitorum superficialis arch

Carpal tunnel

Sensory distribution

Ulnar n. C8-T1

Compression sites

Thoracic outlet

Cubital tunnel

Ulnar tunnel

Sensory distribution

Radial n. C5-C8

High compression in arm

Radial tunnel

Wrist

Sensory distribution

Motor and sensory functions of each n. assessed individually throughout entire upper extremity to delineate level of compression or entrapment

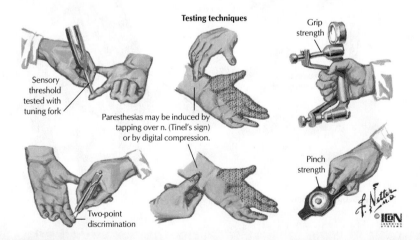

Testing techniques

Sensory threshold tested with tuning fork

Paresthesias may be induced by tapping over n. (Tinel's sign) or by digital compression.

Two-point discrimination

Grip strength

Pinch strength

Compression injury to radial, median, and ulnar nerves may occur at several sites along each of these nerves' courses down the arm and forearm. The next series of pages offers an applied review of the anatomy and clinical presentation of several common neuropathies. Refer to muscle tables presented previously for review of muscle action and anticipated functional weakness.

Clinical Correlation

Anatomy on pp. 185, 189

Digital Nerve Compression

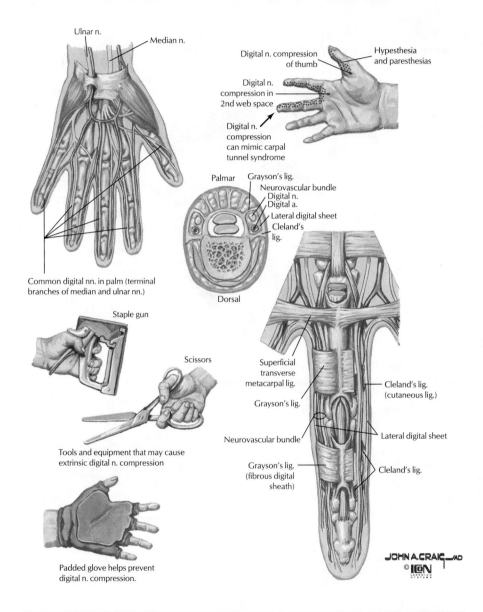

Ulnar n.

Median n.

Digital n. compression of thumb

Hypesthesia and paresthesias

Digital n. compression in 2nd web space

Digital n. compression can mimic carpal tunnel syndrome

Common digital nn. in palm (terminal branches of median and ulnar nn.)

Palmar

Grayson's lig.

Neurovascular bundle
Digital n.
Digital a.

Lateral digital sheet

Cleland's lig.

Dorsal

Staple gun

Scissors

Tools and equipment that may cause extrinsic digital n. compression

Padded glove helps prevent digital n. compression.

Superficial transverse metacarpal lig.

Grayson's lig.

Neurovascular bundle

Grayson's lig. (fibrous digital sheath)

Cleland's lig. (cutaneous lig.)

Lateral digital sheet

Cleland's lig.

JOHN A.CRAIG—AD
©ICN

Proper palmar digital nerves are terminal branches of the median and ulnar nerves in the hand. They course along lateral aspects of each digit, anterior (palmar side) to palmar digital arteries. These nerves are sensory and may be injured by trauma, casts or splints, gripping objects tightly, repetitive movements such as those used by musicians, and athletic activities.

Embryology: Appendicular Skeleton

Mesenchymal precartilage primordia of axial and appendicular skeletons at 5 weeks

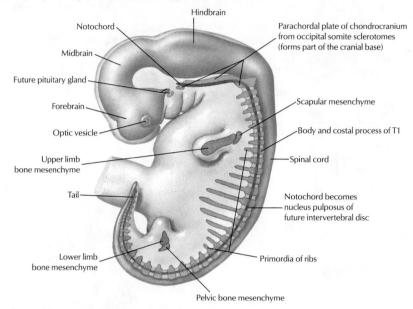

Hindbrain

Notochord

Parachordal plate of chondrocranium from occipital somite sclerotomes (forms part of the cranial base)

Midbrain

Future pituitary gland

Forebrain

Optic vesicle

Upper limb bone mesenchyme

Tail

Lower limb bone mesenchyme

Scapular mesenchyme

Body and costal process of T1

Spinal cord

Notochord becomes nucleus pulposus of future intervertebral disc

Primordia of ribs

Pelvic bone mesenchyme

Precartilage mesenchymal cell condensations of appendicular skeleton at 6th week

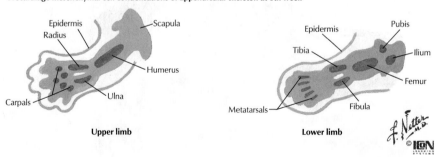

Epidermis
Radius
Scapula
Humerus
Carpals
Ulna

Upper limb

Epidermis
Tibia
Pubis
Ilium
Femur
Fibula
Metatarsals

Lower limb

Along the embryonic axis, mesenchyme derived from sclerotomes forms the axial skeleton and gives rise to the skull and spinal column. The appendicular skeleton forms from mesenchyme derived from somatopleure that condenses to form cartilaginous precursors of limb bones. Upper limb bones then develop by endochondral ossification from cartilaginous precursors (except the clavicle, which develops by intramembranous ossification).

Embryology: Neuromuscular Development

Segmental somites give rise to myotomes that form collections of mesoderm dorsally (epimeres, epaxial) that become innervated by dorsal rami of spinal nerves. These epaxial muscles form intrinsic back muscles. Ventral mesodermal collections form hypomeres (hypaxial) that are innervated by ventral rami of spinal nerves. Hypaxial muscles in the limbs divide into ventral (flexor) and dorsal (extensor) muscles.

Somatic development

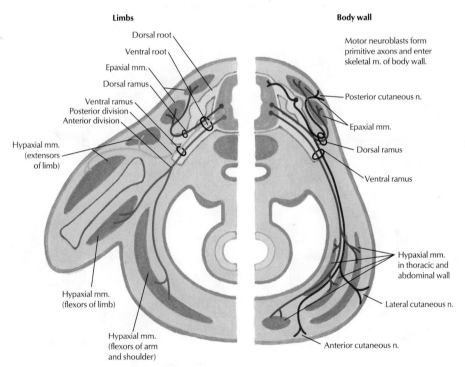

Limbs

Dorsal root
Ventral root
Epaxial mm.
Dorsal ramus
Ventral ramus
Posterior division
Anterior division

Hypaxial mm.
(extensors
of limb)

Hypaxial mm.
(flexors of limb)

Hypaxial mm.
(flexors of arm
and shoulder)

Body wall

Motor neuroblasts form
primitive axons and enter
skeletal m. of body wall.

Posterior cutaneous n.

Epaxial mm.

Dorsal ramus

Ventral ramus

Hypaxial mm.
in thoracic and
abdominal wall

Lateral cutaneous n.

Anterior cutaneous n.

Somatic nervous system innervates somatopleure (body wall).

JOHN A. CRAIG—AD
© ICN

Embryology: Limb Bud Rotation

Initially, as limb buds grow out from the embryonic trunk, the ventral muscle mass (future flexors) faces medially and the dorsal mass (future extensors) faces laterally. With continued growth and differentiation, upper limbs rotate 90° laterally, so that in anatomical position, the ventral flexor muscle compartment faces anteriorly and the dorsal extensor muscle compartment faces posteriorly. Lower limbs rotate 90° medially and are thus 180° out of phase with upper limbs (elbow faces anteriorly and knee faces posteriorly). Thus, in upper limbs, the flexors of the shoulder, elbow, and wrist/fingers are positioned anteriorly, and extensor muscles of the same joints are posteriorly aligned.

Changes in position of limbs before birth

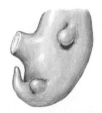
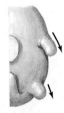

At 5 weeks. Upper and lower limbs have formed as finlike appendages pointing laterally and caudally.

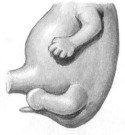
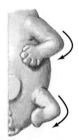

At 6 weeks. Limbs bend anteriorly, so elbows and knees point laterally, palms and soles face trunk.

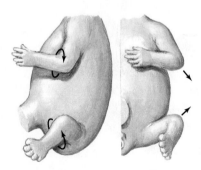
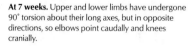

At 7 weeks. Upper and lower limbs have undergone 90° torsion about their long axes, but in opposite directions, so elbows point caudally and knees cranially.

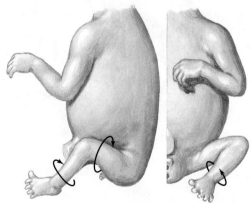

At 8 weeks. Torsion of lower limbs results in twisted or "barber pole" arrangement of their cutaneous innervation.

Embryology: Limb Rotation and Dermatomes

Although the dermatome distribution on the trunk is fairly linear horizontally, some spiraling occurs on the limbs, especially on the lower limb. The upper limb is more uniform, with dermatomes (C4-T2) that closely parallel myotome innervation from the brachial plexus (C5-T1) (a small contributing branch from C4 and T2 to the brachial plexus is normally observed).

Changes in ventral dermatome pattern (cutaneous sensory nerve distribution) during limb development

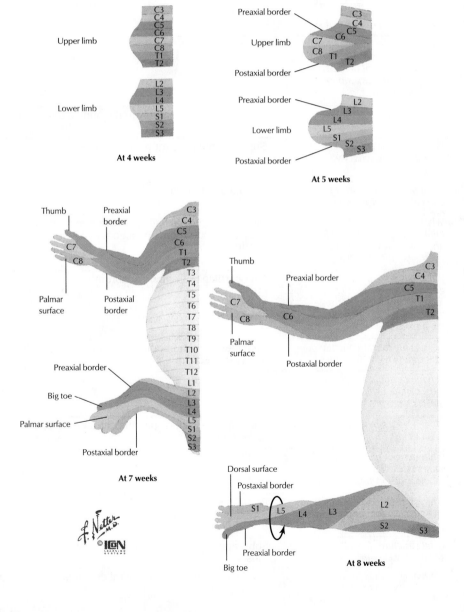

Review Questions

What surface anatomy feature lies atop the shoulder and what muscles attach to this feature?	Acromion. The trapezius and deltoid muscles have attachments to the acromion.
Which superficial vein drains the lateral aspect of the forearm and arm?	Cephalic vein, which then drains into the axillary vein proximally.
Which vein is commonly used for venipuncture?	Median cubital vein in the cubital fossa.
What is the first bone to ossify but the last one to fuse?	Clavicle.
All of the bones of the upper limb develop by endochondral ossification except one, which develops by intramembranous ossification. Which one?	Clavicle.
What is the most commonly fractured bone in children?	Clavicle. Most commonly in the middle third of the bone.
Posteriorly, the spine of the scapula divides what two fossae?	Supraspinatus and infraspinatus fossae.
What are the two parts of the coracoclavicular ligament?	Conoid and trapezoid.
What kind (classification) of joint is the glenohumeral joint, and what movements are possible at this joint?	Multiaxial synovial ball-and-socket joint, capable of flexion, extension, abduction, adduction, and circumduction.
What feature of the shallow glenoid cavity helps to "deepen" this socket for articulation with the head of the humerus?	Fibrocartilaginous glenoid labrum.
What is the most frequently dislocated joint in humans?	Shoulder (glenohumeral) joint. Commonly, in the anterior direction.
Tendonitis about the shoulder most commonly involves which muscle tendon?	Supraspinatus.
What muscles make up the rotator cuff?	Subscapularis, supraspinatus, infraspinatus, and teres minor.
What nerve is particularly vulnerable to injury in a shoulder dislocation?	Axillary.
Which muscle flexes, adducts, and medially rotates the arm at the shoulder?	Pectoralis major.
What structures form the posterior wall of the axilla?	Subscapularis, teres major, and latissimus dorsi muscles.
What major branches arise from the third part of the axillary artery?	Anterior and posterior humeral circumflex, and subscapular.

Review Questions

What arteries contribute to the anastomosis around the scapula?	Dorsal scapular, suprascapular, and subscapular.
What regions drain lymph into axillary lymph nodes?	Upper limb and anterior chest wall, especially the breast (75%).
What is the origin of the fascia comprising the axillary sheath?	Prevertebral fascia.
For each nerve listed, identify the muscles innervated:	
Axillary:	Deltoid and teres minor
Dorsal scapular:	Levator scapular and rhomboids
Medial pectoral:	Pectoralis minor and major
Upper subscapular:	Subscapularis
Lower subscapular:	Subscapularis and teres major
Long thoracic:	Serratus anterior
Thoracodorsal:	Latissimus dorsi
What are the five terminal branches of the brachial plexus?	Axillary, musculocutaneous, radial, median, and ulnar nerves.
What is the most common benign soft tissue tumor?	Lipoma.
What nerve innervates muscles that flex the forearm at the elbow?	Musculocutaneous.
Which arm muscle flexes at the elbow and is a powerful supinator?	Biceps brachii.
What muscle or muscles extend the forearm at the elbow, and which nerve innervates them?	Triceps (all three heads) and anconeus. All are innervated by the radial nerve.
Tapping the triceps tendon checks the integrity of which spinal cord levels? Biceps tendon?	C7 and C8 (radial nerve). C5 and C6 (musculocutaneous nerve).
What artery courses with median and ulnar nerves in the arm?	Brachial.
Fracture of the midshaft of the humerus places what nerve at risk of entrapment?	Radial.
What kind of union occurs between the radius and ulna along their length?	Radioulnar fibrous (syndesmosis) joint united by the interosseous membrane.
At the proximal radioulnar (uniaxial synovial pivot) joint, what ligament keeps the radial head in the radial notch of the ulna?	Anular.
Dislocation of the elbow occurs most frequently in which direction?	Posteriorly.

Review Questions

In a Monteggia fracture (ulnar fracture), what nerve may be at risk of injury?	Posterior interosseous.
What common site of origin is shared by superficial muscles in the anterior compartment of the forearm?	Medial epicondyle of the humerus.
What muscles of the anterior forearm compartment are not innervated by the median nerve?	Flexor carpi ulnaris and ulnar half of the flexor digitorum profundus (ulnar nerve).
What are the primary actions of each of these muscles? *Flexor carpi radialis:* *Flexor digitorum superficialis:* *Flexor digitorum profundus:* *Brachioradialis:* *Extensor carpi ulnaris:* *Extensor digitorum:* *Extensor pollicis brevis:* *Abductor pollicis longus:*	 Flex and abduct hand at wrist Flex middle phalanges of medial four digits Flex distal phalanges of medial four digits Flex forearm at elbow Extend and adduct hand at wrist Extend medial four digits at metacarpophalangeal (MCP) joint Extend proximal phalanx of thumb at MCP joint Abduct and extend thumb at MCP joint
What are the actions and innervation of muscles of the posterior forearm compartment?	Extensors of wrist and/or digits and supinator of the forearm; radial nerve.
How are bone fragments displaced in a fracture of the middle or distal radius?	Proximal fragment is kept in the neutral position (anatomical position) by the pronator teres and supinator muscles, but distal fragment is pronated by action of the pronator quadratus muscle.
Which carpal lies deep to the anatomical snuffbox and is frequently fractured by falls on an outstretched hand?	Scaphoid.
What kind of joint is the wrist joint, and what movements occur there?	Radiocarpal (biaxial synovial ellipsoid) joint between the distal radius and the scaphoid, lunate, and triquetrum; flexion, extension, abduction, adduction, and circumduction.
What is a Colles' fracture?	A common extension-compression fracture of the distal radius that results in a typical silver-fork or dinner-fork deformity.
What ligaments reinforce the MCP joint (biaxial condyloid synovial joint)?	Capsule, radial and ulnar collaterals, and palmar (volar) plate.
What ligament prevents hyperextension of proximal and distal interphalangeal joints?	Palmar (volar) plate.
What are the action and innervation of the adductor pollicis muscle?	Adducts thumb toward middle digit; supplied by the ulnar nerve.
What are the origin and innervation of the first and second lumbrical muscles?	Lateral two tendons of the flexor digitorum profundus; supplied by the median nerve.

Review Questions

What muscles flex the MCP joints and extend the proximal and distal interphalangeal joints of the middle three digits?	Lumbrical and interosseous.
The ability to hold a slip of paper between the extended middle and ring fingers tests the action of what muscles and integrity of what nerve?	Palmar interossei muscles (adduction: PAD); ulnar nerve.
What nerve innervates the thenar eminence muscles?	Median (recurrent branch).
Which artery is the major contributor to the superficial palmar arch?	Ulnar.
What is the carpal tunnel?	Osseofascial tunnel consisting of the carpal arch and overlying flexor retinaculum. It contains nine muscle tendons and the median nerve.
Identify two potential spaces that may become infected in the hand.	Thenar (anterior to adductor pollicis) and midpalmar.
What finger injury is characterized by a stretched or torn extensor tendon?	Mallet finger, a common baseball injury.
What can cause fracture of the neck of a metacarpal?	Blow to the fist, often called a boxer's fracture.
What kind of finger injury can result in a boutonnière deformity if not properly treated?	Ventral (palmar or volar) dislocation, or fracture, of the middle phalanx with avulsion of the central part of the extensor tendon.
Rheumatoid arthritis most often affects which joints of the body?	The small wrist and finger joints.
Injury to the long thoracic nerve may result in what functional deficit?	Weakness of the serratus anterior muscle, resulting in winging of the scapula and an inability to pull the scapula forward against the posterior thoracic wall.

Where on the hand would you test sensation for each of the following nerves?
   Median nerve:
   Ulnar nerve:
   Radial nerve:
	
	Palmar (volar) tip of the index finger
	Palmar (volar) tip of the little finger
	Dorsal web space between the thumb and index finger

What deficits would you expect with injury to the proximal radial nerve in the arm?	Weakened extension at the elbow, wrist (wrist drop), and metacarpal finger joints, and weakened supination.

For each of the following nerves, identify the site of compression neuropathy related to the nerve's course through a muscle.
   Radial (deep branch):
   Ulnar nerve:
   Median nerve:
	
	Supinator (radial tunnel)
	Flexor carpi ulnaris (cubital tunnel)
	Pronator teres in proximal forearm
	Flexor digitorum superficialis

Review Questions

Injury of what nerve is responsible for each of the following presentations?	
Thenar atrophy:	Medial nerve
Hypothenar atrophy:	Ulnar nerve
Claw hand:	Ulnar nerve
Wrist drop:	Radial nerve
First dorsal interosseous atrophy:	Ulnar nerve
Paresthesia along lateral forearm:	Musculocutaneous nerve
Paresthesia over lateral deltoid:	Axillary nerve
Weakened finger adduction:	Ulnar nerve
Winging of scapula:	Long thoracic nerve
Tinel's sign:	Median nerve
What is the somatopleure?	The portion of the somite that gives rise to mesenchyme that will become the cartilaginous precursors of the upper limb bones.
Which part of the myotome is innervated by the ventral ramus of a spinal nerve?	The hypomere (hypaxial muscles). These include all the muscles of the upper limb.
Why is it important to understand limb bud rotation in the embryo?	Limb bud rotation helps in understanding why flexor muscles come to occupy the anterior compartments of the arm and forearm, and extensors the posterior compartment.
How does the upper limb bud rotate compared with the lower limb bud?	The upper bud rotates 90° laterally, and the lower bud rotates 90° medially. Hence, the big toe is medial and the thumb is lateral in anatomical position.
What dermatome overlies each of the following structures or features?	
Middle finger:	C7
Shoulder:	C5-6
Little finger:	C8
Elbow:	C7-8
Medial arm:	T1

4

Lower Limb

Introduction The lower limb supports the body's weight and moves the body by integrating its muscle actions. Its components are the gluteal region, thigh, leg, and foot. Clinically, it is convenient to divide the limb into functional muscle compartments and to assess the nerves innervating each compartment's muscles. When one is standing still, the joints of the limb "lock" to conserve the muscles' energy, thus allowing prolonged erect standing.

Surface Anatomy: Key Landmarks

Inguinal ligament: folded, inferior edge of the external abdominal oblique aponeurosis that separates abdominal region from thigh (Poupart's ligament)
Greater trochanter: point of the hip and attachment site for several gluteal muscles
Quadriceps femoris: muscle mass of the anterior thigh, composed of four muscles that extend the leg at the knee (rectus femoris and three vastus muscles)
Patella: kneecap
Popliteal fossa: region posterior to the knee
Gastrocnemius muscles: muscle mass that forms the calf
Calcaneal (Achilles') tendon: prominent tendon of several calf muscles
Small saphenous vein: drains blood from the lateral dorsal venous arch and posterior leg (calf) into the popliteal vein posterior to the knee
Great saphenous vein: drains blood from the medial dorsal venous arch, leg, and thigh into the femoral vein just inferior to the inguinal ligament

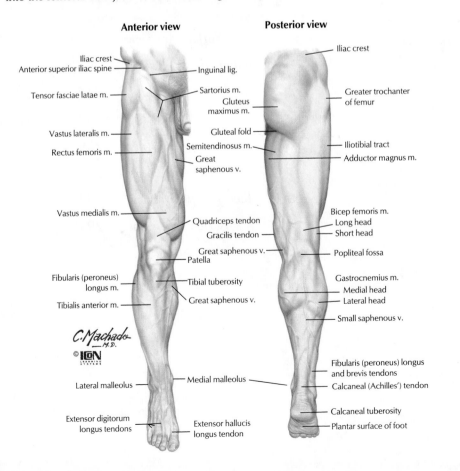

Anterior view

Posterior view

Iliac crest
Anterior superior iliac spine
Inguinal lig.
Tensor fasciae latae m.
Sartorius m.
Gluteus maximus m.
Vastus lateralis m.
Gluteal fold
Rectus femoris m.
Semitendinosus m.
Great saphenous v.
Vastus medialis m.
Quadriceps tendon
Gracilis tendon
Great saphenous v.
Patella
Fibularis (peroneus) longus m.
Tibial tuberosity
Tibialis anterior m.
Great saphenous v.

C. Machado
M.D.
© ICON
LEARNING SYSTEMS

Lateral malleolus
Medial malleolus
Extensor digitorum longus tendons
Extensor hallucis longus tendon

Iliac crest
Greater trochanter of femur
Iliotibial tract
Adductor magnus m.
Bicep femoris m.
Long head
Short head
Popliteal fossa
Gastrocnemius m.
Medial head
Lateral head
Small saphenous v.
Fibularis (peroneus) longus and brevis tendons
Calcaneal (Achilles') tendon
Calcaneal tuberosity
Plantar surface of foot

Surface Anatomy: Superficial Veins and Nerves

Superficial veins drain blood toward the heart and communicate with deep veins that parallel arteries of the lower limb. When vigorous muscle contraction compresses the deep veins, some of the venous blood is shunted into superficial veins and returned to the heart. These veins have valves to aid venous return. Corresponding cutaneous nerves are terminal sensory branches of major lower limb nerves that arise from lumbar (L1-L4) and sacral (L4-S4) plexuses.

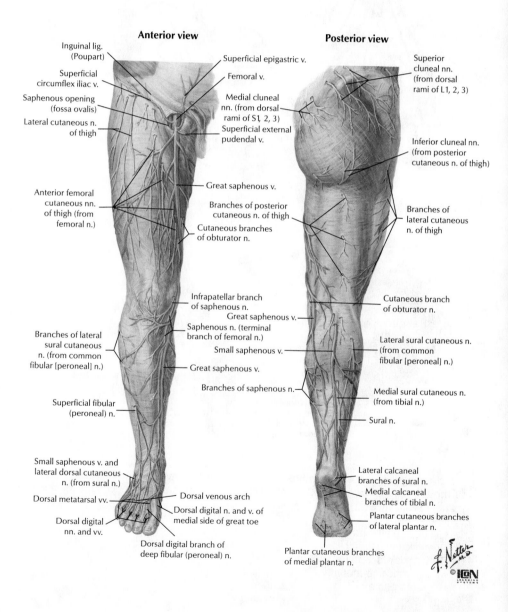

Anterior view

Posterior view

Inguinal lig. (Poupart)

Superficial circumflex iliac v.

Saphenous opening (fossa ovalis)

Lateral cutaneous n. of thigh

Superficial epigastric v.

Femoral v.

Medial cluneal nn. (from dorsal rami of S1, 2, 3)

Superficial external pudendal v.

Superior cluneal nn. (from dorsal rami of L1, 2, 3)

Inferior cluneal nn. (from posterior cutaneous n. of thigh)

Anterior femoral cutaneous nn. of thigh (from femoral n.)

Great saphenous v.

Branches of posterior cutaneous n. of thigh

Cutaneous branches of obturator n.

Branches of lateral cutaneous n. of thigh

Branches of lateral sural cutaneous n. (from common fibular [peroneal] n.)

Superficial fibular (peroneal) n.

Infrapatellar branch of saphenous n.

Great saphenous v.

Saphenous n. (terminal branch of femoral n.)

Small saphenous v.

Great saphenous v.

Branches of saphenous n.

Cutaneous branch of obturator n.

Lateral sural cutaneous n. (from common fibular [peroneal] n.)

Medial sural cutaneous n. (from tibial n.)

Sural n.

Small saphenous v. and lateral dorsal cutaneous n. (from sural n.)

Dorsal metatarsal vv.

Dorsal digital nn. and vv.

Dorsal venous arch

Dorsal digital n. and v. of medial side of great toe

Dorsal digital branch of deep fibular (peroneal) n.

Lateral calcaneal branches of sural n.

Medial calcaneal branches of tibial n.

Plantar cutaneous branches of lateral plantar n.

Plantar cutaneous branches of medial plantar n.

Clinical Correlation

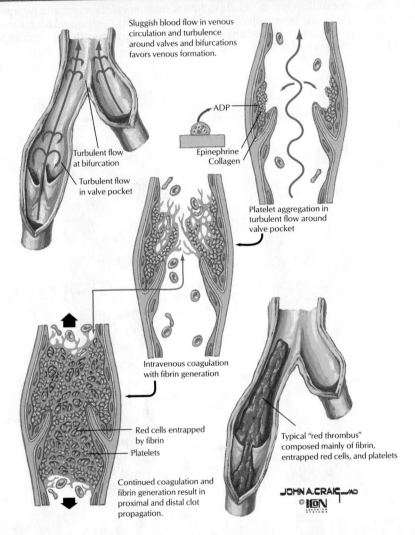

Sluggish blood flow in venous circulation and turbulence around valves and bifurcations favors venous formation.

ADP

Turbulent flow at bifurcation

Epinephrine
Collagen

Turbulent flow in valve pocket

Platelet aggregation in turbulent flow around valve pocket

Intravenous coagulation with fibrin generation

Red cells entrapped by fibrin

Platelets

Typical "red thrombus" composed mainly of fibrin, entrapped red cells, and platelets

Continued coagulation and fibrin generation result in proximal and distal clot propagation.

JOHN A.CRAIG—AD
©ICN

Although deep venous thrombosis (DVT) may occur anywhere in the body, veins of the lower limb are most often involved. Three cardinal events account for the pathogenesis and risk of DVT:
- Stasis
- Venous wall injury
- Hypercoagulability

Clinical risk factors for DVT include:
- Postsurgical immobility
- Vessel trauma
- Infection
- Paralysis
- Malignancy
- Pregnancy

Hip and Gluteal Region: Bones

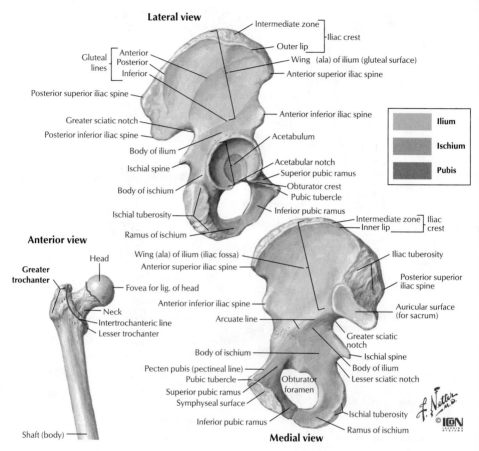

Lateral view

Intermediate zone
Iliac crest
Outer lip
Wing (ala) of ilium (gluteal surface)
Anterior superior iliac spine

Gluteal lines — Anterior, Posterior, Inferior

Posterior superior iliac spine

Greater sciatic notch

Posterior inferior iliac spine

Body of ilium

Ischial spine

Body of ischium

Ischial tuberosity

Ramus of ischium

Anterior inferior iliac spine
Acetabulum
Acetabular notch
Superior pubic ramus
Obturator crest
Pubic tubercle
Inferior pubic ramus

	Ilium
	Ischium
	Pubis

Anterior view

Head
Greater trochanter
Neck
Intertrochanteric line
Lesser trochanter
Shaft (body)

Intermediate zone — Iliac crest
Inner lip

Wing (ala) of ilium (iliac fossa)
Anterior superior iliac spine
Fovea for lig. of head
Anterior inferior iliac spine
Arcuate line
Body of ischium
Pecten pubis (pectineal line)
Pubic tubercle
Superior pubic ramus
Symphyseal surface
Obturator foramen
Inferior pubic ramus

Iliac tuberosity
Posterior superior iliac spine
Auricular surface (for sacrum)
Greater sciatic notch
Ischial spine
Body of ilium
Lesser sciatic notch
Ischial tuberosity
Ramus of ischium

Medial view

FEATURE	CHARACTERISTICS
Coxal (Hip) Bone	Fusion of three bones on each side to form the pelvis, which articulates with the sacrum to form the pelvic girdle
Ilium	Body fused to ischium and pubis, all meeting in the acetabulum (socket for articulation with femoral head) Ala (wing): weak spot of ilium
Ischium	Body fused with other two bones; ramus fused with pubis
Pubis	Body fused with other two bones; ramus fused with ischium
Femur (Proximal)	
Long bone	Longest bone in the body and very strong
Head	Point of articulation with acetabulum of coxal bone
Neck	Common fracture site
Greater trochanter	Point of the hip; attachment site for several gluteal muscles
Lesser trochanter	Attachment site of iliopsoas tendon (strong hip flexor)

Hip and Gluteal Region: Joint and Ligaments

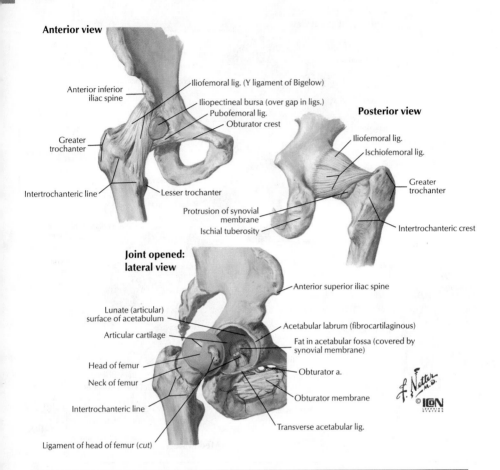

Anterior view

Anterior inferior iliac spine

Iliofemoral lig. (Y ligament of Bigelow)

Iliopectineal bursa (over gap in ligs.)

Pubofemoral lig.

Obturator crest

Greater trochanter

Posterior view

Iliofemoral lig.

Ischiofemoral lig.

Greater trochanter

Intertrochanteric line

Lesser trochanter

Protrusion of synovial membrane

Ischial tuberosity

Intertrochanteric crest

Joint opened: lateral view

Anterior superior iliac spine

Lunate (articular) surface of acetabulum

Articular cartilage

Acetabular labrum (fibrocartilaginous)

Fat in acetabular fossa (covered by synovial membrane)

Head of femur

Neck of femur

Obturator a.

Intertrochanteric line

Obturator membrane

Ligament of head of femur (*cut*)

Transverse acetabular lig.

LIGAMENT	ATTACHMENT	COMMENT
Hip (Multiaxial Synovial Ball-and-Socket) Joint		
Capsular	Acetabular margin to femoral neck	Encloses femoral head and part of neck; acts in flexion, extension, abduction, adduction, circumduction
Iliofemoral	Iliac spine and acetabulum to intertrochanteric line	Is strongest ligament; forms inverted Y (of Bigelow); limits hyperextension and lateral rotation
Ischiofemoral	Acetabulum to femoral neck posteriorly	Limits extension and medial rotation; is weaker ligament
Pubofemoral	Pubic ramus to lower femoral neck	Limits extension and abduction
Labrum	Acetabulum	Fibrocartilage, deepens socket
Transverse acetabular	Acetabular notch interiorly	Cups acetabulum to form a socket for femoral head
Ligament of head of femur	Acetabular notch and transverse ligament to femoral head	Artery to femoral head runs in ligament

Hip and Gluteal Region: Arteries of the Joint

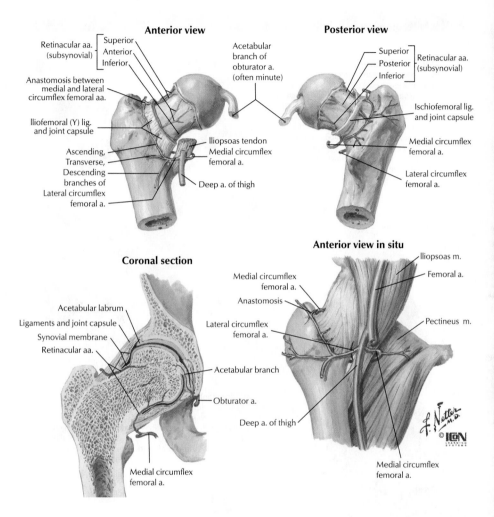

Anterior view

Retinacular aa. (subsynovial) — Superior, Anterior, Inferior

Anastomosis between medial and lateral circumflex femoral aa.

Iliofemoral (Y) lig. and joint capsule

Ascending, Transverse, Descending branches of Lateral circumflex femoral a.

Acetabular branch of obturator a. (often minute)

Iliopsoas tendon

Medial circumflex femoral a.

Deep a. of thigh

Posterior view

Superior, Posterior, Inferior — Retinacular aa. (subsynovial)

Ischiofemoral lig. and joint capsule

Medial circumflex femoral a.

Lateral circumflex femoral a.

Coronal section

Acetabular labrum

Ligaments and joint capsule

Synovial membrane

Retinacular aa.

Acetabular branch

Obturator a.

Deep a. of thigh

Medial circumflex femoral a.

Anterior view in situ

Iliopsoas m.

Femoral a.

Medial circumflex femoral a.

Anastomosis

Lateral circumflex femoral a.

Pectineus m.

Medial circumflex femoral a.

ARTERY	COURSE AND STRUCTURES SUPPLIED
Medial circumflex	Usually arises from deep artery of thigh; branches supply femoral head and neck; passes posterior to iliopsoas muscle tendon
Lateral circumflex	Usually arises from deep artery of the thigh
Acetabular branch	Arises from obturator artery; runs in ligament of head of femur; supplies femoral head
Gluteal branches (superior and inferior)	Form anastomoses with medial and lateral femoral circumflex branches

The arteries form a rich anastomosis around the hip joint.

Clinical Correlation

Congenital Hip Dislocation
Anatomy on pp. 207–209

Ortolani's (reduction) test
With baby relaxed and content on firm surface, hips and knees flexed to 90°. Hips examined one at a time. Examiner grasps baby's thigh with middle finger over greater trochanter and lifts thigh to bring femoral head from its dislocated posterior position to opposite the acetabulum. Simultaneously, thigh gently abducted, reducing femoral head into acetabulum. In positive finding, examiner senses reduction by palpable, nearly audible "clunk."

"Clunk"

Barlow's (dislocation) test
Reverse of Ortolani's test. If femoral head is in acetabulum at time of examination, Barlow's test is performed to discover any hip instability. Baby's thigh grasped as above and adducted with gentle downward pressure. Dislocation is palpable as femoral head slips out of acetabulum. Diagnosis confirmed with Ortolani's test.

In the United States, approximately 1.5 in 1000 infants are born with congenital hip dislocation. With early diagnosis and treatment, approximately 96% of affected children have normal hip function. Girls are affected more often than boys. Approximately 60% of affected children are firstborns, which may suggest that unstretched uterine and abdominal walls limit fetal movement. Ortolani's test of hip abduction confirms the diagnosis.

Clinical Correlation

Degenerative Joint Disease, Early Changes   *Anatomy on pp. 207–209*

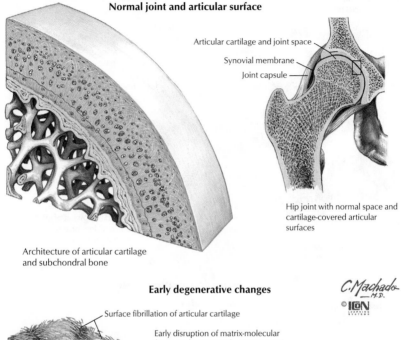

Normal joint and articular surface

Articular cartilage and joint space

Synovial membrane

Joint capsule

Architecture of articular cartilage and subchondral bone

Hip joint with normal space and cartilage-covered articular surfaces

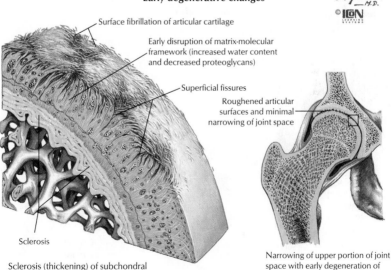

Early degenerative changes

C. Machado
—M.D.
© ICN

Surface fibrillation of articular cartilage

Early disruption of matrix-molecular framework (increased water content and decreased proteoglycans)

Superficial fissures

Roughened articular surfaces and minimal narrowing of joint space

Sclerosis

Sclerosis (thickening) of subchondral bone early sign of degeneration

Narrowing of upper portion of joint space with early degeneration of articular cartilage

Degenerative joint disease, a catch-all term for osteoarthritis, degenerative arthritis, osteoarthrosis, or hypertrophic arthritis, is characterized by progressive loss of articular cartilage and failure of repair. Osteoarthritis can affect any synovial joint but most often involves the foot, knee, hip, spine, and hand.

Clinical Correlation

Degenerative Joint Disease, Late Changes *Anatomy on pp. 207–209*

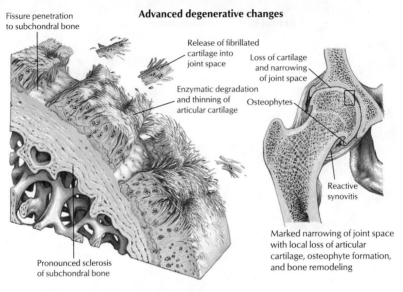

Advanced degenerative changes

Fissure penetration to subchondral bone

Release of fibrillated cartilage into joint space

Loss of cartilage and narrowing of joint space

Enzymatic degradation and thinning of articular cartilage

Osteophytes

Reactive synovitis

Pronounced sclerosis of subchondral bone

Marked narrowing of joint space with local loss of articular cartilage, osteophyte formation, and bone remodeling

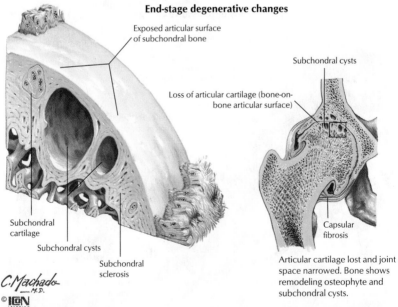

End-stage degenerative changes

Exposed articular surface of subchondral bone

Subchondral cysts

Loss of articular cartilage (bone-on-bone articular surface)

Subchondral cartilage

Subchondral cysts

Subchondral sclerosis

Capsular fibrosis

Articular cartilage lost and joint space narrowed. Bone shows remodeling osteophyte and subchondral cysts.

Osteoarthritis of the hip often develops slowly and leads to a painful antalgic shuffling gait. Although the pain is most often felt over the gluteal region and the proximal anterior and lateral thigh and groin area, it can be referred to the anterior mid-thigh and anterior and medial aspect of the knee. This pain is conveyed by sensory branches of the femoral nerve.

Hip and Gluteal Region: Sacral and Coccygeal Plexuses

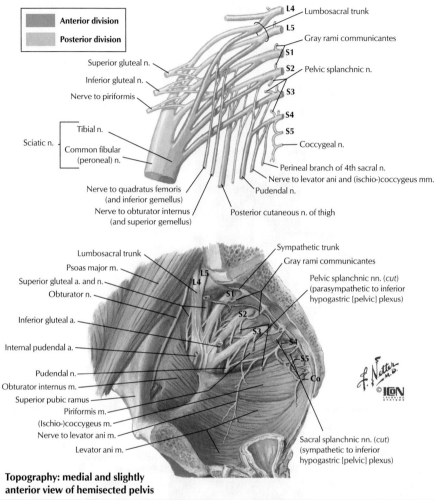

Anterior division

Posterior division

L4

Lumbosacral trunk

L5

Gray rami communicantes

S1

S2 Pelvic splanchnic n.

Superior gluteal n.

Inferior gluteal n.

S3

Nerve to piriformis

S4

S5

Tibial n.

Sciatic n.

Common fibular
(peroneal) n.

Coccygeal n.

Perineal branch of 4th sacral n.

Nerve to levator ani and (ischio-)coccygeus mm.

Pudendal n.

Nerve to quadratus femoris
(and inferior gemellus)

Nerve to obturator internus
(and superior gemellus)

Posterior cutaneous n. of thigh

Lumbosacral trunk

Psoas major m.

Superior gluteal a. and n.

Obturator n.

Inferior gluteal a.

Internal pudendal a.

Pudendal n.

Obturator internus m.

Superior pubic ramus

Piriformis m.

(Ischio-)coccygeus m.

Nerve to levator ani m.

Levator ani m.

Sympathetic trunk

Gray rami communicantes

Pelvic splanchnic nn. (cut)
(parasympathetic to inferior
hypogastric [pelvic] plexus)

L5
L4

S1

S2

S3

S4

S5

Co

Sacral splanchnic nn. (cut)
(sympathetic to inferior
hypogastric [pelvic] plexus)

**Topography: medial and slightly
anterior view of hemisected pelvis**

DIVISION AND NERVE	INNERVATION
Anterior	
Pudendal	Supplies motor and sensory innervation to perineum
Tibial	Innervates posterior thigh muscles, posterior leg muscles, and sole of foot; with common fibular nerve, it forms sciatic nerve (largest nerve in the body)
Posterior	
Superior gluteal	Innervates gluteus medius and minimus muscles
Inferior gluteal	Innervates gluteus maximus muscle
Common fibular	Portion of sciatic nerve (with tibial) that innervates lateral and anterior muscle compartments of leg

The sacral plexus (L4-S4) is illustrated; only major branches are summarized in the table.

Hip and Gluteal Region: Muscles

Superficial dissection

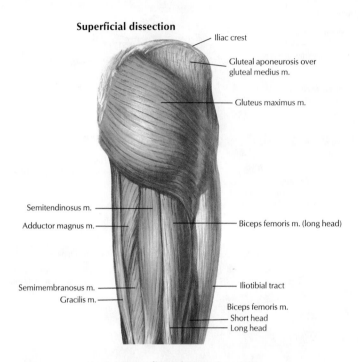

Iliac crest

Gluteal aponeurosis over gluteal medius m.

Gluteus maximus m.

Semitendinosus m.

Adductor magnus m.

Biceps femoris m. (long head)

Semimembranosus m.

Gracilis m.

Iliotibial tract

Biceps femoris m.
Short head
Long head

Deep dissection

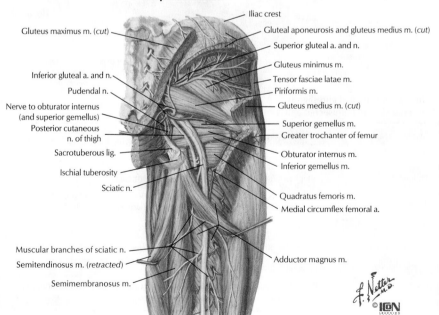

Gluteus maximus m. (*cut*)

Inferior gluteal a. and n.

Pudendal n.

Nerve to obturator internus
(and superior gemellus)

Posterior cutaneous
n. of thigh

Sacrotuberous lig.

Ischial tuberosity

Sciatic n.

Muscular branches of sciatic n.

Semitendinosus m. (*retracted*)

Semimembranosus m.

Iliac crest

Gluteal aponeurosis and gluteus medius m. (*cut*)

Superior gluteal a. and n.

Gluteus minimus m.

Tensor fasciae latae m.

Piriformis m.

Gluteus medius m. (*cut*)

Superior gemellus m.

Greater trochanter of femur

Obturator internus m.

Inferior gemellus m.

Quadratus femoris m.

Medial circumflex femoral a.

Adductor magnus m.

Hip and Gluteal Region: Muscles (continued)

MUSCLE	PROXIMAL ATTACHMENT (ORIGIN)	DISTAL ATTACHMENT (INSERTION)	INNERVATION	MAIN ACTIONS
Gluteus maximus	Ilium posterior to posterior gluteal line, dorsal surface of sacrum and coccyx, and sacrotuberous ligament	Most fibers end in iliotibial tract that inserts into lateral condyle of tibia; some fibers insert on gluteal tuberosity of femur	Inferior gluteal nerve	Extends thigh at the hip and assists in its lateral rotation; steadies thigh and assists in raising trunk from flexed position
Gluteus medius	External surface of ilium	Lateral surface of greater trochanter	Superior gluteal nerve	Abducts and medially rotates thigh at hip; steadies pelvis on leg when opposite leg is raised
Gluteus minimus	External surface of ilium	Anterior surface of greater trochanter	Superior gluteal nerve	Abducts and medially rotates thigh at hip; steadies pelvis on leg when opposite leg is raised
Piriformis	Anterior surface of sacrum and sacrotuberous ligament	Superior border of greater trochanter	Branches of ventral rami S1 and S2	Laterally rotates extended thigh at hip and abducts flexed thigh at hip; steadies femoral head in acetabulum
Obturator internus	Pelvic surface of obturator membrane and surrounding bones	Medial surface of greater trochanter	Nerve to obturator internus	Laterally rotates extended thigh at hip and abducts flexed thigh at hip; steadies femoral head in acetabulum
Gemelli, superior and inferior	*Superior*: ischial spine *Inferior*: ischial tuberosity	Medial surface of greater trochanter	*Superior gemellus*: same nerve supply as obturator internus *Inferior gemellus*: same nerve supply as quadratus femoris	Laterally rotate extended thigh at the hip and abduct flexed thigh at the hip; steady femoral head in acetabulum
Quadratus femoris	Lateral border of ischial tuberosity	Quadrate tubercle on intertrochanteric crest of femur and inferior to it	Nerve to quadratus femoris	Laterally rotates thigh at hip; steadies femoral head in acetabulum

Clinical Correlation

Intracapsular Femoral Neck Fracture   Anatomy on pp. 208, 209, 217

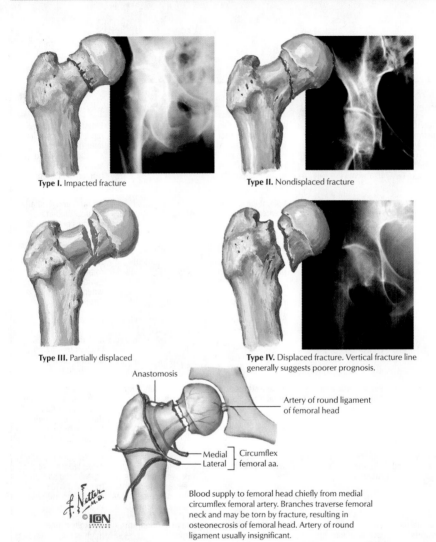

Type I. Impacted fracture

Type II. Nondisplaced fracture

Type III. Partially displaced

Type IV. Displaced fracture. Vertical fracture line generally suggests poorer prognosis.

Anastomosis

Artery of round ligament of femoral head

Medial ⎤ Circumflex
Lateral ⎦ femoral aa.

Blood supply to femoral head chiefly from medial circumflex femoral artery. Branches traverse femoral neck and may be torn by fracture, resulting in osteonecrosis of femoral head. Artery of round ligament usually insignificant.

Femoral neck fractures are common injuries. In the young, the fracture often results from trauma; in the elderly, the cause is often related to osteoporosis and associated with a fall. The Garden classification identifies four fracture types:

I: impaction of superior portion of femoral neck (incomplete fracture)
II: nondisplaced fracture (complete fracture)
III: partial displacement between femoral head and neck
IV: complete displacement between femoral head and neck

The occurrence of complications related to nonunion and avascular necrosis of the femoral head increases from type I to IV.

Thigh: Bones

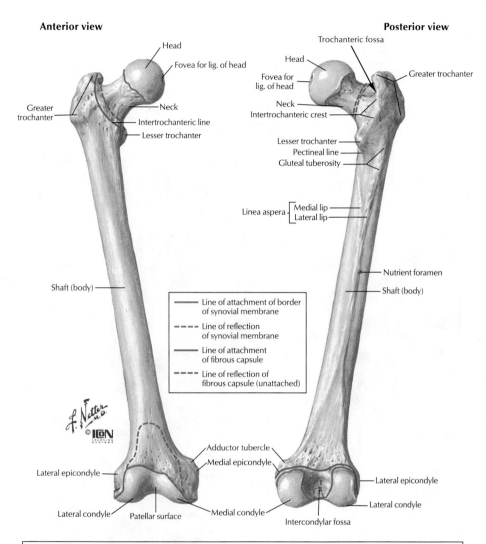

Anterior view

Head
Fovea for lig. of head
Greater trochanter
Neck
Intertrochanteric line
Lesser trochanter
Shaft (body)
Lateral epicondyle
Lateral condyle
Patellar surface
Medial condyle

Posterior view

Trochanteric fossa
Head
Greater trochanter
Fovea for lig. of head
Neck
Intertrochanteric crest
Lesser trochanter
Pectineal line
Gluteal tuberosity
Linea aspera { Medial lip / Lateral lip
Nutrient foramen
Shaft (body)
Adductor tubercle
Medial epicondyle
Lateral epicondyle
Lateral condyle
Intercondylar fossa

——— Line of attachment of border of synovial membrane
- - - - Line of reflection of synovial membrane
——— Line of attachment of fibrous capsule
- - - - Line of reflection of fibrous capsule (unattached)

FEATURE	CHARACTERISTICS
Femur	
Long bone	Longest bone in the body; very strong
Head	Point of articulation with acetabulum of coxal bone
Neck	Common fracture site
Greater trochanter	Point of hip; attachment site for several gluteal muscles
Lesser trochanter	Attachment site of iliopsoas tendon (strong hip flexor)
Distal condyles	Medial and lateral (smaller) sites that articulate with tibial condyles
Patella	Sesamoid bone (largest) embedded in quadriceps femoris tendon

Thigh: Anterior Compartment Muscles

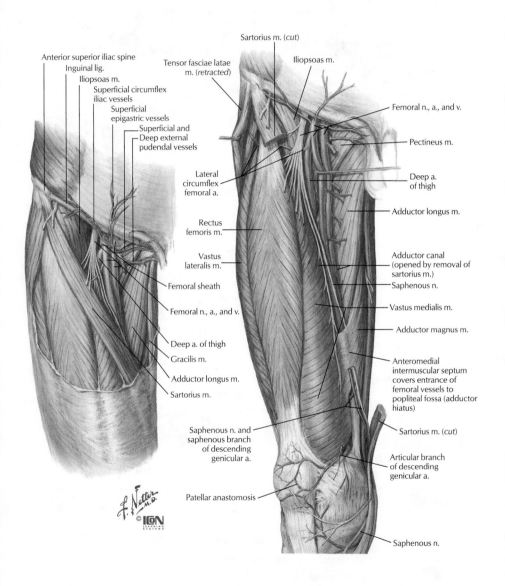

Anterior superior iliac spine
Inguinal lig.
Iliopsoas m.
Superficial circumflex iliac vessels
Superficial epigastric vessels
Superficial and Deep external pudendal vessels

Sartorius m. (cut)

Tensor fasciae latae m. (retracted)

Iliopsoas m.

Femoral n., a., and v.

Pectineus m.

Deep a. of thigh

Adductor longus m.

Lateral circumflex femoral a.

Rectus femoris m.

Vastus lateralis m.

Femoral sheath

Femoral n., a., and v.

Deep a. of thigh

Gracilis m.

Adductor longus m.

Sartorius m.

Adductor canal (opened by removal of sartorius m.)

Saphenous n.

Vastus medialis m.

Adductor magnus m.

Anteromedial intermuscular septum covers entrance of femoral vessels to popliteal fossa (adductor hiatus)

Sartorius m. (cut)

Articular branch of descending genicular a.

Saphenous n. and saphenous branch of descending genicular a.

Patellar anastomosis

Saphenous n.

Thigh: Anterior Compartment Muscles (continued)

MUSCLE	PROXIMAL ATTACHMENT (ORIGIN)	DISTAL ATTACHMENT (INSERTION)	INNERVATION	MAIN ACTIONS
Psoas major (iliopsoas)	Sides of T12-L5 vertebrae and disks between them; transverse processes of all lumbar vertebrae	Lesser trochanter of femur	Ventral rami of lumbar nerves (L1-L3)	Acts jointly with iliacus in flexing thigh at hip joint and in stabilizing hip joint
Iliacus (iliopsoas)	Iliac crest, iliac fossa, ala of sacrum, and anterior sacroiliac ligaments	Tendon of psoas major, lesser trochanter, and femur	Femoral nerve	Acts jointly with psoas major in flexing thigh at hip joint and in stabilizing hip joint
Tensor fasciae latae	Anterior superior iliac spine and anterior iliac crest	Iliotibial tract that attaches to lateral condyle of tibia	Superior gluteal nerve	Abducts, medially rotates, and flexes thigh at hip; helps to keep knee extended
Sartorius	Anterior superior iliac spine and superior part of notch inferior to it	Superior part of medial surface of tibia	Femoral nerve	Flexes, abducts, and laterally rotates thigh at hip joint; flexes knee joint

Quadriceps Femoris

MUSCLE	PROXIMAL ATTACHMENT (ORIGIN)	DISTAL ATTACHMENT (INSERTION)	INNERVATION	MAIN ACTIONS
Rectus femoris	Anterior inferior iliac spine and ilium superior to acetabulum	Base of patella and by patellar ligament to tibial tuberosity	Femoral nerve	Extends leg at knee joint; rectus femoris also steadies hip joint and helps iliopsoas to flex thigh at hip
Vastus lateralis	Greater trochanter and lateral lip of linea aspera of femur	Base of patella and by patellar ligament to tibial tuberosity	Femoral nerve	Extends leg at knee joint
Vastus medialis	Intertrochanteric line and medial lip of linea aspera of femur	Base of patella and by patellar ligament to tibial tuberosity	Femoral nerve	Extends leg at knee joint
Vastus intermedius	Anterior and lateral surfaces of femoral shaft	Base of patella and by patellar ligament to tibial tuberosity	Femoral nerve	Extends leg at knee joint

Thigh: Medial Compartment Muscles

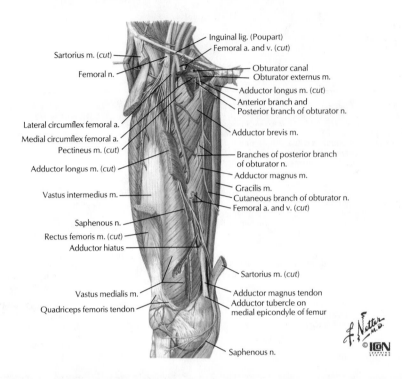

Sartorius m. (*cut*)
Femoral n.
Lateral circumflex femoral a.
Medial circumflex femoral a.
Pectineus m. (*cut*)
Adductor longus m. (*cut*)
Vastus intermedius m.
Saphenous n.
Rectus femoris m. (*cut*)
Adductor hiatus
Vastus medialis m.
Quadriceps femoris tendon

Inguinal lig. (Poupart)
Femoral a. and v. (*cut*)
Obturator canal
Obturator externus m.
Adductor longus m. (*cut*)
Anterior branch and
Posterior branch of obturator n.
Adductor brevis m.
Branches of posterior branch
of obturator n.
Adductor magnus m.
Gracilis m.
Cutaneous branch of obturator n.
Femoral a. and v. (*cut*)
Sartorius m. (*cut*)
Adductor magnus tendon
Adductor tubercle on
medial epicondyle of femur
Saphenous n.

MUSCLE	PROXIMAL ATTACHMENT (ORIGIN)	DISTAL ATTACHMENT (INSERTION)	INNERVATION	MAIN ACTIONS
Pectineus	Superior ramus of pubis	Pectineal line of femur, just inferior to lesser trochanter	Femoral nerve; may receive a branch from obturator nerve	Adducts and flexes thigh at hip; assists with medial rotation of thigh
Adductor longus	Body of pubis inferior to pubic crest	Middle third of linea aspera of femur	Obturator nerve	Adducts thigh at hip
Adductor brevis	Body and inferior ramus of pubis	Pectineal line and proximal part of linea aspera of femur	Obturator nerve	Adducts thigh at hip and to some extent flexes it
Adductor magnus	Inferior ramus of pubis, ramus of ischium, and ischial tuberosity	Gluteal tuberosity, linea aspera, medial supracondylar line (adductor part), and adductor tubercle of femur (hamstring part)	*Adductor part*: obturator nerve *Hamstring part*: tibial part of sciatic nerve	Adducts thigh at hip; *adductor part*: also flexes thigh at hip; *hamstring part*: extends thigh
Gracilis	Body and inferior ramus of pubis	Superior part of medial surface of tibia	Obturator nerve	Adducts thigh at hip, flexes leg at knee, and helps to rotate it medially
Obturator externus	Margins of obturator foramen and obturator membrane	Trochanteric fossa of femur	Obturator nerve	Rotates thigh laterally at hip; steadies femoral head in acetabulum

Thigh: Posterior Compartment Muscles

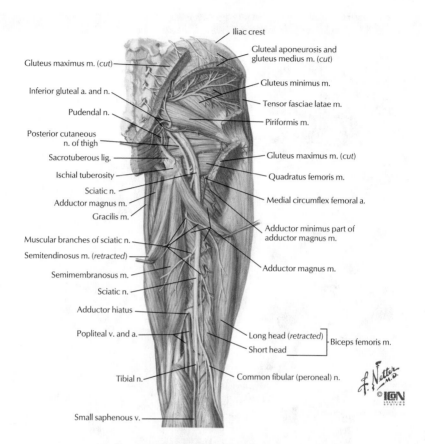

Iliac crest

Gluteal aponeurosis and gluteus medius m. (*cut*)

Gluteus maximus m. (*cut*)

Gluteus minimus m.

Inferior gluteal a. and n.

Tensor fasciae latae m.

Pudendal n.

Piriformis m.

Posterior cutaneous n. of thigh

Sacrotuberous lig.

Gluteus maximus m. (*cut*)

Ischial tuberosity

Quadratus femoris m.

Sciatic n.

Adductor magnus m.

Medial circumflex femoral a.

Gracilis m.

Adductor minimus part of adductor magnus m.

Muscular branches of sciatic n.

Semitendinosus m. (*retracted*)

Adductor magnus m.

Semimembranosus m.

Sciatic n.

Adductor hiatus

Popliteal v. and a.

Long head (*retracted*)

Short head } Biceps femoris m.

Tibial n.

Common fibular (peroneal) n.

Small saphenous v.

MUSCLE	PROXIMAL ATTACHMENT (ORIGIN)	DISTAL ATTACHMENT (INSERTION)	INNERVATION	MAIN ACTIONS
Semitendinosus	Ischial tuberosity	Medial surface of superior part of tibia	Tibial division of sciatic nerve	Extends thigh at hip; flexes leg at knee and rotates it medially; with flexed hip and knee, extends trunk
Semimembranosus	Ischial tuberosity	Posterior part of medial condyle of tibia	Tibial division of sciatic nerve	Extends thigh at hip; flexes leg at knee and rotates it medially; with flexed hip and knee, extends trunk
Biceps femoris	*Long head*: ischial tuberosity *Short head*: linea aspera and lateral supracondylar line of femur	Lateral side of head of fibula; tendon at this site split by fibular collateral ligament of knee	*Long head*: tibial division of sciatic nerve *Short head*: common fibular (peroneal) division of sciatic nerve	Flexes leg at knee and rotates it laterally; extends thigh at hip (e.g., when starting to walk)

Clinical Correlation

Diagnosis of Hip, Buttock, and Back Pain   *Anatomy on pp. 214, 221*

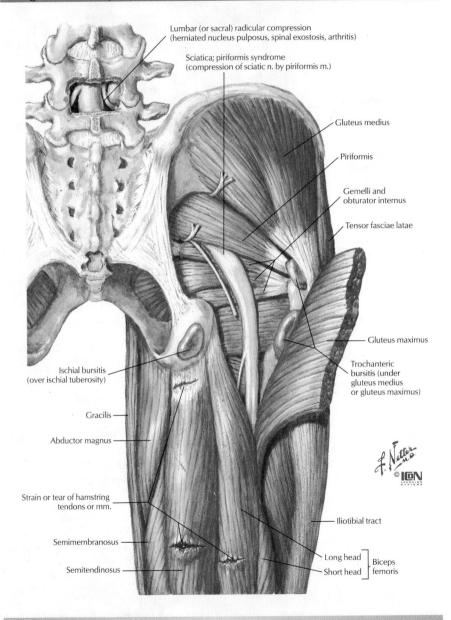

Lumbar (or sacral) radicular compression
(herniated nucleus pulposus, spinal exostosis, arthritis)

Sciatica; piriformis syndrome
(compression of sciatic n. by piriformis m.)

Gluteus medius

Piriformis

Gemelli and
obturator internus

Tensor fasciae latae

Gluteus maximus

Trochanteric
bursitis (under
gluteus medius
or gluteus maximus)

Ischial bursitis
(over ischial tuberosity)

Gracilis

Abductor magnus

Strain or tear of hamstring
tendons or mm.

Semimembranosus

Semitendinosus

Iliotibial tract

Long head ⎤ Biceps
Short head ⎦ femoris

Athletically active individuals may report hip pain when an injury is actually related to the lumbar spine (herniated disk), buttocks (bursitis or hamstring injury), or
pelvic region (intrapelvic disorder). Careful follow-up should examine all potential
causes of the pain to determine whether it is referred and thus originates from another source.

Thigh: Lumbar Plexus (L1-4)

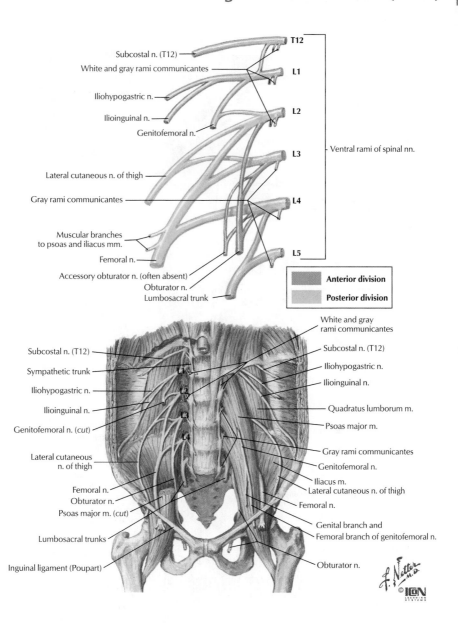

Subcostal n. (T12)

White and gray rami communicantes

Iliohypogastric n.

Ilioinguinal n.

Genitofemoral n.

Lateral cutaneous n. of thigh

Gray rami communicantes

Muscular branches to psoas and iliacus mm.

Femoral n.

Accessory obturator n. (often absent)

Obturator n.

Lumbosacral trunk

T12
L1
L2
L3
L4
L5

Ventral rami of spinal nn.

Anterior division
Posterior division

White and gray rami communicantes

Subcostal n. (T12)
Sympathetic trunk
Iliohypogastric n.
Ilioinguinal n.
Genitofemoral n. (cut)
Lateral cutaneous n. of thigh
Femoral n.
Obturator n.
Psoas major m. (cut)
Lumbosacral trunks
Inguinal ligament (Poupart)

Subcostal n. (T12)
Iliohypogastric n.
Ilioinguinal n.
Quadratus lumborum m.
Psoas major m.
Gray rami communicantes
Genitofemoral n.
Iliacus m.
Lateral cutaneous n. of thigh
Femoral n.
Genital branch and Femoral branch of genitofemoral n.
Obturator n.

DIVISION: NERVE	INNERVATION
Anterior: obturator	Passes through the obturator foramen and innervates medial compartment muscles of thigh
Posterior: femoral	Passes deep to the inguinal ligament, lateral to the femoral sheath, and innervates iliopsoas and anterior compartment muscles of thigh

Only the major branches are summarized in the table.

Thigh: Key Arteries

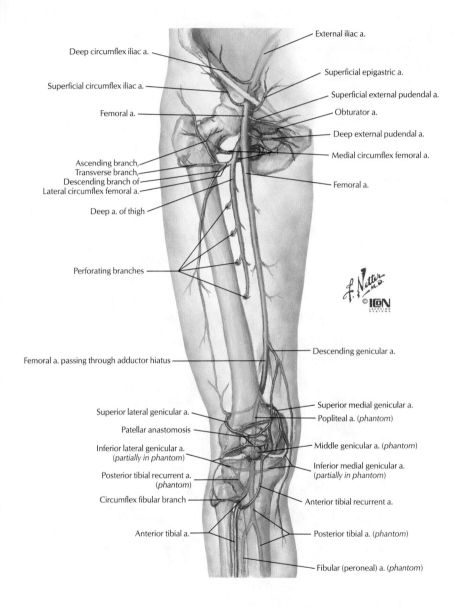

Deep circumflex iliac a.

External iliac a.

Superficial circumflex iliac a.

Superficial epigastric a.

Femoral a.

Superficial external pudendal a.

Obturator a.

Deep external pudendal a.

Ascending branch,
Transverse branch,
Descending branch of
Lateral circumflex femoral a.

Medial circumflex femoral a.

Femoral a.

Deep a. of thigh

Perforating branches

Descending genicular a.

Femoral a. passing through adductor hiatus

Superior lateral genicular a.

Superior medial genicular a.
Popliteal a. (*phantom*)

Patellar anastomosis

Inferior lateral genicular a.
(*partially in phantom*)

Middle genicular a. (*phantom*)

Inferior medial genicular a.
(*partially in phantom*)

Posterior tibial recurrent a.
(*phantom*)

Circumflex fibular branch

Anterior tibial recurrent a.

Anterior tibial a.

Posterior tibial a. (*phantom*)

Fibular (peroneal) a. (*phantom*)

ARTERY	COURSE AND STRUCTURES SUPPLIED
Obturator	Arises from internal iliac artery (pelvis); has anterior and posterior branches; passes through obturator foramen
Femoral	Continuation of external iliac artery with numerous branches to perineum, hip, thigh, and knee
Deep artery of thigh	Arises from femoral artery; supplies hip and thigh

Clinical Correlation

Revascularization
Anatomy on p. 224

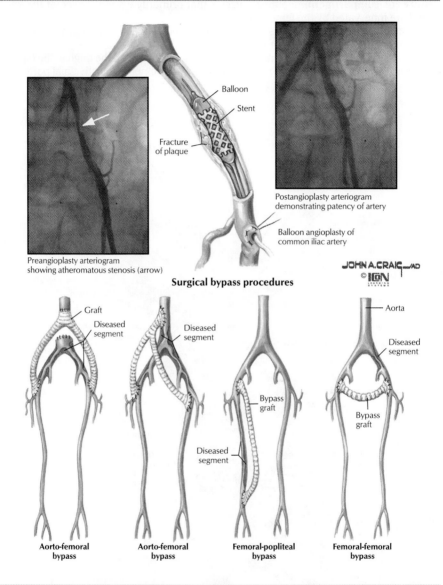

Balloon

Stent

Fracture
of plaque

Postangioplasty arteriogram
demonstrating patency of artery

Balloon angioplasty of
common iliac artery

Preangioplasty arteriogram
showing atheromatous stenosis (arrow)

JOHN A. CRAIG—MD
©ICON
LEARNING
SYSTEMS

Surgical bypass procedures

Graft

Diseased
segment

Diseased
segment

Aorta

Diseased
segment

Bypass
graft

Bypass
graft

Diseased
segment

**Aorto-femoral
bypass**

**Aorto-femoral
bypass**

**Femoral-popliteal
bypass**

**Femoral-femoral
bypass**

Peripheral vascular disease (PVD) and claudication can usually be managed medically by reducing associated risk factors. However, in patients who are refractory to medical management, several invasive options exist:
- **Percutaneous angioplasty**: balloon dilation (with or without an endovascular stent) for recanalization of a stenosed artery (percutaneous revascularization)
- **Surgical bypass**: bypassing a diseased segment with a graft (1-3% operative mortality)

Thigh: Serial Cross Sections

Intermuscular septa (lateral, medial, posterior) divide the thigh into three sections:

Anterior compartment: contains muscles that primarily extend the leg at the knee and are innervated by the femoral nerve

Medial compartment: contains muscles that primarily adduct the thigh at the hip and are innervated by the obturator nerve

Posterior compartment: contains muscles that primarily extend the thigh at the hip and flex the leg at the knee and are innervated by the sciatic nerve (mostly tibial portion)

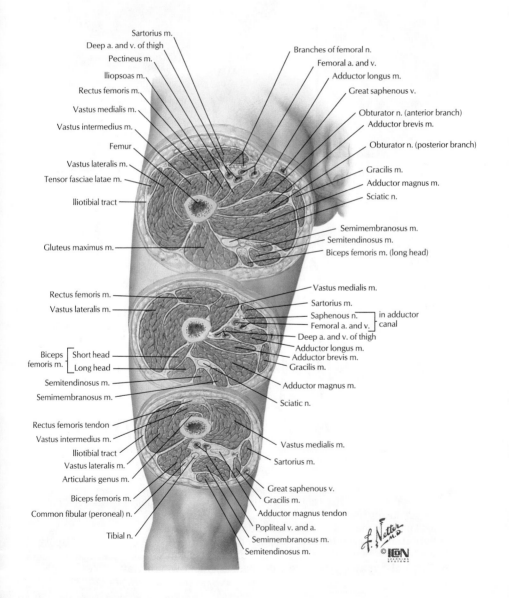

Sartorius m.
Deep a. and v. of thigh
Pectineus m.
Iliopsoas m.
Rectus femoris m.
Vastus medialis m.
Vastus intermedius m.
Femur
Vastus lateralis m.
Tensor fasciae latae m.
Iliotibial tract
Gluteus maximus m.

Branches of femoral n.
Femoral a. and v.
Adductor longus m.
Great saphenous v.
Obturator n. (anterior branch)
Adductor brevis m.
Obturator n. (posterior branch)
Gracilis m.
Adductor magnus m.
Sciatic n.
Semimembranosus m.
Semitendinosus m.
Biceps femoris m. (long head)

Rectus femoris m.
Vastus lateralis m.
Biceps [Short head
femoris m. [Long head
Semitendinosus m.
Semimembranosus m.

Vastus medialis m.
Sartorius m.
Saphenous n.   ] in adductor
Femoral a. and v.] canal
Deep a. and v. of thigh
Adductor longus m.
Adductor brevis m.
Gracilis m.
Adductor magnus m.
Sciatic n.

Rectus femoris tendon
Vastus intermedius m.
Iliotibial tract
Vastus lateralis m.
Articularis genus m.
Biceps femoris m.
Common fibular (peroneal) n.
Tibial n.

Vastus medialis m.
Sartorius m.
Great saphenous v.
Gracilis m.
Adductor magnus tendon
Popliteal v. and a.
Semimembranosus m.
Semitendinosus m.

Clinical Correlation

Fractures of the Shaft and Distal Femur   *Anatomy on pp. 12, 217*

Shaft fractures

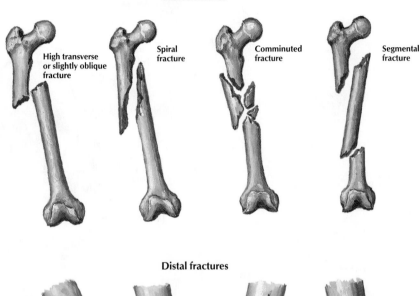

High transverse
or slightly oblique
fracture

Spiral
fracture

Comminuted
fracture

Segmental
fracture

Distal fractures

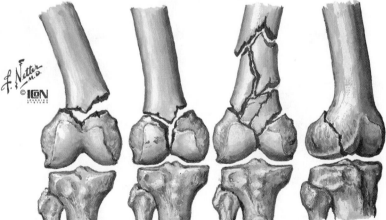

Transverse supra-
condylar fracture

Intercondylar (T or Y)
fracture

Comminuted fracture
extending into shaft

Fracture of single
condyle (may occur in
frontal or oblique plane)

Femoral shaft fractures occur in all age groups but are especially common in young and elderly persons. Spiral fractures usually occur from torsional forces rather than direct forces. Fractures of the distal femur are divided into two groups on the basis of whether they involve the joint surface. If reduction and fixation of intraarticular fractures are not satisfactory, osteoarthritis is a common posttraumatic complication.

Clinical Correlation

Pressure (Decubitus) Ulcers   *Anatomy on pp. 204, 208, 234, 238, 252*

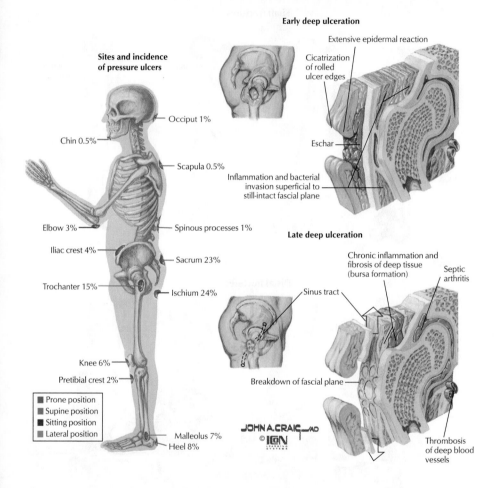

Early deep ulceration

Extensive epidermal reaction

Cicatrization of rolled ulcer edges

Eschar

Inflammation and bacterial invasion superficial to still-intact fascial plane

Sites and incidence of pressure ulcers

Occiput 1%

Chin 0.5%

Scapula 0.5%

Elbow 3%

Spinous processes 1%

Late deep ulceration

Iliac crest 4%

Sacrum 23%

Trochanter 15%

Ischium 24%

Chronic inflammation and fibrosis of deep tissue (bursa formation)

Septic arthritis

Sinus tract

Knee 6%

Pretibial crest 2%

Breakdown of fascial plane

■ Prone position
■ Supine position
■ Sitting position
■ Lateral position

Malleolus 7%
Heel 8%

JOHN A.CRAIG—MD
©ICN

Thrombosis of deep blood vessels

Pressure ulcers (bedsores) are common complications in patients confined to beds or wheelchairs. They form when soft tissue is compressed between a bony eminence (e.g., greater trochanter) and the bed or wheelchair. Comatose, paraplegic, or debilitated patients cannot sense discomfort caused by pressure from prolonged contact with hard surfaces. Four stages of these ulcers are

I: changes in skin temperature, consistency, or sensation; persistent redness

II: partial-thickness skin loss, similar to an abrasion with a shallow crater or blister

III: full-thickness skin loss with subcutaneous tissue damage and a deep crater

IV: full-thickness skin loss with necrosis or damage to muscle, bone, or adjacent structures

Clinical Correlation

Multiple Myeloma

Anatomy on pp. 207, 217, 246

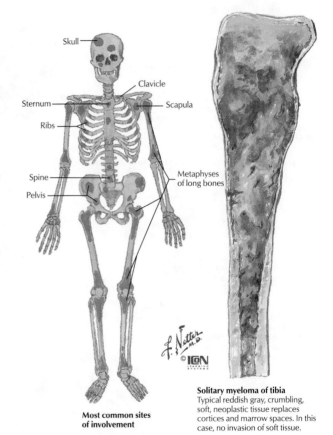

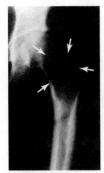

Anteroposterior view of proximal femur. Vague radiolucent lesion (arrows).

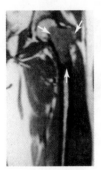

Coronal MRI. Lesion (same as above) has gray signal (arrows) in contrast to brighter signal of marrow fat.

Skull

Clavicle

Sternum

Scapula

Ribs

Spine

Pelvis

Metaphyses of long bones

Most common sites of involvement

Solitary myeloma of tibia
Typical reddish gray, crumbling, soft, neoplastic tissue replaces cortices and marrow spaces. In this case, no invasion of soft tissue.

Multiple myeloma, a tumor of plasma cells, is the most common malignant type of primary bone tumor. This painful tumor is sensitive to radiation therapy, and new chemotherapeutic agents and bone marrow transplantation offer hope for improved survival. Fever, weight loss, fatigue, anemia, thrombocytopenia, and renal failure are associated with this cancer, which usually occurs in middle age.

Clinical Correlation

Surgical Approach to Total Hip Replacement

Anatomy on pp. 209, 214

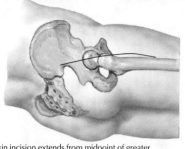

1. Skin incision extends from midpoint of greater trochanter downward along line of femur and upward about same distance toward posterior superior iliac spine. Deep fascia and iliotibial tract incised in same line.

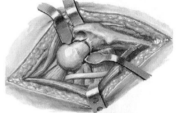

Vastus lateralis m.
Tensor fasciae latae m.
Iliotibial tract
Gluteus medius m.
Gluteus maximus m.
Piriformis m.
Superior gemellus m.
Quadratus femoris m.
Inferior gemellus m.
Sciatic n.
Obturator internus m.

2. Fibers of gluteus maximus muscle separated by blunt dissection, its femoral insertion partially detached. Piriformis and short lateral rotator muscles exposed with care to avoid sciatic nerve (usually obscured by fat).

Posterior capsule
Gluteus minimus m.
Medial femoral circumflex a.
Quadratus femoris m.

3. Gluteus medius muscle retracted; piriformis, gemellus, and obturator internus muscles divided close to their insertion into greater trochanter. Quadratus femoris and obturator externus muscles partially or totally detached. Medial femoral circumflex artery identified and cauterized.

4. Fully exposed femoral head and neck supported with superior and inferior retractors.

Note: Various procedures are used successfully.

5. To expose acetabulum, femur with cut neck retracted anteriorly. Gluteus medius and minimus muscles retracted with pin. Posterior capsule and short lateral rotator muscles retracted with spiked retractor; inferior retractor placed under transverse acetabular ligament. Anterior capsule may also be cut to increase exposure.

Surgical replacement of a joint, or arthroplasty, has revolutionized treatment of once-crippling diseases such as osteoarthritis and rheumatoid arthritis. Because the hip is a major weight-bearing joint and has a wide range of motion in three planes (flexion-extension, abduction-adduction, lateral-medial rotation), it is often involved in degenerative joint disease. Total hip replacement surgery requires thorough knowledge of adjacent anatomy of the hip, gluteal region, and thigh, as well as understanding of biomechanics of this synovial joint.

Clinical Correlation

Acetabular Reconstruction and Total Hip Replacement

Anatomy on pp. 208, 209

Preoperative view

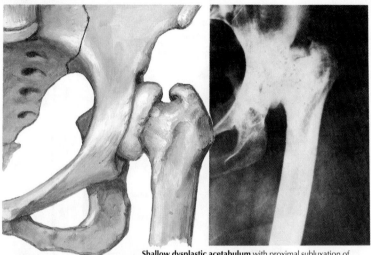

Shallow dysplastic acetabulum with proximal subluxation of femoral head and superolateral deficiency of acetabulum

Postoperative view

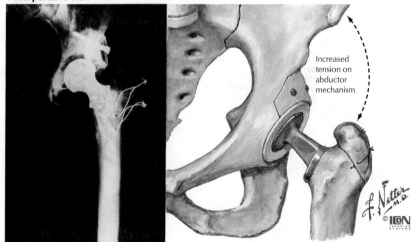

Increased tension on abductor mechanism

Total hip replacement with reinforcement of superior acetabulum with bone graft from excised femoral head. Bone graft held in place with screws. Limb slightly lengthened and tension in abductor muscle mass increased.

An acetabulum can be dysplastic and deficient, which makes the socket of this ball-and-socket joint too shallow for optimal articulation and function. In such cases, the acetabulum may be reconstructed with bone grafts as part of total hip replacement surgery.

Leg: Bones

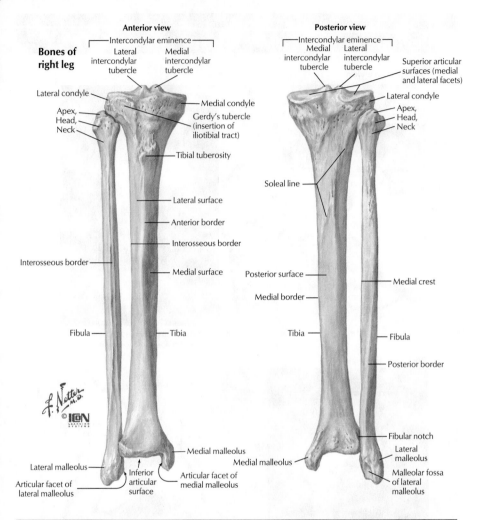

Anterior view

Bones of
right leg

Intercondylar eminence
Lateral intercondylar tubercle
Medial intercondylar tubercle

Lateral condyle
Apex,
Head,
Neck

Medial condyle
Gerdy's tubercle (insertion of iliotibial tract)

Tibial tuberosity

Lateral surface

Anterior border

Interosseous border

Interosseous border

Medial surface

Fibula

Tibia

Lateral malleolus

Articular facet of lateral malleolus

Inferior articular surface

Medial malleolus

Articular facet of medial malleolus

Posterior view

Intercondylar eminence
Medial intercondylar tubercle
Lateral intercondylar tubercle

Superior articular surfaces (medial and lateral facets)

Lateral condyle
Apex,
Head,
Neck

Soleal line

Posterior surface

Medial crest

Medial border

Tibia

Fibula

Posterior border

Fibular notch

Medial malleolus

Lateral malleolus

Malleolar fossa of lateral malleolus

FEATURE	CHARACTERISTICS
Tibia	
Long bone	Large, weight-bearing bone
Proximal facets	Large plateau for articulation with femoral condyles
Tibial tuberosity	Insertion site for patellar ligament
Inferior articular surface	Surface for cupping talus at the ankle joint
Medial malleolus	Prominence on medial aspect of ankle
Fibula	
Long bone	Slender bone, primarily for muscle attachment
Neck	Possible damage to common fibular nerve if fracture occurs here

Clinical Correlation

Tibial Fractures   *Anatomy on pp. 12, 232*

Tibial plateau fracture

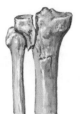

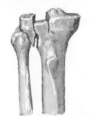

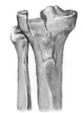

I. Split fracture of lateral tibial plateau

II. Split fracture of lateral condyle plus depression of tibial plateau

III. Depression of lateral tibia plateau without split fracture

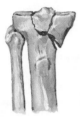

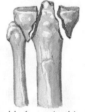

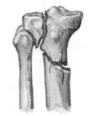

IV. Comminuted split fracture of media tibial plateau and tibial spine

V. Bicondylar fracture involving both tibial plateaus with widening

VI. Fracture of lateral tibial plateau with separation of metaphyseal-diaphyseal junction

Fracture of shaft of tibia

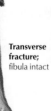

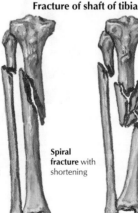

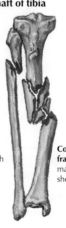

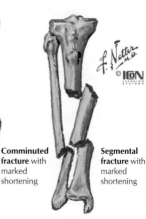

Transverse fracture; fibula intact

Spiral fracture with shortening

Comminuted fracture with marked shortening

Segmental fracture with marked shortening

Six types of tibial plateau fractures are recognized, most of which involve the lateral tibial condyle (plateau), result from direct trauma, and, because they involve the articular surface, must be stabilized. Fractures of the tibial shaft are the most common fractures of a long bone. Because the tibia is largely subcutaneous along its medial border, many such fractures are open injuries. Often, both the tibia and fibula are fractured.

Leg: Knee Joint and Muscle-Tendon Support

Lateral view

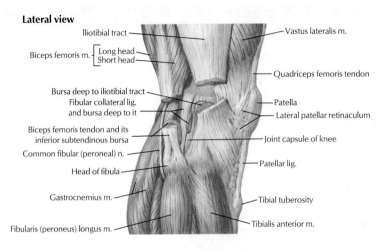

Iliotibial tract
Biceps femoris m. {Long head / Short head}
Bursa deep to iliotibial tract
Fibular collateral lig. and bursa deep to it
Biceps femoris tendon and its inferior subtendinous bursa
Common fibular (peroneal) n.
Head of fibula
Gastrocnemius m.
Fibularis (peroneus) longus m.

Vastus lateralis m.
Quadriceps femoris tendon
Patella
Lateral patellar retinaculum
Joint capsule of knee
Patellar lig.
Tibial tuberosity
Tibialis anterior m.

Medial view

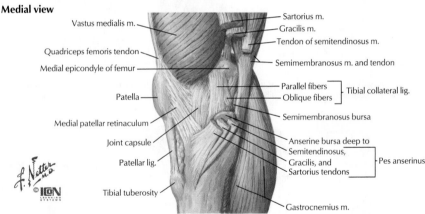

Vastus medialis m.
Quadriceps femoris tendon
Medial epicondyle of femur
Patella
Medial patellar retinaculum
Joint capsule
Patellar lig.
Tibial tuberosity

Sartorius m.
Gracilis m.
Tendon of semitendinosus m.
Semimembranosus m. and tendon
Parallel fibers / Oblique fibers } Tibial collateral lig.
Semimembranosus bursa
Anserine bursa deep to Semitendinosus, Gracilis, and Sartorius tendons } Pes anserinus
Gastrocnemius m.

Externally, the knee joint is stabilized laterally and medially by the attachment of tendons.

MUSCLE OR TENDON	COMMENT
Lateral Aspect	
Biceps femoris	Posterolateral support, attaching to fibular head
Gastrocnemius (lateral)	Support somewhat more posteriorly
Iliotibial tract	Lateral support and stabilization
Popliteus	Located posterolaterally beneath the fibular collateral ligament
Medial Aspect	
Semimembranosus	Posteromedial support
Gastrocnemius (medial)	Support somewhat more posteriorly
Pes anserinus	Semitendinosus, gracilis, and sartorius (looks like a goose's foot) tendons, attaching to medial tibial condyle

Clinical Correlation

Patellar Injuries

Anatomy on pp. 234, 236

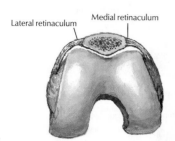
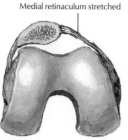
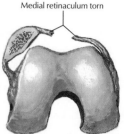

Lateral retinaculum   Medial retinaculum   Medial retinaculum stretched   Medial retinaculum torn

Skyline view. Normally, patella rides in grove between medial and lateral femoral condyles.

In subluxation, patella deviates laterally because of weakness of vastus medialis muscle and tightness of lateral retinaculum.

In dislocation, patella is displaced completely out of intercondylar groove.

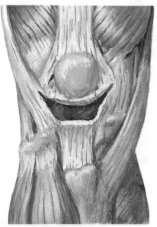
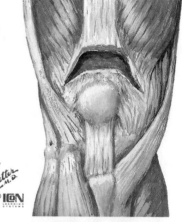

Patellar ligament rupture
Rupture of patellar ligament at inferior margin of patella

Quadriceps tendon rupture
Rupture of quadriceps femoris tendon at superior margin of patella

Subluxation of the patella, usually laterally, is a fairly common occurrence, especially in adolescent girls and young women. It often presents with tenderness along the medial patellar aspect and atrophy of the quadriceps tendon, especially the oblique portion medially derived from the vastus medialis. Patellar tendon rupture usually occurs just inferior to the patella as a result of direct trauma in younger people (aged <30 years). Quadriceps tendon rupture occurs mostly in older individuals (aged >60 years), from either minor trauma or age-related degenerative changes, including

- Arthritis
- Arteriosclerosis
- Chronic renal failure
- Corticosteroid therapy
- Diabetes
- Hyperparathyroidism
- Gout

Leg: Knee Joint and Ligaments

In extension: anterior view

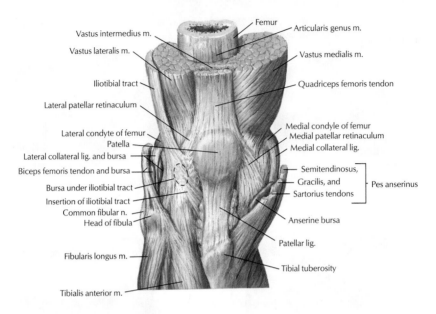

Vastus intermedius m.
Vastus lateralis m.
Iliotibial tract
Lateral patellar retinaculum
Lateral condyle of femur
Patella
Lateral collateral lig. and bursa
Biceps femoris tendon and bursa
Bursa under iliotibial tract
Insertion of iliotibial tract
Common fibular n.
Head of fibula
Fibularis longus m.
Tibialis anterior m.

Femur
Articularis genus m.
Vastus medialis m.
Quadriceps femoris tendon
Medial condyle of femur
Medial patellar retinaculum
Medial collateral lig.
Semitendinosus,
Gracilis, and   Pes anserinus
Sartorius tendons
Anserine bursa
Patellar lig.
Tibial tuberosity

In extension: posterior view   In flexion: anterior view

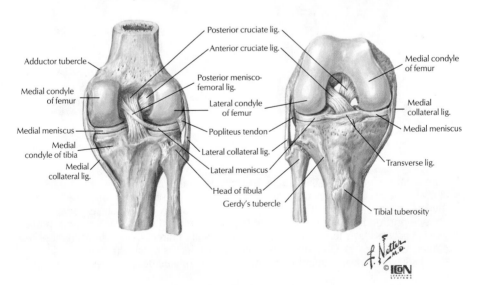

Adductor tubercle
Medial condyle of femur
Medial meniscus
Medial condyle of tibia
Medial collateral lig.

Posterior cruciate lig.
Anterior cruciate lig.
Posterior menisco-femoral lig.
Lateral condyle of femur
Popliteus tendon
Lateral collateral lig.
Lateral meniscus
Head of fibula
Gerdy's tubercle

Medial condyle of femur
Medial collateral lig.
Medial meniscus
Transverse lig.
Tibial tuberosity

Leg: Knee Joint and Ligaments (continued)

The knee is the most sophisticated joint in the body and participates in flexion, extension, and some gliding and medial rotation when it is flexed. With full extension, the femur rotates medially on the tibia, and ligaments tighten.

LIGAMENT	ATTACHMENT	COMMENT
Knee (Biaxial Condylar Synovial) Joint		
Capsule	Surrounds femoral and tibial condyles and patella	Is fibrous, weak (offers little support); flexion, extension, some gliding and medial rotation
Extracapsular Ligaments		
Tibial collateral	Medial femoral epicondyle to medical tibial condyle	Limits extension and abduction of leg; attached to medial meniscus
Fibular collateral	Lateral femoral epicondyle to fibular head	Limits extension and adduction of leg; overlies popliteus tendon
Patellar	Patella to tibial tuberosity	Acts in extension of quadriceps tendon
Arcuate popliteal	Fibular head to capsule	Passes over popliteus muscle
Oblique popliteal	Semimembranosus tendon to posterior knee	Limits hyperextension and lateral rotation
Intracapsular Ligaments		
Medial meniscus	Interarticular area of tibia, lies over medial facet, attached to tibial collateral	Is semicircular (C shaped); acts as cushion; often torn
Lateral meniscus	Interarticular area of tibia, lies over lateral facet	Is more circular and smaller than medial meniscus; acts as cushion
Anterior cruciate	Anterior intercondylar tibia to lateral femoral condyle	Prevents posterior slipping of femur on tibia; torn in hyperextension
Posterior cruciate	Posterior intercondylar tibia to medial femoral condyle	Prevents anterior slipping of femur on tibia; shorter and stronger than anterior cruciate
Transverse	Anterior aspect of menisci	Binds and stabilizes menisci
Posterior meniscofemoral (of Wrisberg)	Posterior lateral meniscus to medial femoral condyle	Is strong
Patellofemoral (Biaxial Synovial Saddle) Joint		
Quadriceps tendon	Muscles to superior patella	Is part of extension mechanism
Patellar	Patella to tibial tuberosity	Acts in extension of quadriceps tendon; patella stabilized by medial and lateral ligament (retinaculum) attachment to tibia and femur

Leg: Knee Joint Bursae

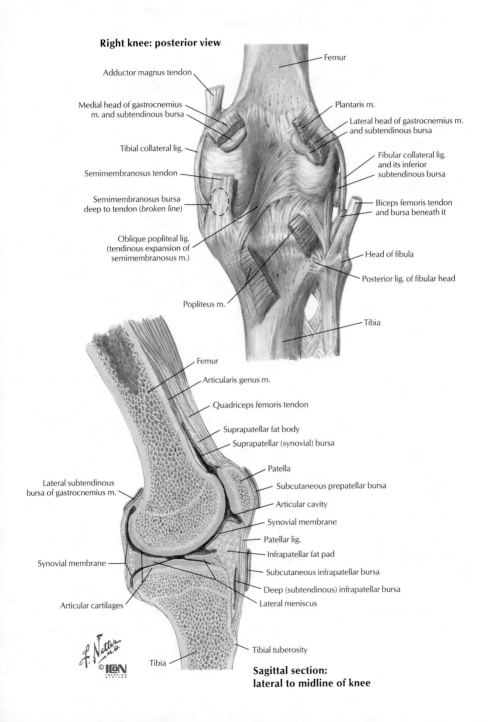

Right knee: posterior view

Adductor magnus tendon

Medial head of gastrocnemius m. and subtendinous bursa

Tibial collateral lig.

Semimembranosus tendon

Semimembranosus bursa deep to tendon (*broken line*)

Oblique popliteal lig. (tendinous expansion of semimembranosus m.)

Popliteus m.

Femur

Plantaris m.

Lateral head of gastrocnemius m. and subtendinous bursa

Fibular collateral lig. and its inferior subtendinous bursa

Biceps femoris tendon and bursa beneath it

Head of fibula

Posterior lig. of fibular head

Tibia

Femur

Articularis genus m.

Quadriceps femoris tendon

Suprapatellar fat body

Suprapatellar (synovial) bursa

Patella

Subcutaneous prepatellar bursa

Articular cavity

Synovial membrane

Patellar lig.

Infrapatellar fat pad

Subcutaneous infrapatellar bursa

Deep (subtendinous) infrapatellar bursa

Lateral meniscus

Lateral subtendinous bursa of gastrocnemius m.

Synovial membrane

Articular cartilages

Tibial tuberosity

Tibia

Sagittal section: lateral to midline of knee

Leg: Knee Joint Bursae (continued)

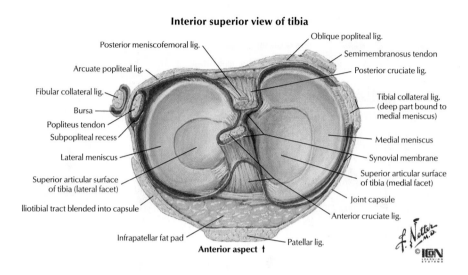

Interior superior view of tibia

Posterior meniscofemoral lig.

Oblique popliteal lig.

Semimembranosus tendon

Arcuate popliteal lig.

Posterior cruciate lig.

Fibular collateral lig.

Tibial collateral lig. (deep part bound to medial meniscus)

Bursa

Popliteus tendon

Subpopliteal recess

Medial meniscus

Lateral meniscus

Synovial membrane

Superior articular surface of tibia (lateral facet)

Superior articular surface of tibia (medial facet)

Iliotibial tract blended into capsule

Joint capsule

Anterior cruciate lig.

Infrapatellar fat pad

Patellar lig.

Anterior aspect ↑

Because of the number of muscle tendons running across the knee joint, several bursae protect underlying structures from friction. The first four bursae listed communicate with the synovial cavity of the knee joint.

BURSA	LOCATION
Suprapatellar	Between quadriceps tendon and femur
Popliteus	Between popliteus tendon and lateral tibial condyle
Anserine	Between pes anserinus and tibia and tibial collateral ligament
Subtendinous	Deep to heads of the gastrocnemius muscles
Semimembranosus	Deep to the tendon of the semimembranosus muscle
Prepatellar	Between skin and patella
Subcutaneous infrapatellar	Between skin and tibial tuberosity
Deep infrapatellar	Between patellar ligament and tibia

Clinical Correlation

Rupture of the Anterior Cruciate Ligament

Anatomy on pp. 236, 238, 239

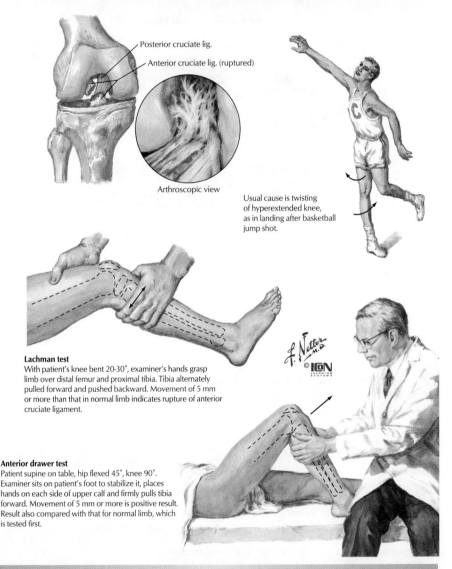

Posterior cruciate lig.

Anterior cruciate lig. (ruptured)

Arthroscopic view

Usual cause is twisting of hyperextended knee, as in landing after basketball jump shot.

Lachman test
With patient's knee bent 20-30°, examiner's hands grasp limb over distal femur and proximal tibia. Tibia alternately pulled forward and pushed backward. Movement of 5 mm or more than that in normal limb indicates rupture of anterior cruciate ligament.

Anterior drawer test
Patient supine on table, hip flexed 45°, knee 90°. Examiner sits on patient's foot to stabilize it, places hands on each side of upper calf and firmly pulls tibia forward. Movement of 5 mm or more is positive result. Result also compared with that for normal limb, which is tested first.

Rupture of the anterior cruciate ligament (ACL) is a common athletic injury usually related to sharp turns, when the knee is twisted while the foot is firmly on the ground. The patient may hear a popping sound and feel a tearing sensation associated with acute pain. Joint stability can be assessed by using the Lachman and anterior drawer tests. With an ACL injury, the tibia moves anteriorly (the ACL normally limits knee hyperextension) in the latter test and back and forth in the former.

Clinical Correlation

Sprains of Knee Ligaments

Anatomy on pp. 234-239

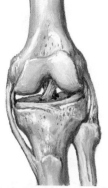
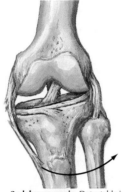
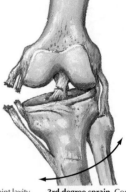

1st-degree sprain. Localized joint pain and tenderness but no joint laxity

2nd-degree sprain. Detectable joint laxity plus localized pain and tenderness

3rd-degree sprain. Complete disruption of ligaments and gross joint instability

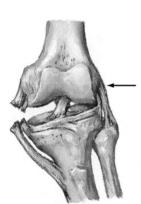

Valgus stress may rupture tibial collateral and capsular ligaments.

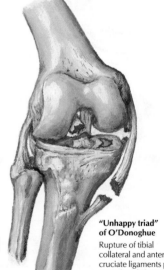

"Unhappy triad" of O'Donoghue

Rupture of tibial collateral and anterior cruciate ligaments plus tear of medial meniscus

Ligament injuries—sprains—of the knee are common in athletes and can be characterized as
- **First degree:** ligament stretched but little if any tearing
- **Second degree:** partial tearing of ligament with joint laxity
- **Third degree:** complete rupture of ligament; unstable joint

Damage to the tibial collateral ligament may also involve a tear of the medial meniscus, because the meniscus is attached to the ligament. The "unhappy triad"—tears of these structures and the ACL—is usually the result of a direct blow to the lateral aspect of the knee with the foot on the ground.

Clinical Correlation

Tears of the Meniscus
Anatomy on pp. 236, 239

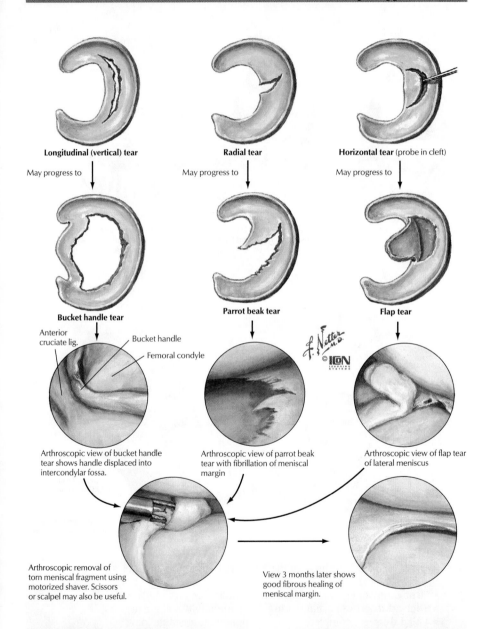

Longitudinal (vertical) tear

Radial tear

Horizontal tear (probe in cleft)

May progress to

May progress to

May progress to

Bucket handle tear

Parrot beak tear

Flap tear

Anterior cruciate lig.

Bucket handle

Femoral condyle

Arthroscopic view of bucket handle tear shows handle displaced into intercondylar fossa.

Arthroscopic view of parrot beak tear with fibrillation of meniscal margin

Arthroscopic view of flap tear of lateral meniscus

Arthroscopic removal of torn meniscal fragment using motorized shaver. Scissors or scalpel may also be useful.

View 3 months later shows good fibrous healing of meniscal margin.

The fibrocartilaginous menisci are often torn when the knee undergoes a twisting injury. Patients report pain at the joint line, and the involved knee "gives way" when flexed or extended. Rupture of the tibial collateral ligament often involves a medial meniscus tear because of their attachment to each other.

Clinical Correlation

Osgood-Schlatter Disease

Anatomy on pp. 234, 236, 238

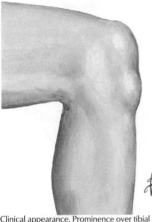

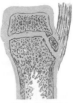
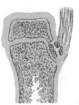

Normal insertion of patellar ligament of ossifying tibial tuberosity

In Osgood-Schlatter disease, superficial portion of tuberosity pulled away, forming separate bone fragments

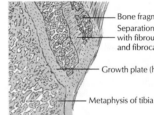

Bone fragment

Separation filled with fibrous tissue and fibrocartilage

Growth plate (hyaline cartilage)

Metaphysis of tibia

High-power magnification of involved area

Clinical appearance. Prominence over tibial tuberosity due partly to soft-tissue swelling and partly to avulsed fragments

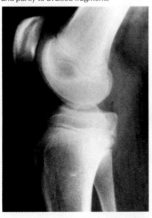

Radiograph shows separation of superficial portion of tibial tuberosity.

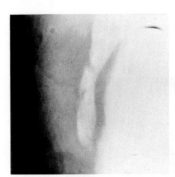

Focal radiograph shows fragment at site of insertion of patellar ligament.

Osgood-Schlatter disease (OSD) is a partial avulsion of the tibial tuberosity. During normal fetal development, the tuberosity develops as a distinct anterior segment of the epiphysis of the proximal tibia. After birth, this segment develops its own growth plate composed mostly of fibrocartilage instead of hyaline cartilage, the fibrocartilage perhaps serving as a strategy to handle the tensile stress placed on the tuberosity by the patellar ligament. The tuberosity normally ossifies and joins with the tibial epiphysis, but in OSD, repetitive stress on the tuberosity may cause it to separate (avulse) from the tibia. The avulsed fragment continues to grow, with the intervening space filled with new bone or fibrous connective tissue so that the tibial tuberosity is enlarged. At times, a painful prominence occurs. OSD is usually more common in children who engage in vigorous physical activity than in less active children.

Clinical Correlation

Osteoarthritis of the Knee
Anatomy on pp. 236, 238, 239

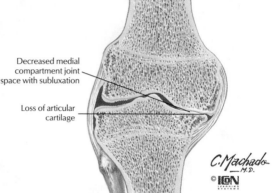

Decreased medial compartment joint space with subluxation

Loss of articular cartilage

Knee with osteoarthritis exhibits varus deformity, medial subluxation, loss of articular cartilage, and osteophyte formation.

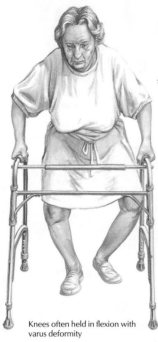

Knees often held in flexion with varus deformity

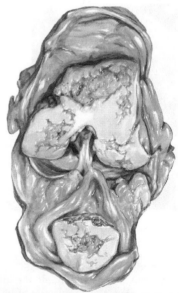

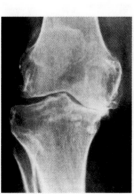

Radiograph. Varus deformity and medial subluxation of knee

Opened knee joint. Severe erosion of articular cartilage with minimal synovial change

Osteoarthritis of the knee, like the hip disorder, is a painful condition that is associated with activity, but other causes, including changes in weather, may also precipitate painful episodes. Stiffness after inactivity and a decreased range of motion are common. With time, subluxation of the knee may occur with a varum (bowleg) deformity.

Clinical Correlation

Septic Bursitis and Septic Arthritis   *Anatomy on pp. 208, 234, 238, 239*

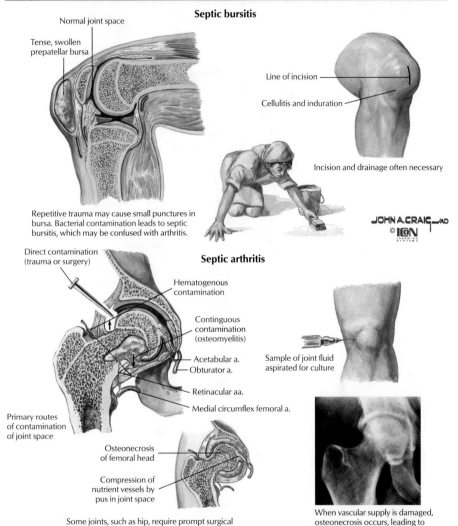

Septic bursitis

Normal joint space

Tense, swollen prepatellar bursa

Line of incision

Cellulitis and induration

Incision and drainage often necessary

Repetitive trauma may cause small punctures in bursa. Bacterial contamination leads to septic bursitis, which may be confused with arthritis.

JOHN A.CRAIG—AD
©ICN

Direct contamination (trauma or surgery)

Septic arthritis

Hematogenous contamination

Contiguous contamination (osteomyelitis)

Acetabular a.
Obturator a.

Sample of joint fluid aspirated for culture

Retinacular aa.

Medial circumflex femoral a.

Primary routes of contamination of joint space

Osteonecrosis of femoral head

Compression of nutrient vessels by pus in joint space

Some joints, such as hip, require prompt surgical decompression to avoid damage to vascular supply.

When vascular supply is damaged, osteonecrosis occurs, leading to collapse of femoral head.

Humans have more than 150 bursae in subcutaneous tissues. With increased irritation, these bursae, which are lined with synovium and contain synovial fluid, produce more fluid until significant swelling or bacterial infection or both occur, the result being septic bursitis, characterized by
- Heat over the affected area
- Swelling
- Local tenderness
- Limited range of motion

Septic arthritis occurs when infection gains entry to the joint space. If initial therapy fails, surgical débridement and lengthy antibiotic treatment may be needed.

Leg: Tibiofibular Joints and Ligaments

Anterior view with ligament attachments

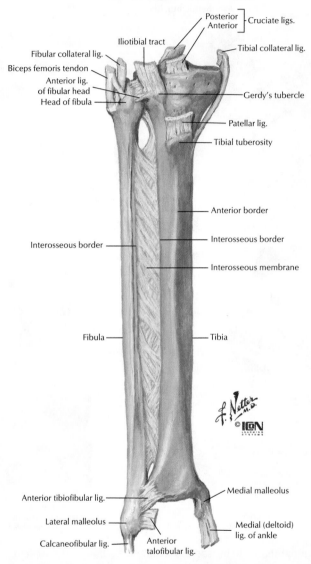

Posterior
Anterior } Cruciate ligs.

Iliotibial tract

Fibular collateral lig.

Biceps femoris tendon

Anterior lig. of fibular head

Head of fibula

Tibial collateral lig.

Gerdy's tubercle

Patellar lig.

Tibial tuberosity

Anterior border

Interosseous border

Interosseous border

Interosseous membrane

Interosseous membrane

Fibula

Tibia

Anterior tibiofibular lig.

Medial malleolus

Lateral malleolus

Medial (deltoid) lig. of ankle

Calcaneofibular lig.

Anterior talofibular lig.

LIGAMENT	ATTACHMENT	COMMENT
Proximal Tibiofibular (Plane Synovial) Joint		
Anterior and posterior ligaments of fibular head	Fibular head to lateral tibia	Anterior ligament wider and stronger than posterior ligament; some gliding movement
Interosseous membrane	Lateral tibia to medial fibula	Firm attachment to both bones

Leg: Posterior Compartment Muscles, Deep Layer

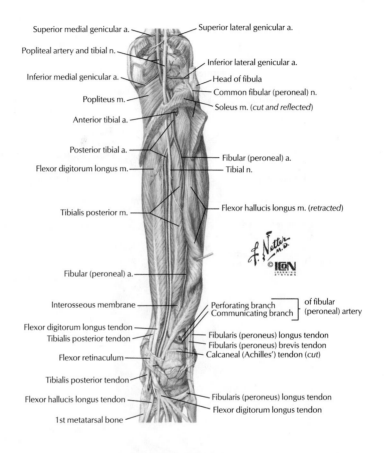

Superior medial genicular a.
Popliteal artery and tibial n.
Inferior medial genicular a.
Popliteus m.
Anterior tibial a.
Posterior tibial a.
Flexor digitorum longus m.
Tibialis posterior m.

Superior lateral genicular a.
Inferior lateral genicular a.
Head of fibula
Common fibular (peroneal) n.
Soleus m. (cut and reflected)
Fibular (peroneal) a.
Tibial n.
Flexor hallucis longus m. (retracted)

Fibular (peroneal) a.
Interosseous membrane
Flexor digitorum longus tendon
Tibialis posterior tendon
Flexor retinaculum
Tibialis posterior tendon
Flexor hallucis longus tendon
1st metatarsal bone

Perforating branch } of fibular
Communicating branch } (peroneal) artery
Fibularis (peroneus) longus tendon
Fibularis (peroneus) brevis tendon
Calcaneal (Achilles') tendon (cut)
Fibularis (peroneus) longus tendon
Flexor digitorum longus tendon

MUSCLE	PROXIMAL ATTACHMENT (ORIGIN)	DISTAL ATTACHMENT (INSERTION)	INNERVATION	MAIN ACTIONS
Popliteus	Lateral epicondyle of femur and lateral meniscus	Posterior surface of tibia, superior to soleal line	Tibial nerve	Weakly flexes leg at knee and unlocks it
Flexor hallucis longus	Inferior two thirds of posterior surface of fibula and inferior interosseous membrane	Base of distal phalanx of great toe (big toe)	Tibial nerve	Flexes great toe at all joints and plantar-flexes foot at ankle; supports longitudinal arches of foot
Flexor digitorum longus	Medial part of posterior surface of tibia inferior to soleal line, and from fascia covering tibialis posterior	Bases of distal phalanges of lateral four digits	Tibial nerve	Flexes lateral four digits and plantar-flexes foot at ankle; supports longitudinal arches of foot
Tibialis posterior	Interosseous membrane, posterior surface of tibia inferior to soleal line, and posterior surface of fibula	Tuberosity of navicular, cuneiform, and cuboid and bases of metatarsals 2, 3, and 4	Tibial nerve	Plantar-flexes foot at ankle and inverts foot

Leg: Posterior Compartment Muscles, Superficial and Intermediate

Intermediate dissection

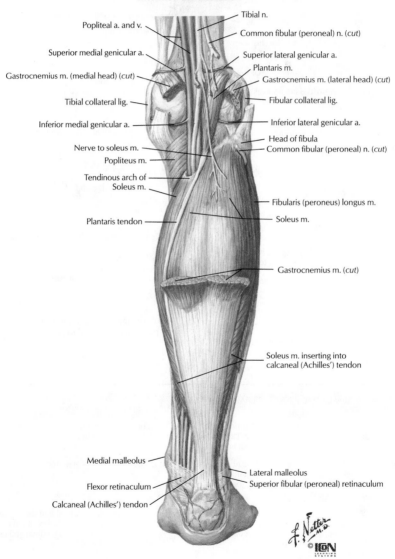

Popliteal a. and v.

Superior medial genicular a.

Gastrocnemius m. (medial head) (cut)

Tibial collateral lig.

Inferior medial genicular a.

Nerve to soleus m.

Popliteus m.

Tendinous arch of Soleus m.

Plantaris tendon

Medial malleolus

Flexor retinaculum

Calcaneal (Achilles') tendon

Tibial n.

Common fibular (peroneal) n. (cut)

Superior lateral genicular a.

Plantaris m.

Gastrocnemius m. (lateral head) (cut)

Fibular collateral lig.

Inferior lateral genicular a.

Head of fibula

Common fibular (peroneal) n. (cut)

Fibularis (peroneus) longus m.

Soleus m.

Gastrocnemius m. (cut)

Soleus m. inserting into calcaneal (Achilles') tendon

Lateral malleolus

Superior fibular (peroneal) retinaculum

Leg: Posterior Compartment Muscles, Superficial and Intermediate (continued)

Superficial dissection

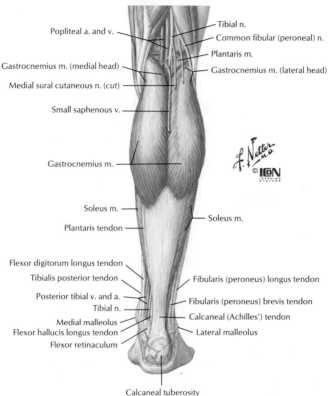

Popliteal a. and v.

Gastrocnemius m. (medial head)

Medial sural cutaneous n. (*cut*)

Small saphenous v.

Gastrocnemius m.

Soleus m.

Plantaris tendon

Flexor digitorum longus tendon

Tibialis posterior tendon

Posterior tibial v. and a.

Tibial n.

Medial malleolus

Flexor hallucis longus tendon

Flexor retinaculum

Tibial n.

Common fibular (peroneal) n.

Plantaris m.

Gastrocnemius m. (lateral head)

Soleus m.

Fibularis (peroneus) longus tendon

Fibularis (peroneus) brevis tendon

Calcaneal (Achilles') tendon

Lateral malleolus

Calcaneal tuberosity

MUSCLE	PROXIMAL ATTACHMENT (ORIGIN)	DISTAL ATTACHMENT (INSERTION)	INNERVATION	MAIN ACTIONS
Gastroc-nemius	*Lateral head*: lateral aspect of lateral condyle of femur *Medial head*: popliteal surface of femur, superior to medial condyle	Posterior surface of calcaneus via calcaneal tendon	Tibial nerve	Plantar-flexes foot at ankle; raises heel during walking; flexes leg at knee joint
Soleus	Posterior aspect of head of fibula, superior fourth of posterior surface of fibula, soleal line, and medial border of tibia	Posterior surface of calcaneus via calcaneal tendon	Tibial nerve	Plantar-flexes foot at ankle; steadies leg on foot
Plantaris	Inferior end of lateral supracondylar line of femur and oblique popliteal ligament	Posterior surface of calcaneus via calcaneal tendon (tendo calcaneus)	Tibial nerve	Weakly assists gastrocnemius in plantar-flexing foot at ankle and flexing knee

Leg: Anterior Compartment Muscles

Superficial dissection

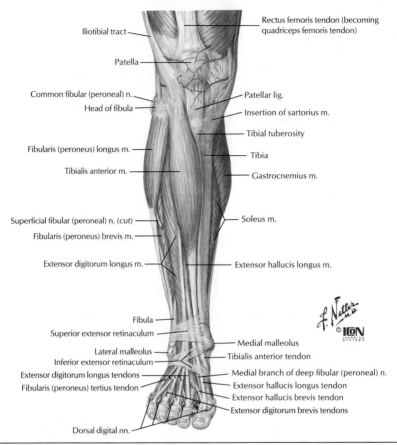

Iliotibial tract

Rectus femoris tendon (becoming quadriceps femoris tendon)

Patella

Common fibular (peroneal) n.

Head of fibula

Patellar lig.

Insertion of sartorius m.

Tibial tuberosity

Fibularis (peroneus) longus m.

Tibialis anterior m.

Tibia

Gastrocnemius m.

Superficial fibular (peroneal) n. (cut)

Fibularis (peroneus) brevis m.

Soleus m.

Extensor digitorum longus m.

Extensor hallucis longus m.

Fibula

Superior extensor retinaculum

Lateral malleolus

Inferior extensor retinaculum

Extensor digitorum longus tendons

Fibularis (peroneus) tertius tendon

Medial malleolus

Tibialis anterior tendon

Medial branch of deep fibular (peroneal) n.

Extensor hallucis longus tendon

Extensor hallucis brevis tendon

Extensor digitorum brevis tendons

Dorsal digital nn.

MUSCLE	PROXIMAL ATTACHMENT (ORIGIN)	DISTAL ATTACHMENT (INSERTION)	INNERVATION	MAIN ACTIONS
Tibialis anterior	Lateral condyle and superior half of lateral surface of tibia	Medial and inferior surfaces of medial cuneiform and base of first metatarsal	Deep fibular (peroneal) nerve	Dorsiflexes foot at ankle and inverts foot
Extensor hallucis longus	Middle part of anterior surface of fibula and interosseous membrane	Dorsal aspect of base of distal phalanx of great toe	Deep fibular (peroneal) nerve	Extends great toe and dorsiflexes foot at ankle
Extensor digitorum longus	Lateral condyle of tibia and superior three fourths of anterior surface of interosseous membrane and fibula	Middle and distal phalanges of lateral four digits	Deep fibular (peroneal) nerve	Extends lateral four digits and dorsiflexes foot at ankle
Fibularis (peroneus) tertius	Inferior third of anterior surface of fibula and interosseous membrane	Dorsum of base of fifth metatarsal	Deep fibular (peroneal) nerve	Dorsiflexes foot at ankle and aids in eversion of foot

Leg: Anterior Compartment Muscles (continued)

Deeper dissection

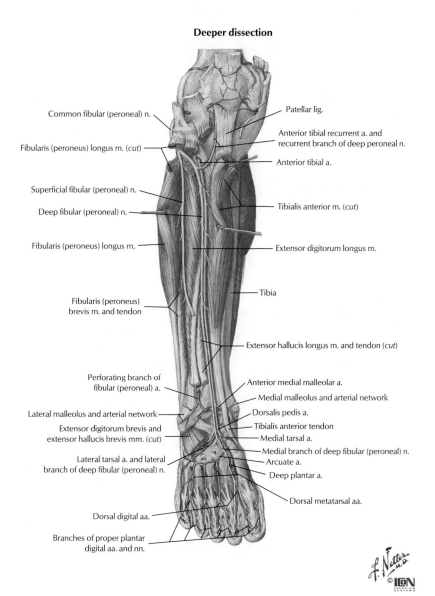

Common fibular (peroneal) n.

Fibularis (peroneus) longus m. (*cut*)

Superficial fibular (peroneal) n.

Deep fibular (peroneal) n.

Fibularis (peroneus) longus m.

Fibularis (peroneus) brevis m. and tendon

Perforating branch of fibular (peroneal) a.

Lateral malleolus and arterial network

Extensor digitorum brevis and extensor hallucis brevis mm. (*cut*)

Lateral tarsal a. and lateral branch of deep fibular (peroneal) n.

Dorsal digital aa.

Branches of proper plantar digital aa. and nn.

Patellar lig.

Anterior tibial recurrent a. and recurrent branch of deep peroneal n.

Anterior tibial a.

Tibialis anterior m. (*cut*)

Extensor digitorum longus m.

Tibia

Extensor hallucis longus m. and tendon (*cut*)

Anterior medial malleolar a.

Medial malleolus and arterial network

Dorsalis pedis a.

Tibialis anterior tendon

Medial tarsal a.

Medial branch of deep fibular (peroneal) n.

Arcuate a.

Deep plantar a.

Dorsal metatarsal aa.

Leg: Lateral Compartment Muscles

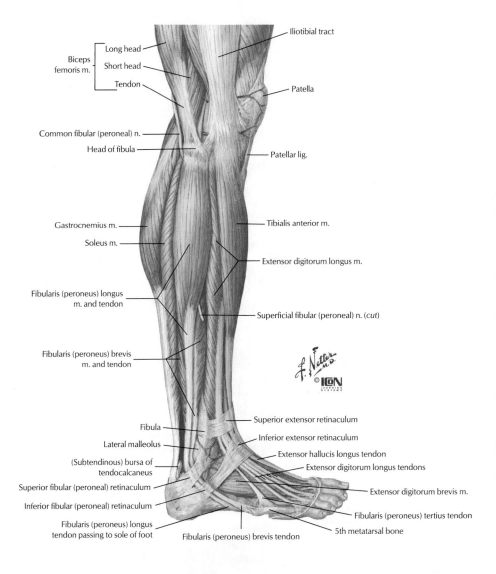

MUSCLE	PROXIMAL ATTACHMENT (ORIGIN)	DISTAL ATTACHMENT (INSERTION)	INNERVATION	MAIN ACTIONS
Fibularis (peroneus) longus	Head and superior two thirds of lateral surface of fibula	Base of first metatarsal and medial cuneiform	Superficial fibular (peroneal) nerve	Everts foot and weakly plantar-flexes foot at ankle
Fibularis (peroneus) brevis	Inferior two thirds of lateral surface of fibula	Dorsal surface of tuberosity on lateral side of fifth metatarsal	Superficial fibular (peroneal) nerve	Everts foot and weakly plantar-flexes foot at ankle

Leg: Cross Section

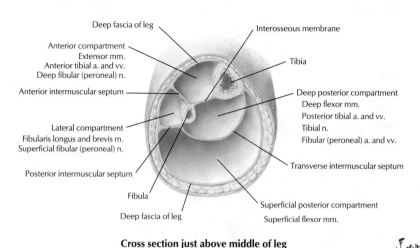

Deep fascia of leg

Interosseous membrane

Anterior compartment
Extensor mm.
Anterior tibial a. and vv.
Deep fibular (peroneal) n.

Tibia

Anterior intermuscular septum

Deep posterior compartment
Deep flexor mm.
Posterior tibial a. and vv.
Tibial n.
Fibular (peroneal) a. and vv.

Lateral compartment
Fibularis longus and brevis m.
Superficial fibular (peroneal) n.

Posterior intermuscular septum

Transverse intermuscular septum

Fibula

Superficial posterior compartment
Superficial flexor mm.

Deep fascia of leg

Cross section just above middle of leg

Tibialis anterior m.

Anterior tibial a. and vv. and
deep fibular (peroneal) n.

Extensor hallucis longus m.

Tibia

Extensor digitorum longus m.

Interosseous membrane

Superficial fibular (peroneal) n.

Great saphenous v. and saphenous n.

Anterior intermuscular septum

Fibularis (peroneus) longus m.

Tibialis posterior m.

Fibularis (peroneus) brevis m.

Flexor digitorum longus m.

Posterior intermuscular septum

Fibula

Fibular (peroneal) a. and vv.

Posterior tibial a. and vv. and tibial n.

Lateral sural cutaneous n.

Flexor hallucis longus m.

Transverse intermuscular septum

Plantaris tendon

Soleus m.

Gastrocnemius m. (medial head)
Medial sural cutaneous n.

Gastrocnemius muscle (lateral head)

Small saphenous v.

The interosseous membrane and intermuscular septa divide the leg into three compartments (the posterior being subdivided into superficial and deep compartments). The compartments may be summarized as follows:

Posterior: muscles that plantar flex and invert the foot at the ankle and flex the toes, are innervated by the tibial nerve, and are supplied by the posterior tibial artery

Anterior: muscles that dorsiflex (extend) and invert/evert the foot at the ankle and extend the toes, are innervated by the deep fibular nerve, and are supplied by the anterior tibial artery

Lateral: muscles that plantar-flex and evert the foot at the ankle, are innervated by the superficial fibular nerve, and are supplied by the fibular artery

Clinical Correlation

Genu Varum and Valgum

Anatomy on pp. 234, 236, 250

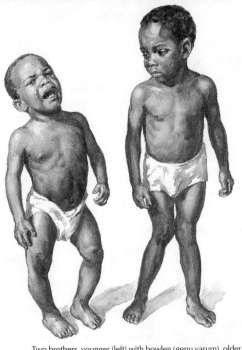

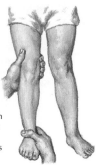

Laxity of knee ligaments demonstrated with passive adduction and abduction, which easily brings limb into proper alignment

Two brothers, younger (left) with bowleg (genu varum), older (right) with knock-knee (genu valgum). In both children, limbs eventually became normally aligned without corrective treatment.

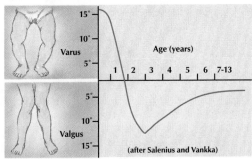

Graph depicts normal developmental changes in tibiofemoral angle. Substantial deviation suggests pathologic cause such as rickets, Blount's disease, or other disorders requiring specific treatment.

The knee of a standing patient should look symmetrical and level. The tibia normally has a slight valgus angulation when compared with the femur (valgus is a term used to describe the bone distal to the examined joint; a valgus angulation refers to a slight lateral angle). Excessive valgus angulation is called genu valgum, or knock-knee, and an excessive varus angulation is called genu varum, or bowleg. The etiology of these deformities, which occur in growing children, is often related to rickets, skeletal dysplasia, or trauma. Most resolve without treatment.

Clinical Correlation

Osteosarcoma of the Tibia
Anatomy on p. 232

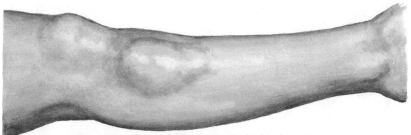

Osteosarcoma of proximal tibia presents as localized, tender prominence.

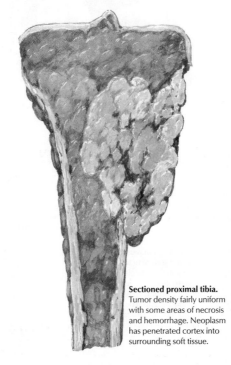

Sectioned proximal tibia.
Tumor density fairly uniform
with some areas of necrosis
and hemorrhage. Neoplasm
has penetrated cortex into
surrounding soft tissue.

Osteosarcoma is the most common malignant bone tumor of mesenchymal origin. It is more common in males and usually occurs before the age of 30 years, often in the distal femur or proximal tibia. Other sites include the proximal humerus, proximal femur, and pelvis. Most tumors appear in the metaphysis of long bones at areas of greatest growth. The tumors often invade cortical bone in this region because of its rich vascular supply and then infiltrate surrounding soft tissue. These tumors are aggressive and require immediate treatment.

Clinical Correlation

Shin Splints   *Anatomy on p. 247*

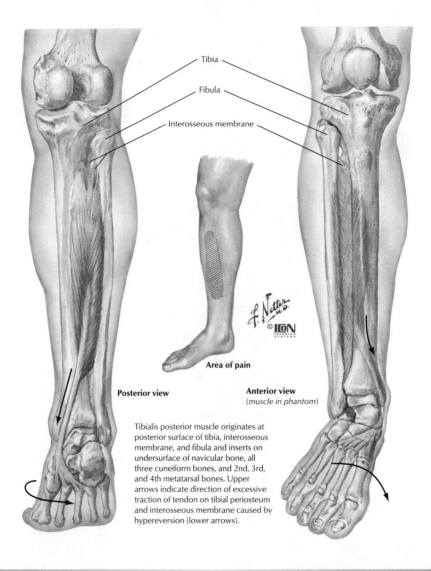

Tibia

Fibula

Interosseous membrane

Area of pain

Posterior view

Anterior view
(muscle in phantom)

Tibialis posterior muscle originates at posterior surface of tibia, interosseous membrane, and fibula and inserts on undersurface of navicular bone, all three cuneiform bones, and 2nd, 3rd, and 4th metatarsal bones. Upper arrows indicate direction of excessive traction of tendon on tibial periosteum and interosseous membrane caused by hypereversion (lower arrows).

Shin splints refers to pain along the inner distal two thirds of the tibial shaft and is a common syndrome in athletes. The primary cause is repetitive pulling of the tibialis posterior tendon as one pushes off the foot during running. Stress on the muscle occurs at its attachment to the tibia and interosseous membrane. Chronic conditions can produce periostitis and bone remodeling or lead to stress fractures. Pain, which usually begins as soreness after running, can worsen and occur while walking or climbing stairs.

Clinical Correlation

Exertional Compartment Syndromes   *Anatomy on pp. 250-252*

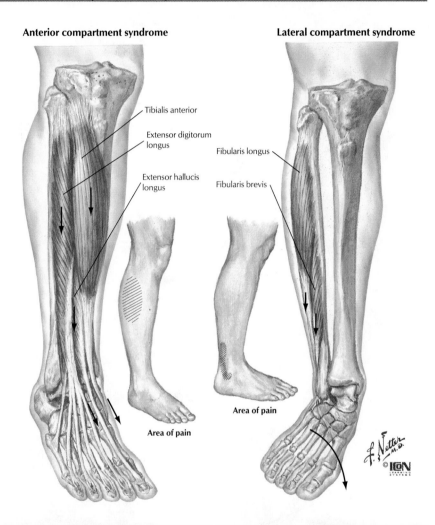

Anterior compartment syndrome

- Tibialis anterior
- Extensor digitorum longus
- Extensor hallucis longus

Area of pain

Lateral compartment syndrome

- Fibularis longus
- Fibularis brevis

Area of pain

Anterior (tibial) compartment syndrome (or anterior or lateral shin splints) occurs from excessive contraction of anterior compartment muscles; pain over these muscles radiates down the ankle and dorsum of the foot overlying the extensor tendons. Lateral compartment syndrome occurs in people with excessively mobile ankle joints in which hypereversion irritates lateral compartment muscles. These conditions are usually chronic, and expansion of the compartment may lead to nerve and vessel compression. In the acute syndrome (rapid, unrelenting expansion), the compartment may have to be opened surgically (fasciotomy) to relieve pressure. The five *P*s of acute anterior compartment syndrome are

- Pain
- Pallor
- Paresis (footdrop)
- Paresthesia
- Pulseless (variable)

Clinical Correlation

Achilles' Tendonitis and Bursitis   *Anatomy on pp. 248, 249, 261*

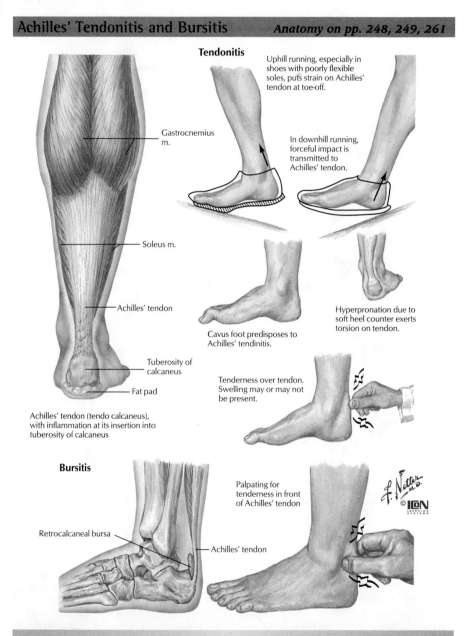

Tendonitis

Uphill running, especially in shoes with poorly flexible soles, puts strain on Achilles' tendon at toe-off.

In downhill running, forceful impact is transmitted to Achilles' tendon.

Gastrocnemius m.

Soleus m.

Achilles' tendon

Tuberosity of calcaneus

Fat pad

Achilles' tendon (tendo calcaneus), with inflammation at its insertion into tuberosity of calcaneus

Cavus foot predisposes to Achilles' tendinitis.

Hyperpronation due to soft heel counter exerts torsion on tendon.

Tenderness over tendon. Swelling may or may not be present.

Bursitis

Retrocalcaneal bursa

Achilles' tendon

Palpating for tenderness in front of Achilles' tendon

Tendonitis of the calcaneal (Achilles') tendon is a painful inflammation that often occurs in runners who run on hills or uneven surfaces. Repetitive stress on the tendon occurs as the heel strikes the ground and when plantarflexion lifts the foot and toes. Tendon rupture is a serious injury, as the avascular tendon heals slowly. Retrocalcaneal bursitis, an inflammation of the subtendinous bursa between the overlying tendon and the calcaneus, presents as a tender area just anterior to the tendon attachment.

Ankle and Foot: Bones of the Ankle

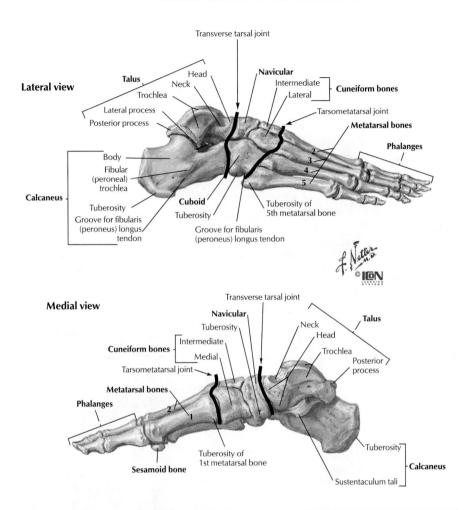

Transverse tarsal joint

Lateral view

Talus
Head
Neck
Trochlea
Lateral process
Posterior process

Navicular
Intermediate
Lateral } **Cuneiform bones**

Tarsometatarsal joint
Metatarsal bones

Phalanges

Body
Fibular (peroneal) trochlea
Calcaneus
Tuberosity
Groove for fibularis (peroneus) longus tendon

Cuboid
Tuberosity

Groove for fibularis (peroneus) longus tendon

Tuberosity of 5th metatarsal bone

Medial view

Transverse tarsal joint

Navicular
Tuberosity
Intermediate
Medial

Neck
Head
Trochlea
Talus
Posterior process

Cuneiform bones {

Tarsometatarsal joint
Metatarsal bones
Phalanges

Sesamoid bone

Tuberosity of 1st metatarsal bone

Tuberosity } **Calcaneus**

Sustentaculum tali

FEATURE	CHARACTERISTICS
Talus (ankle bone)	Transfers weight from tibia to foot; no muscle attachment
Trochlea	Articulates with tibia and fibula
Head	Articulates with navicular bone
Calcaneus (heel bone)	Articulates with talus superiorly and cuboid anteriorly
Sustentaculum tali	Medial shelf that supports talar head
Navicular	Boat shaped, between talar head and three cuneiforms
Tuberosity	If large, can cause medial pain in tight-fitting shoe
Cuboid	Most lateral tarsal bone
Groove	For fibularis (peroneus) longus tendon
Cuneiform	Three wedge-shaped bones

Tarsal bones are in red type.

Ankle and Foot: Bones of the Foot

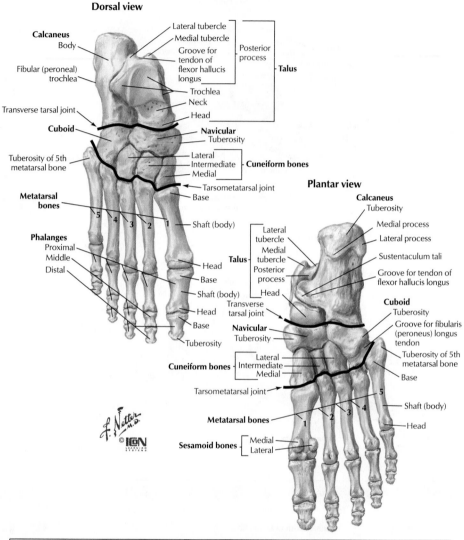

Dorsal view

Calcaneus
Body
Fibular (peroneal) trochlea
Transverse tarsal joint
Cuboid
Tuberosity of 5th metatarsal bone
Metatarsal bones
Phalanges
Proximal
Middle
Distal

Lateral tubercle
Medial tubercle
Groove for tendon of flexor hallucis longus
Posterior process
Talus
Trochlea
Neck
Head
Navicular
Tuberosity
Lateral
Intermediate
Medial
Cuneiform bones
Tarsometatarsal joint
Base
Shaft (body)
5 4 3 2 1
Head
Base
Shaft (body)
Head
Base
Tuberosity

Plantar view

Calcaneus
Tuberosity
Medial process
Lateral process
Sustentaculum tali
Groove for tendon of flexor hallucis longus
Cuboid
Tuberosity
Groove for fibularis (peroneus) longus tendon
Tuberosity of 5th metatarsal bone
Base
Shaft (body)
Head

Talus
Lateral tubercle
Medial tubercle
Posterior process
Head
Transverse tarsal joint
Navicular
Tuberosity
Cuneiform bones
Lateral
Intermediate
Medial
Tarsometatarsal joint
Metatarsal bones
5 4 3 2 1
Sesamoid bones
Medial
Lateral

FEATURE	CHARACTERISTICS
Metatarsals	
Numbered 1-5, from great toe (big toe) to little toe	Possess base, shaft, and head Fibularis brevis tendon inserts on fifth metatarsal
Two sesamoid bones	Associated with flexor hallucis brevis tendons
Phalanges	
Three for each digit except great toe	Possess base, shaft, and head Termed proximal, middle, and distal Stubbed fifth toe common injury

Ankle and Foot: Tendon Sheaths of the Ankle

Synovial sheaths provide protection and lubrication for muscle tendons passing from the leg into the foot. Various fibrous bands (retinacula) tether tendons at the ankle:

Flexor retinaculum: medial malleolus to calcaneus (plantar flexor tendons)
Extensor retinaculum: superior and inferior bands (dorsiflexor tendons)
Fibular retinacula: superior and inferior bands (fibularis tendons of lateral compartment)

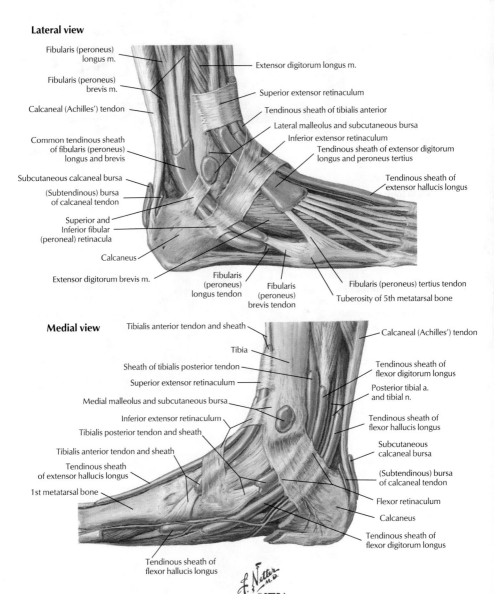

Lateral view

Fibularis (peroneus) longus m.

Fibularis (peroneus) brevis m.

Calcaneal (Achilles') tendon

Common tendinous sheath of fibularis (peroneus) longus and brevis

Subcutaneous calcaneal bursa

(Subtendinous) bursa of calcaneal tendon

Superior and Inferior fibular (peroneal) retinacula

Calcaneus

Extensor digitorum brevis m.

Fibularis (peroneus) longus tendon

Fibularis (peroneus) brevis tendon

Extensor digitorum longus m.

Superior extensor retinaculum

Tendinous sheath of tibialis anterior

Lateral malleolus and subcutaneous bursa

Inferior extensor retinaculum

Tendinous sheath of extensor digitorum longus and peroneus tertius

Tendinous sheath of extensor hallucis longus

Fibularis (peroneus) tertius tendon

Tuberosity of 5th metatarsal bone

Medial view

Tibialis anterior tendon and sheath

Tibia

Sheath of tibialis posterior tendon

Superior extensor retinaculum

Medial malleolus and subcutaneous bursa

Inferior extensor retinaculum

Tibialis posterior tendon and sheath

Tibialis anterior tendon and sheath

Tendinous sheath of extensor hallucis longus

1st metatarsal bone

Tendinous sheath of flexor hallucis longus

Calcaneal (Achilles') tendon

Tendinous sheath of flexor digitorum longus

Posterior tibial a. and tibial n.

Tendinous sheath of flexor hallucis longus

Subcutaneous calcaneal bursa

(Subtendinous) bursa of calcaneal tendon

Flexor retinaculum

Calcaneus

Tendinous sheath of flexor digitorum longus

Ankle and Foot: Ankle Joints and Ligaments

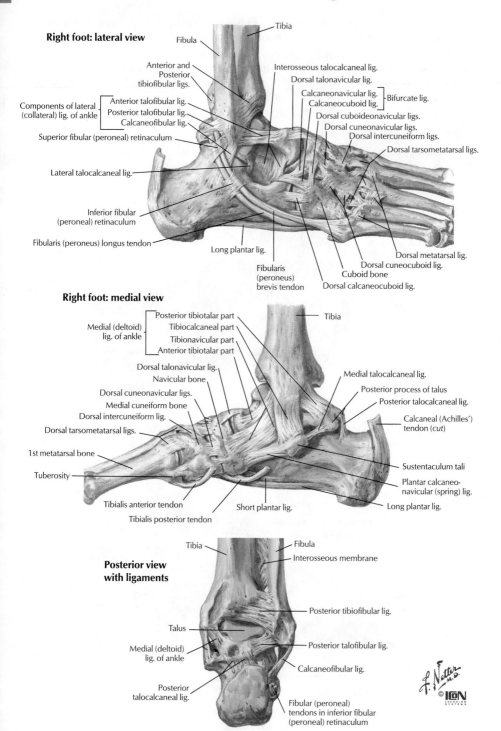

Right foot: lateral view

Tibia
Fibula
Anterior and Posterior tibiofibular ligs.
Interosseous talocalcaneal lig.
Dorsal talonavicular lig.
Calcaneonavicular lig.
Calcaneocuboid lig. — Bifurcate lig.
Components of lateral (collateral) lig. of ankle:
Anterior talofibular lig.
Posterior talofibular lig.
Calcaneofibular lig.
Dorsal cuboideonavicular ligs.
Dorsal cuneonavicular ligs.
Dorsal intercuneiform ligs.
Superior fibular (peroneal) retinaculum
Dorsal tarsometatarsal ligs.
Lateral talocalcaneal lig.
Inferior fibular (peroneal) retinaculum
Dorsal metatarsal lig.
Fibularis (peroneus) longus tendon
Dorsal cuneocuboid lig.
Cuboid bone
Long plantar lig.
Fibularis (peroneus) brevis tendon
Dorsal calcaneocuboid lig.

Right foot: medial view

Medial (deltoid) lig. of ankle:
Posterior tibiotalar part
Tibiocalcaneal part
Tibionavicular part
Anterior tibiotalar part
Tibia
Dorsal talonavicular lig.
Navicular bone
Medial talocalcaneal lig.
Posterior process of talus
Posterior talocalcaneal lig.
Dorsal cuneonavicular ligs.
Medial cuneiform bone
Dorsal intercuneiform lig.
Dorsal tarsometatarsal ligs.
Calcaneal (Achilles') tendon (cut)
1st metatarsal bone
Sustentaculum tali
Tuberosity
Plantar calcaneonavicular (spring) lig.
Tibialis anterior tendon
Short plantar lig.
Long plantar lig.
Tibialis posterior tendon

Posterior view with ligaments

Tibia
Fibula
Interosseous membrane
Posterior tibiofibular lig.
Talus
Posterior talofibular lig.
Medial (deltoid) lig. of ankle
Calcaneofibular lig.
Posterior talocalcaneal lig.
Fibular (peroneal) tendons in inferior fibular (peroneal) retinaculum

Ankle and Foot: Ankle Joints and Ligaments (continued)

LIGAMENT	ATTACHMENT	COMMENT
Distal Tibiofibular (Fibrous [Syndesmosis]) Joint		
Anterior tibiofibular	Anterior distal tibia and fibula	Runs obliquely
Posterior tibiofibular	Posterior distal tibia and fibula	Is weaker than anterior ligament
Inferior transverse	Medial malleolus to fibula	Is deep continuation of posterior ligament
Talocrural (Uniaxial Synovial Hinge [Ginglymus]) Joint		
Capsule	Tibia to talus	Functions in plantarflexion and dorsiflexion
Medial (deltoid)	Medial malleolus to talus, calcaneus, and navicular	Limits eversion of foot; maintains medial long arch; has four parts
Lateral (collateral)	Lateral malleolus to talus and calcaneus	Is weak and often sprained; resists inversion of foot; has three parts
INTERTARSAL JOINTS *Talocalcaneal (Subtalar Plane Synovial) Joints*		
Capsule	Margins of articulation	Functions in inversion and eversion
Talocalcaneal	Talus to calcaneus	Has medial, lateral, and posterior parts
Interosseous talocalcaneal	Talus to calcaneus	Is strong; binds bones together
Talocalcaneonavicular (Partial Ball-and-Socket Synovial) Joint		
Capsule	Encloses part of joint	Functions in gliding and rotational movements
Plantar calcaneonavicular	Sustentaculum tali to navicular	Is strong plantar support for head of talus (called spring ligament)
Dorsal talonavicular	Talus to navicular	Is dorsal support to talus
Calcaneocuboid (Plane Synovial) Joint		
Capsule	Encloses joint	Functions in inversion and eversion
Calcaneocuboid	Calcaneus to cuboid	Are dorsal, plantar (short plantar, strong), and long plantar ligaments

Cuboideonavicular, cuneonavicular, intercuneiform, and cuneocuboid joints: dorsal, plantar, and interosseous ligaments are present, but little movement occurs at these joints, and they have little clinical significance.

Ankle and Foot: Foot Joints and Ligaments

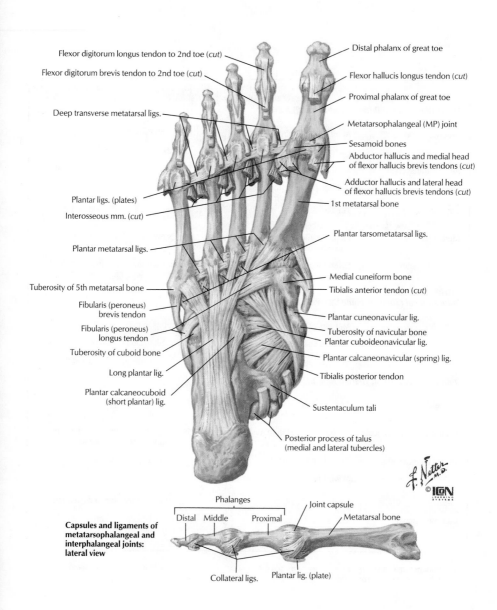

Flexor digitorum longus tendon to 2nd toe (*cut*)

Flexor digitorum brevis tendon to 2nd toe (*cut*)

Deep transverse metatarsal ligs.

Plantar ligs. (plates)

Interosseous mm. (*cut*)

Plantar metatarsal ligs.

Tuberosity of 5th metatarsal bone

Fibularis (peroneus) brevis tendon

Fibularis (peroneus) longus tendon

Tuberosity of cuboid bone

Long plantar lig.

Plantar calcaneocuboid (short plantar) lig.

Distal phalanx of great toe

Flexor hallucis longus tendon (*cut*)

Proximal phalanx of great toe

Metatarsophalangeal (MP) joint

Sesamoid bones

Abductor hallucis and medial head of flexor hallucis brevis tendons (*cut*)

Adductor hallucis and lateral head of flexor hallucis brevis tendons (*cut*)

1st metatarsal bone

Plantar tarsometatarsal ligs.

Medial cuneiform bone

Tibialis anterior tendon (*cut*)

Plantar cuneonavicular lig.

Tuberosity of navicular bone
Plantar cuboideonavicular lig.

Plantar calcaneonavicular (spring) lig.

Tibialis posterior tendon

Sustentaculum tali

Posterior process of talus (medial and lateral tubercles)

Phalanges

Joint capsule

Metatarsal bone

Distal   Middle   Proximal

Capsules and ligaments of metatarsophalangeal and interphalangeal joints: lateral view

Collateral ligs.   Plantar lig. (plate)

Ankle and Foot: Foot Joints and Ligaments (continued)

LIGAMENT	ATTACHMENT	COMMENT
Tarsometatarsal (Plane Synovial) Joints		
Capsule	Encloses joint	Functions in gliding or sliding movements
Tarsometatarsal	Tarsals to metatarsals	Are dorsal, plantar, interosseous ligaments
Intermetatarsal (Plane		
Capsule	Base of metatarsals	Provides little movement, supports transverse arch
Intermetatarsal	Adjacent metatarsals	Are dorsal, plantar, interosseous ligaments
Deep transverse	Adjacent metatarsals	Connect adjacent heads
Metatarsophalangeal (Multiaxial Condyloid Synovial) Joints		
Capsule	Encloses joint	Functions in flexion, extension, some abduction and adduction, and circumduction
Collateral	Metatarsal heads to base of proximal phalanges	Are strong ligaments
Plantar (plates)	Plantar side of capsule	Are part of weight-bearing surface
Interphalangeal (Uniaxial Hinge Synovial) Joints		
Capsule	Encloses each joint	Functions in flexion and extension
Collateral	Head of one to base of other	Support the capsule
Plantar (plates)	Plantar side of capsule	Support the capsule

Clinical Correlation

Classification of Ankle Fractures   *Anatomy on pp. 260, 262*

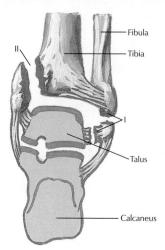

Fibula
Tibia

II

I

Talus

Calcaneus

Supination-adduction (SA)

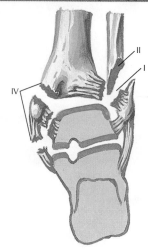

II

IV
I

Supination-external rotation (SER)

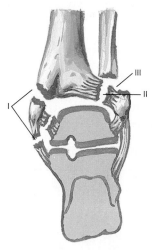

III

II

I

Pronation-abduction (PA)

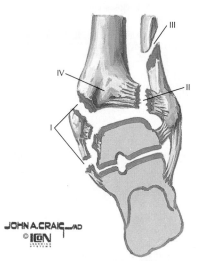

III

IV
II

I

JOHN A.CRAIG—AD
©ICN

Pronation-external rotation (PER)

Ankle fractures are common in all age groups. Ankle fractures may be grouped according to the Lauge-Hansen classification into four types with subdivided stages:
- **Supination-adduction (SA)**: stages I and II; usually stable
- **Supination-external rotation (SER)**: stages I-IV; usually unstable or displaced
- **Pronation-abduction (PA)**: stages I-III; perfect symmetrical mortise reduction needed
- **Pronation-external rotation (PER)**: stages I-IV; must also correct fibular length

Clinical Correlation

Rotational Fractures

Anatomy on pp. 246, 260-263

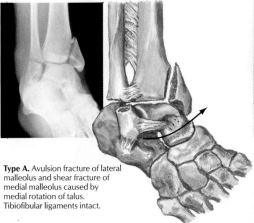

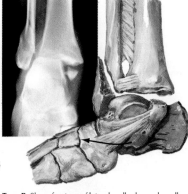

Type A. Avulsion fracture of lateral malleolus and shear fracture of medial malleolus caused by medial rotation of talus. Tibiofibular ligaments intact.

Type B. Shear fracture of lateral malleolus and small avulsion fracture of medial malleolus caused by lateral rotation of talus. Tibiofibular ligaments intact or only partially torn.

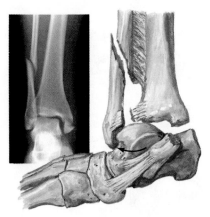

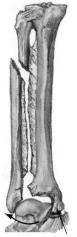

Maisonneuve fracture. Complete disruption of tibiofibular syndesmosis with diastasis caused by external rotation of talus and transmission of force to proximal fibula, resulting in high fracture of fibula. Interosseous membrane torn longitudinally.

Torn deltoid lig.

Type C. Disruption of tibiofibular ligaments with diastasis of syndesmosis caused by external rotation of talus. Force transmitted to fibula results in oblique fracture at higher level. In this case, avulsion of medial malleolus has also occurred.

Most ankle injuries are caused by twisting, so that the talus rotates in the frontal plane and impinges on either the lateral or medial malleolus, which causes it to fracture and places tension on supporting ligaments of the opposite side. Three types are recognized:

A: medial rotation of the talus

B: lateral rotation of the talus

C: injury extends proximally, with tibiofibular ligament and interosseous membrane being torn (a variant is the Maisonneuve fracture)

Clinical Correlation

Fractures of the Calcaneus
Anatomy on pp. 259, 260, 262

Extraarticular fracture of calcaneus

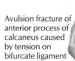
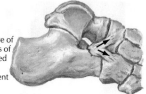
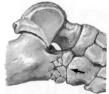

Avulsion fracture of anterior process of calcaneus caused by tension on bifurcate ligament

Comminuted fracture of anterior process of calcaneus due to compression by cuboid in forceful abduction of forefoot

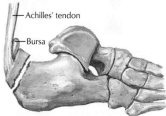

Achilles' tendon

Bursa

Avulsion fracture of tuberosity of calcaneus due to sudden, violent contraction of Achilles' tendon

Fracture of medial process of tuberosity of calcaneus

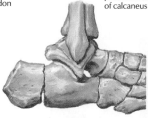

Fracture of sustentaculum tali

Fracture of body of calcaneus with no involvement of subtalar articulation

Intraarticular fracture of calcaneus

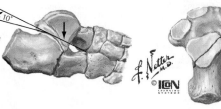

Primary fracture line
Talus driven down into calcaneus, usually by fall and landing on heel

Primary fracture line runs across posterior facet, forming anteromedial and posterolateral fragments.

Calcaneal fractures (the most common tarsal fracture) are extraarticular or intraarticular. Extraarticular fractures include

- Anterior process fracture (stress on bifurcate ligament caused by landing on an adducted, plantar-flexed foot)
- Avulsion fracture of the calcaneal tuberosity (sudden, forceful contraction of gastrocnemius and soleus muscles)
- Fracture of the sustentaculum tali (jumping and landing on an inverted foot)
- Fracture of the body (jumping and landing on a heel)

However, approximately 75% of all calcaneal fractures are intraarticular (forceful landing on a heel); the talus is driven down into the calcaneus, which cannot withstand the force because it is cancellous bone.

Clinical Correlation

Fractures of the Talar Neck   *Anatomy on pp. 259, 260, 262, 278*

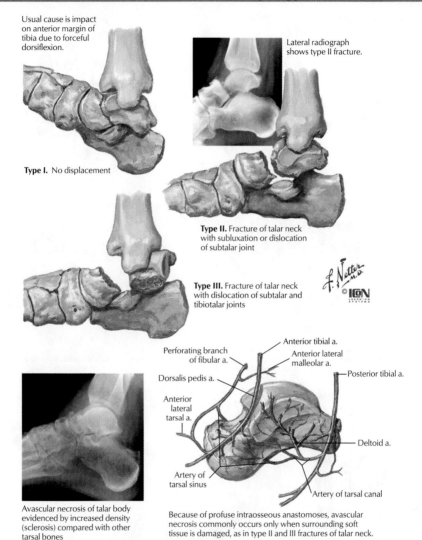

Usual cause is impact on anterior margin of tibia due to forceful dorsiflexion.

Type I. No displacement

Lateral radiograph shows type II fracture.

Type II. Fracture of talar neck with subluxation or dislocation of subtalar joint

Type III. Fracture of talar neck with dislocation of subtalar and tibiotalar joints

Perforating branch of fibular a.

Anterior tibial a.

Anterior lateral malleolar a.

Dorsalis pedis a.

Posterior tibial a.

Anterior lateral tarsal a.

Deltoid a.

Artery of tarsal sinus

Artery of tarsal canal

Avascular necrosis of talar body evidenced by increased density (sclerosis) compared with other tarsal bones

Because of profuse intraosseous anastomoses, avascular necrosis commonly occurs only when surrounding soft tissue is damaged, as in type II and III fractures of talar neck.

The talar neck is the most common site for fractures of this tarsal. Injury usually results from direct trauma or landing on the foot after a fall from a great height. The foot is hyperdorsiflexed so that the neck impinges on the distal tibia. The three types of fractures are

I: nondisplaced

II: neck fracture with subluxation or dislocation of the subtalar joint

III: neck fracture with dislocation of the subtalar and tibiotalar joints

These fractures can lead to avascular necrosis of the talus body because most of the blood supply to the talus passes through the talar neck.

Clinical Correlation

Metatarsal and Phalangeal Injuries   *Anatomy on pp. 260, 262, 264*

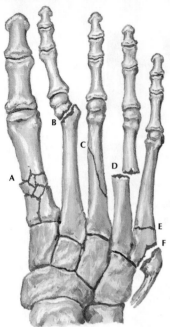

Types of fractures of metatarsal: A. comminuted fracture, B. displaced neck fracture, C. oblique fracture, D. displaced transverse fracture, E. fracture of base of 5th metatarsal, F. avulsion of tuberosity of 5th metatarsal

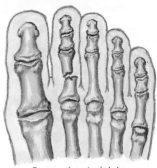

Fracture of proximal phalanx

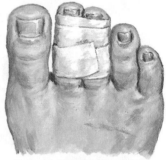

Fracture of phalanx splinted by taping to adjacent toe (buddy taping)

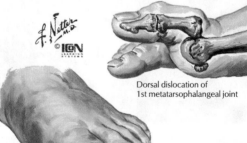

Dorsal dislocation of 1st metatarsophalangeal joint

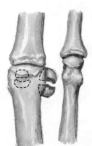

Fracture of sesamoid bones (must be differentiated from congenital bipartite sesamoid bones)

Crush injury of great toe

Direct trauma to the foot can result in fractures of the metatarsals and phalanges. These fractures can usually be treated with immobilization, because the fragments are often not displaced. Avulsion fractures of the fifth metatarsal are common to this bone and occur as a result of stresses placed on the fibularis brevis tendon during muscle contraction. Dislocation of the first metatarsal is common in athletes and ballet dancers because of repeated hyperdorsiflexion.

Ankle and Foot: Muscles of the Dorsum of the Foot

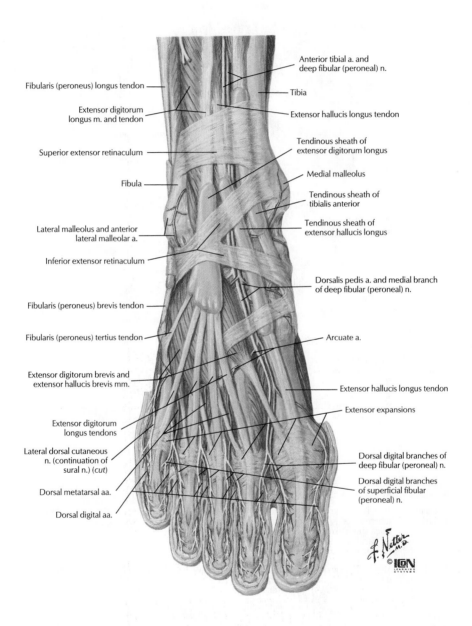

Fibularis (peroneus) longus tendon

Extensor digitorum longus m. and tendon

Superior extensor retinaculum

Fibula

Lateral malleolus and anterior lateral malleolar a.

Inferior extensor retinaculum

Fibularis (peroneus) brevis tendon

Fibularis (peroneus) tertius tendon

Extensor digitorum brevis and extensor hallucis brevis mm.

Extensor digitorum longus tendons

Lateral dorsal cutaneous n. (continuation of sural n.) (cut)

Dorsal metatarsal aa.

Dorsal digital aa.

Anterior tibial a. and deep fibular (peroneal) n.

Tibia

Extensor hallucis longus tendon

Tendinous sheath of extensor digitorum longus

Medial malleolus

Tendinous sheath of tibialis anterior

Tendinous sheath of extensor hallucis longus

Dorsalis pedis a. and medial branch of deep fibular (peroneal) n.

Arcuate a.

Extensor hallucis longus tendon

Extensor expansions

Dorsal digital branches of deep fibular (peroneal) n.

Dorsal digital branches of superficial fibular (peroneal) n.

Ankle and Foot: Muscles of the Sole (First Layer)

Superficial dissection

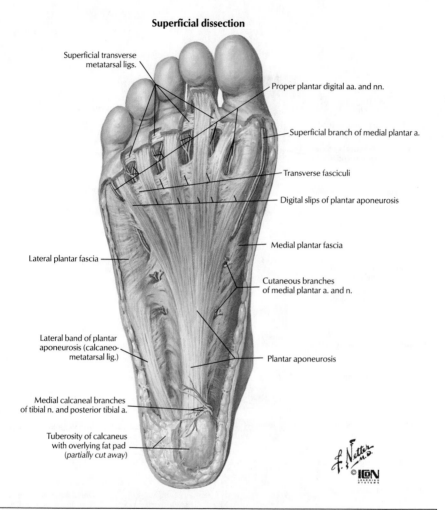

Superficial transverse metatarsal ligs.

Proper plantar digital aa. and nn.

Superficial branch of medial plantar a.

Transverse fasciculi

Digital slips of plantar aponeurosis

Medial plantar fascia

Lateral plantar fascia

Cutaneous branches of medial plantar a. and n.

Lateral band of plantar aponeurosis (calcaneo-metatarsal lig.)

Plantar aponeurosis

Medial calcaneal branches of tibial n. and posterior tibial a.

Tuberosity of calcaneus with overlying fat pad (*partially cut away*)

MUSCLE	PROXIMAL ATTACHMENT (ORIGIN)	DISTAL ATTACHMENT (INSERTION)	INNERVATION	MAIN ACTIONS
Abductor hallucis	Medial tubercle of tuberosity of calcaneus, flexor retinaculum, and plantar aponeurosis	Medial side of base of proximal phalanx of first digit	Medial plantar nerve	Abducts and flexes great toe
Flexor digitorum brevis	Medial tubercle of tuberosity of calcaneus, plantar aponeurosis, and intermuscular septa	Both sides of middle phalanges of lateral four digits	Medial plantar nerve	Flexes lateral four digits
Abductor digiti minimi	Medial and lateral tubercles of tuberosity of calcaneus, plantar aponeurosis, and intermuscular septa	Lateral side of base of proximal phalanx of fifth digit	Lateral plantar nerve	Abducts and flexes little toe

Ankle and Foot: Muscles of the Sole (First Layer) (continued)

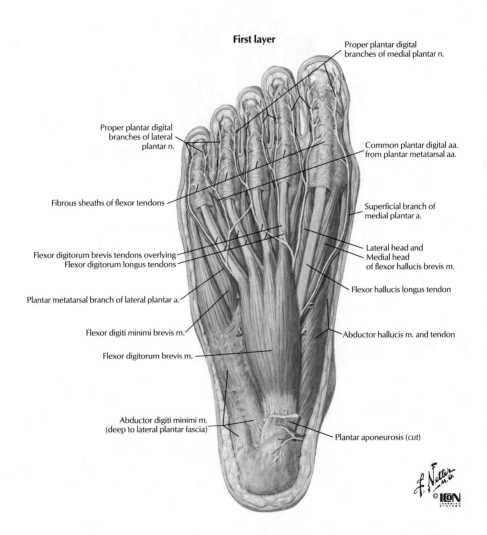

First layer

Proper plantar digital branches of medial plantar n.

Proper plantar digital branches of lateral plantar n.

Common plantar digital aa. from plantar metatarsal aa.

Fibrous sheaths of flexor tendons

Superficial branch of medial plantar a.

Flexor digitorum brevis tendons overlying Flexor digitorum longus tendons

Lateral head and Medial head of flexor hallucis brevis m.

Flexor hallucis longus tendon

Plantar metatarsal branch of lateral plantar a.

Flexor digiti minimi brevis m.

Abductor hallucis m. and tendon

Flexor digitorum brevis m.

Abductor digiti minimi m. (deep to lateral plantar fascia)

Plantar aponeurosis (*cut*)

Ankle and Foot: Muscles of the Sole (Second and Third Layers)

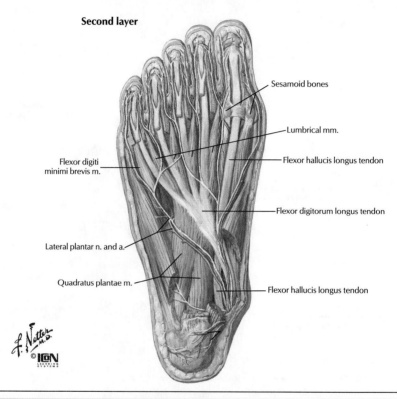

Second layer

Sesamoid bones

Lumbrical mm.

Flexor digiti minimi brevis m.

Flexor hallucis longus tendon

Flexor digitorum longus tendon

Lateral plantar n. and a.

Quadratus plantae m.

Flexor hallucis longus tendon

MUSCLE	PROXIMAL ATTACHMENT (ORIGIN)	DISTAL ATTACHMENT (INSERTION)	INNERVATION	MAIN ACTIONS
Quadratus plantae	Medial surface and lateral margin of plantar surface of calcaneus	Posterolateral margin of tendon of flexor digitorum longus	Lateral plantar nerve	Assist flexor digitorum longus in flexing lateral four digits
Lumbricals	Tendons of flexor digitorum longus	Medial aspect of expansion over lateral four digits	*Medial one*: medial plantar nerve *Lateral three*: lateral plantar nerve	Flex proximal phalanges and extend middle and distal phalanges of lateral four digits
Flexor hallucis brevis	Plantar surfaces of cuboid and lateral cuneiforms	Both sides of base of proximal phalanx of first digit	Medial plantar nerve	Flexes proximal phalanx of great toe
Adductor hallucis	*Oblique head*: bases of metatarsals 2-4 *Transverse head*: plantar ligaments of metatarsophalangeal joints	Tendons of both heads attach to lateral side of base of proximal phalanx of first digit	Deep branch of lateral plantar nerve	Adducts great toe; assists in maintaining transverse arch of foot
Flexor digiti minimi brevis	Base of fifth metatarsal	Base of proximal phalanx of fifth digit	Superficial branch of lateral plantar nerve	Flexes proximal phalanx of little toe, thereby assisting with its flexion

Ankle and Foot: Muscles of the Sole (Second and Third Layers) (continued)

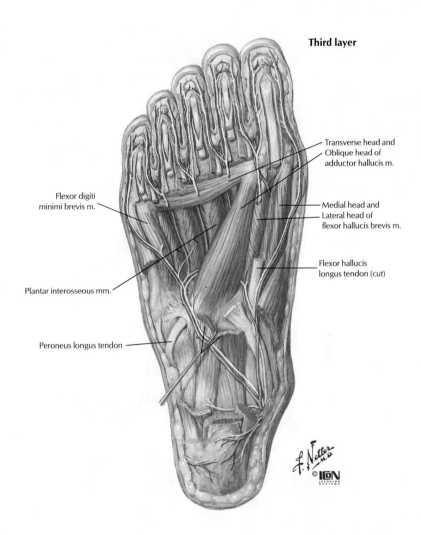

Third layer

Transverse head and
Oblique head of
adductor hallucis m.

Flexor digiti
minimi brevis m.

Medial head and
Lateral head of
flexor hallucis brevis m.

Flexor hallucis
longus tendon (cut)

Plantar interosseous mm.

Peroneus longus tendon

Ankle and Foot: Deep Muscles and Arteries of Foot

Arteries of the dorsal foot are branches of the dorsalis pedis artery (from the anterior tibial), which divides into the
- Medial and lateral tarsal arteries
- Arcuate artery
- Deep plantar artery
- Dorsal metatarsal arteries
- Dorsal digital arteries

MUSCLE	PROXIMAL ATTACHMENT (ORIGIN)	DISTAL ATTACHMENT (INSERTION)	INNERVATION	MAIN ACTIONS
Plantar interossei (three muscles)	Bases and medial sides of metatarsals 3-5	Medial sides of bases of proximal phalanges of digits 3-5	Lateral plantar nerve	Adduct digits (2-4) and flex metatarsophalangeal joints
Dorsal interossei (four muscles)	Adjacent sides of metatarsals 1-5	*First*: medial side of proximal phalanx of second digit *Second to fourth*: lateral sides of digits 2-4	Lateral plantar nerve	Abduct digits and flex metatarsophalangeal joints

Dorsal view

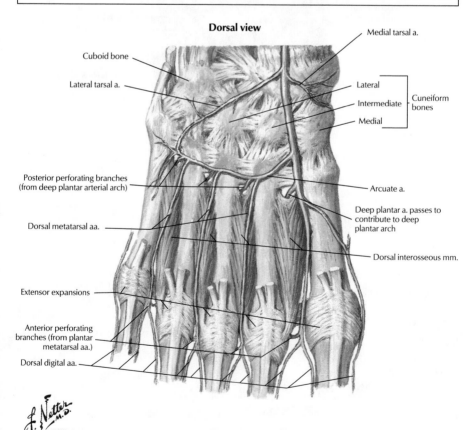

Cuboid bone

Lateral tarsal a.

Posterior perforating branches (from deep plantar arterial arch)

Dorsal metatarsal aa.

Extensor expansions

Anterior perforating branches (from plantar metatarsal aa.)

Dorsal digital aa.

Medial tarsal a.

Lateral
Intermediate   Cuneiform bones
Medial

Arcuate a.

Deep plantar a. passes to contribute to deep plantar arch

Dorsal interosseous mm.

Ankle and Foot: Deep Muscles and Arteries of Foot (continued)

Plantar view

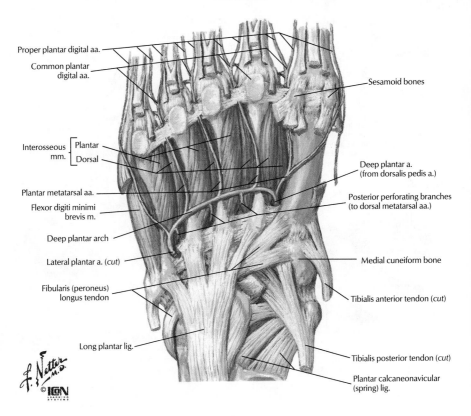

Proper plantar digital aa.

Common plantar digital aa.

Interosseous mm. — Plantar / Dorsal

Plantar metatarsal aa.

Flexor digiti minimi brevis m.

Deep plantar arch

Lateral plantar a. (*cut*)

Fibularis (peroneus) longus tendon

Long plantar lig.

Sesamoid bones

Deep plantar a. (from dorsalis pedis a.)

Posterior perforating branches (to dorsal metatarsal aa.)

Medial cuneiform bone

Tibialis anterior tendon (*cut*)

Tibialis posterior tendon (*cut*)

Plantar calcaneonavicular (spring) lig.

Ankle and Foot: Arteries and Nerves of the Sole

The arteries of the plantar surface of the foot (sole) are continuations of the posterior tibial artery of the leg and give rise to medial and lateral plantar arteries. The medial plantar artery divides into superficial and deep branches; the lateral plantar artery forms the deep plantar arch and anastomoses with the deep plantar from the dorsum of the foot. From the deep plantar arch arise the four plantar metatarsal arteries and their common digital branches. The medial and lateral plantar nerves innervate the sole and arise from the tibial nerve.

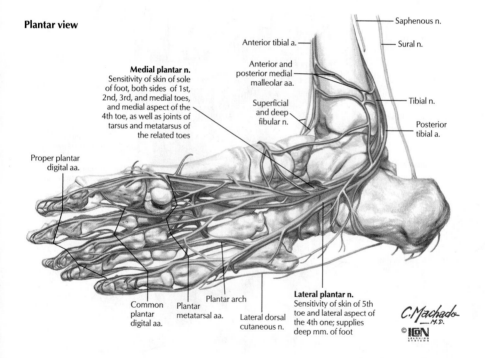

Plantar view

Saphenous n.

Anterior tibial a.

Sural n.

Medial plantar n.
Sensitivity of skin of sole of foot, both sides of 1st, 2nd, 3rd, and medial toes, and medial aspect of the 4th toe, as well as joints of tarsus and metatarsus of the related toes

Anterior and posterior medial malleolar aa.

Superficial and deep fibular n.

Tibial n.

Posterior tibial a.

Proper plantar digital aa.

Common plantar digital aa.

Plantar metatarsal aa.

Plantar arch

Lateral dorsal cutaneous n.

Lateral plantar n.
Sensitivity of skin of 5th toe and lateral aspect of the 4th one; supplies deep mm. of foot

C. Machado
—M.D.

© ICN

Clinical Correlation

Congenital Club Foot

Anatomy on pp. 250, 262, 271

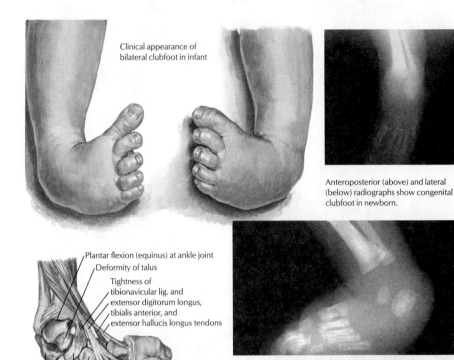

Clinical appearance of
bilateral clubfoot in infant

Anteroposterior (above) and lateral
(below) radiographs show congenital
clubfoot in newborn.

Plantar flexion (equinus) at ankle joint
Deformity of talus
Tightness of
tibionavicular lig. and
extensor digitorum longus,
tibialis anterior, and
extensor hallucis longus tendons

Inversion of
calcaneus

Extreme varus position
of forefoot bones

Lateral radiograph
demonstrates
severe clubfoot
complicated by
extreme plantar
flexion of forefoot
in newborn.

Congenital club foot (congenital equinovarus) is a structural defect in which the entire foot is plantar-flexed (equinus) and the hindfoot and forefoot are inverted (varus). This deformity has a strong genetic link; males are more frequently affected, but females often have a more severe deformity. The bones not only are misaligned with each other but also may have an abnormal shape and size. Thus, after correction, the true club foot is smaller than normal. Management may be conservative or may require splinting or casting or even surgery.

Clinical Correlation

Toe Deformities
Anatomy on pp. 260, 273

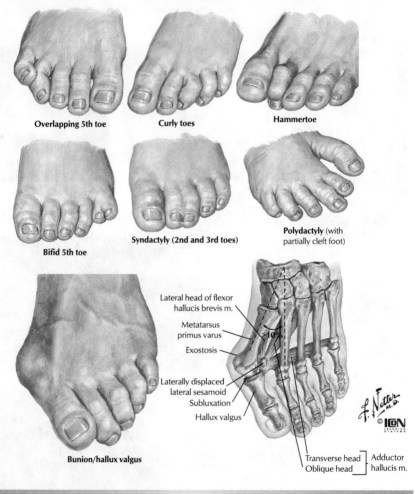

Overlapping 5th toe

Curly toes

Hammertoe

Bifid 5th toe

Syndactyly (2nd and 3rd toes)

Polydactyly (with partially cleft foot)

Lateral head of flexor hallucis brevis m.

Metatarsus primus varus

Exostosis

Laterally displaced lateral sesamoid

Subluxation

Hallux valgus

Bunion/hallux valgus

Transverse head ⎤ Adductor
Oblique head ⎦ hallucis m.

DEFECT	COMMENT
Overlapping fifth toe	Common familial deformity
Curly toes	Familial deformity, usually from hypoplasia or absence of intrinsic muscles of affected toes
Hammer toe	Proximal interphalangeal joint flexion deformity associated with poorly fitting shoes
Bifid fifth toe	May share common phalanx
Syndactyly	Web deformity (also occurs in the hand)
Cleft foot	Often associated with cleft hand, lip, and palate
Hallux valgus	Bunion, often in women from wearing narrow shoes
Turf toe	Hyperextension of great toe, common in football players (not shown)

Clinical Correlation

Plantar Fasciitis   *Anatomy on pp. 262, 264, 272*

Heel spur syndrome

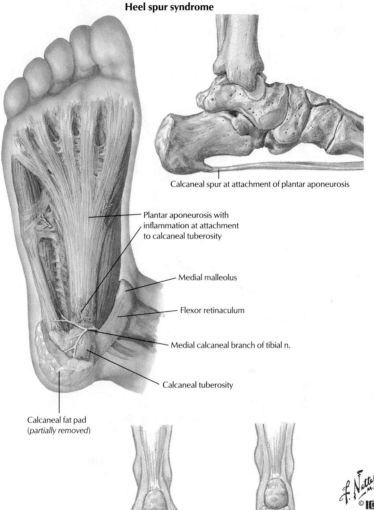

Calcaneal spur at attachment of plantar aponeurosis

Plantar aponeurosis with inflammation at attachment to calcaneal tuberosity

Medial malleolus

Flexor retinaculum

Medial calcaneal branch of tibial n.

Calcaneal tuberosity

Calcaneal fat pad (*partially removed*)

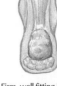

Loose-fitting heel counter in running shoe allows calcaneal fat pad to spread at heel strike, increasing transmission of impact to heel.

Firm, well-fitting heel counter maintains compactness of fat pad, which buffers force of impact.

Plantar fasciitis (heel spur syndrome) is a common cause of heel pain, especially in joggers, and results from inflammation of plantar aponeurosis (fascia) at its point of attachment to the calcaneus. A bony spur may develop with this condition, but the inflammation causes most of the pain, which is mediated by the medial calcaneal branch of the tibial nerve.

Clinical Correlation

Common Foot Infections
Anatomy on pp. 204, 271

Ingrown toenail

Area of excision

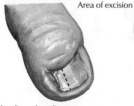

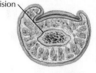

En bloc excision includes nail matrix.

Broken lines show lines of incision for excision of lateral ¹/₄ of toenail, nail bed, and matrix.

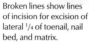

After excision, wound allowed to granulate

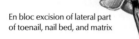

En bloc excision of lateral part of toenail, nail bed, and matrix

D. Mascaro
© ICN

Pain and swelling due to deep infection of central plantar space

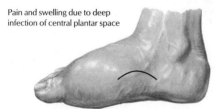

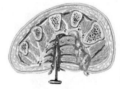

Puncture wound or perforating ulcer may penetrate deep central plantar spaces, leading to abscess.

Incision site for drainage of central plantar spaces

Distal and lateral subungual onychomycosis (DLSO)

DLSO may be found with tinea pedis.

C. Machado
_M.D._
© ICN

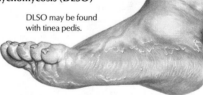

DLSO due to *Trichophyton rubrum*

Additional clinical features of DLSO

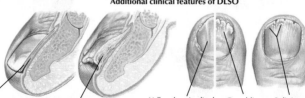

Onycholysis (detachment of the nail from its bed)

Subungual hyperkeratosis

Yellow longitudinal spikes

Crumbling

Splitting

CONDITION	COMMENT
Ingrown toenail	Usually great toe, medial or lateral aspect; can lead to an inflamed area that becomes secondarily infected
Onychomycosis	Fungal nail infection, which makes a toenail thick and brittle
Puncture wound	Common injury; can lead to deep infection; requires check of tetanus status

Clinical Correlation

Diabetic Foot Lesions
Anatomy on pp. 271, 274-278

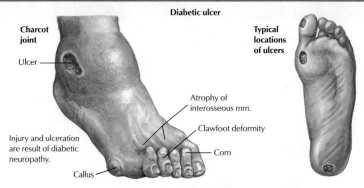

Diabetic ulcer

Charcot joint

Ulcer

Injury and ulceration are result of diabetic neuropathy.

Callus

Atrophy of interosseous mm.

Clawfoot deformity

Corn

Typical locations of ulcers

Infection

Cross section through forefoot shows abscess in central plantar space. Infection due to impaired immune response, skin defects, and poor perfusion.

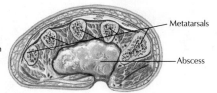

Metatarsals

Abscess

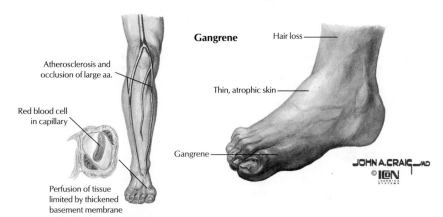

Gangrene   Hair loss

Atherosclerosis and occlusion of large aa.

Red blood cell in capillary

Thin, atrophic skin

Gangrene

Perfusion of tissue limited by thickened basement membrane

JOHN A.CRAIG—MD
©ICN

Diabetes mellitus (DM), a common complex metabolic disorder characterized by hyperglycemia, affects approximately 17 million people in the United States. The skin is one of many organ systems affected, especially skin of the leg and foot. Microvascular disease may result in decreased cutaneous blood flow, peripheral sensory neuropathy may render the skin susceptible to injury and may blunt healing, and hyperglycemia predisposes the extremity to increased occurrence of bacterial and fungal infections. Associated complications in the lower limb include Charcot joint (progressive destructive arthropathy caused by neuropathy), ulceration, infection, gangrene, and amputation. DM accounts for most of the nontraumatic foot and lower leg amputations, which total more than 80,000 per year.

Clinical Correlation

Neuropathy and Fungal Infections in the Diabetic Foot

Anatomy on pp. 271, 274-278, 290

Neuropathy

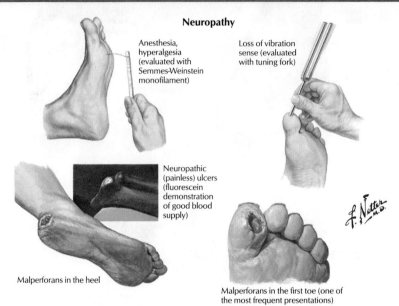

Anesthesia, hyperalgesia (evaluated with Semmes-Weinstein monofilament)

Loss of vibration sense (evaluated with tuning fork)

Neuropathic (painless) ulcers (fluorescein demonstration of good blood supply)

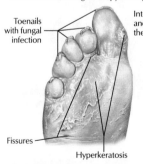

Malperforans in the heel

Malperforans in the first toe (one of the most frequent presentations)

Fungal infection

Fungal infections of the nails and skin are common in patients with diabetes. With foot involvement, accompanying minor skin lesions can be the portal of infection, which can result in chronic wounds and even amputations. Excellent foot care and antifungal therapy are important preventative measures in the setting of advanced diabetic neuropathy.

Toenails with fungal infection

Interdigital tinea pedis and fissures under the toes

Amputation, the most disabling consequence of diabetic neuropathy, results from deep infection, which develops in the setting of the "insensate foot."

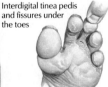

Toenail with fungal infection, showing sharp, irregular edges

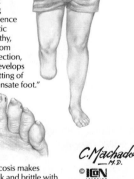

Fissures

Hyperkeratosis

Dysfunction of sweat glands, observed among patients with autonomic neuropathy, can cause local changes to the skin that can favor the occurrence of cracks, fissures, and ulcers that are potential portals of entry for bacteria.

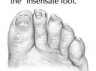

Onychomycosis makes toenails thick and brittle with sharp edges that can injure the skin on adjacent toes.

Peripheral neuropathy is common at distal sites such as the leg and foot and predispose patients to numbness or dysesthesias (burning or tingling sensations) that may lead to injury. Likewise, fungal infections of the toenails and skin often accompany other distal complications of DM.

Arterial Occlusive Disease
Anatomy on pp. 224, 247, 271

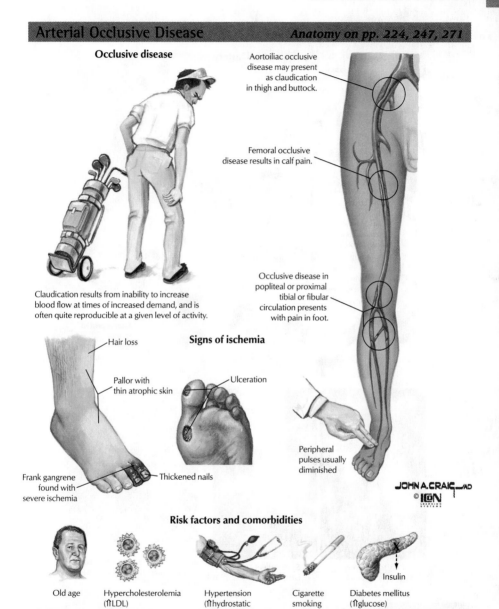

Occlusive disease

Aortoiliac occlusive disease may present as claudication in thigh and buttock.

Femoral occlusive disease results in calf pain.

Occlusive disease in popliteal or proximal tibial or fibular circulation presents with pain in foot.

Claudication results from inability to increase blood flow at times of increased demand, and is often quite reproducible at a given level of activity.

Signs of ischemia

Hair loss

Pallor with thin atrophic skin

Ulceration

Peripheral pulses usually diminished

Frank gangrene found with severe ischemia

Thickened nails

JOHN A. CRAIG—AD
©ICN

Risk factors and comorbidities

Old age

Hypercholesterolemia (⇑LDL)

Hypertension (⇑hydrostatic pressure)

Cigarette smoking

Diabetes mellitus (⇑glucose)

Insulin

Atherosclerosis can affect not only the coronary and cerebral vasculature but also the arteries that supply the kidneys, intestines, and lower limbs. The resulting arterial stenosis (narrowing) or occlusion in the leg leads to peripheral vascular disease (PVD), a disorder largely associated with increasing age. PVD produces symptoms of claudication, which should be a warning sign of atherosclerosis elsewhere that may produce myocardial infarction and stroke.

Clinical Correlation

Gout
Anatomy on pp. 259, 260

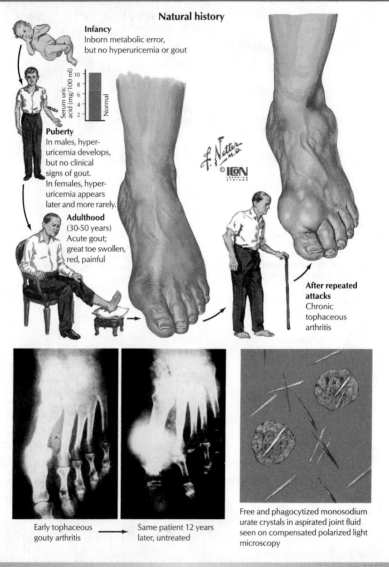

Natural history

Infancy
Inborn metabolic error, but no hyperuricemia or gout

Puberty
In males, hyperuricemia develops, but no clinical signs of gout. In females, hyperuricemia appears later and more rarely.

Adulthood
(30-50 years)
Acute gout; great toe swollen, red, painful

After repeated attacks
Chronic tophaceous arthritis

Early tophaceous gouty arthritis ⟶ Same patient 12 years later, untreated

Free and phagocytized monosodium urate crystals in aspirated joint fluid seen on compensated polarized light microscopy

Uric acid (ionized urate in plasma) is a by-product of purine metabolism and is largely eliminated from the body by renal secretion and excretion. An abnormally increased serum urate concentration may lead to gout. Gout is a disease caused by precipitation of sodium urate crystals within the joint synovial or tenosynovial spaces, which produces inflammation. Approximately 85-90% of clinical gout is caused by underexcretion of urate by kidneys and may be due to genetic or renal disease or diseases that affect renal function. Chronic gout presents with deforming arthritis that affects the hands, wrists, feet (especially the great toe), knees, and shoulders.

Nerve Summary: Femoral Nerve

The femoral nerve innervates muscles in the anterior compartment of the thigh, which are largely extensors of the leg at the knee. The patellar tendon reflex (L3-4) (knee extension) tests the integrity of this nerve. Major cutaneous branches include the separate lateral cutaneous nerve of the thigh and, from the femoral nerve directly, the
• Anterior cutaneous branches to the anterior thigh
• Saphenous nerve (terminal branch of femoral) to the medial knee, leg, and ankle

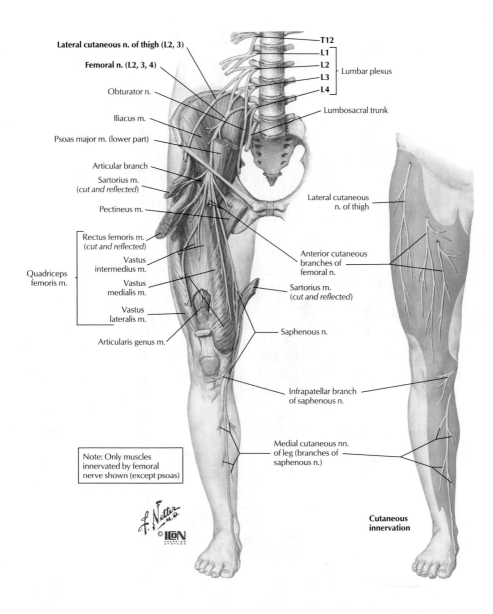

Lateral cutaneous n. of thigh (L2, 3)

Femoral n. (L2, 3, 4)

Obturator n.

Iliacus m.

Psoas major m. (lower part)

Articular branch

Sartorius m.
(cut and reflected)

Pectineus m.

Rectus femoris m.
(cut and reflected)

Vastus intermedius m.

Vastus medialis m.

Vastus lateralis m.

Articularis genus m.

Quadriceps femoris m.

T12
L1
L2
L3
L4

Lumbar plexus

Lumbosacral trunk

Lateral cutaneous n. of thigh

Anterior cutaneous branches of femoral n.

Sartorius m. (cut and reflected)

Saphenous n.

Infrapatellar branch of saphenous n.

Medial cutaneous nn. of leg (branches of saphenous n.)

Note: Only muscles innervated by femoral nerve shown (except psoas)

Cutaneous innervation

Nerve Summary: Obturator Nerve

The obturator nerve innervates muscles of the medial compartment of the thigh, which are largely adductors of the thigh at the hip. The nerve divides into superficial and deep branches on both sides of the obturator externus and adductor brevis muscles. A small field of cutaneous innervation exists on the medial thigh. Injury to this nerve usually occurs inside the pelvis and can lead to weakened adduction of the thigh.

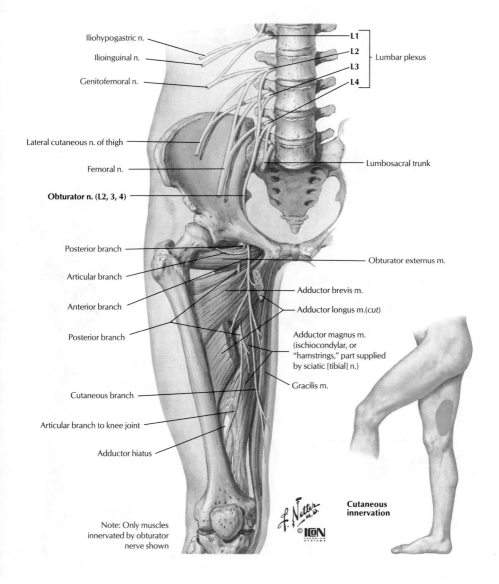

Iliohypogastric n.

Ilioinguinal n.

Genitofemoral n.

Lateral cutaneous n. of thigh

Femoral n.

Obturator n. (L2, 3, 4)

Posterior branch

Articular branch

Anterior branch

Posterior branch

Cutaneous branch

Articular branch to knee joint

Adductor hiatus

L1

L2

L3

L4

Lumbar plexus

Lumbosacral trunk

Obturator externus m.

Adductor brevis m.

Adductor longus m.(cut)

Adductor magnus m.
(ischiocondylar, or
"hamstrings," part supplied
by sciatic [tibial] n.)

Gracilis m.

Note: Only muscles
innervated by obturator
nerve shown

Cutaneous
innervation

Nerve Summary: Sciatic Nerve

The sciatic nerve is the largest nerve in the body and is composed of the tibial and common fibular (peroneal) nerves. The sciatic nerve innervates muscles of the posterior compartment of the thigh (tibial component), which are largely extensors of the thigh at the hip and flexors of the leg at the knee. It also innervates all muscles below the knee, via its tibial and common fibular components.

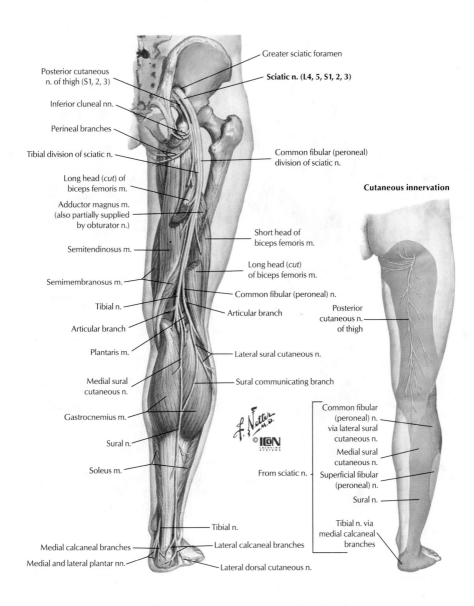

Posterior cutaneous n. of thigh (S1, 2, 3)

Inferior cluneal nn.

Perineal branches

Tibial division of sciatic n.

Long head (*cut*) of biceps femoris m.

Adductor magnus m. (also partially supplied by obturator n.)

Semitendinosus m.

Semimembranosus m.

Tibial n.

Articular branch

Plantaris m.

Medial sural cutaneous n.

Gastrocnemius m.

Sural n.

Soleus m.

Medial calcaneal branches

Medial and lateral plantar nn.

Greater sciatic foramen

Sciatic n. (L4, 5, S1, 2, 3)

Common fibular (peroneal) division of sciatic n.

Short head of biceps femoris m.

Long head (*cut*) of biceps femoris m.

Common fibular (peroneal) n.

Articular branch

Lateral sural cutaneous n.

Sural communicating branch

From sciatic n.

Tibial n.

Lateral calcaneal branches

Lateral dorsal cutaneous n.

Cutaneous innervation

Posterior cutaneous n. of thigh

Common fibular (peroneal) n. via lateral sural cutaneous n.

Medial sural cutaneous n.

Superficial fibular (peroneal) n.

Sural n.

Tibial n. via medial calcaneal branches

Nerve Summary: Tibial Nerve

The tibial nerve, the larger of the two components of the sciatic nerve, innervates muscles of the posterior compartment of the leg and all muscles of the plantar foot. These muscles are largely plantar flexors, some with inversion function as well. A lesion to this nerve may result in loss of plantarflexion and weakened inversion of the foot, and thus a shuffling gait. The Achilles' tendon reflex (S1-2) (plantarflexion) tests this nerve.

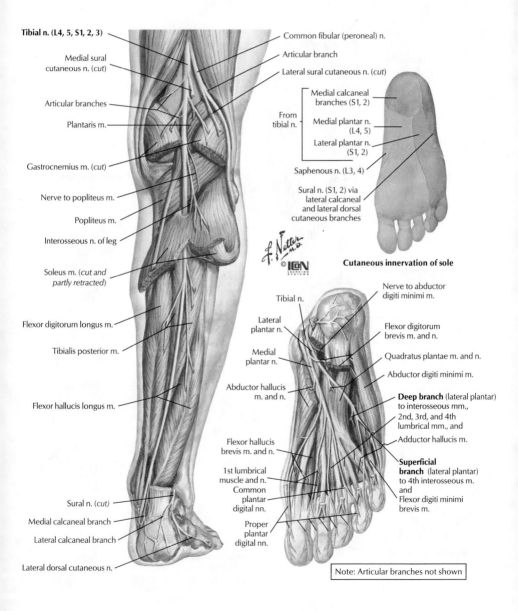

Tibial n. (L4, 5, S1, 2, 3)

Medial sural cutaneous n. (cut)

Articular branches

Plantaris m.

Gastrocnemius m. (cut)

Nerve to popliteus m.

Popliteus m.

Interosseous n. of leg

Soleus m. (cut and partly retracted)

Flexor digitorum longus m.

Tibialis posterior m.

Flexor hallucis longus m.

Sural n. (cut)

Medial calcaneal branch

Lateral calcaneal branch

Lateral dorsal cutaneous n.

Common fibular (peroneal) n.

Articular branch

Lateral sural cutaneous n. (cut)

Medial calcaneal branches (S1, 2)

From tibial n.   Medial plantar n. (L4, 5)

Lateral plantar n. (S1, 2)

Saphenous n. (L3, 4)

Sural n. (S1, 2) via lateral calcaneal and lateral dorsal cutaneous branches

Cutaneous innervation of sole

Tibial n.

Lateral plantar n.

Medial plantar n.

Abductor hallucis m. and n.

Flexor hallucis brevis m. and n.

1st lumbrical muscle and n.
Common plantar digital nn.

Proper plantar digital nn.

Nerve to abductor digiti minimi m.

Flexor digitorum brevis m. and n.

Quadratus plantae m. and n.

Abductor digiti minimi m.

Deep branch (lateral plantar) to interosseous mm., 2nd, 3rd, and 4th lumbrical mm., and Adductor hallucis m.

Superficial branch (lateral plantar) to 4th interosseous m. and Flexor digiti minimi brevis m.

Note: Articular branches not shown

Nerve Summary: Common Fibular (Peroneal) Nerve

The common fibular nerve innervates muscles of the lateral compartment of the leg (everts the foot) via its superficial branch and muscles of the anterior compartment of the leg and dorsum of the foot via its deep branch. These muscles are largely dorsiflexors. Footdrop and steppage gait may occur if this nerve or its deep branch is injured. The nerve is most vulnerable to injury as it passes around the fibular head.

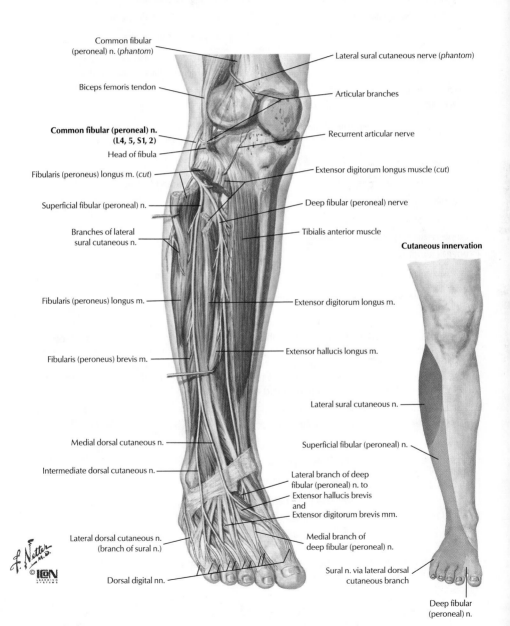

Common fibular (peroneal) n. (phantom)

Biceps femoris tendon

Common fibular (peroneal) n. (L4, 5, S1, 2)

Head of fibula

Fibularis (peroneus) longus m. (cut)

Superficial fibular (peroneal) n.

Branches of lateral sural cutaneous n.

Fibularis (peroneus) longus m.

Fibularis (peroneus) brevis m.

Medial dorsal cutaneous n.

Intermediate dorsal cutaneous n.

Lateral dorsal cutaneous n. (branch of sural n.)

Dorsal digital nn.

Lateral sural cutaneous nerve (phantom)

Articular branches

Recurrent articular nerve

Extensor digitorum longus muscle (cut)

Deep fibular (peroneal) nerve

Tibialis anterior muscle

Cutaneous innervation

Extensor digitorum longus m.

Extensor hallucis longus m.

Lateral sural cutaneous n.

Superficial fibular (peroneal) n.

Lateral branch of deep fibular (peroneal) n. to Extensor hallucis brevis and Extensor digitorum brevis mm.

Medial branch of deep fibular (peroneal) n.

Sural n. via lateral dorsal cutaneous branch

Deep fibular (peroneal) n.

Nerve Summary: Muscle Actions and Gait

A summary of actions of major muscles on joints of the lower limb follows. This list is not exhaustive (the muscle tables provide more detail).

HIP

Flex: iliopsoas, rectus femoris, sartorius

Extend: hamstrings, gluteus maximus

Abduct: gluteus medius and minimus

Rotate medially: gluteus medius and minimus

Rotate laterally: obturator internus, gemelli, piriformis

Adduct: adductor group of muscles

KNEE

Flex: hamstrings, gracilis, sartorius

Extend: quadriceps femoris

Rotate medially: semitendinosus, semimembranosus

Rotate laterally: biceps femoris

ANKLE

Plantarflex: gastrocnemius, soleus, tibialis posterior, flexor digitorum longus, flexor hallucis longus

Dorsiflex: tibialis anterior, extensor digitorum longus, extensor hallucis longus, fibularis tertius

INTERTARSAL

Evert: fibularis longus, brevis, tertius

Invert: tibialis anterior and posterior

METATARSOPHALANGEAL

Flex: interossei and lumbricals

Extend: extensor digitorum longus, brevis

Abduct: dorsal interossei

Adduct: plantar interossei

INTERPHALANGEAL

Flex: flexor digitorum longus, brevis

Extend: extensor digitorum longus, brevis

The gait cycle involves both a swing phase and a stance phase (foot is weight-bearing). The swing phase occurs from toe-off (TO) and acceleration to the midswing (MSW) to deceleration and the heel strike (HS), when the foot meets the ground. The stance phase occurs from heel strike (HS) to flat foot (FF) to midstance (MST) to the push-off (toe-off [TO]). The major muscles involved are summarized below:

GAIT CYCLE	MUSCLES INVOLVED IN ACTION
TO to MSW	Quadriceps femoris, then hamstrings (knee) and iliopsoas, adductors (hip)
TO to HS	Tibialis anterior and fibularis (peroneal) muscles (ankle)
HS to FF	Tibialis anterior and fibularis (peroneal) muscles (ankle)
HS to MST	Quadriceps femoris and gluteus maximus (hip)
MST to TO	Gastrocnemius and soleus (ankle)
HS to TO*	Gluteus medius and minimus

*These muscles abduct on the weight-bearing limb to minimize pelvic tilting. Evidence of pelvic tilting (a gluteal lurch) is a positive Trendelenburg sign.

Nerve Summary: Dermatomes

The spiral dermatome pattern of the lower limb is the result of embryonic rotation of the limb. Key dermatomes include

Inguinal region: L1
Anterior knee: L4
Second toe: L5

Zones of autonomous sensory testing and spinal cord levels involved in primary movements of the joints are illustrated.

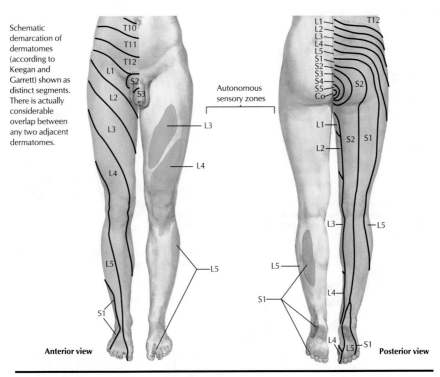

Schematic demarcation of dermatomes (according to Keegan and Garrett) shown as distinct segments. There is actually considerable overlap between any two adjacent dermatomes.

Anterior view

Autonomous sensory zones

Posterior view

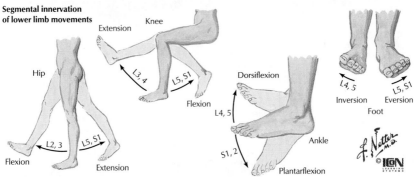

Segmental innervation of lower limb movements

Embryology: Lower Limb Rotation

While the upper limb rotates 90° laterally, the lower limb rotates approximately 90° medially so that the knee and elbow are oriented approximately 180° from each other. The thumb lies laterally in anatomical position, with the great toe medially. Knee, ankle, and toe flexor muscles are on the posterior aspect of the lower limb, and knee, ankle, and toe extensor muscles are on the ventral aspect. The hip is unaffected, so hip flexors are anterior and extensors are posterior. This limb rotation pattern produces a spiral (barber pole) arrangement of the dermatomes as one moves distally along the limb.

Changes in position of limbs before birth

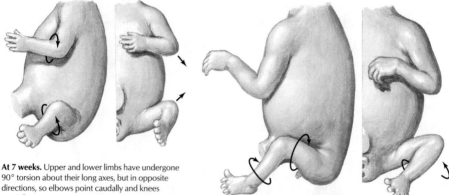

At 7 weeks. Upper and lower limbs have undergone 90° torsion about their long axes, but in opposite directions, so elbows point caudally and knees cranially.

At 8 weeks. Torsion of lower limbs results in twisted or "barber pole" arrangement of their cutaneous innervation.

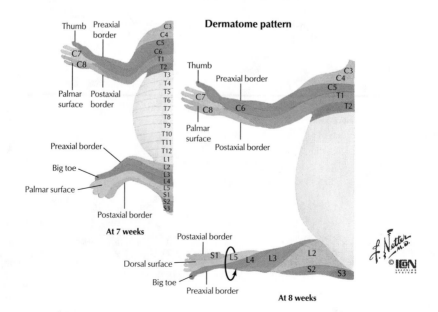

Dermatome pattern

At 7 weeks

At 8 weeks

Review Questions

Where does the small saphenous vein terminate?	It drains venous blood from the lateral dorsal venous arch and calf into the popliteal vein posterior to the knee.
What are the three cardinal events associated with DVT?	Stasis, venous wall injury, and hypercoagulability.
What three bones fuse to form the coxal (hip) bone?	Ilium, ischium, and pubis. All come together in the acetabulum.
Which hip joint ligament is the strongest?	Iliofemoral, which forms an inverted Y ligament (of Bigelow) that limits hyperextension.
What is the major blood supply to the femoral head?	Primarily the retinacular arteries of the medial and lateral femoral circumflex, and the acetabular branch of the obturator artery, which runs in the ligament of the femoral head (less important in adults).
What test is used to assess a congenital dislocation of the hip?	Ortolani's (reduction) test. Hip instability is tested with Barlow's test.
What nerve innervates the major hip abductor muscles?	Superior gluteal. Weakness of abductors (gluteus medius and minimus) on the weight-bearing limb can lead to a gluteal lurch during walking, and this is known as a positive Trendelenburg sign.
What is the primary function of the gluteus maximus muscle?	Strongest extensor of the thigh at the hip. Especially important when walking uphill, climbing stairs, or rising from a sitting position.
What are two components of the sciatic nerve?	Tibial and common fibular nerves.
What are major risks with a type IV femoral neck fracture (complete displacement)?	Nonunion and avascular necrosis of the femoral head.
What powerful flexor of the thigh at the hip attaches to the lesser trochanter?	Iliopsoas muscle.
What muscles flex the thigh at the hip and extend the leg at the knee?	Tensor fascia lata and rectus femoris.
What nerve innervates muscles of the anterior compartment of the thigh?	Femoral (L2-L4). These muscles are largely extensors of the leg at the knee.
What is the principal function of muscles of the medial compartment of the thigh?	Adduction of the thigh at the hip. Many also help to flex the thigh at the hip.
What are the hamstring muscles?	Semitendinosus, semimembranosus, and long head of the biceps femoris. They extend the thigh at the hip and flex the leg at the knee.

Review Questions

How does the femoral nerve gain access to the thigh?	It passes deep to the inguinal ligament, lateral to the femoral sheath (which contains the femoral artery and vein and inguinal lymph nodes). The inguinal lymph nodes are the major collection point for all lymph drained from the lower limb.
How does the femoral artery reach the popliteal fossa (region posterior to the knee)?	It passes through the adductor hiatus (an aperture in the tendon of insertion of the adductor magnus muscle) to reach the popliteal fossa, where it becomes the popliteal artery.
As pertains to the lower limb, what are the two most common sites for pressure ulcers?	Ischium (tuberosity) and greater trochanter.
What is the most malignant type of primary bone tumor?	Multiple myeloma, a malignant tumor of plasma cells.
What is the weight-bearing bone of the leg?	Tibia. The fibula is largely a bone for muscle attachment.
What is the most common fracture in long bones?	Fracture of the tibial shaft. These fractions are often open injuries.
What is the pes anserinus?	Attachment arrangement of the tendons of the semitendinosus, gracilis, and sartorius muscles to the medial tibial condyle (looks like a goose's foot).
What type of joint is the knee?	Biaxial condylar synovial joint, the most complex joint in the body.
Which four bursae surrounding the knee joint also communicate with its synovial cavity?	Suprapatellar, popliteus, anserine, and subtendinous (gastrocnemius) bursae.
How does one test for an ACL injury?	Anterior drawer sign, where the tibia moves anteriorly in relation to the femur. The ACL normally prevents hyperextension of the knee and is injured more than the posterior cruciate ligament.
What is the unhappy triad?	Injury to the ACL, tibial collateral ligament, and medial meniscus.
What is Osgood-Schlatter disease?	A partial avulsion of the tibial tuberosity, more common in physically active children.
What typical presentation of the legs is seen with chronic osteoarthritis of the knee?	Subluxation of the knee with a genu varum, or bowleg, deformity.
What is the arterial blood supply to muscles of the anterior compartment of the leg?	Anterior tibial.
Where do most of the malignant osteosarcomas occur?	In the metaphysis of the long bones where the greatest growth occurs.

Review Questions

What nerve innervates each of the following muscles?

Gastrocnemius	Tibial
Fibularis longus:	Superficial fibular
Tibialis anterior:	Deep fibular
Plantaris:	Tibial
Extensor hallucis longus:	Deep fibular
Flexor digitorum brevis:	Medial plantar (from tibial)
Soleus:	Tibial
Abductor digiti minimi:	Lateral plantar (from tibial)
Plantar and dorsal interossei:	Lateral plantar (from tibial)

What muscle is most often implicated in shin splints?	Tibialis posterior where it attaches along the tibia and interosseous membrane.
What are the five Ps of acute anterior compartment syndrome?	Pain, pallor, paresis (foot drop), paresthesia, and pulseless.
How is the weight of the body transferred to the foot?	Weight is transferred through the talus (ankle bone).
How is the joint between the talus and tibia classified?	Talocrural joint, a uniaxial synovial hinge (ginglymus) joint.
What important ankle ligament limits eversion of the foot?	Medial (deltoid) ligament (has four parts). However, the weaker lateral (collateral) ligament is most often sprained, because it resists inversion of the foot.
What is the spring ligament, and why is it important?	Plantar calcaneonavicular ligament. It supports the head of the talus and medial longitudinal arch of the foot. It is fairly elastic—hence its name.
Which tarsal bone is fractured most often?	Calcaneus. Most are intraarticular fractures in which the talus is driven down on the calcaneus, as in a fall from a great height, with a landing on the heel.
What complication may occur with talar neck fractures?	Avascular necrosis of the body of the talus, because most of the blood supply to the talus passes through the talar neck.
What is the function of the dorsal interossei?	Abduct digits and flex metatarsophalangeal joints.
What is the blood supply to the sole of the foot?	Medial and lateral plantar arteries derived from the posterior tibial artery.
What muscles act during the stance phase of gait from the time the heel strikes (HS) the ground to the flat foot (FF) stance?	HS to FF involves contraction of the tibialis anterior (and other dorsiflexors) to dorsiflex the foot at HS and then slowly relax it to the FF stance. Ankle eversion (fibularis muscles) also occurs with this movement. Patients with weakened dorsiflexors (deep fibular nerve problem) may slap their foot to the ground after the HS phase instead of executing a smooth landing. The gluteus maximus also helps to maintain hip extension and keeps the body from tilting forward.

Review Questions

Describe the following clinical conditions:

Club foot:	Plantar-flexed at ankle with an inverted (varus) foot
Hammer toe:	Proximal interphalangeal joint flexion deformity from poorly fitting shoes
Hallux valgus:	Bunion, with valgus deformity of the great toe
Plantar fasciitis:	Heel spur syndrome; inflammation of plantar aponeurosis
Onychomycosis:	Fungal infection, which makes toenails thick and brittle
Charcot joint:	Arthropathy of the ankle caused by neuropathy, often related to diabetic foot
Claudication:	Limping related to muscle ischemia from atherosclerosis
Gout:	Joint inflammation from deposition of urate in synovial space
Shuffling gait:	Weakened plantarflexion and inversion (tibial nerve problem)
Footdrop:	Weakened dorsiflexion (common or deep fibular nerve problem)
Genu valgum:	Knock-knee; excessive valgus angulation of the tibia
Pes cavus:	Unusually high median longitudinal arch
How does the lower limb rotate in utero compared with the upper limb?	Rotates medially 90° while the upper limb rotates laterally 90°. Thus, the limbs are 180° out of phase with one another (knee anterior and big toe medial versus elbow posterior and thumb lateral).

5

Thorax

Introduction Ribs and muscles encase the thorax, protecting the vital heart and lungs and assisting in breathing. The thoracic cavity is divided into two separate pleural cavities and an intervening mediastinum (middle septum).

Surface Anatomy: Key Landmarks

Jugular (suprasternal) notch: notch marking the level of the second thoracic vertebra
Sternal angle (of Louis): articulation between the manubrium and body of the sternum; dividing line separating the superior and inferior mediastinum; site of articulation of the second pair of ribs; useful for counting intercostal spaces
Nipple (in males): marks the T4 dermatome and approximate level of the dome of the diaphragm on the right side
Xiphoid process: inferior extent of the sternum and anterior attachment point of the diaphragm

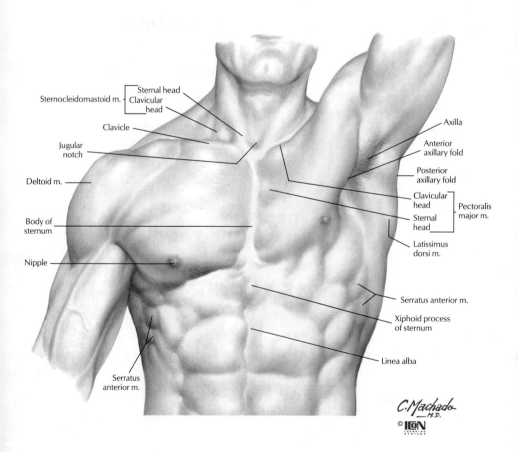

Surface Anatomy: Female Breast

The breast extends from approximately the second to the sixth ribs and from the sternum medially to the midaxillary line. Mammary gland tissue lies in the superficial fascia, is a modified sweat gland, and is supported by strands of fibrous tissue called suspensory ligaments (of Cooper). The nipple usually lies at approximately the level of the fourth intercostal space and is surrounded by the pigmented areola. Gland lobules drain into lactiferous ducts that open on the nipple surface.

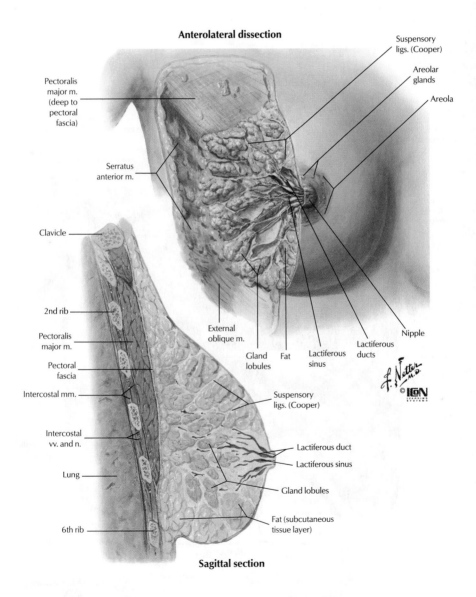

Anterolateral dissection

Suspensory ligs. (Cooper)

Areolar glands

Areola

Pectoralis major m. (deep to pectoral fascia)

Serratus anterior m.

Clavicle

2nd rib

Pectoralis major m.

External oblique m.

Nipple

Lactiferous ducts

Pectoral fascia

Gland lobules   Fat   Lactiferous sinus

Intercostal mm.

Suspensory ligs. (Cooper)

Intercostal vv. and n.

Lactiferous duct

Lactiferous sinus

Lung

Gland lobules

6th rib

Fat (subcutaneous tissue layer)

Sagittal section

Surface Anatomy: Lymphatics and Vessels of the Breast

Lymph drains from the glandular tissue to the subareolar lymphatic plexus and then to axillary lymph nodes (approximately 75%) or to infraclavicular, pectoral, or parasternal (internal thoracic) nodes (it may also drain to the opposite breast). Arteries supplying the breast include the

- Anterior intercostal branches of internal thoracic (mammary) artery
- Lateral thoracic artery (branch of axillary artery)
- Thoracodorsal artery (branch of axillary artery)

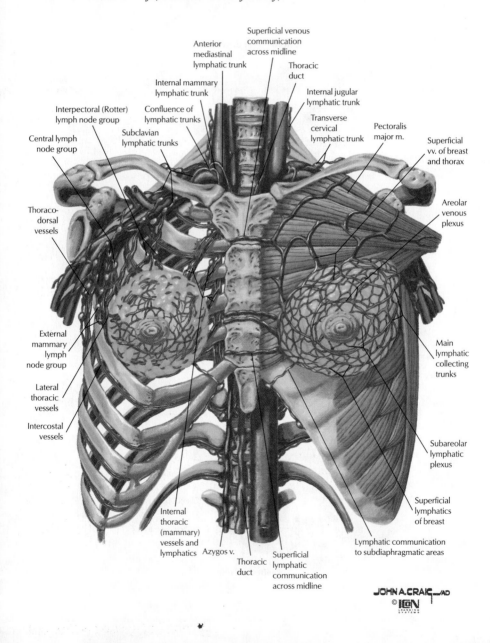

JOHN A.CRAIG—AD
©ICN

Clinical Correlation

Examination of the Breast   *Anatomy on pp. 301, 302*

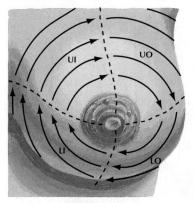

Breast is palpated systematically, either quadrant by quadrant or in increasing or decreasing circles.

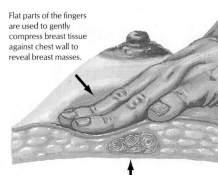

Flat parts of the fingers are used to gently compress breast tissue against chest wall to reveal breast masses.

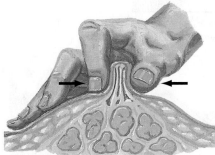

Nipple is squeezed gently to detect bleeding or discharge.

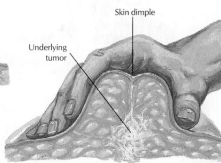

Skin dimple

Underlying tumor

Molding of the breast about a mass may elicit skin dimpling.

For clinical purposes, the breast is divided into quadrants:
• **UI**: upper inner
• **UO**: upper outer (includes the axillary tail [of Spence])
• **LI**: lower inner
• **LO**: lower outer
Via a uniform pattern of examination, by quadrants or in a rotary fashion, the entire breast is gently palpated by compression against the chest wall. Each nipple is examined for elasticity and discharge.

Clinical Correlation

Fibrocystic Change and Fibroadenoma   *Anatomy on pp. 301, 302*

Fibrocystic disease

Multiple, well-demarcated cysts within breast tissue

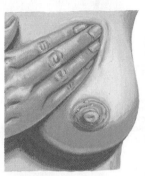

Often detected on self-examination as a mass that may fluctuate in size in different phases of the menstrual cycle

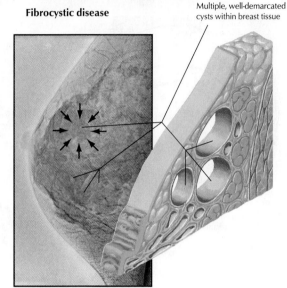

Vascular shadow

Fibroadenoma

Connective tissue shadows

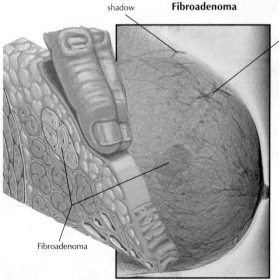

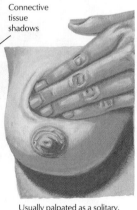

Usually palpated as a solitary, smooth, firm, well-demarcated nodule

Fibroadenoma

JOHN A.CRAIG—MD
©ICN

Fibrocystic change (disease) is a general term covering a large group of benign conditions (occurring in approximately 80% of women) that are often related to cyclic changes in maturation and involution of glandular tissue. Fibroadenoma, the second most common tumor of the breast after carcinoma, is a benign neoplasm of glandular epithelium and is usually accompanied by a significant increase in connective tissue stroma. Both conditions present as palpable masses and warrant follow-up evaluation.

Clinical Correlation

Clinical Signs of Breast Cancer 1 · *Anatomy on pp. 301, 302*

Vascular signs

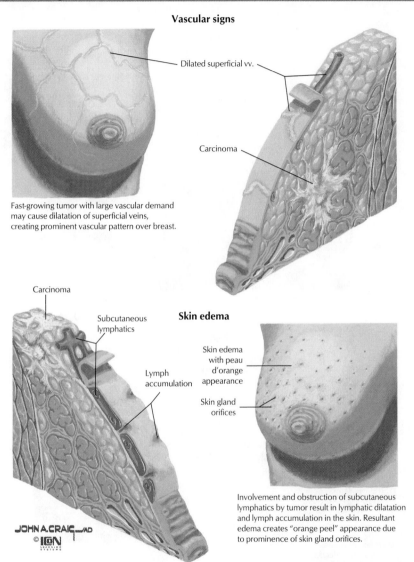

Fast-growing tumor with large vascular demand may cause dilatation of superficial veins, creating prominent vascular pattern over breast.

Dilated superficial vv.

Carcinoma

Carcinoma

Subcutaneous lymphatics

Skin edema

Lymph accumulation

Skin edema with peau d'orange appearance

Skin gland orifices

Involvement and obstruction of subcutaneous lymphatics by tumor result in lymphatic dilatation and lymph accumulation in the skin. Resultant edema creates "orange peel" appearance due to prominence of skin gland orifices.

JOHN A.CRAIG—AD
© ICN

Breast cancer is the most common malignancy in women (approximately 200,000 US cases per year). Approximately two thirds of all cases occur in postmenopausal women.

TYPE	COMMENT
Invasive	A neoplasm that includes infiltrating ductal carcinoma (approximately 70-80%), invasive lobular carcinoma (5-10%), tubular carcinoma (10-20%), and other forms
Noninvasive	A heterogeneous group of proliferative lesions with diverse malignant potential that includes ductal carcinoma in situ (DCIS)

Clinical Correlation

Clinical Signs of Breast Cancer 2   *Anatomy on pp. 301, 302*

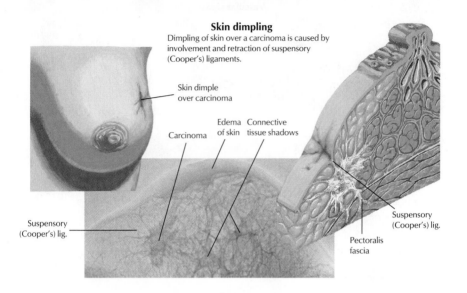

Skin dimpling
Dimpling of skin over a carcinoma is caused by involvement and retraction of suspensory (Cooper's) ligaments.

Skin dimple over carcinoma

Carcinoma   Edema of skin   Connective tissue shadows

Suspensory (Cooper's) lig.

Suspensory (Cooper's) lig.

Pectoralis fascia

JOHN A. CRAIG—MD
© ICON

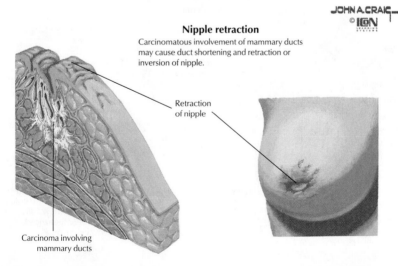

Nipple retraction
Carcinomatous involvement of mammary ducts may cause duct shortening and retraction or inversion of nipple.

Retraction of nipple

Carcinoma involving mammary ducts

Approximately 50% of cancers develop in the upper outer quadrant; metastatic involvement of lymph nodes usually occurs in the axilla, because 75% of lymph from the breast drains to axillary nodes. By use of an isotope injected into the tumor region, the first lymph node (sentinel node) draining the area can be identified and excised to evaluate for metastatic disease. Distant sites of metastasis include

- Lungs and pleura
- Liver
- Bones
- Brain

Clinical Correlation

Mastectomy and Lumpectomy   *Anatomy on pp. 301, 302, 310*

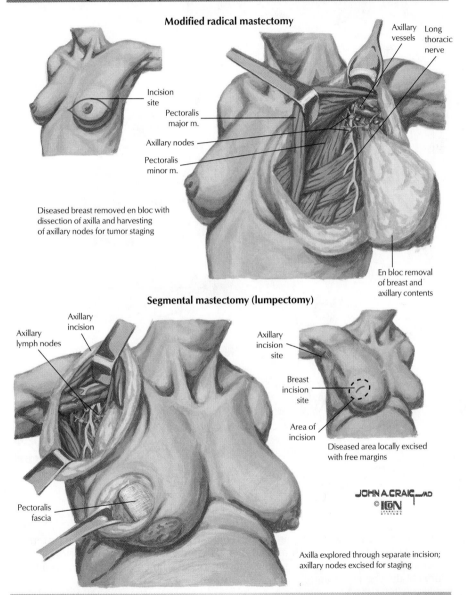

Modified radical mastectomy

Axillary vessels

Long thoracic nerve

Incision site

Pectoralis major m.

Axillary nodes

Pectoralis minor m.

Diseased breast removed en bloc with dissection of axilla and harvesting of axillary nodes for tumor staging

En bloc removal of breast and axillary contents

Segmental mastectomy (lumpectomy)

Axillary lymph nodes

Axillary incision

Axillary incision site

Breast incision site

Area of incision

Diseased area locally excised with free margins

Pectoralis fascia

JOHN A.CRAIG—MD
© ICN

Axilla explored through separate incision; axillary nodes excised for staging

Surgical management includes either segmental mastectomy, commonly known as lumpectomy, with or without sentinel node biopsy, or modified radical mastectomy. In the latter procedure, the breast, axillary nodes, and nipple with areola are resected. Care must be exercised to spare the long thoracic nerve (innervates the serratus anterior muscle) and thoracodorsal nerve (innervates the latissimus dorsi muscle). Postoperative chemotherapy, tamoxifen, radiation therapy, or a combination may be included as part of management.

Thoracic Wall: Thoracic Cage (Skeleton)

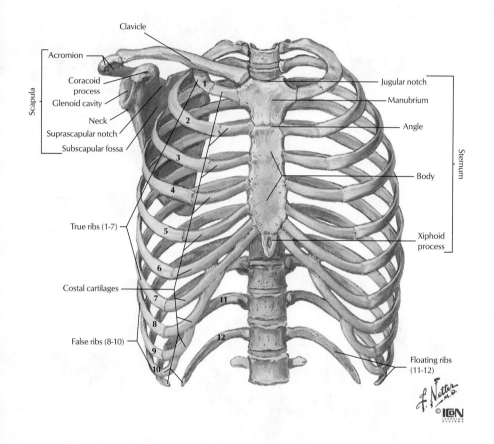

Clavicle

Acromion

Coracoid process

Glenoid cavity

Neck

Suprascapular notch

Subscapular fossa

Scapula

True ribs (1-7)

Costal cartilages

False ribs (8-10)

Jugular notch

Manubrium

Angle

Body

Xiphoid process

Sternum

Floating ribs (11-12)

The thoracic cage, which is part of the axial skeleton, includes the midline sternum and 12 pairs of ribs, each with a head, neck, tubercle, and body. The pectoral girdle, which includes the clavicle and scapula, forms the attachment of the upper limb to the thorax at the shoulder joint.

FEATURE	CHARACTERISTICS
Sternum	Long flat bone: composed of the manubrium, body, and xiphoid process
True ribs	Ribs 1-7: articulate with the sternum directly
False ribs	Ribs 8-10: articulate to costal cartilages of the ribs above
Floating ribs	Ribs 11 and 12: articulate with vertebrae only

Thoracic Wall: Joints of the Thoracic Cage

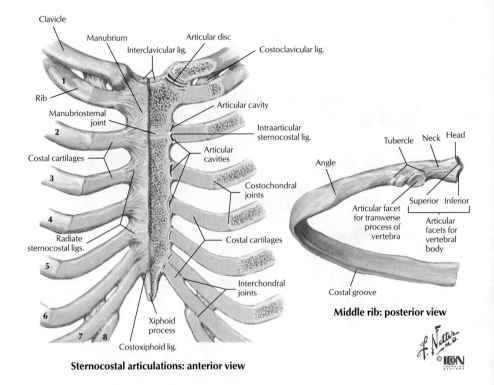

Sternocostal articulations: anterior view

Middle rib: posterior view

Articulation of the ribs with thoracic vertebrae is reviewed in Chapter 2 (Back).

LIGAMENT	ATTACHMENT	COMMENT
Sternoclavicular (Saddle-Type Synovial) Joint with an Articular Disc		
Capsule	Clavicle and manubrium	Allows elevation, depression, protraction, retraction, circumduction
Sternoclavicular	Clavicle and manubrium	Consists of anterior and posterior ligaments
Interclavicular	Between both clavicles	Connects two sternoclavicular joints
Costoclavicular	Clavicle to first rib	Anchors clavicle to first rib
Sternocostal (Primary Cartilaginous [Synchondroses]) Joints		
First sternocostal	First rib to manubrium	Allows no movement at this joint
Radiate sternocostal	Ribs 2-7 with sternum	Permit some gliding or sliding movement at these synovial plane joints
Costochondral (Primary Cartilaginous) Joints		
Cartilage	Costal cartilage to rib	Allow no movement at these joints
Interchondral (Synovial Plane) Joints		
Interchondral	Between costal cartilages	Allow some gliding movement

Thoracic Wall: Muscles of the Anterior Wall

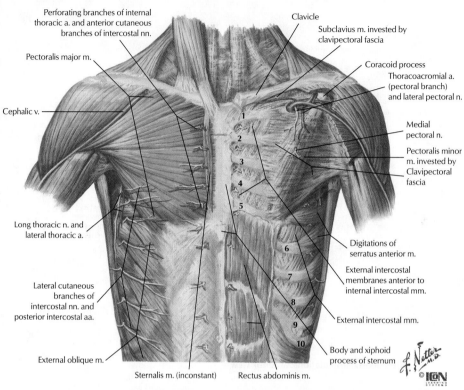

Perforating branches of internal thoracic a. and anterior cutaneous branches of intercostal nn.

Pectoralis major m.

Cephalic v.

Long thoracic n. and lateral thoracic a.

Lateral cutaneous branches of intercostal nn. and posterior intercostal aa.

External oblique m.

Sternalis m. (inconstant)

Rectus abdominis m.

Clavicle

Subclavius m. invested by clavipectoral fascia

Coracoid process

Thoracoacromial a. (pectoral branch) and lateral pectoral n.

Medial pectoral n.

Pectoralis minor m. invested by Clavipectoral fascia

Digitations of serratus anterior m.

External intercostal membranes anterior to internal intercostal mm.

External intercostal mm.

Body and xiphoid process of sternum

On the right, the pectoralis major and serratus anterior muscles are shown (see Chapter 3 [Upper Limb]); on the left, the pectoralis major has been removed.

MUSCLE	SUPERIOR ATTACHMENT (ORIGIN)	INFERIOR ATTACHMENT (INSERTION)	INNERVATION	MAIN ACTIONS
External intercostal	Inferior border of rib	Superior border of rib below	Intercostal nerve	Elevate ribs
Internal intercostal	Inferior border of rib	Superior border of rib below	Intercostal nerve	Elevate ribs (upper four and five); others depress ribs
Innermost intercostal	Inferior border of rib	Superior border of rib below	Intercostal nerve	Probably elevate ribs
Transversus thoracis	Posterior surface of lower sternum	Internal surface of costal cartilages 2-6	Intercostal nerve	Depress ribs
Subcostal	Internal surface of lower rib near their angles	Superior borders of second or third ribs below	Intercostal nerve	Elevate ribs
Levator costarum	Transverse processes of C7 and T1-T11	Subjacent ribs between tubercle and angle	Dorsal primary rami of C8-T11	Elevate ribs

All intercostal muscles keep intercostal spaces rigid, thereby preventing them from bulging out during expiration and being drawn in during respiration. The role of individual intercostal muscles and accessory muscles of respiration in moving the ribs is difficult to interpret despite many electromyographic studies.

Thoracic Wall: Vessels and Muscles of the Internal Wall

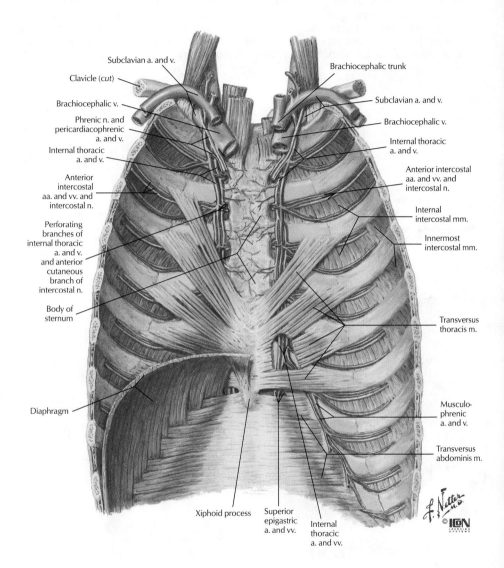

Subclavian a. and v.

Clavicle (*cut*)

Brachiocephalic v.

Phrenic n. and pericardiacophrenic a. and v.

Internal thoracic a. and v.

Anterior intercostal aa. and vv. and intercostal n.

Perforating branches of internal thoracic a. and v. and anterior cutaneous branch of intercostal n.

Body of sternum

Diaphragm

Xiphoid process

Superior epigastric a. and vv.

Internal thoracic a. and vv.

Brachiocephalic trunk

Subclavian a. and v.

Brachiocephalic v.

Internal thoracic a. and v.

Anterior intercostal aa. and vv. and intercostal n.

Internal intercostal mm.

Innermost intercostal mm.

Transversus thoracis m.

Musculo-phrenic a. and v.

Transversus abdominis m.

ARTERY	COURSE
Internal thoracic	Arises from subclavian and terminates by dividing into superior epigastric and musculophrenic arteries
Intercostals	Anterior and posterior segments that arise from internal thoracic and aorta, respectively, and anastomose
Subcostal	From aorta, courses inferior to the 12th rib
Pericardiacophrenic	From internal thoracic and accompanies phrenic nerve

Thoracic Wall: Intercostal Nerves and Vessels

Intercostal nerves are the primary ventral rami of the first 11 thoracic spinal nerves. The 12th thoracic nerve gives rise to the subcostal nerve, which courses inferior to the 12th rib. The intercostal vein, artery, and nerve (spells VAN) run in the ribs' costal grooves between the internal and innermost intercostal muscles. The nerves give rise to lateral and anterior cutaneous branches and branches innervating the intercostal muscles.

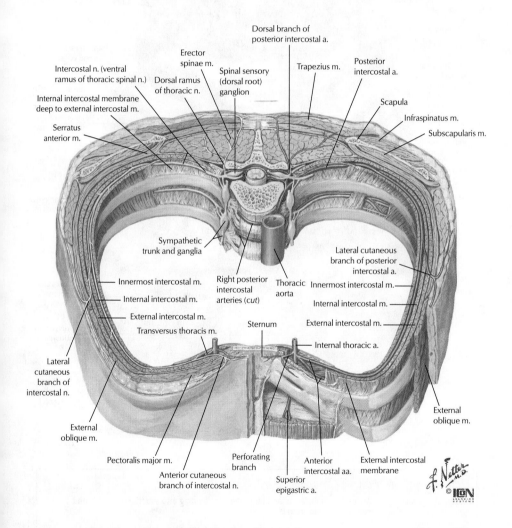

Clinical Correlation

Thoracic Cage Injuries
Anatomy on pp. 308, 309, 312

Simple

- Costovertebral dislocation (any level)
- Transverse rib fracture
- Oblique rib fracture
- Overriding rib fracture
- Chondral fracture
- Costochondral separation
- Condrosternal separation
- Sternal fracture

Complicated

- Traumatization of pleura and of lung (pneumothorax, lung contusion, subcutaneous emphysema)
- Multiple rib fractures (stove-in or flail chest)
- Tear of blood vessels (hemothorax)
- Compound by missle (may be deflected) or by puncture wound
- Injury to heart or to great vessels

Intercostal nerve block to relieve pain of fractured ribs

Optimal point to inject is angle of rib because rib is here most easily palpable.

6 cm

10 cm

Sites for injection
1. Angle of rib (preferred)
2. Posterior axillary line
3. Anterior axillary line
4. Infiltration of fracture site
5. Parasternal

Needle introduced to contact lower border of rib (**1**), withdrawn slightly, directed caudad, advanced 1/8 in. to slip under rib and enter intercostal space (**2**). To avoid pneumothorax, aspirate before injecting anesthetic.

Thoracic cage injuries result from trauma and often involve rib fractures (the 1st, 11th, and 12th ribs are usually spared), crush injuries (with rib fractures), and penetrating chest wounds (gunshot and stab). Pain caused by rib fractures, which is often intense because of expansion and contraction of the rib cage during respiration, may be treated by intercostal nerve block.

Pleura and Lungs: Anterior Topography

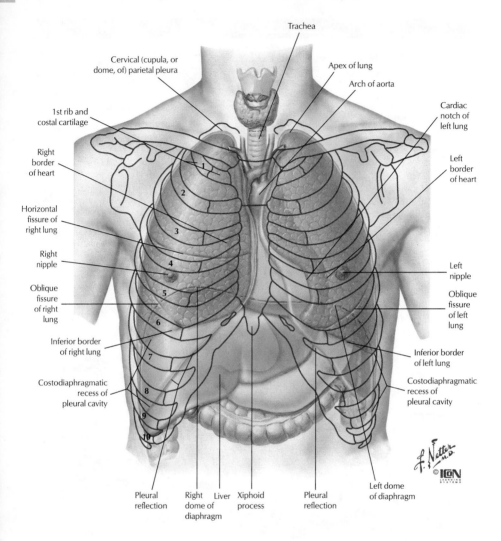

Trachea

Cervical (cupula, or dome, of) parietal pleura

Apex of lung

Arch of aorta

Cardiac notch of left lung

1st rib and costal cartilage

Right border of heart

Left border of heart

Horizontal fissure of right lung

Right nipple

Left nipple

Oblique fissure of right lung

Oblique fissure of left lung

Inferior border of right lung

Inferior border of left lung

Costodiaphragmatic recess of pleural cavity

Costodiaphragmatic recess of pleural cavity

Left dome of diaphragm

Pleural reflection

Right dome of diaphragm

Liver

Xiphoid process

Pleural reflection

The lungs reside in the pleural cavity (right and left), which is a potential space between the investing visceral pleura and the parietal pleura that lines the interior aspect of the thoracic wall.

FEATURE	DEFINITION
Cupula	Dome of cervical parietal pleura extending above the first rib
Parietal pleura	Membrane that in descriptive terms includes costal, mediastinal, diaphragmatic, and cervical (cupula) pleura
Pleural reflections	Points at which parietal pleural reflects off one surface and extends onto another (e.g., costal to diaphragmatic)
Pleural recesses	Reflection points at which lung does not fully extend into the pleural space (e.g., costodiaphragmatic and costomediastinal)

Pleura and Lungs: Posterior Topography

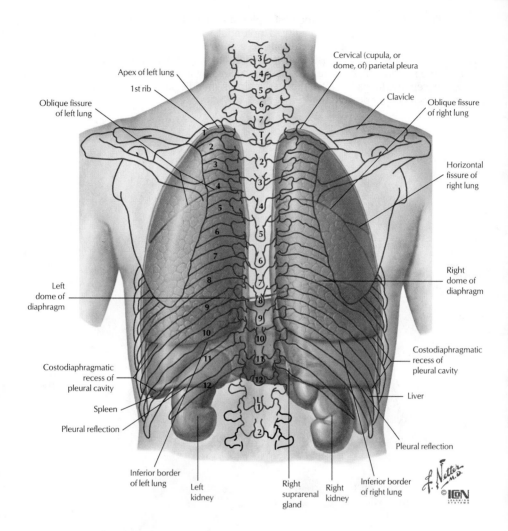

The lungs lie adjacent to parietal pleura inferiorly to the sixth costal cartilage (note the cardiac notch on the left side on page 314). Beyond this point, the lungs do not occupy the full extent of the pleural space during quiet respiration, and these points are important if one needs to access the pleural cavity without injuring the lungs.

LANDMARK	MARGIN OF LUNG	MARGIN OF PLEURA
Midclavicular line	6th rib	8th rib
Midaxillary line	8th rib	10th rib
Midscapular line	10th rib	12th rib

Pleura and Lungs: Lungs In Situ

This illustration shows part of the costal pleura removed to reveal the lungs, invested in visceral pleura. The pleural cavity, a potential space, normally contains a small amount of serous fluid that lubricates surfaces and reduces friction during respiration. The parietal pleura is very sensitive to pain, but few pain fibers innervate the visceral pleura. The region between the two pleural cavities, which contains all other thoracic viscera except the lungs, is called the mediastinum (middle septum). The left side of the neck shows a deeper dissection.

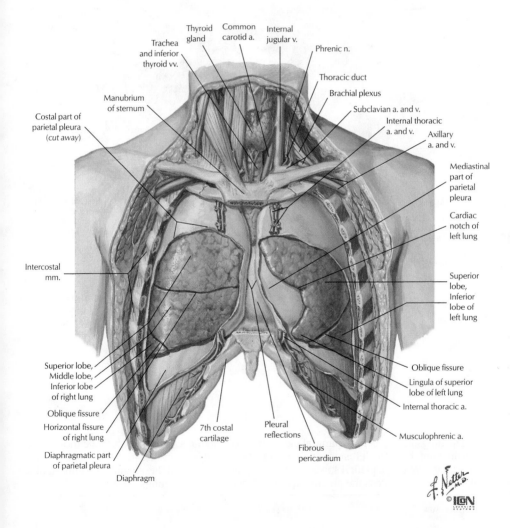

Pleura and Lungs: Features of the Medial Aspect of the Lungs

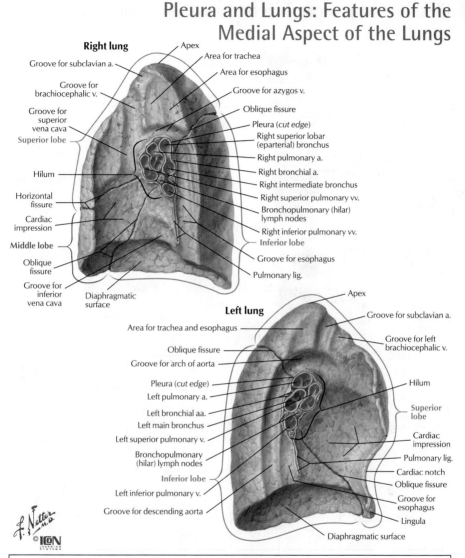

Right lung

Apex
Area for trachea
Area for esophagus
Groove for azygos v.
Oblique fissure
Pleura (*cut edge*)
Right superior lobar (eparterial) bronchus
Right pulmonary a.
Right bronchial a.
Right intermediate bronchus
Right superior pulmonary vv.
Bronchopulmonary (hilar) lymph nodes
Right inferior pulmonary vv.
Inferior lobe
Groove for esophagus
Pulmonary lig.

Groove for subclavian a.
Groove for brachiocephalic v.
Groove for superior vena cava
Superior lobe
Hilum
Horizontal fissure
Cardiac impression
Middle lobe
Oblique fissure
Groove for inferior vena cava
Diaphragmatic surface

Left lung

Apex
Groove for subclavian a.
Groove for left brachiocephalic v.
Hilum
Superior lobe
Cardiac impression
Pulmonary lig.
Cardiac notch
Oblique fissure
Groove for esophagus
Lingula
Diaphragmatic surface

Area for trachea and esophagus
Oblique fissure
Groove for arch of aorta
Pleura (*cut edge*)
Left pulmonary a.
Left bronchial aa.
Left main bronchus
Left superior pulmonary v.
Bronchopulmonary (hilar) lymph nodes
Inferior lobe
Left inferior pulmonary v.
Groove for descending aorta

FEATURE	CHARACTERISTICS
Lobes	Three lobes (superior, middle, inferior) in right lung; two in left
Horizontal fissure	Only on right lung, extends along line of fourth rib
Oblique fissure	On both lungs, extends from T2 vertebra to sixth costal cartilage
Impressions	Made by adjacent structures, in fixed lungs
Hilum	Points at which structures (bronchus, vessels, nerves, lymphatics) enter or leave lungs
Lingula	Tongue-shaped feature of left lung
Cardiac notch	Indentation for the heart, in left lung
Pulmonary ligament	Double layer of parietal pleura hanging from the hilum that marks reflection of visceral pleura to parietal pleura
Bronchopulmonary segment	10 functional segments in each lung supplied by a segmental bronchus and a segmental artery from the pulmonary artery

Pleura and Lungs: Trachea and Bronchi

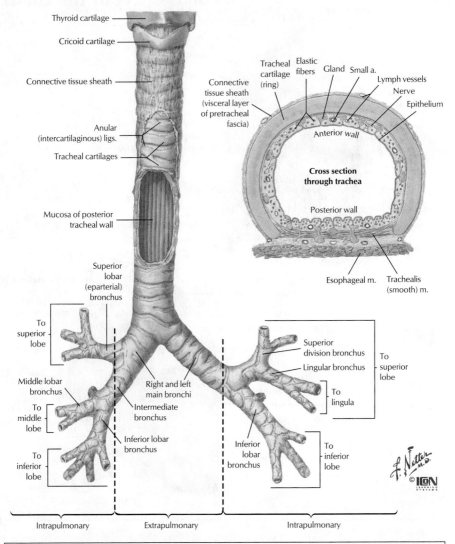

Thyroid cartilage

Cricoid cartilage

Connective tissue sheath

Anular (intercartilaginous) ligs.

Tracheal cartilages

Mucosa of posterior tracheal wall

Connective tissue sheath (visceral layer of pretracheal fascia)

Tracheal cartilage (ring) Elastic fibers Gland Small a.

Lymph vessels

Nerve

Epithelium

Anterior wall

Cross section through trachea

Posterior wall

Esophageal m.   Trachealis (smooth) m.

Superior lobar (eparterial) bronchus

To superior lobe

Middle lobar bronchus

To middle lobe

To inferior lobe

Right and left main bronchi

Intermediate bronchus

Inferior lobar bronchus

Superior division bronchus

Lingular bronchus

To superior lobe

To lingula

Inferior lobar bronchus

To inferior lobe

Intrapulmonary   Extrapulmonary   Intrapulmonary

FEATURE	CHARACTERISTICS
Trachea	Is approximately 5 inches long and 1 inch in diameter; courses inferiorly anterior to esophagus and posterior to aortic arch
Cartilaginous rings	Are 16-20 C-shaped rings
Bronchus	Divides into right and left main (primary) bronchi at the level of the sternal angle of Louis
Right bronchus	Is shorter, wider, and more vertical than left bronchus; aspirated foreign objects more likely to pass into this bronchus
Carina	Is internal, keel-like cartilage at bifurcation of trachea
Secondary bronchi	Supply lobes of each lung (three on right, two on left)
Tertiary bronchi	Supply bronchopulmonary segments (10 for each lung)

Clinical Correlation

Bronchiectasis
Anatomy on pp. 317, 318

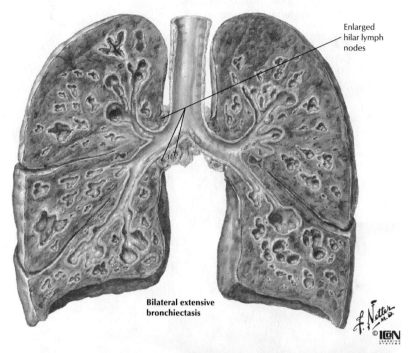

Enlarged hilar lymph nodes

Bilateral extensive bronchiectasis

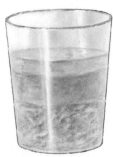

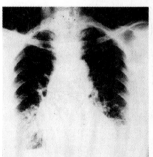

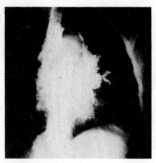

Profuse mucopurulent sputum, foul-smelling, settling into layers characteristic of severe bronchiectasis

PA x-ray film: peribronchial fibrosis in both lung bases

Left bronchogram reveals cystic bronchial dilation

Bronchiectasis is a disease characterized by chronic bronchial dilation caused by congenital or acquired destruction of muscular and elastic supporting tissue. Destruction usually results from inflammation and fibrosis related to intermittent healing. Chronic cough and purulent sputum production are common. Predisposing factors include infections, bronchial obstruction, anatomical defects, hereditary defects (immotile cilia), and recurrent aspiration pneumonias and/or inhalation of irritants.

Clinical Correlation

Bronchogenic Carcinoma
Anatomy on pp. 316-318

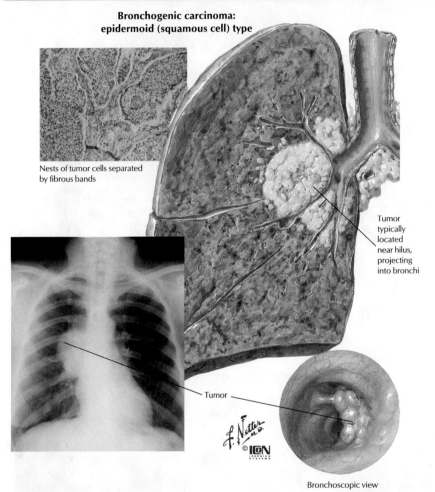

Bronchogenic carcinoma: epidermoid (squamous cell) type

Nests of tumor cells separated by fibrous bands

Tumor typically located near hilus, projecting into bronchi

Tumor

Bronchoscopic view

Lung cancer is the leading cause of cancer-related death. It arises either from alveolar lining cells of the lung parenchyma or from epithelium of the tracheobronchial tree. The World Health Organization (WHO) classification of lung carcinoma includes

- Squamous cell carcinoma (most common; usually arises in main bronchi near the hilum)
- Small cell carcinoma (rapidly growing tumor; more common in men)
- Adenocarcinoma (including the bronchoalveolar type, which grows along alveoli and bronchioles)
- Large cell anaplastic carcinoma (multinucleated, poorly differentiated cells)
- Adenosquamous carcinoma (tumor showing glandular and squamous cell differentiation)
- Carcinoid (small, slow-growing tumors)
- Bronchial gland carcinoma (e.g., mucoepidermoid)
- Other types

Clinical Correlation

Pancoast and Superior Vena Cava Syndromes

Anatomy on pp. 316, 317, 322, 339

Pancoast syndrome (superior sulcus tumor)

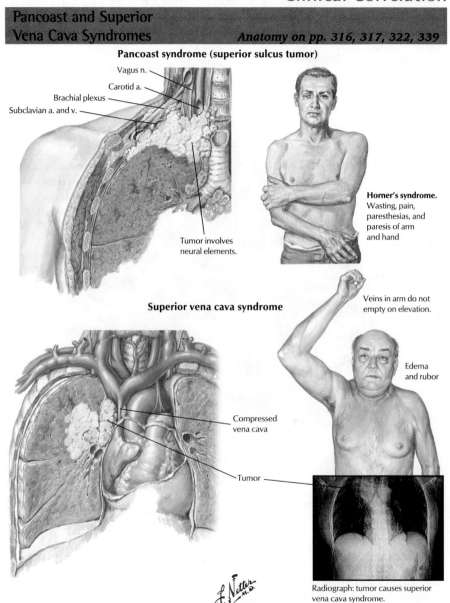

Vagus n.

Carotid a.

Brachial plexus

Subclavian a. and v.

Tumor involves neural elements.

Horner's syndrome. Wasting, pain, paresthesias, and paresis of arm and hand

Superior vena cava syndrome

Veins in arm do not empty on elevation.

Edema and rubor

Compressed vena cava

Tumor

Radiograph: tumor causes superior vena cava syndrome.

Bronchogenic carcinoma may impinge on adjacent anatomical structures. In Pancoast syndrome, tumor may spread to involve the sympathetic trunk, which compromises sympathetic tone to the head and leads to Horner's syndrome (myosis, ptosis, anhydrosis, flushing). Neurovascular components passing into the upper limb may be affected, with resulting paresthesia (in neck, head, shoulder, and limb, 90% in the ulnar nerve distribution). In superior vena cava (SVC) syndrome, tumor impinges on various structures, which leads to a sensation of fullness in the head and neck, headache, blurred vision, facial edema, enlarged neck veins, and dyspnea.

Pleura and Lungs: Superior Mediastinum

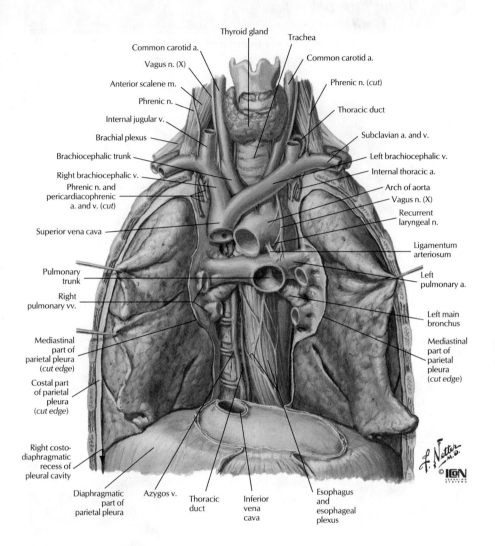

The region from the first rib and extending inferiorly to the sternal angle (T4-T5 vertebrae posteriorly) is called the superior mediastinum (middle septum).

FEATURE	DEFINITION
Contents	SVC, brachiocephalic veins, aortic arch, thoracic (lymphatic) duct, trachea, esophagus, thymus, vagus, and phrenic nerves
Superior thoracic aperture	Boundary that conveys many structures noted above between the neck and thorax; called thoracic outlet by clinicians
Thoracic outlet syndrome	Compression of one or more of the structures passing through the outlet, e.g., subclavian artery compressed between first rib and clavicle, or by an exceptionally long transverse process of C7

Pleura and Lungs: Transverse Section T5-6

Contents of the upper portion of the thorax and proximal arm are seen in this transverse section at the level of the T5-6 intervertebral disc, just inferior to the sternal angle and superior mediastinum. Note especially the pulmonary trunk division, SVC on the right, ascending aorta (about to become the aortic arch at the sternal angle), main bronchi, esophagus, and, posteriorly, thoracic lymphatic duct. Also, observe that the two pleural sacs containing the lungs do not cross the midline or communicate with each other.

Transverse Section: T5-6 Intervertebral Disc

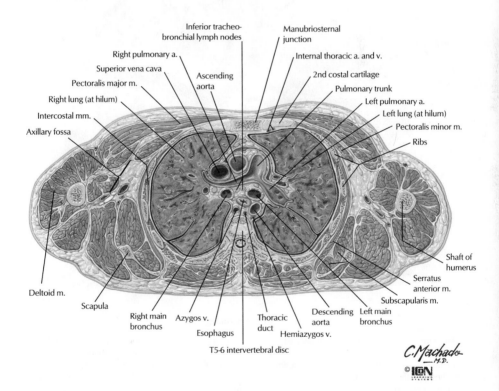

Inferior tracheo-
bronchial lymph nodes

Manubriosternal
junction

Right pulmonary a.

Internal thoracic a. and v.

Superior vena cava

Ascending
aorta

2nd costal cartilage

Pectoralis major m.

Pulmonary trunk

Right lung (at hilum)

Left pulmonary a.

Left lung (at hilum)

Intercostal mm.

Pectoralis minor m.

Axillary fossa

Ribs

Shaft of
humerus

Serratus
anterior m.

Deltoid m.

Subscapularis m.

Scapula

Right main
bronchus

Azygos v.

Thoracic
duct

Descending
aorta

Left main
bronchus

Esophagus

Hemiazygos v.

T5-6 intervertebral disc

C.Machado
—M.D.

© ICON

Pleura and Lungs: Lymphatics

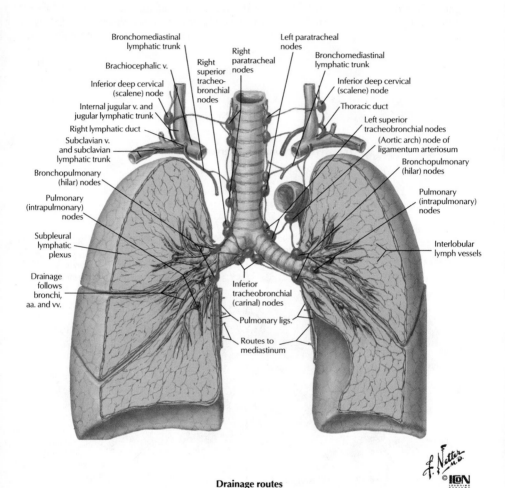

Bronchomediastinal
lymphatic trunk

Brachiocephalic v.

Inferior deep cervical
(scalene) node

Internal jugular v. and
jugular lymphatic trunk

Right lymphatic duct

Subclavian v.
and subclavian
lymphatic trunk

Bronchopulmonary
(hilar) nodes

Pulmonary
(intrapulmonary)
nodes

Subpleural
lymphatic
plexus

Drainage
follows
bronchi,
aa. and vv.

Right
superior
tracheo-
bronchial
nodes

Right
paratracheal
nodes

Left paratracheal
nodes

Bronchomediastinal
lymphatic trunk

Inferior deep cervical
(scalene) node

Thoracic duct

Left superior
tracheobronchial nodes
(Aortic arch) node of
ligamentum arteriosum

Bronchopulmonary
(hilar) nodes

Pulmonary
(intrapulmonary)
nodes

Interlobular
lymph vessels

Inferior
tracheobronchial
(carinal) nodes

Pulmonary ligs.

Routes to
mediastinum

Drainage routes

Right lung: All lobes drain to pulmonary and broncho-pulmonary (hilar) nodes, then to inferior tracheobronchial (carinal) nodes, right superior tracheobronchial nodes, and to right paratracheal nodes on way to brachiocephalic vein via bronchomediastinal lymphatic trunk and/or inferior deep cervical (scalene) node.

Left lung: Superior lobe drains to pulmonary and bronchopulmonary (hilar) nodes, inferior tracheobronchial (carinal) nodes, left superior tracheobronchial nodes, left paratracheal nodes and/or (aortic arch) node of ligamentum arteriosum, then to brachiocephalic vein via left bronchomediastinal trunk and thoracic duct. Left inferior lobe drains also to pulmonary and bronchopulmonary (hilar) nodes and to inferior tracheobronchial (carinal) nodes, but then mostly to right superior tracheobronchial nodes, where it follows same route as lymph from right lung.

Clinical Correlation

Sources of Pulmonary Emboli
Anatomy on pp. 322, 340, 368

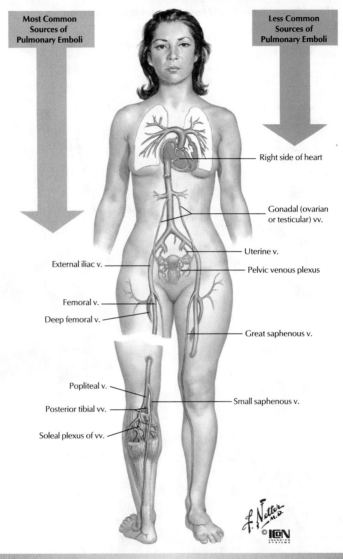

Most Common
Sources of
Pulmonary Emboli

Less Common
Sources of
Pulmonary Emboli

Right side of heart

Gonadal (ovarian
or testicular) vv.

Uterine v.

External iliac v.

Pelvic venous plexus

Femoral v.

Deep femoral v.

Great saphenous v.

Popliteal v.

Small saphenous v.

Posterior tibial vv.

Soleal plexus of vv.

The lungs naturally filter venous clots larger than circulating blood cells and can usually accommodate small clots because of their fibrinolytic ("clot buster") mechanisms. However, pulmonary embolism (PE) is the cause of death in 10-15% of hospitalized patients. Approximately 95% of the time, thromboemboli originate from deep leg veins. Major causes of PE include venous stasis (caused by bed rest, for example), trauma (fractures or tissue injury), and coagulation disorders (inherited or acquired); these three causes are known as Virchow's triad. Other contributors to PE include postoperative and postpartum immobility and some hormone medications that increase the risk of blood clots.

Clinical Correlation

Pulmonary Embolism
Anatomy on pp. 322, 340

Embolism of lesser degree without infarction

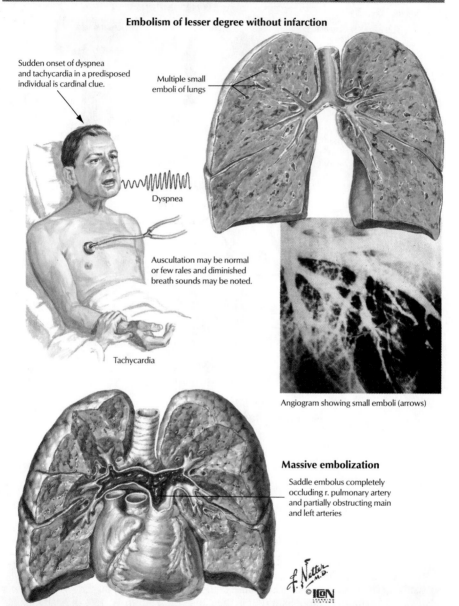

Sudden onset of dyspnea and tachycardia in a predisposed individual is cardinal clue.

Multiple small emboli of lungs

Dyspnea

Auscultation may be normal or few rales and diminished breath sounds may be noted.

Tachycardia

Angiogram showing small emboli (arrows)

Massive embolization

Saddle embolus completely occluding r. pulmonary artery and partially obstructing main and left arteries

Although 60-80% of PEs are silent because of small size, larger emboli may obstruct medium-sized vessels and lead to infarction or even obstruction of the pulmonary trunk (saddle embolus). PE without infarction is common and manifested by tachypnea, anxiety, dyspnea, and vague substernal pressure. Saddle embolus is an emergency that can precipitate acute cor pulmonale (right-sided heart failure) and circulatory collapse.

Clinical Correlation

Pneumothorax

Anatomy on pp. 314, 315, 322

Tension pneumothorax
Pathophysiology

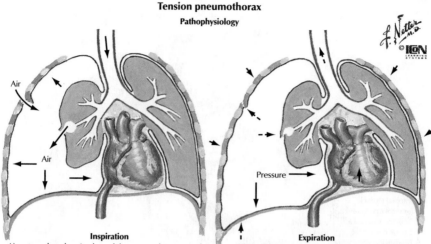

Inspiration

Air enters pleural cavity through lung wound or ruptured bleb (or occasionally via penetrating chest wound) with valvelike opening. Ipsilateral lung collapses and mediastinum shifts to opposite side, compressing lung.

Expiration

Intrapleural pressure rises, closing valvelike opening, thus preventing escape of pleural air. Pressure is thus progressively increased with each breath. Mediastinal and tracheal shifts are augmented, diaphragm is depressed, and venous return is impaired.

Clinical manifestations

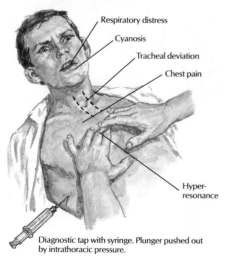

- Respiratory distress
- Cyanosis
- Tracheal deviation
- Chest pain
- Hyper-resonance

Diagnostic tap with syringe. Plunger pushed out by intrathoracic pressure.

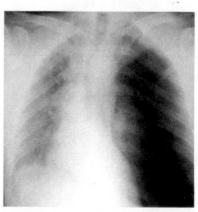

Left-sided tension pneumothorax. Lung collapsed, mediastinum and trachea deviated to opposite lung.

Chest trauma (stab wound or fractured rib) may lacerate the chest wall and the parietal and visceral pleura, which causes a tension pneumothorax that results in a partially or completely collapsed lung on the affected side.

Clinical Correlation

Hemothorax *Anatomy on pp. 314, 315, 322*

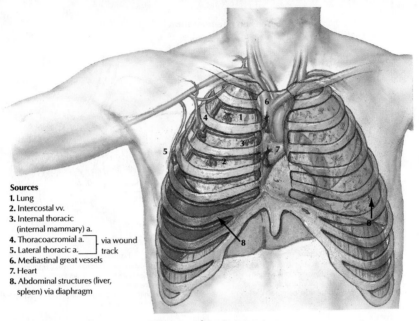

Sources
1. Lung
2. Intercostal vv.
3. Internal thoracic (internal mammary) a.
4. Thoracoacromial a. ⎤ via wound
5. Lateral thoracic a. ⎦ track
6. Mediastinal great vessels
7. Heart
8. Abdominal structures (liver, spleen) via diaphragm

Degrees and management

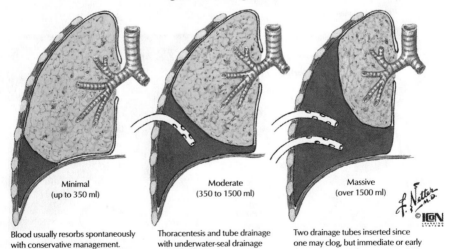

Minimal
(up to 350 ml)

Blood usually resorbs spontaneously with conservative management. Thoracentesis rarely necessary.

Moderate
(350 to 1500 ml)

Thoracentesis and tube drainage with underwater-seal drainage usually suffices.

Massive
(over 1500 ml)

Two drainage tubes inserted since one may clog, but immediate or early thoracotomy may be necessary to arrest bleeding.

Accumulation of blood in the pleural cavity transforms this potential space into a real space capable of accommodating a large volume. Blood in this cavity does not clot well because of the smooth pleural surfaces and defibrinating action of respiratory movements.

Clinical Correlation

Chest Drainage Tubes

Anatomy on pp. 311, 312, 314

Techniques for introduction of chest drainage tubes

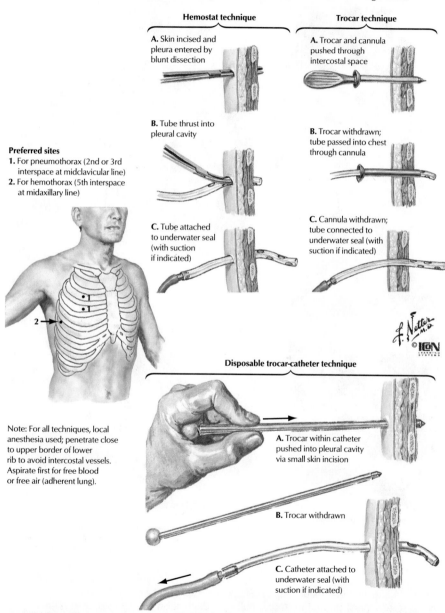

Hemostat technique

A. Skin incised and pleura entered by blunt dissection

B. Tube thrust into pleural cavity

C. Tube attached to underwater seal (with suction if indicated)

Trocar technique

A. Trocar and cannula pushed through intercostal space

B. Trocar withdrawn; tube passed into chest through cannula

C. Cannula withdrawn; tube connected to underwater seal (with suction if indicated)

Preferred sites
1. For pneumothorax (2nd or 3rd interspace at midclavicular line)
2. For hemothorax (5th interspace at midaxillary line)

Note: For all techniques, local anesthesia used; penetrate close to upper border of lower rib to avoid intercostal vessels. Aspirate first for free blood or free air (adherent lung).

Disposable trocar-catheter technique

A. Trocar within catheter pushed into pleural cavity via small skin incision

B. Trocar withdrawn

C. Catheter attached to underwater seal (with suction if indicated)

A chest tube provides a way to evacuate air or fluids (blood, pus, chyle) from the pleural cavity, thus reapposing parietal and visceral pleura and enhancing the patient's ability to breathe normally.

Clinical Correlation

Silicosis, Asbestosis, and Mesothelioma   *Anatomy on pp. 308, 322*

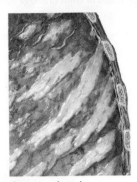

Plumonary asbestosis. pleural plaques

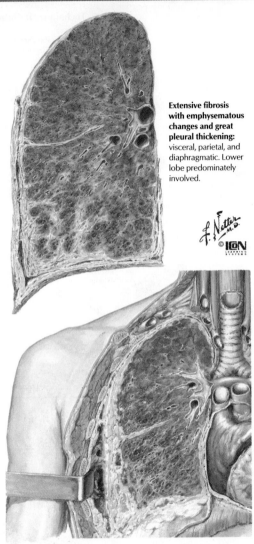

Extensive fibrosis with emphysematous changes and great pleural thickening: visceral, parietal, and diaphragmatic. Lower lobe predominately involved.

Complicated silicosis. Massive fibrosis and conglomerate nodulation. Pleura thickened, nodulated, and adhesive.

Mesothelioma of pleura. Neoplastic growth encasing right lung, infiltrating interlobar fissure, and invading parietal pleura and pericardium. Hemorrhagic fluid in remainder of pleural cavity. Asbestosis of lung.

Silicosis, the most common occupational disease in the world, is caused by inhalation of crystalline silicon dioxide (silica). Silica particles collect in terminal airways, which leads to fibroblast proliferation and collagen deposition. Asbestosis, also an occupational disease, is linked to interstitial fibrosis, bronchogenic carcinoma, pleural effusion, fibrous plaque formation, and mesotheliomas. Malignant mesothelioma is a rare cancer that often arises from pleura; 50% of patients have a history of asbestos exposure, with the disease occurring 25-40 years after initial exposure.

Clinical Correlation

Causes of Chronic Cough

Anatomy on pp. 322, 352

Causes of chronic cough

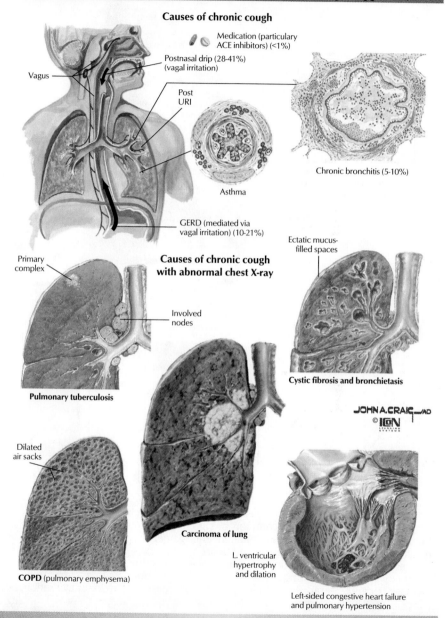

Medication (particulary ACE inhibitors) (<1%)

Postnasal drip (28-41%) (vagal irritation)

Vagus

Post URI

Asthma

Chronic bronchitis (5-10%)

GERD (mediated via vagal irritation) (10-21%)

Causes of chronic cough with abnormal chest X-ray

Primary complex

Involved nodes

Ectatic mucus-filled spaces

Cystic fibrosis and bronchietasis

Pulmonary tuberculosis

Dilated air sacks

COPD (pulmonary emphysema)

Carcinoma of lung

L. ventricular hypertrophy and dilation

Left-sided congestive heart failure and pulmonary hypertension

JOHN A. CRAIG—AD
© ICON

Although an acute cough often signals an upper respiratory viral infection, a chronic cough may indicate a more serious underlying illness. Chronic cough itself has clinical consequences, including conjunctival bleeding, epistaxis, vomiting, stress urinary incontinence, rib fractures, disc herniation, hernias, esophageal rupture, and cardiac arrhythmias.

Clinical Correlation

Chronic Obstructive Pulmonary Disease   *Anatomy on pp. 316, 317*

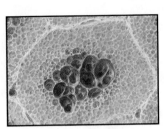

Magnified section. Distended, inter-communicating, saclike spaces in central area of acini.

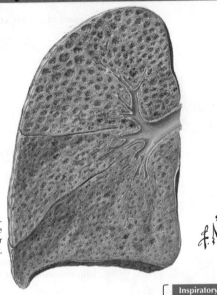

Gross specimen. Involvement tends to be most marked in upper part of lung.

Maximum expiratory flow-volume curves

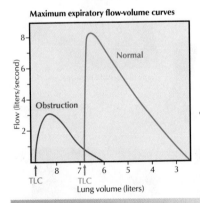

Flow (liters/second)

Normal

Obstruction

Lung volume (liters)

TLC increased largely because of increased RV and FRC. VC usually decreased but may be normal.

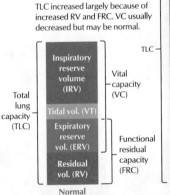

Total lung capacity (TLC)

Inspiratory reserve volume (IRV)

Tidal vol. (VT)

Expiratory reserve vol. (ERV)

Residual vol. (RV)

Vital capacity (VC)

Functional residual capacity (FRC)

Normal

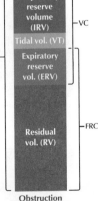

Inspiratory reserve volume (IRV)

Tidal vol. (VT)

Expiratory reserve vol. (ERV)

Residual vol. (RV)

VC

TLC

FRC

Obstruction

Chronic obstructive pulmonary disease (COPD) is a broad classification of obstructive lung diseases, the two most common being chronic bronchitis and emphysema. Emphysema is characterized by permanent enlargement of airspaces at and distal to respiratory bronchioles and destruction of bronchiole walls by inflammation. Hence, lung compliance increases, and decreased elastic recoil results in airway collapse during expiration. Total lung capacity (TLC) and functional residual capacity (FRC) increase because of trapped air in lungs, which increases the work of expiration, as patients try to force air from the lungs (leads to a barrel-chested appearance). Smoking is a major risk factor. The three main types of emphysema are

- Centriacinar (centrilobular) with involvement of central and proximal acini, usually in upper lung zones
- Panacinar with acini uniformly enlarged, mostly in lower lung zones
- Distal acinar with distal acini involvement, usually near visceral pleura and along lobar septa

Clinical Correlation

Cor Pulmonale Caused by COPD   *Anatomy on pp. 316, 340, 351*

Elevation of pulmonary artery pressure — Systolic / Diastolic

Reduction of pulmonary arterial bed (loss of vessels plus reflex hypoxic vasoconstriction)

Normal readings <25 <10

Venous distention

X-ray film showing typical enlarged pulmonary artery shadows and outflow tract of right ventricle

Hypertrophy and dilatation of right ventricle, leading to hypertrophy and dilatation of right atrium and to tricuspid insufficiency terminally

Bulge of septum to left may impair left ventricular filling (reverse Bernheim phenomenon)

Hematocrit increased

Enlargement of liver (passive congestion)

Normal   Cor pulmonale

Peripheral edema

In COPD, total cross-sectional area of the pulmonary vasculature decreases because of pathologic destruction and pulmonary vasospasm, which leads to pulmonary hypertension. The work of the right ventricle thus increases and may result in hypertrophy and dilation. A patient with cor pulmonale (right-sided heart failure) has distended neck veins that do not collapse on inspiration, hepatic engorgement (tender and enlarged), pitting edema of the limbs, increased hematocrit (from chronic hypoxemia), and prominent pulmonary vessels on a posteroanterior chest x-ray film.

Clinical Correlation

Idiopathic Pulmonary Fibrosis   *Anatomy on pp. 316, 317*

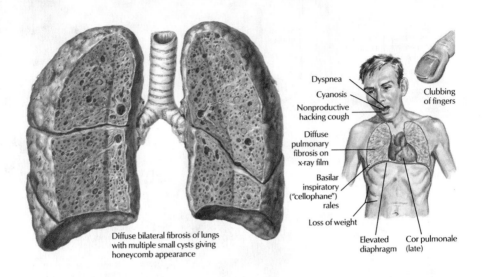

Dyspnea
Cyanosis
Nonproductive hacking cough
Diffuse pulmonary fibrosis on x-ray film
Basilar inspiratory ("cellophane") rales
Loss of weight

Clubbing of fingers

Elevated diaphragm   Cor pulmonale (late)

Diffuse bilateral fibrosis of lungs with multiple small cysts giving honeycomb appearance

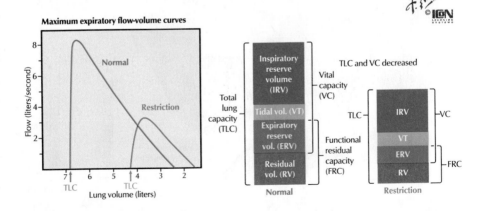

Maximum expiratory flow-volume curves

Flow (liters/second)

Normal

Restriction

Lung volume (liters)

TLC   TLC

Total lung capacity (TLC)

Inspiratory reserve volume (IRV)

Vital capacity (VC)

Tidal vol. (VT)

Expiratory reserve vol. (ERV)

Functional residual capacity (FRC)

Residual vol. (RV)

Normal

TLC and VC decreased

TLC

IRV — VC

VT

ERV — FRC

RV

Restriction

Chronic restrictive lung diseases (approximately 15% of noninfectious lung diseases) include a diverse group of disorders with reduced compliance (more pressure required to inflate stiffened lungs), chronic inflammation, and fibrosis. Virtually all lung volumes, especially TLC and vital capacity (VC), are reduced. Idiopathic pulmonary fibrosis is a poorly understood interstitial fibrotic disorder that leads to hypoxemia and cyanosis. Males are affected more than females; most patients are aged 30-50 years at diagnosis. Some unknown injurious agent (environmental or occupational) first causes alveolitis and initiates an immune response, which leads to epithelial cell injury and the fibrogenic response. Median survival time is 4-5 years.

Clinical Correlation

Lung Abscess

Anatomy on pp. 314-318

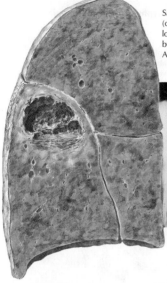

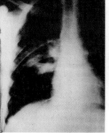

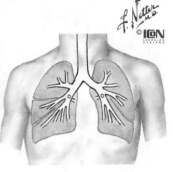

Sagittal section of lung with abscess (cavity in superior segment of lower lobe containing fluid and surrounded by fibrous tissue and pneumonic patches). Also pleural thickening over abscess.

PA x-ray film showing an abscess cavity with fluid level in superior segment of right lower lobe

Right main bronchus is more in line with trachea than is the left, so that aspiration is more likely and incidence of abscess is greater on right side.

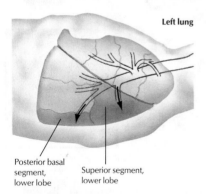

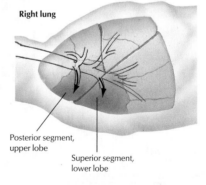

Left lung   **Right lung**

Posterior segment, upper lobe

Posterior basal segment, lower lobe

Superior segment, lower lobe

Superior segment, lower lobe

Although left lung is less commonly affected, superior and posterior basal segments are most vulnerable on that side.

In supine position, posterior segment of right upper lobe and superior segment of lower lobe are most vulnerable to aspirational abscess.

Lung abscess is a localized inflammatory disorder of the parenchyma that is characterized by necrosis surrounded by pneumonitis. Abscess can be a consequence of
- Aspiration of infective agents (during anesthesia, coma, seizure, or alcoholic intoxication)
- Aspiration of gastric contents
- Complications of acute bacterial pneumonia
- Bronchial obstruction
- Septic embolism (from septic thrombophlebitis or endocarditis)

Abscess formation usually occurs in the right lung because the right main bronchus is wider, shorter, and more vertical than the left one.

Clinical Correlation

Pneumonia   *Anatomy on p. 317*

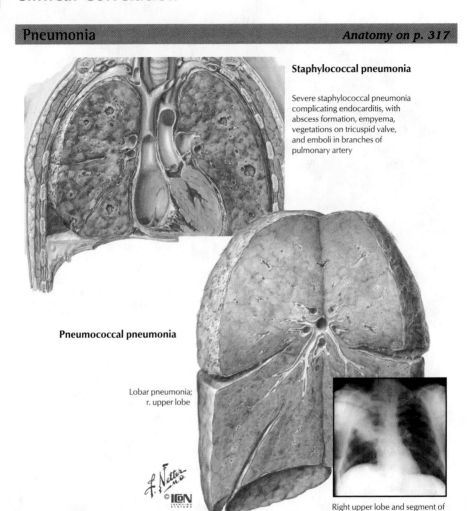

Staphylococcal pneumonia

Severe staphylococcal pneumonia
complicating endocarditis, with
abscess formation, empyema,
vegetations on tricuspid valve,
and emboli in branches of
pulmonary artery

Pneumococcal pneumonia

Lobar pneumonia;
r. upper lobe

Right upper lobe and segment of
right lower lobe pneumonia

Lungs are continually exposed to infectious agents, and infections, in the form of pneumonia, account for one sixth of all deaths in the United States. Patients often present with respiratory symptoms such as cough, sputum production, and shortness of breath, often with fever and chills. Infants and elderly persons are especially vulnerable to pneumococcal pneumonia, as are individuals with congestive heart failure (CHF), COPD, diabetes, or alcoholism. Staphylococcal pneumonia often occurs after a viral respiratory illness (incidence increases after an influenza outbreak).

PATHOGEN	FREQUENCY (%)	PATHOGEN	FREQUENCY (%)
Streptococcus pneumoniae (pneumococcal pneumonia)	20-60	Gram-negative bacilli	3-10
Mixed flora (aspiration pneumonia)	6-10	*Staphylococcus aureus*	3-5
Chlamydia pneumoniae	4-6	*Legionella pneumophila*	2-8
Haemophilus influenzae	3-10	*Mycoplasma pneumoniae*	1-6

Clinical Correlation

Dissemination of Tuberculosis   *Anatomy on pp. 317, 318, 324*

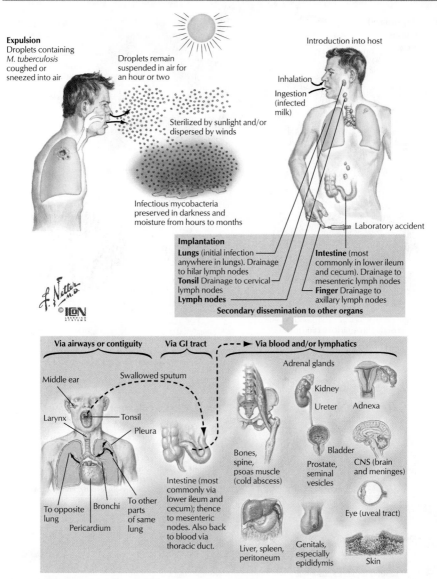

Expulsion
Droplets containing *M. tuberculosis* coughed or sneezed into air

Droplets remain suspended in air for an hour or two

Introduction into host

Inhalation

Ingestion (infected milk)

Sterilized by sunlight and/or dispersed by winds

Infectious mycobacteria preserved in darkness and moisture from hours to months

Laboratory accident

Implantation
Lungs (initial infection anywhere in lungs). Drainage to hilar lymph nodes
Tonsil Drainage to cervical lymph nodes
Lymph nodes

Intestine (most commonly in lower ileum and cecum). Drainage to mesenteric lymph nodes
Finger Drainage to axillary lymph nodes

Secondary dissemination to other organs

Via airways or contiguity   **Via GI tract**   **Via blood and/or lymphatics**

Middle ear   Swallowed sputum

Adrenal glands

Kidney

Ureter   Adnexa

Larynx   Tonsil

Pleura

Bladder

Bones, spine, psoas muscle (cold abscess)

Prostate, seminal vesicles

CNS (brain and meninges)

To opposite lung   Bronchi   To other parts of same lung

Pericardium

Intestine (most commonly via lower ileum and cecum); thence to mesenteric nodes. Also back to blood via thoracic duct.

Eye (uveal tract)

Liver, spleen, peritoneum

Genitals, especially epididymis

Skin

Tuberculosis (TB) is a communicable granulomatous disease caused by *Mycobacterium tuberculosis*. TB causes 6% of all deaths worldwide (much less in the United States) and thrives when poverty, crowding, and chronic debilitating illness are prevalent. TB is disseminated through the air by small droplet nuclei (particles that contain *M. tuberculosis* bacilli). As they grow, bacilli elicit a cellular immune response; however, before cellular immunity develops, bacilli spread via lymphatics to pulmonary hilar lymph nodes and via blood to other organ systems.

Clinical Correlation

Pulmonary Tuberculosis   *Anatomy on pp. 317, 324*

Initial (primary) tuberculous complex

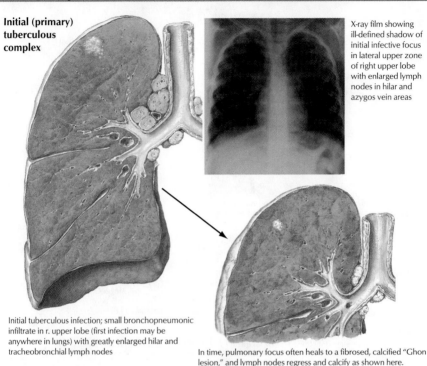

X-ray film showing ill-defined shadow of initial infective focus in lateral upper zone of right upper lobe with enlarged lymph nodes in hilar and azygos vein areas

Initial tuberculous infection; small bronchopneumonic infiltrate in r. upper lobe (first infection may be anywhere in lungs) with greatly enlarged hilar and tracheobronchial lymph nodes

In time, pulmonary focus often heals to a fibrosed, calcified "Ghon lesion," and lymph nodes regress and calcify as shown here.

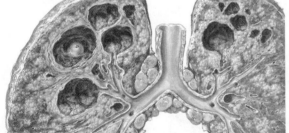

Pulmonary tuberculosis extensive cavitary disease

Multiple cavities in both lungs with erosion into bronchi plus caseous pneumonitis and fibrosis throughout. One cavity in right lung contains an eroded aneurysmal blood vessel (Rasmussen), which is common cause of hemorrhage.

Primary TB develops in previously unexposed and unsensitized individuals; significant disease develops in approximately 5% of these individuals. Reactivation or secondary TB arises in previously sensitized persons. Primary lesions often occur in distal alveoli of the lower part of the upper lobe or upper portion of the lower lobe, near the pleura. Hilar nodes are commonly affected, with caseation. Reactivation TB is usually located in apicoposterior segments of the upper lobes, with more than 70% of these patients having upper lobe infiltrates typical of reactivation. Cavitation may occur with erosion into the airways, which leads to sputum production and further dissemination.

Pleura and Lungs: Autonomic Nerves in the Thorax

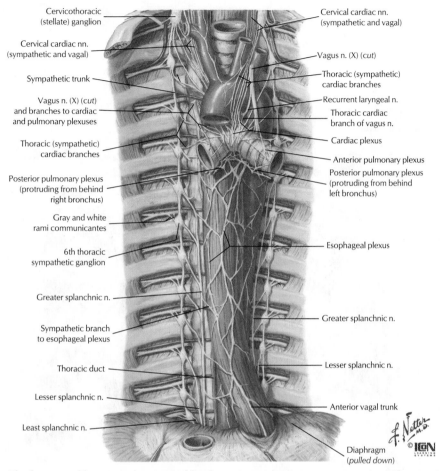

Cervicothoracic (stellate) ganglion

Cervical cardiac nn. (sympathetic and vagal)

Sympathetic trunk

Vagus n. (X) (cut) and branches to cardiac and pulmonary plexuses

Thoracic (sympathetic) cardiac branches

Posterior pulmonary plexus (protruding from behind right bronchus)

Gray and white rami communicantes

6th thoracic sympathetic ganglion

Greater splanchnic n.

Sympathetic branch to esophageal plexus

Thoracic duct

Lesser splanchnic n.

Least splanchnic n.

Cervical cardiac nn. (sympathetic and vagal)

Vagus n. (X) (cut)

Thoracic (sympathetic) cardiac branches

Recurrent laryngeal n.

Thoracic cardiac branch of vagus n.

Cardiac plexus

Anterior pulmonary plexus

Posterior pulmonary plexus (protruding from behind left bronchus)

Esophageal plexus

Greater splanchnic n.

Lesser splanchnic n.

Anterior vagal trunk

Diaphragm (pulled down)

The lungs and heart are innervated by the autonomic nervous system (see Chapter 1 [Introduction]). Sympathetics dilate bronchi and increase heart rate and force of contraction; parasympathetics have opposite effects.

NERVE OR PLEXUS	INNERVATION
Parasympathetics	Fibers that course in vagus nerve (preganglionic efferents)
Sympathetics	Fibers that arise from upper portion of thoracic spinal cord (T1-T4) and synapse in sympathetic chain ganglia
Pulmonary plexus	Anterior and posterior plexuses: synapse location for parasympathetics
Cardiac plexus	Synapse location for parasympathetics
Cervical cardiac nerves	Postganglionic sympathetics: ascend sympathetic chain and then course to cardiac and pulmonary plexuses
Thoracic cardiac nerves	Postganglionic sympathetics: course directly from sympathetic chain to cardiac and pulmonary plexuses
Visceral afferents	Pain fibers: course retrograde in sympathetics to dorsal root ganglion (cell bodies) and into dorsal horn of T1-T4 spinal cord; fibers for stretch, irritant, chemoreceptor, and cough-mediated sensations: course with glossopharyngeal or vagus nerve to brainstem

Pericardium and Heart: Heart In Situ

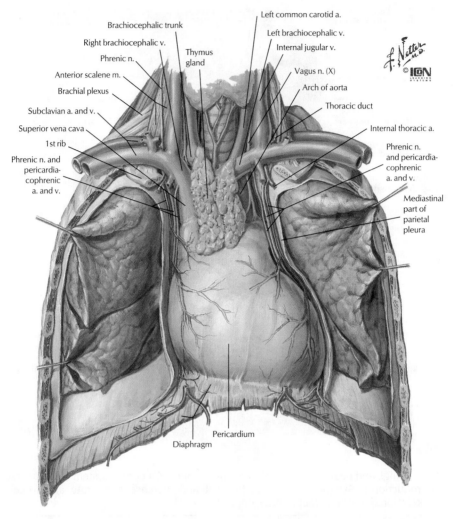

Brachiocephalic trunk

Left common carotid a.

Right brachiocephalic v.

Left brachiocephalic v.

Phrenic n.

Thymus gland

Internal jugular v.

Anterior scalene m.

Vagus n. (X)

Brachial plexus

Arch of aorta

Subclavian a. and v.

Thoracic duct

Superior vena cava

Internal thoracic a.

1st rib

Phrenic n. and pericardiacophrenic a. and v.

Phrenic n. and pericardiacophrenic a. and v.

Mediastinal part of parietal pleura

Pericardium

Diaphragm

The heart is enclosed within a fibroserous sac called the pericardium (see table below). The pericardial cavity is the potential space between the two serous layers of the pericardium and contains a thin film of serous lubricating fluid to reduce friction of the beating heart. The pericardium and heart occupy the middle mediastinum.

FEATURE	DEFINITION
Fibrous pericardium	Tough, outer layer that reflects onto great vessels
Serous pericardium	Layer that lines inner aspect of fibrous pericardium (parietal layer); reflects onto heart as epicardium (visceral layer)
Innervation	Phrenic nerve (C3-5) for conveying pain; vasomotor innervation via sympathetics
Transverse sinus	Space posterior to aorta and pulmonary trunk; can clamp vessels with fingers in this sinus and above
Oblique sinus	Pericardial space posterior to heart

Clinical Correlation

Pericarditis *Anatomy on p. 340*

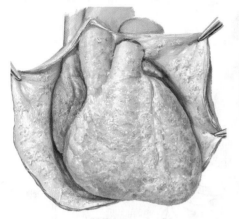

Mild fibrinous pericarditis

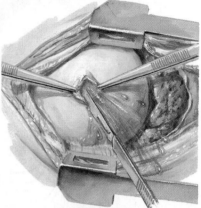

Pericardial effusion. Pleuropericardial window being created and biopsy specimen taken via incision in 5th left intercostal space

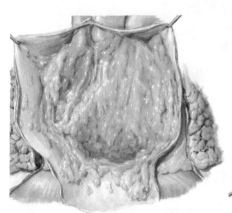

Purulent pericarditis

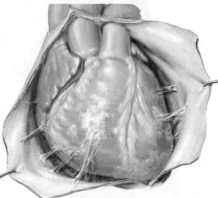

Adhesive pericarditis

Diseases of the pericardium involve inflammatory conditions (pericarditis) and effusions (fluid accumulation in the pleural cavity). The usual cause of primary disease is a virus, although bacteria and fungi are also causative agents. Uremia (in renal failure) is the most common systemic disorder associated with pericarditis. Findings of pericarditis include

- Atypical chest pain
- High-pitched friction rub
- Effusion caused by inflammation (mimics cardiac tamponade)
- Exudate associated with acute disease: fibrous (with uremia or a viral etiology) or fibrinopurulent (when bacterial etiology)

Clinical Correlation

Cardiac Tamponade   *Anatomy on pp. 340, 366*

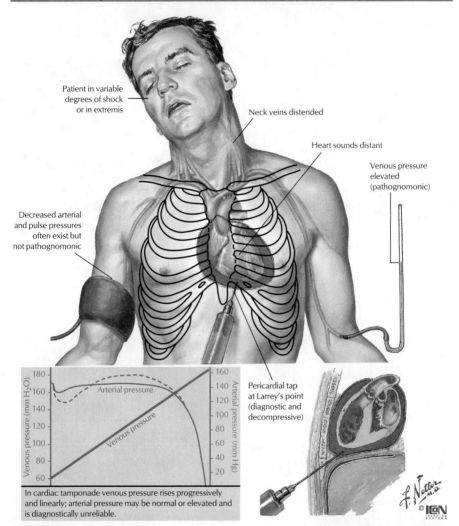

Patient in variable degrees of shock or in extremis

Neck veins distended

Heart sounds distant

Venous pressure elevated (pathognomonic)

Decreased arterial and pulse pressures often exist but not pathognomonic

Pericardial tap at Larrey's point (diagnostic and decompressive)

In cardiac tamponade venous pressure rises progressively and linearly; arterial pressure may be normal or elevated and is diagnostically unreliable.

Cardiac tamponade can result from fluid accumulation or bleeding into the pericardial cavity (hemopericardium). Bleeding may be caused by a ruptured aortic aneurysm, ruptured myocardial infarct, or penetrating injury, which compromises the beating heart and decreases venous return and cardiac output. Signs and symptoms include

- Tachycardia
- Hypotension*
- Muffled heart sounds*
- Jugular venous distention (Kussmaul's sign)* (lack of expected decline in jugular venous pressure with inspiration)
- Increased pulsus paradoxus

*Beck's triad

Pericardium and Heart:
Coronary Arteries and Cardiac Veins

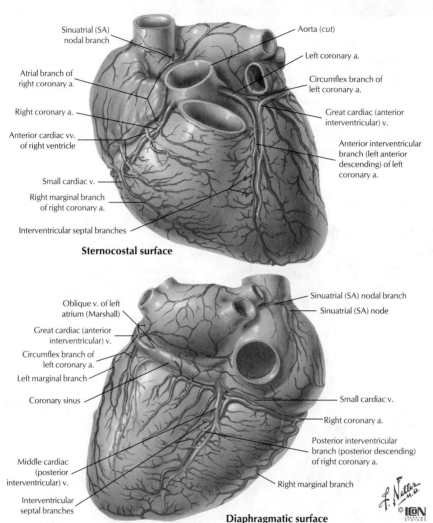

Sinuatrial (SA) nodal branch

Aorta (*cut*)

Left coronary a.

Atrial branch of right coronary a.

Circumflex branch of left coronary a.

Right coronary a.

Great cardiac (anterior interventricular) v.

Anterior cardiac vv. of right ventricle

Anterior interventricular branch (left anterior descending) of left coronary a.

Small cardiac v.

Right marginal branch of right coronary a.

Interventricular septal branches

Sternocostal surface

Oblique v. of left atrium (Marshall)

Sinuatrial (SA) nodal branch

Sinuatrial (SA) node

Great cardiac (anterior interventricular) v.

Circumflex branch of left coronary a.

Left marginal branch

Coronary sinus

Small cardiac v.

Right coronary a.

Posterior interventricular branch (posterior descending) of right coronary a.

Middle cardiac (posterior interventricular) v.

Interventricular septal branches

Right marginal branch

Diaphragmatic surface

VESSEL	COURSE
Right coronary artery	Consists of major branches: sinuatrial (SA) nodal, right marginal, posterior interventricular (posterior descending), atrioventricular (AV) nodal
Left coronary artery	Consists of major branches: circumflex, anterior interventricular (left anterior descending) (LAD), left marginal
Great cardiac vein	Parallels LAD artery and drains into coronary sinus
Middle cardiac vein	Parallels posterior descending artery and drains into coronary sinus
Small cardiac vein	Parallels right marginal artery and drains into coronary sinus
Anterior cardiac veins	Are several small veins that drain directly into right atrium
Smallest cardiac veins	Drain through the cardiac wall directly into all four heart chambers

Clinical Correlation

Angiogenesis
Anatomy on p. 343

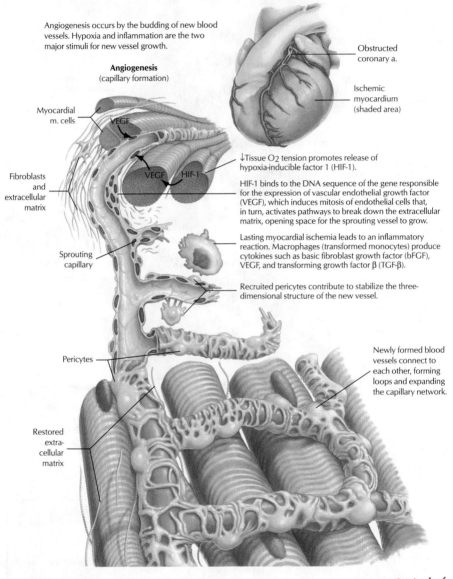

Angiogenesis occurs by the budding of new blood vessels. Hypoxia and inflammation are the two major stimuli for new vessel growth.

Angiogenesis
(capillary formation)

Myocardial m. cells

VEGF

Fibroblasts and extracellular matrix

VEGF   HIF-1

Sprouting capillary

Pericytes

Restored extra-cellular matrix

Obstructed coronary a.

Ischemic myocardium (shaded area)

↓Tissue O_2 tension promotes release of hypoxia-inducible factor 1 (HIF-1).

HIF-1 binds to the DNA sequence of the gene responsible for the expression of vascular endothelial growth factor (VEGF), which induces mitosis of endothelial cells that, in turn, activates pathways to break down the extracellular matrix, opening space for the sprouting vessel to grow.

Lasting myocardial ischemia leads to an inflammatory reaction. Macrophages (transformed monocytes) produce cytokines such as basic fibroblast growth factor (bFGF), VEGF, and transforming growth factor β (TGF-β).

Recruited pericytes contribute to stabilize the three-dimensional structure of the new vessel.

Newly formed blood vessels connect to each other, forming loops and expanding the capillary network.

C. Machado
—M.D.

© ICN
LEARNING
SYSTEMS

Revascularization after an ischemic episode, bypass surgery, or percutaneous coronary intervention is vital for establishing new vessels (angiogenesis) and for creating anastomoses with existing vessels. The mechanism of angiogenesis is illustrated here.

Clinical Correlation

Acute Coronary Syndromes
Anatomy on p. 343

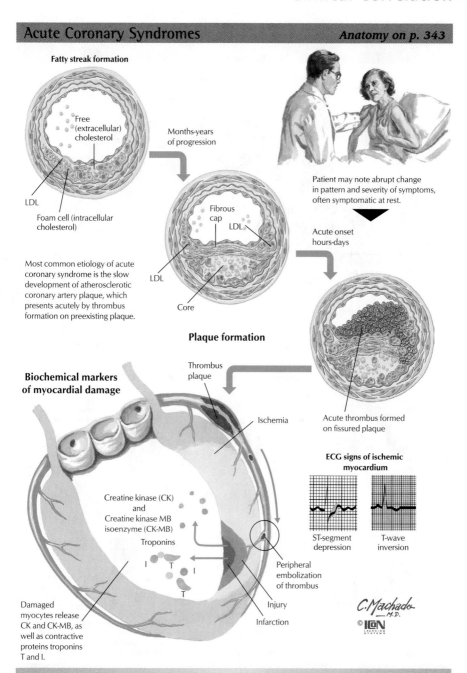

Fatty streak formation

Free (extracellular) cholesterol

LDL

Foam cell (intracellular cholesterol)

Most common etiology of acute coronary syndrome is the slow development of atherosclerotic coronary artery plaque, which presents acutely by thrombus formation on preexisting plaque.

Months-years of progression

Fibrous cap

LDL

LDL

Core

Plaque formation

Patient may note abrupt change in pattern and severity of symptoms, often symptomatic at rest.

Acute onset hours-days

Acute thrombus formed on fissured plaque

Biochemical markers of myocardial damage

Thrombus plaque

Ischemia

Creatine kinase (CK) and Creatine kinase MB isoenzyme (CK-MB)

Troponins

I   T   I

T

Damaged myocytes release CK and CK-MB, as well as contractive proteins troponins T and I.

Peripheral embolization of thrombus

Injury

Infarction

ECG signs of ischemic myocardium

ST-segment depression

T-wave inversion

C. Machado, M.D.
©ICN

Acute coronary syndromes involve signs and symptoms that are associated with a spectrum of disorders including transient ischemia, recurrent or unstable angina, non–Q-wave myocardial infarction (MI), or transmural/Q-wave MI. Electrocardiographic findings include ST-segment and T-wave changes.

Clinical Correlation

Cardiovascular Disease in the Elderly and in Women
Anatomy on p. 343

Cardiovascular disease in the elderly

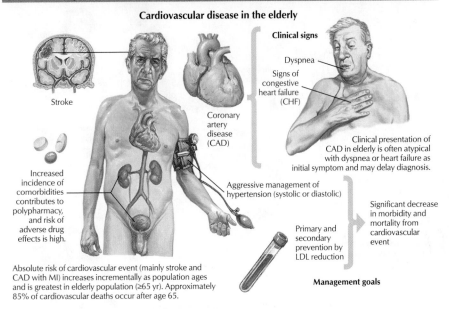

Stroke

Increased incidence of comorbidities contributes to polypharmacy, and risk of adverse drug effects is high.

Coronary artery disease (CAD)

Clinical signs

Dyspnea

Signs of congestive heart failure (CHF)

Clinical presentation of CAD in elderly is often atypical with dyspnea or heart failure as initial symptom and may delay diagnosis.

Aggressive management of hypertension (systolic or diastolic)

Primary and secondary prevention by LDL reduction

Significant decrease in morbidity and mortality from cardiovascular event

Management goals

Absolute risk of cardiovascular event (mainly stroke and CAD with MI) increases incrementally as population ages and is greatest in elderly population (≥65 yr). Approximately 85% of cardiovascular deaths occur after age 65.

Cardiovascular disease in women

Risk factors

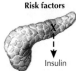

Insulin

Diabetes in women is a more powerful risk factor than in men, associated with 3-7 times increase in CHD development.

Smoking is a stronger risk factor for MI in middle-aged women than men.

Hormone replacement is contraindicated as cardioprotection in postmenopausal women.

Treatment of dyslipidemias (⬆LDL, ⬇HDL, ⬆triglycerides) offers reduction in cardiovascular event risk.

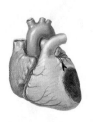

Cardiovascular disease is leading cause of death in both men and women. More women die of cardiovascular disease than of breast cancer.

C. Machado
—M.D.

©ICON
LEARNING
SYSTEMS

Clinical presentation

Women may present with "heartburn"-type symptoms due to CHD.

Back pain is a common "anginal equivalent" in women.

Fatigue and dyspnea on exertion with decreased exercise tolerance are common complaints.

CHD symptoms reported by women often differ from those reported by men. These vague or confusing symptoms may contribute to a delayed or missed diagnosis.

With the aging of the US population, cardiovascular disease among the elderly and women is a major health problem, especially with the notable increase in obesity and diabetes. The incidence has decreased in elderly men but remains unchanged in women. Some more common manifestations of cardiovascular disease are illustrated.

Clinical Correlation

Angina Pectoris

Anatomy on pp. 339, 343

Pain of myocardial ischemia

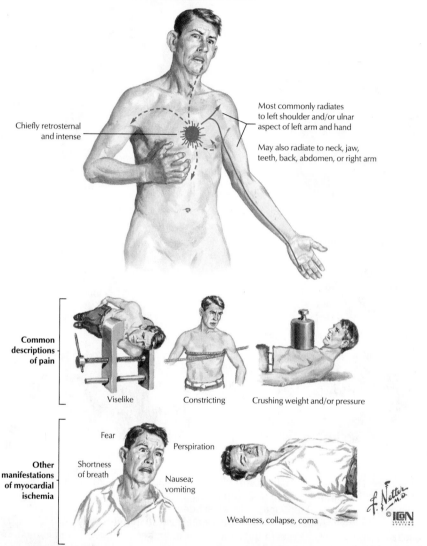

Chiefly retrosternal and intense

Most commonly radiates to left shoulder and/or ulnar aspect of left arm and hand

May also radiate to neck, jaw, teeth, back, abdomen, or right arm

Common descriptions of pain

Viselike   Constricting   Crushing weight and/or pressure

Other manifestations of myocardial ischemia

Fear

Perspiration

Shortness of breath

Nausea; vomiting

Weakness, collapse, coma

Angina pectoris is the sensation caused by myocardial ischemia and is usually described as pressure, discomfort, or feeling of choking in the left chest or substernal region that radiates to the left shoulder and arm as well as the neck, jaw and teeth, abdomen, and back. The pain also may radiate to the right arm. This radiating pattern is an example of referred pain in which visceral afferents from the heart enter the upper thoracic spinal cord along with somatic afferents, both converging in the spinal cord's dorsal horn. Interpretation of the visceral pain may initially be confused with somatic sensations from the same cord levels.

Clinical Correlation

Myocardial Infarction   *Anatomy on p. 343*

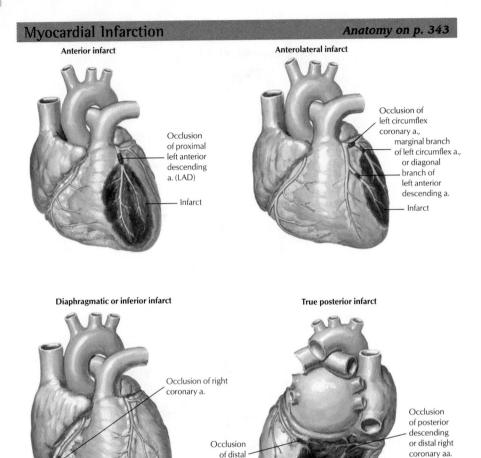

Anterior infarct

Occlusion of proximal left anterior descending a. (LAD)

Infarct

Anterolateral infarct

Occlusion of left circumflex coronary a., marginal branch of left circumflex a., or diagonal branch of left anterior descending a.

Infarct

Diaphragmatic or inferior infarct

Occlusion of right coronary a.

Occlusion of distal circumflex a.

Infarct

True posterior infarct

Occlusion of posterior descending or distal right coronary aa.

Infarct

    MI affects more than 1 million Americans per year, and more than 40% who have an MI in a given year die from it. Coronary atherosclerosis and coronary thrombosis, the major causes of MI, precipitate local ischemia and necrosis of a defined myocardial area. Necrosis usually occurs approximately 20-30 minutes after coronary artery occlusion. MI usually begins in the subendocardium because this region is the most poorly perfused of the ventricular wall.

ARTERY OCCLUDED	FREQUENCY AND AFFECTED AREA
LAD	40-50%; affects anterior and apical left ventricle and anterior two thirds of interventricular septum (IVS)
Right coronary	30-40%; affects posterior wall of left ventricle, posterior one third of IVS (if right-dominant coronary circulation)
Left circumflex	15-20%; affects lateral wall of left ventricle (can also affect posterior wall if left-dominant coronary circulation)

Clinical Correlation

Coronary Bypass
Anatomy on pp. 308, 311, 340, 343

Myocardial revascularization employing both internal thoracic arteries

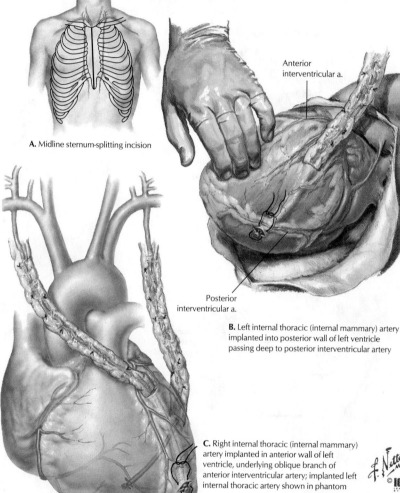

A. Midline sternum-splitting incision

Anterior
interventricular a.

Posterior
interventricular a.

B. Left internal thoracic (internal mammary) artery
implanted into posterior wall of left ventricle
passing deep to posterior interventricular artery

C. Right internal thoracic (internal mammary)
artery implanted in anterior wall of left
ventricle, underlying oblique branch of
anterior interventricular artery; implanted left
internal thoracic artery shown in phantom

Coronary bypass offers a surgical approach for revascularization with either saphenous vein grafts (great saphenous vein harvested from a lower limb) or internal thoracic (mammary) artery (ITA) implants (radial artery is also used). Bilateral ITA implants are indicated when two sites of revascularization are required, usually when patients have diffuse disease that involves the left ventricle. Advantages of ITA implants are that they are arterial grafts, do not have valves, are a better match size for native vessels than are veins, and are easy to harvest. Also, they have low vasoconstrictor sensitivity and high vasodilator sensitivity, among other properties, which lead to very high long-term patency compared with the 7- to 9-year patency of vein grafts.

Clinical Correlation

Saphenous Vein Graft Disease
Anatomy on pp. 343, 367

Percutaneous coronary intervention: vascular access

Distal protection device

Aorta

Guide catheter

Saphenous v. graft

Stenotic lesion

Guide wire in left coronary a.

Guide catheter

LAD

Brachial a.

Femoral a.

Guide catheter

Stenotic lesion

Native vessel

Occlusion balloon inflated

Stent delivery catheter with its balloon inflated and the stent expanded

Stent in place

Aspiration catheter aspirating atherosclerotic debris

C. Machado
M.D.

© ICN

Saphenous vein graft disease after coronary artery bypass grafting is a long-term complication. Patients often present with angina; the venous graft is characterized by a diffuse, friable plaque and often a thrombus with the potential to embolize distally. Percutaneous coronary intervention provides access to the graft, which is often obtained via the femoral artery. By this method, one may introduce distal protection and thrombectomy devices, such as balloons for expansion or stents, which reduce the incidence of occlusion, embolization, and infarctions in these patients with ischemia.

Pericardium and Heart: Right Atrium and Ventricle

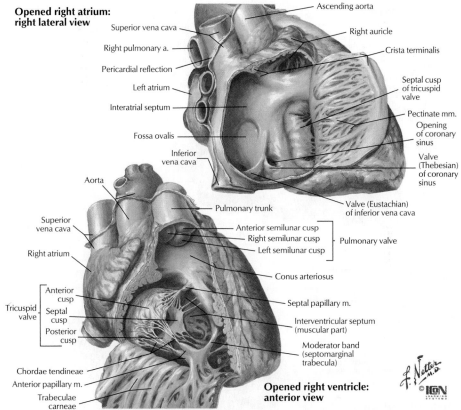

Opened right atrium: right lateral view

Ascending aorta
Superior vena cava
Right auricle
Right pulmonary a.
Crista terminalis
Pericardial reflection
Left atrium
Septal cusp of tricuspid valve
Interatrial septum
Pectinate mm.
Fossa ovalis
Opening of coronary sinus
Inferior vena cava
Valve (Thebesian) of coronary sinus
Aorta
Valve (Eustachian) of inferior vena cava
Superior vena cava
Pulmonary trunk
Right atrium
Anterior semilunar cusp
Right semilunar cusp
Left semilunar cusp
Pulmonary valve
Conus arteriosus
Anterior cusp
Septal papillary m.
Tricuspid valve — Septal cusp
Interventricular septum (muscular part)
Posterior cusp
Moderator band (septomarginal trabecula)
Chordae tendineae
Anterior papillary m.
Trabeculae carneae

Opened right ventricle: anterior view

General features and function of the heart are reviewed in Chapter 1 (Introduction).

FEATURE	DEFINITION
Right Atrium	
Auricle	Pouchlike appendage of atrium; embryonic heart tube derivative
Pectinate muscles	Ridges of myocardium inside auricle
Crista terminalis	Ridge that runs from the inferior (IVC) to superior (SVC) vena cava openings; its superior extent marks the site of the SA node
Fossa ovalis	Depression in interatrial septum; former site of foramen ovale
Atrial openings	One each for SVC, IVC, and coronary sinus (venous return from cardiac veins)
Right Ventricle	
Trabeculae carneae	Irregular ridges of ventricular myocardium
Papillary muscles	Anterior, posterior, and septal projections of myocardium extending into ventricular cavity; prevent valve leaflet prolapse
Chordae tendineae	Fibrous cords that connect papillary muscles to valve leaflets
Moderator band	Muscular band that conveys AV bundle from septum to base of ventricle at site of anterior papillary muscle
Ventricular openings	One to pulmonary trunk through pulmonary valve; one to receive blood from right atrium through tricuspid valve

Pericardium and Heart: Left Atrium and Ventricle

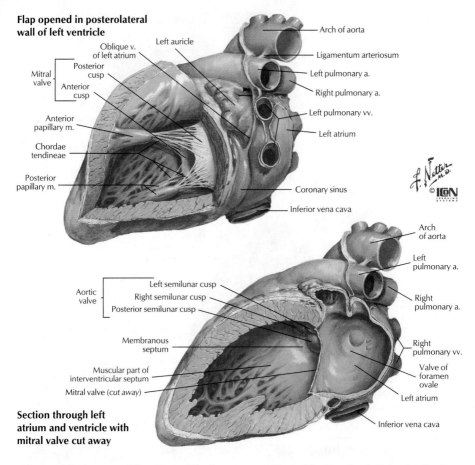

Flap opened in posterolateral wall of left ventricle

- Arch of aorta
- Left auricle
- Oblique v. of left atrium
- Ligamentum arteriosum
- Mitral valve
  - Posterior cusp
  - Anterior cusp
- Left pulmonary a.
- Right pulmonary a.
- Left pulmonary vv.
- Anterior papillary m.
- Left atrium
- Chordae tendineae
- Posterior papillary m.
- Coronary sinus
- Inferior vena cava

- Arch of aorta
- Left pulmonary a.
- Aortic valve
  - Left semilunar cusp
  - Right semilunar cusp
  - Posterior semilunar cusp
- Right pulmonary a.
- Membranous septum
- Right pulmonary vv.
- Muscular part of interventricular septum
- Valve of foramen ovale
- Mitral valve (cut away)
- Left atrium
- Inferior vena cava

Section through left atrium and ventricle with mitral valve cut away

General features and function of the heart are reviewed in Chapter 1 (Introduction).

FEATURE	DEFINITION
Left Atrium	
Auricle	Small appendage representing primitive embryonic atrium whose wall has pectinate muscle
Atrial wall	Wall slightly thicker than thin-walled right atrium
Atrial openings	Usually four openings for four pulmonary veins
Left Ventricle	
Papillary muscles	Anterior and posterior muscles, larger than those of right ventricle
Chordae tendineae	Fibrous cords that connect papillary muscles to valve leaflets
Ventricular wall	Wall much thicker than that of right ventricle
Membranous septum	Very thin superior portion of IVS and site of most ventricular septal defects (VSDs)
Ventricular openings	One to aorta through aortic valve; one to receive blood from left atrium through mitral valve

Pericardium and Heart: Valves and Fibrous Skeleton

Heart in diastole:
viewed from base with atria removed

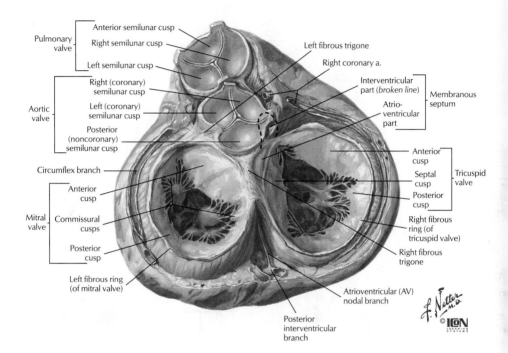

Pulmonary valve
- Anterior semilunar cusp
- Right semilunar cusp
- Left semilunar cusp

Aortic valve
- Right (coronary) semilunar cusp
- Left (coronary) semilunar cusp
- Posterior (noncoronary) semilunar cusp

Circumflex branch

Mitral valve
- Anterior cusp
- Commissural cusps
- Posterior cusp

Left fibrous ring (of mitral valve)

Left fibrous trigone

Right coronary a.

Interventricular part (*broken line*)
Atrio-ventricular part
Membranous septum

Anterior cusp
Septal cusp
Posterior cusp
Tricuspid valve

Right fibrous ring (of tricuspid valve)

Right fibrous trigone

Atrioventricular (AV) nodal branch

Posterior interventricular branch

The heart has four valves that, along with the myocardium, attach to fibrous rings of dense collagen that make up the fibrous skeleton of the heart. The first heart sound (S_1) results from the closing of the mitral and tricuspid valves, whereas the second sound (S_2) results from the closing of the aortic and pulmonic valves.

VALVE	CHARACTERISTIC
Tricuspid	(Right AV) Between right atrium and ventricle, has three cusps
Pulmonary	(Semilunar) Between the right ventricle and pulmonary trunk, possesses three semilunar cusps (leaflets)
Mitral	(Bicuspid) Between left atrium and ventricle, has two cusps
Aortic	(Semilunar) Between left ventricle and aorta, possesses three semilunar cusps

Clinical Correlation

Cardiac Auscultation   *Anatomy on pp. 300, 308, 314, 351, 352*

Precordial areas of auscultation

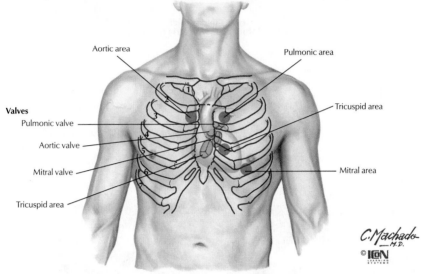

Aortic area

Pulmonic area

Valves

Pulmonic valve

Aortic valve

Mitral valve

Tricuspid area

Tricuspid area

Mitral area

C. Machado
—M.D.

© ICN
LEARNING SYSTEMS

Diagrams of several murmurs

Innocent murmur

S_1 S_2

Systolic murmur from increased pulmonic flow followed by fixed, widely split S_2 (atrial septal defect)

S_1 ES $A_2\,P_2$

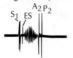

Murmur and ejection click (pulmonary hypertension)

S_1 EC S_2

Systolic murmur (chronic mitral regurgitation) with S_3 and S_4 (dilated cardiomyopathy)

S_4 S_1 S_2 S_3

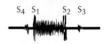

Holosystolic murmur (IVSD or mitral or tricuspid regurgitation)

S_1 S_2

Continuous murmur (patent ductus arteriosus)

S_1 S_2

Diastolic murmur (aortic or pulmonary regurgitation)

S_1 S_2

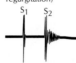

Long diastolic murmur following opening snap (mitral stenosis)

S_1 S_2 OS

Auscultation of the heart requires not only an understanding of the heart sounds (normal and abnormal) but also knowledge of the optimal location to detect them. Sounds are heard best by auscultating the area where turbulent blood flow radiates, i.e., distal to the valve the blood has just passed through.

AREA	COMMENT
Aortic	Upper right sternal border; aortic stenosis
Pulmonary	Upper left sternal border to below left clavicle; second heart sound, pulmonary valve murmurs, VSD murmur, continuous murmur of patent ductus arteriosus (PDA)
Tricuspid	Left fourth intercostal space; tricuspid and aortic regurgitation
Mitral	Left fifth intercostal space, apex; first heart sound, murmurs of mitral or aortic valves, third and fourth heart sounds

Clinical Correlation

Common portals of bacterial entry in bacterial endocarditis

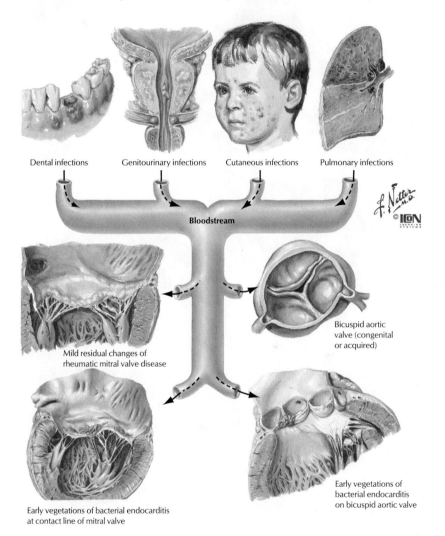

Dental infections   Genitourinary infections   Cutaneous infections   Pulmonary infections

Bloodstream

Mild residual changes of
rheumatic mitral valve disease

Bicuspid aortic
valve (congenital
or acquired)

Early vegetations of bacterial endocarditis
at contact line of mitral valve

Early vegetations of
bacterial endocarditis
on bicuspid aortic valve

Common predisposing lesions

Infective endocarditis (IE) is an infection of the cardiac valves (often previously damaged) or the endocardial surface that results in an infectious colonization and formation of a thrombotic mass, termed vegetation. Any microorganism may cause IE, although most cases are due to bacteria (usually streptococci). The mitral and aortic valves are most often involved. Fever and heart murmurs (approximately 85% of patients have murmurs) are common. Predisposing factors include cardiac abnormalities (congenital or acquired), valve replacement surgery, and intravenous drug abuse.

Clinical Correlation

Thickened stenotic mitral valve: anterior cusp has typical convexity; enlarged left atrium; "jet lesion" on left ventricular wall

Stenosis and insufficiency (fusion of all commissures)

Calcific stenosis

Great hyper-trophy of left ventricle in aortic stenosis

Elongation of left ventricle with tension on chordae tendineae, which may prevent full closure of mitral valve

CONDITION	COMMENT
Aortic stenosis	Leads to left ventricular overload and hypertrophy; caused by rheumatic heart disease (RHD), calcific stenosis, congenital bicuspid valve (1-2%)
Aortic regurgitation (insufficiency)	Caused by congenitally malformed leaflets, RHD, IE, ankylosing spondylitis, Marfan's syndrome, aortic root dilation
Mitral stenosis	Leads to left atrial dilation; usually caused by RHD
Mitral regurgitation (insufficiency)	Caused by abnormalities of valve leaflets, rupture of papillary muscle or chordae tendineae, papillary muscle fibrosis, IE, left ventricular enlargement

Clinical Correlation

Mitral Valve Prolapse
Anatomy on pp. 352, 353

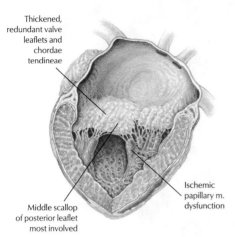

Thickened, redundant valve leaflets and chordae tendineae

Middle scallop of posterior leaflet most involved

Ischemic papillary m. dysfunction

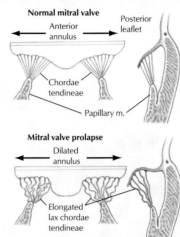

Normal mitral valve

Anterior annulus

Posterior leaflet

Chordae tendineae

Papillary m.

Mitral valve prolapse

Dilated annulus

Elongated lax chordae tendineae

Increased annulus length, leaflet area, and elongated chordae tendineae allow "buckling" or prolapse of valve leaflets into left atrium during systole.

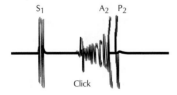

Late systolic murmur following midsystolic click (mitral prolapse)

S₁   A₂ P₂

Click

S. Moon, M.S.
© ICON

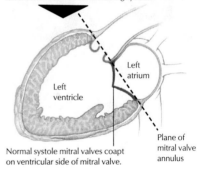

Left atrium

Left ventricle

Plane of mitral valve annulus

Normal systole mitral valves coapt on ventricular side of mitral valve.

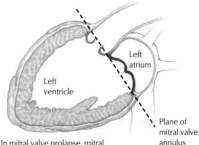

Left atrium

Left ventricle

Plane of mitral valve annulus

In mitral valve prolapse, mitral valve leaflets coapt on atrial side of the plane of the mitral annulus. Some mitral regurgitation may be present.

Mitral valve prolapse is the most common type of congenital heart disease in adults (4-5%) and is often asymptomatic. Cardiac auscultation is the key to clinical diagnosis.

Clinical Correlation

Systemic Lupus Erythematosus
Anatomy on pp. 352, 353

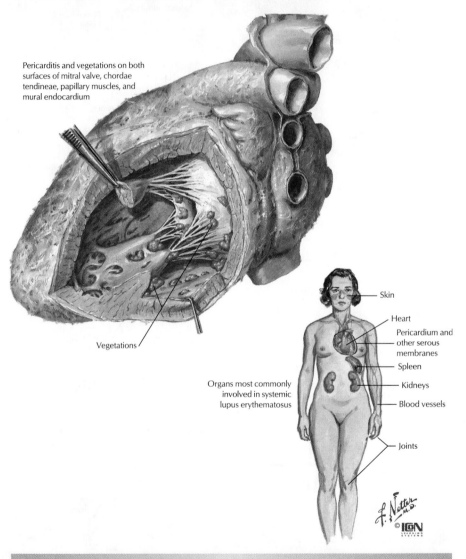

Pericarditis and vegetations on both surfaces of mitral valve, chordae tendineae, papillary muscles, and mural endocardium

Vegetations

Organs most commonly involved in systemic lupus erythematosus

Skin

Heart

Pericardium and other serous membranes

Spleen

Kidneys

Blood vessels

Joints

Systemic lupus erythematosus (SLE), a chronic inflammatory autoimmune disease that is clinically unpredictable, remitting, and relapsing, can involve any organ but mainly affects the skin, joints, heart, kidney, and nervous system. SLE shows a striking female predominance, an incidence as high as 1 case/2500 individuals, and peak occurrence between 15 and 40 years of age. SLE results from interactions between genetic factors and environmental triggers including sex hormone metabolism, diet, stress, sunlight exposure, silica exposure, and toxins. Pericarditis, myocarditis, and valvular endocarditis with warty vegetations (verrucae) on valve leaflets (Libman-Sachs endocarditis) may occur (approximately 50% of SLE cases have heart involvement).

Pericardium and Heart: Cardiac Nerves

Parasympathetic fibers (from vagus nerve) and sympathetic fibers (from cervical and thoracic cardiac nerves of the sympathetic trunk, T1-T4) course to the cardiac plexus and innervate the heart. The intrinsic heart rate is usually approximately 100 beats/min, but normal parasympathetic tone maintains the resting rate at approximately 72 beats/min. Phrenic nerves (C3-C5), also seen in this illustration, innervate the diaphragm and convey afferent pain fibers from the pericardium to the spinal cord.

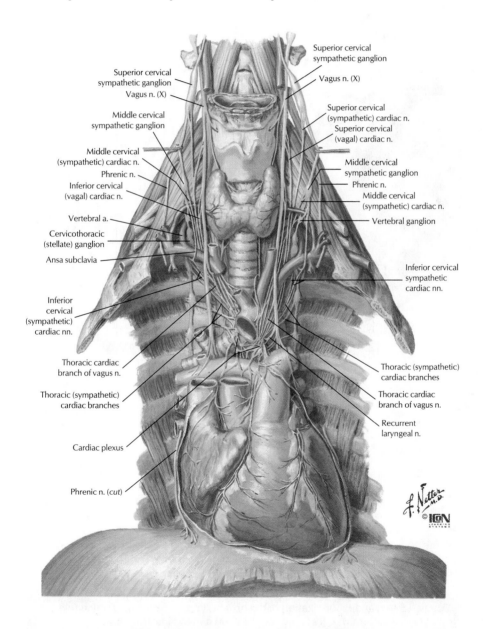

Superior cervical sympathetic ganglion

Superior cervical sympathetic ganglion

Vagus n. (X)

Vagus n. (X)

Middle cervical sympathetic ganglion

Superior cervical (sympathetic) cardiac n.
Superior cervical (vagal) cardiac n.

Middle cervical (sympathetic) cardiac n.

Phrenic n.

Inferior cervical (vagal) cardiac n.

Middle cervical sympathetic ganglion

Phrenic n.

Middle cervical (sympathetic) cardiac n.

Vertebral a.

Vertebral ganglion

Cervicothoracic (stellate) ganglion

Ansa subclavia

Inferior cervical sympathetic cardiac nn.

Inferior cervical (sympathetic) cardiac nn.

Thoracic cardiac branch of vagus n.

Thoracic (sympathetic) cardiac branches

Thoracic (sympathetic) cardiac branches

Thoracic cardiac branch of vagus n.

Recurrent laryngeal n.

Cardiac plexus

Phrenic n. (cut)

Clinical Correlation

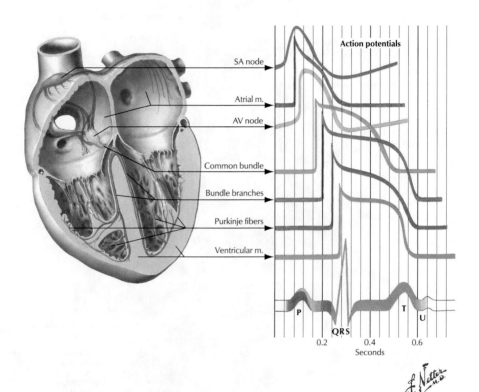

FEATURE	DEFINITION
SA node	Pacemaker of heart; site where action potential is initiated
AV node	Node that receives impulses from SA node and conveys them to the common AV bundle (of His)
Bundle branches	Right and left bundles that convey impulses down either side of IVS to subendocardial Purkinje system

Depolarization and repolarization of the myocardium generate the familiar electro-cardiographic pattern (P, QRS, T waves), as shown in the illustration.

Clinical Correlation

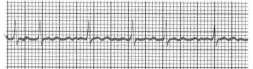

Atrial Fibrillation

Anatomy on pp. 351, 352

Abnormal repetitive impulses (wavelets)

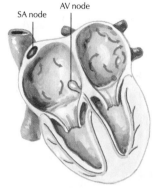

SA node

AV node

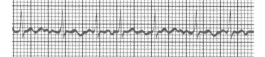

ECG demonstrating fine atrial fibrillation pattern

ECG demonstrating coarse atrial fibrillation pattern

No single mechanism causes atrial fibrillation. Small, multiple re-entrant wavelets may coalesce to form small atrial circuits. Rapid repetitive impulses generated by myocytes located in left atrium near pulmonary vein orifices stimulate atrial fibrillation.

Causes and associated conditions

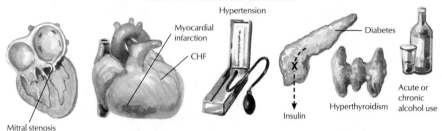

Hypertension

Myocardial infarction

CHF

Diabetes

X

Insulin

Hyperthyroidism

Acute or chronic alcohol use

Mitral stenosis

Electrical intervention options

Cardioversion

Dual chamber pacing
(may include implantable defibrillator)

R
Q S

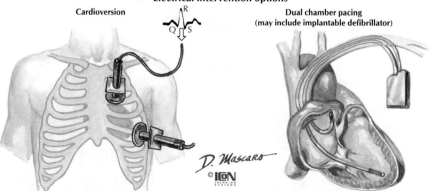

D. Mascaro
© ICN
LEARNING
SYSTEMS

Emergent cardioversion is considered in two circumstances: (1) when onset of atrial fibrillation results in hemodynamic instability in a previously stable patient (manifest as hypotension, angina/myocardial ischemia, or rapid onset of CHF) or (2) when patient with borderline hemodynamic status suddenly develops atrial fibrillation.

Permanent dual chamber pacing should be considered in those with bradycardia at rest or in patients requiring AV nodal ablation to prevent refractory rapid ventricular response.

Atrial fibrillation is the most common arrhythmia (although it is uncommon in children). It affects approximately 4% of people older than 60 years.

Clinical Correlation

Ventricular Tachycardia

Anatomy on pp. 343, 351, 352

Acute management
Patient assessment

Presyncopal

Dyspnea
(pulmonary
edema)

Ventricular
tachycardia

Hypotension

Patient status

Ventricular tachycardia
well tolerated

Presyncope, hypotension,
pulmonary edema

**IV antiarrhythmic
agents**

DC cardioversion
also utilized in
cases refractory
to medical
management

If medical
response poor,
overdrive
pacing with
transvenous
right
ventricular lead

Urgent blood studies
CBC
Electrolytes
(including magnesium)
BUN, creatinine,
cardiac enzymes
Glucose,
toxicology screen
Blood gases if indicated

(Follow-up studies to rule
out myocardial infarction)

VT   DC
      cardioversion

Sinus
rhythm

Primary acute management goal after stabilization of patient is termination of
ventricular tachycardia.

Long-term management

Long-term management with antiarrhythmics
and other pharmacologic agents is often
dictated by diagnosis.

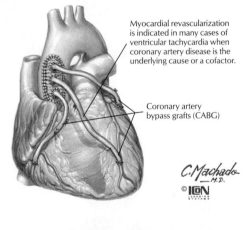

Myocardial revascularization
is indicated in many cases of
ventricular tachycardia when
coronary artery disease is the
underlying cause or a cofactor.

Coronary artery
bypass grafts (CABG)

C. Machado
_M.D.
© ICN

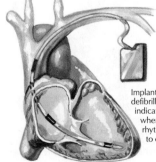

Implantable cardioverter
defibrillator (ICD)
indicated, particularly
when rate and
rhythm are refractory
to other therapies

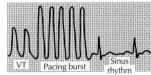

VT   Pacing burst   Sinus
                      rhythm

ECG demonstrating pacing effect on
rhythm

Ventricular tachycardia is a dysrhythmia originating from a ventricular focus with
a heart rate typically greater than 120 beats/min. It is usually associated with coronary
artery disease.

Clinical Correlation

Cardiac Pacemakers   *Anatomy on pp. 340, 351*

**Implantable cardiac pacemaker
(dual-chamber cardiac pacing)**

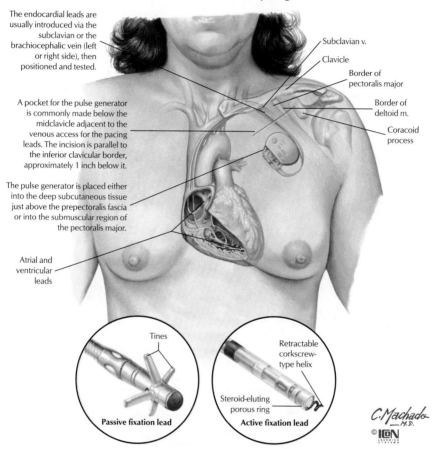

The endocardial leads are usually introduced via the subclavian or the brachiocephalic vein (left or right side), then positioned and tested.

A pocket for the pulse generator is commonly made below the midclavicle adjacent to the venous access for the pacing leads. The incision is parallel to the inferior clavicular border, approximately 1 inch below it.

The pulse generator is placed either into the deep subcutaneous tissue just above the prepectoralis fascia or into the submuscular region of the pectoralis major.

Atrial and ventricular leads

Subclavian v.

Clavicle

Border of pectoralis major

Border of deltoid m.

Coracoid process

Tines

Passive fixation lead

Retractable corkscrew-type helix

Steroid-eluting porous ring

Active fixation lead

C. Machado
—M.D.

©ICN

The leads connecting the pulse generator to the endocardium can be different types: unipolar or bipolar. The unipolar system has a single electrode (cathode, negative pole) in contact with the endocardium, and the anode is the pulse generator itself. The bipolar system lead has both a cathode and an anode at the tip of the same lead. Fixation irritates the myocardium, causing inflammatory reaction. To minimize the inflammatory reaction, most leads have steroid-eluting tips.

Cardiac pacemakers consist of a pulse generator and one or two endocardial leads with an electrode (passive or active fixation lead). The lead is threaded through the subclavian vein, brachiocephalic vein, SVC, and right atrium and is embedded there, or it is threaded into trabeculae carneae of the right ventricular wall. Depending on the device and its programming, the lead may sense as well as pace the cardiac chamber in which it is embedded. In pacing, the electrode impulses generated by the pulse generator depolarize the myocardium and initiate contractions at a prescribed rate.

Clinical Correlation

Cardiac Defibrillators   *Anatomy on pp. 340, 351*

Implantable cardiac defibrillator
(dual-chamber leads)

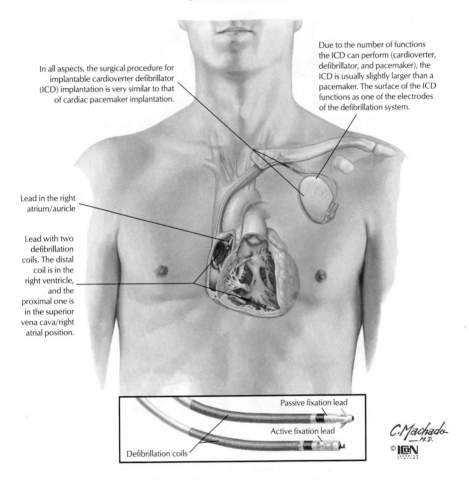

In all aspects, the surgical procedure for implantable cardioverter defibrillator (ICD) implantation is very similar to that of cardiac pacemaker implantation.

Due to the number of functions the ICD can perform (cardioverter, defibrillator, and pacemaker), the ICD is usually slightly larger than a pacemaker. The surface of the ICD functions as one of the electrodes of the defibrillation system.

Lead in the right atrium/auricle

Lead with two defibrillation coils. The distal coil is in the right ventricle, and the proximal one is in the superior vena cava/right atrial position.

Passive fixation lead

Active fixation lead

Defibrillation coils

ICD leads have a tip electrode that can sense the heart rate and deliver an electrical stimulus to pace the heart. The defibrillation coils that are part of ICD leads are not found on standard pacemaker leads. At least one coil (in the right ventricle) is necessary for defibrillation. Some models have a second defibrillation coil, which is positioned in the superior vena cava/right atrium.

Implantable cardioverter defibrillators are used for survivors of sudden cardiac death and patients with sustained ventricular tachycardia or at high risk for development of ventricular arrhythmias (ischemic dilated cardiomyopathy), as well as for other indications. In addition to sensing arrhythmias and providing defibrillation to stop them, the devices can function as pacemakers for postdefibrillation bradycardia or AV dissociation.

Mediastinum

The mediastinum is divided into superior and inferior regions, with the latter subdivided into an anterior (substernal) region, middle (pericardium and heart) region, and posterior (deep to heart) region. The posterior mediastinum contains the
- Esophagus
- Aorta and azygos system of veins
- Lymphatics and thoracic duct
- Nerves (those of autonomic nervous system and spinal nerves)

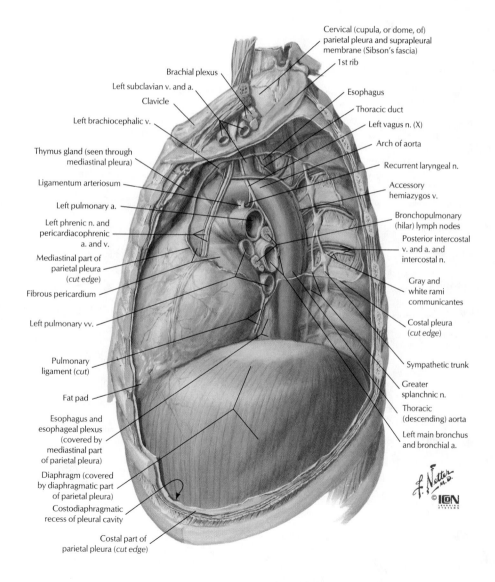

Cervical (cupula, or dome, of) parietal pleura and suprapleural membrane (Sibson's fascia)

1st rib

Brachial plexus

Left subclavian v. and a.

Clavicle

Esophagus

Left brachiocephalic v.

Thoracic duct

Left vagus n. (X)

Thymus gland (seen through mediastinal pleura)

Arch of aorta

Recurrent laryngeal n.

Ligamentum arteriosum

Accessory hemiazygos v.

Left pulmonary a.

Bronchopulmonary (hilar) lymph nodes

Left phrenic n. and pericardiacophrenic a. and v.

Posterior intercostal v. and a. and intercostal n.

Mediastinal part of parietal pleura (cut edge)

Gray and white rami communicantes

Fibrous pericardium

Left pulmonary vv.

Costal pleura (cut edge)

Pulmonary ligament (cut)

Sympathetic trunk

Fat pad

Greater splanchnic n.

Thoracic (descending) aorta

Esophagus and esophageal plexus (covered by mediastinal part of parietal pleura)

Left main bronchus and bronchial a.

Diaphragm (covered by diaphragmatic part of parietal pleura)

Costodiaphragmatic recess of pleural cavity

Costal part of parietal pleura (cut edge)

Mediastinum: Transverse Section T7

This section crosses the level of the inferior portions of the right and left atria (and superior portion of the right ventricle) and demonstrates the lungs in their pleural sacs and the anterior, middle, and posterior subdivisions of the inferior mediastinum. The anterior mediastinum lies substernally and usually contains some fat, and the middle mediastinum contains the pericardium and heart. The posterior mediastinum includes the thoracic nerves, esophagus, aorta, azygos system, and thoracic duct.

Transverse section: level of T7, 3rd interchondral space

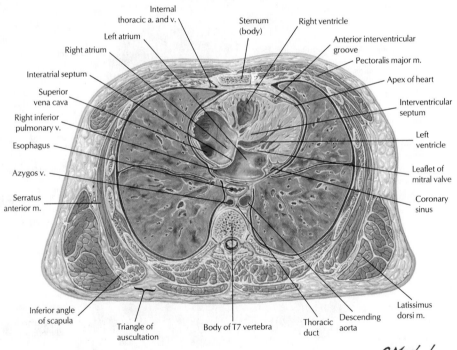

Internal thoracic a. and v.
Sternum (body)
Right ventricle
Left atrium
Anterior interventricular groove
Right atrium
Pectoralis major m.
Interatrial septum
Apex of heart
Superior vena cava
Interventricular septum
Right inferior pulmonary v.
Left ventricle
Esophagus
Leaflet of mitral valve
Azygos v.
Coronary sinus
Serratus anterior m.
Inferior angle of scapula
Latissimus dorsi m.
Triangle of auscultation
Body of T7 vertebra
Thoracic duct
Descending aorta

C. Machado —M.D.
© ICN

Mediastinum: Esophagus and Thoracic Aorta

The esophagus extends from the pharynx (throat) to the stomach and enters the thorax posterior to the trachea. As it descends, it gradually inclines to the left of the median plane, lies anterior to the thoracic aorta, and pierces the diaphragm at the T10 vertebral level. Thoracic aorta branches supply the heart, head and neck, upper limbs, lungs, intercostal spaces, esophagus, pericardium, and superior surface of the diaphragm.

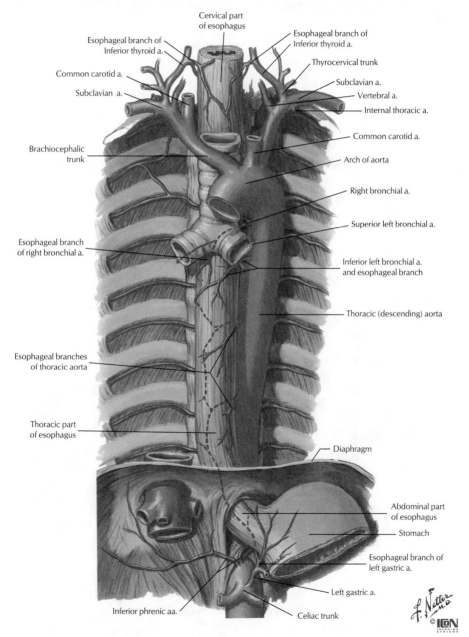

Cervical part of esophagus

Esophageal branch of Inferior thyroid a.

Esophageal branch of Inferior thyroid a.

Thyrocervical trunk

Common carotid a.

Subclavian a.

Subclavian a.

Vertebral a.

Internal thoracic a.

Common carotid a.

Brachiocephalic trunk

Arch of aorta

Right bronchial a.

Superior left bronchial a.

Esophageal branch of right bronchial a.

Inferior left bronchial a. and esophageal branch

Thoracic (descending) aorta

Esophageal branches of thoracic aorta

Thoracic part of esophagus

Diaphragm

Abdominal part of esophagus

Stomach

Esophageal branch of left gastric a.

Left gastric a.

Inferior phrenic aa.

Celiac trunk

Mediastinum: Azygos System of Veins

The azygos venous system drains the posterior thorax and forms an important venous conduit between the IVC and SVC. It is part of the deep venous drainage system seen elsewhere in the body (see Chapter 1 [Introduction]). As in most venous systems, the branches are variable but usually include the azygos vein (with ascending lumbar, subcostal, and intercostal tributaries), hemiazygos vein (with ascending lumbar, subcostal, and intercostal tributaries), and accessory hemiazygos vein (if present, it begins at the fourth intercostal space).

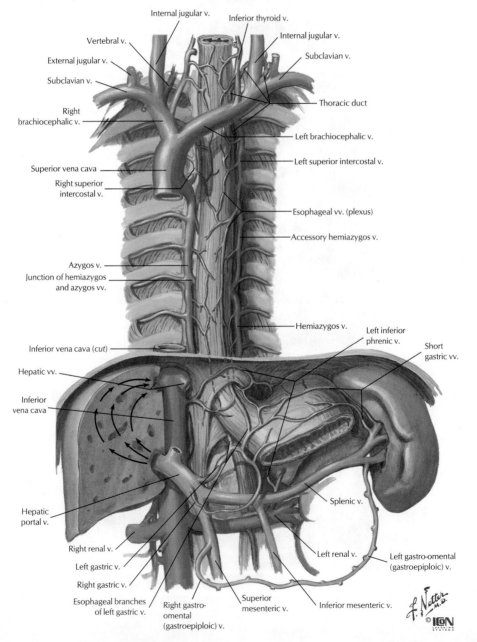

Internal jugular v.
Inferior thyroid v.
Internal jugular v.
Vertebral v.
External jugular v.
Subclavian v.
Subclavian v.
Right brachiocephalic v.
Thoracic duct
Left brachiocephalic v.
Left superior intercostal v.
Superior vena cava
Right superior intercostal v.
Esophageal vv. (plexus)
Accessory hemiazygos v.
Azygos v.
Junction of hemiazygos and azygos vv.
Hemiazygos v.
Left inferior phrenic v.
Short gastric vv.
Inferior vena cava (cut)
Hepatic vv.
Inferior vena cava
Hepatic portal v.
Splenic v.
Right renal v.
Left gastric v.
Left renal v.
Left gastro-omental (gastroepiploic) v.
Right gastric v.
Esophageal branches of left gastric v.
Right gastro-omental (gastroepiploic) v.
Superior mesenteric v.
Inferior mesenteric v.

Mediastinum: Lymphatics

The thoracic lymphatic duct begins in the abdomen at the cisterna chyli (see Chapter 1 [Introduction]), ascends through the posterior mediastinum posterior to the esophagus, crosses to the left of the median plane at approximately T5 to T6, and empties into the venous system at the junction of the left internal jugular and left subclavian veins. Representative thoracic lymph nodes in the left posterior mediastinum are illustrated.

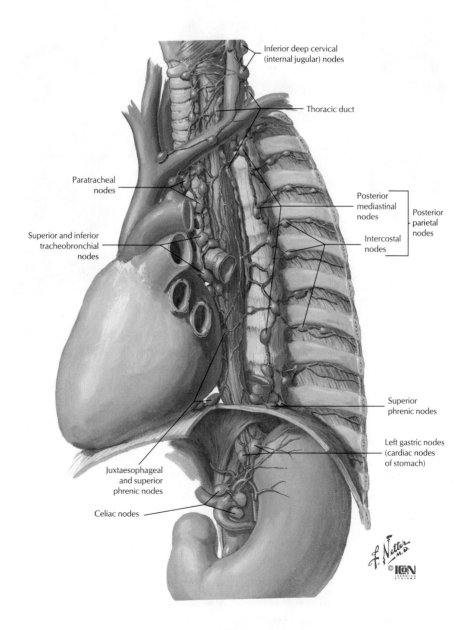

Inferior deep cervical (internal jugular) nodes

Thoracic duct

Paratracheal nodes

Posterior mediastinal nodes

Posterior parietal nodes

Intercostal nodes

Superior and inferior tracheobronchial nodes

Superior phrenic nodes

Left gastric nodes (cardiac nodes of stomach)

Juxtaesophageal and superior phrenic nodes

Celiac nodes

Clinical Correlation

Mediastinal Masses   *Anatomy on pp. 340, 365-367, 369*

Anterior mediastinum

Substernal thyroid gland

Posterior mediastinum

Thymoma

Teratoma

Neurilemoma
Neurofibroma
Ganglioneuroma
Schwann cell tumor

Lymph nodes;
lymphoma

Middle mediastinum

Vascular; aneurysm,
enlarged heart

Bronchogenic
or pericardial cyst

Lymph nodes; lymphoma,
metastatic cancer

Bronchogenic
or pericardial cyst

Esophageal; achalasia,
diverticula

TYPE OF MASS	COMMENT
Anterior Mediastinum (retrosternal pain, cough, dyspnea, SVC syndrome, choking sensation)	
Thymoma	Thymus tumors (<50% malignant), often associated with myasthenia gravis
Thyroid mass	Mass that may cause enlarged gland to extend inferiorly and displace trachea
Teratoma	Benign and malignant tumors of totipotent cells, often containing all three germ cell types (ectoderm, mesoderm, and endoderm)
Lymphoma	Hodgkin's, non-Hodgkin's, and primary mediastinal B-cell tumors
Middle Mediastinum (signs and symptoms similar to those of anterior masses)	
Lymph nodes	Enlarged nodes resulting from infections or malignancy
Aortic aneurysm	Aneurysm that is atherosclerotic in origin, may rupture, and can be in any part of the mediastinum
Vascular dilatation	Enlarged pulmonary artery or cardiomegaly
Cysts	Bronchogenic (at tracheal bifurcation) cysts, pericardial cysts
Posterior Mediastinum (pain, neurologic symptoms, or swallowing difficulty)	
Neurogenic tumors	Tumors of peripheral nerves or sheath cells (e.g., schwannomas)
Esophageal lesions	Diverticula and tumors

Clinical Correlation

Chylothorax   *Anatomy on pp. 314, 322, 365, 369*

Aspiration of milky (chylous) fluid from thoracic cavity (may be reintroduced into body by way of nasogastric tube or by well-monitored intravenous infusion)

Brachiocephalic (innominate) vv.

Superior vena cava

Thoracic duct

Esophagus (*cut away*)

Descending thoracic aorta

Diaphragm

Cisterna chyli

Normal course of thoracic duct

Azygos v.

Ligation of thoracic duct after identification of rupture site by escape of intraabdominally injected dye

Thoracic duct

Chylothorax usually arises from a complication of surgery in the mediastinum, especially vascular surgery of the great vessels. Variations in the anatomy of the thoracic duct probably account for most of the postoperative complications and include
- Dual thoracic ducts
- Numerous lymphovenous anastomoses with azygos and intercostal veins
- Rich supply of lymph nodes and tributaries adjacent to the ligamentum arteriosum

Embryology: Respiratory System

The airway and lungs begin developing during week 4. A laryngotracheal diverticulum appears as an outgrowth of the ventral foregut, just inferior to the last pair of pharyngeal pouches. This diverticulum divides into left and right lung (bronchial) buds, each with a primary bronchus. These buds then divide to form lung lobes. By week 6-7 of development, segmental bronchi develop along with their bronchopulmonary segments (10 in each lung). Endoderm lines the airways; mesoderm forms the lung stroma. At 6 months, alveoli are mature enough for gas exchange, but production of surfactant (which reduces surface tension and prevents alveolar collapse) may not be adequate to support respiration. Therefore, an infant is at great risk if born at this premature time.

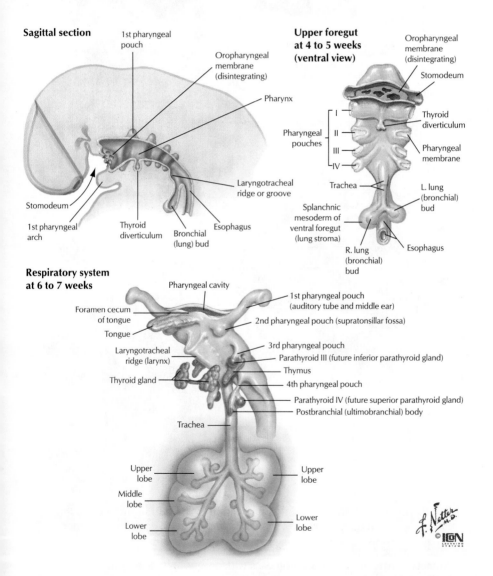

Embryology: Early Vasculature

Toward the end of week 3 of development, the embryo establishes a primitive vascular system to meet the growing need for oxygen and nutrients. Blood leaving the heart enters a series of paired arteries associated with the pharyngeal arches (aortic arches) and then into the aorta. Some blood enters the vitelline vessels to supply the future bowel (yolk sac), and some blood enters the umbilical arteries and passes to the placenta where gases, nutrients, and metabolic wastes are exchanged. The oxygenated blood returns to the embryo via the umbilical vein and courses to the heart.

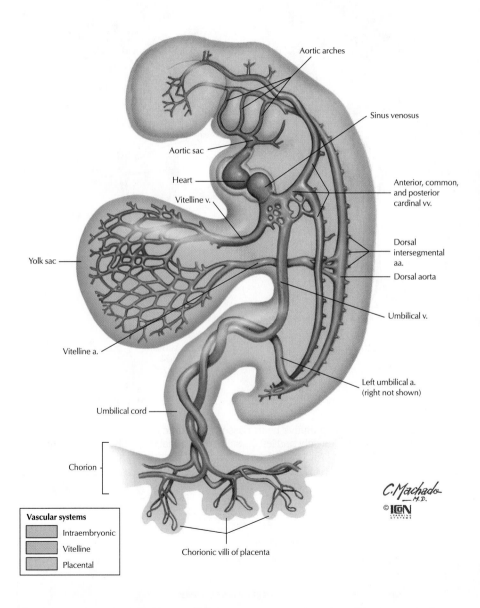

Aortic arches

Sinus venosus

Aortic sac

Heart

Vitelline v.

Anterior, common, and posterior cardinal vv.

Dorsal intersegmental aa.

Dorsal aorta

Yolk sac

Umbilical v.

Vitelline a.

Left umbilical a. (right not shown)

Umbilical cord

Chorion

C. Machado
— M.D.
© ICN
LEARNING
SYSTEMS

Vascular systems

Intraembryonic

Vitelline

Placental

Chorionic villi of placenta

Embryology: Aortic Arches

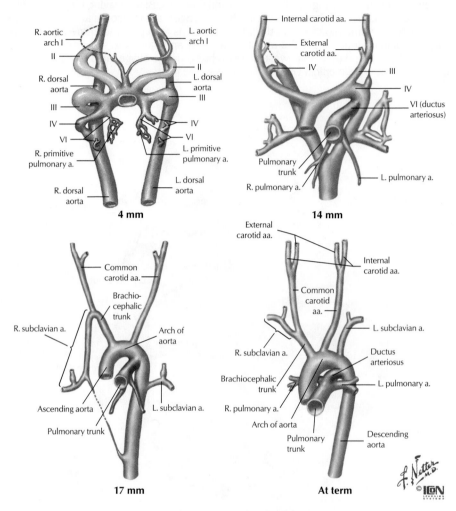

Blood pumped from the primitive heart passes into aortic arches, which are associated with pharyngeal arches. The right and left dorsal aortas caudal to the pharyngeal arches fuse into a single midline aorta. The original six pairs of aortic arches become the following:

ARCH	DERIVATIVE
1	Largely disappears (part of maxillary artery in head)
2	Largely disappears
3	Common and internal carotid arteries
4	Right subclavian artery and aortic arch (on left side only)
5	Disappears
6	Ductus arteriosus and proximal part of pulmonary arteries

Clinical Correlation

Coarctation of the Aorta
Anatomy on pp. 311, 322, 367, 374

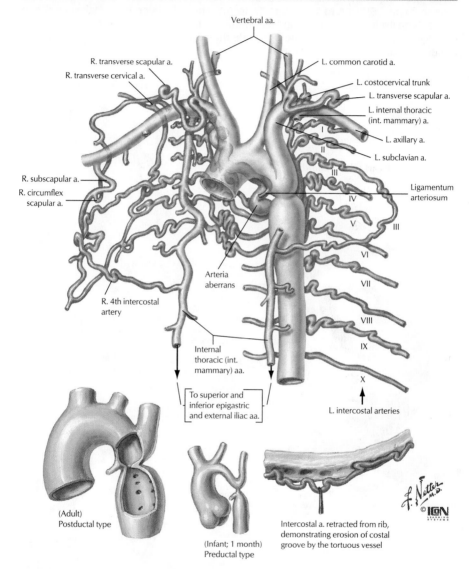

Vertebral aa.

R. transverse scapular a.

R. transverse cervical a.

L. common carotid a.

L. costocervical trunk

L. transverse scapular a.

L. internal thoracic (int. mammary) a.

L. axillary a.

L. subclavian a.

R. subscapular a.

R. circumflex scapular a.

Ligamentum arteriosum

Arteria aberrans

R. 4th intercostal artery

Internal thoracic (int. mammary) aa.

To superior and inferior epigastric and external iliac aa.

L. intercostal arteries

(Adult) Postductal type

(Infant; 1 month) Preductal type

Intercostal a. retracted from rib, demonstrating erosion of costal groove by the tortuous vessel

This coarctation is a congenital narrowing of the aorta, usually near the ligamentum (ductus) arteriosum (preductal, juxtaductal, or postductal). As a result, blood flows via collateral routes, notably into the internal thoracic, epigastric, and scapular branches and intercostal arteries, to gain access to structures distal to the defect (blood flow can be retrograde in these vessels to reach the aorta). The intercostal arteries become dilated and tortuous as they carry more blood at a higher pressure than normal and often erode the costal groove of adjacent ribs.

Embryology: Heart Tube Folding

The primitive heart begins development as a tube (not unlike an artery), receiving blood returning from the embryonic body and pumping it in sequence through the heart tube segments: SV to A to V to BC to TA to AA. This tube eventually makes an S-bend and folds on itself. The original embryonic portions of the adult heart can be seen internally by ridges in the myocardium. These include the pectinate muscles of the atria and the trabeculae carneae of the ventricles.

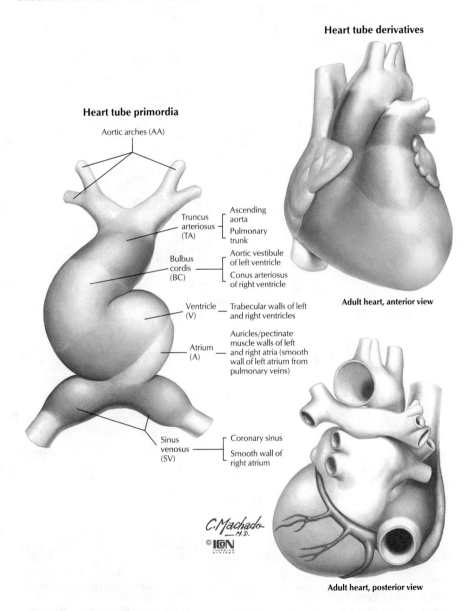

Heart tube derivatives

Heart tube primordia

Aortic arches (AA)

Truncus arteriosus (TA) — Ascending aorta / Pulmonary trunk

Bulbus cordis (BC) — Aortic vestibule of left ventricle / Conus arteriosus of right ventricle

Ventricle (V) — Trabecular walls of left and right ventricles

Atrium (A) — Auricles/pectinate muscle walls of left and right atria (smooth wall of left atrium from pulmonary veins)

Sinus venosus (SV) — Coronary sinus / Smooth wall of right atrium

Adult heart, anterior view

C. Machado
—M.D.
© ICN
LEARNING
SYSTEMS

Adult heart, posterior view

Embryology: Division of the Heart Chambers

Internally, septa grow and divide the atrium and ventricle into right and left chambers. Because most blood does not perfuse the lungs in utero (they are partially collapsed and filled with amniotic fluid), blood in the right atrium passes directly to the left atrium via a small opening in the interatrial septum called the foramen ovale. Any remaining blood is pumped from the right ventricle to the pulmonary trunk and bypasses the lungs by passing into the aortic arch via the ductus arteriosus. The interventricular septum (IVS) grows from the base of the heart cranially and fuses with the endocardial cushion (site of the membranous IVS and common site for VSD).

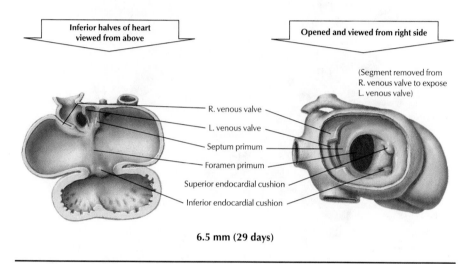

6.5 mm (29 days)

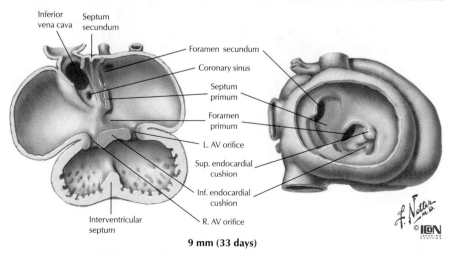

9 mm (33 days)

Clinical Correlation

Transatrial Repair of Ventricular Septal Defect

Anatomy on pp. 351, 352, 377

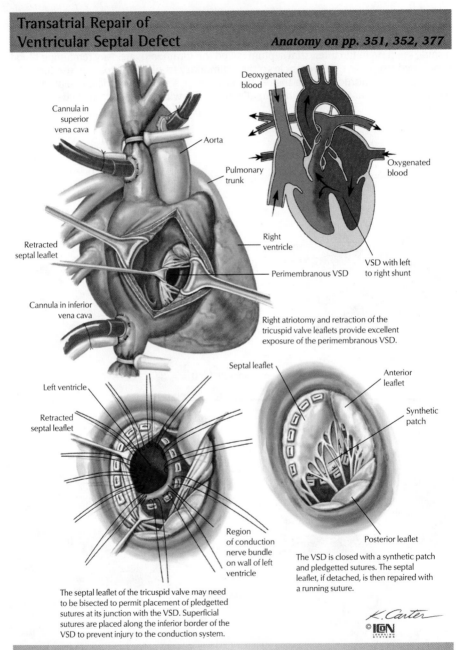

Cannula in superior vena cava

Aorta

Pulmonary trunk

Deoxygenated blood

Oxygenated blood

Right ventricle

VSD with left to right shunt

Perimembranous VSD

Retracted septal leaflet

Cannula in inferior vena cava

Right atriotomy and retraction of the tricuspid valve leaflets provide excellent exposure of the perimembranous VSD.

Septal leaflet

Anterior leaflet

Synthetic patch

Left ventricle

Retracted septal leaflet

Region of conduction nerve bundle on wall of left ventricle

Posterior leaflet

The VSD is closed with a synthetic patch and pledgetted sutures. The septal leaflet, if detached, is then repaired with a running suture.

The septal leaflet of the tricuspid valve may need to be bisected to permit placement of pledgetted sutures at its junction with the VSD. Superficial sutures are placed along the inferior border of the VSD to prevent injury to the conduction system.

K. Carter

© ICN LEARNING SYSTEMS

VSD is the most common congenital heart defect (approximately 1.2/1000 infants, and approximately 30% of all heart defects). The most common site (approximately 80%) is perimembranous; the VSD occurs where the muscular septum and endocardial cushion should fuse (membranous septum). This results in a left-to-right shunt, which may precipitate CHF. The repair illustrated here is via the right atrial approach.

Clinical Correlation

Atrial Septal Defect Repair
Anatomy on pp. 351, 352, 377

The Amplatzer® Septal Occluder is deployed from its delivery sheath forming two discs, one for either side of the septum, and a central waist available in varying diameters to seat on the rims of the atrial septal defect.

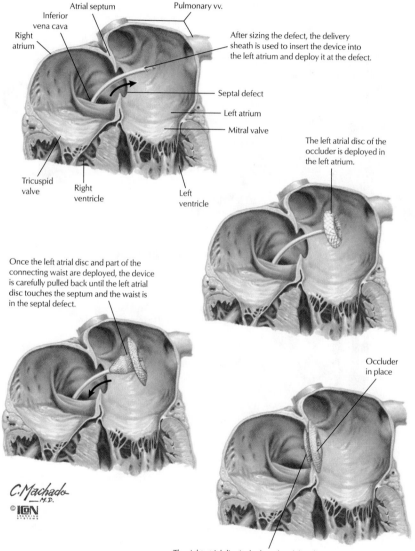

Atrial septum

Inferior vena cava

Right atrium

Pulmonary vv.

After sizing the defect, the delivery sheath is used to insert the device into the left atrium and deploy it at the defect.

Septal defect

Left atrium

Mitral valve

Tricuspid valve

Right ventricle

Left ventricle

The left atrial disc of the occluder is deployed in the left atrium.

Once the left atrial disc and part of the connecting waist are deployed, the device is carefully pulled back until the left atrial disc touches the septum and the waist is in the septal defect.

Occluder in place

C. Machado
—M.D.

© ICON
LEARNING
SYSTEMS

The right atrial disc is deployed and the placement of the occluder is checked by echocardiography. Then, the device is released.

Atrial septal defects make up approximately 10-15% of congenital cardiac anomalies. Repair of these defects (other than fossa ovalis defects) can be surgically achieved by using a relatively new transcatheter approach through the IVC and into the atria, to deploy a septal occluder.

Clinical Correlation

Patent Ductus Arteriosus   *Anatomy on pp. 352, 373, 374*

Patent ductus arteriosus

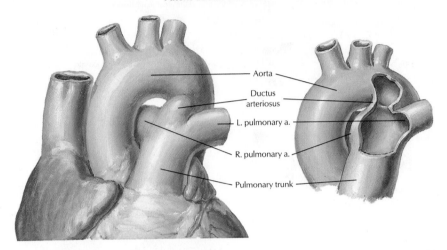

Aorta

Ductus arteriosus

L. pulmonary a.

R. pulmonary a.

Pulmonary trunk

Pathophysiology of patent ductus arteriosus

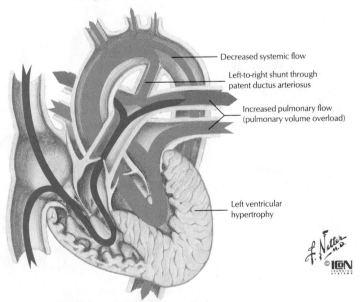

Decreased systemic flow

Left-to-right shunt through patent ductus arteriosus

Increased pulmonary flow (pulmonary volume overload)

Left ventricular hypertrophy

Failure of the ductus arteriosus to close shortly after birth results in a shunt of blood from the aorta into the pulmonary trunk, which may lead to CHF. PDA occurs in approximately 1 in 2000-2500 births (10% of congenital heart defects) and can be treated medically, or surgically if necessary. The latter treatment is by direct surgical ligation or via a less invasive catheter-based device.

Clinical Correlation

Repair of Tetralogy of Fallot   *Anatomy on pp. 351, 352, 374, 377*

Patent ductus arteriosus

Deoxygenated blood

Stenotic pulmonary a.

Ligated ductus arteriosus

Stenotic pulmonary trunk

Oxygenated blood

Stenotic pulmonary valve

VSD with right to left shunt

Aortic and mitral valve seen through VSD

Right ventricular hypertrophy

Hypertrophied right ventricle

GORE-TEX® graft with pledgets

Pulmonary valvotomy followed by pericardial patch to reduce stenosis

Retracted tricuspid valve

Pericardial patch to reduce subpulmonic stenosis

K. Carter

© ICON
LEARNING
SYSTEMS

Tetralogy of Fallot usually results from a maldevelopment of the spiral septum that normally divides the truncus arteriosus into the pulmonary trunk and aorta. This defect involves
• Pulmonary stenosis or narrowing of right ventricular outflow
• Overriding (transposed) aorta
• Right ventricular hypertrophy
• VSD
Surgical repair is done on cardiopulmonary bypass with an aim to close the VSD and provide unobstructed flow into the pulmonary trunk.

Review Questions

What is the sternal angle of Louis, and why is it important?	It is the articulation of the manubrium and body of the sternum, and it marks the dividing point of the superior from the inferior mediastinum. It also overlies the tracheal bifurcation and aortic arch and is useful for counting intercostal spaces (second ribs articulate here).
What is the primary site for lymphatic drainage from the breast?	Axillary lymph nodes (75% of all lymph).
What dermatome overlies the nipple in the male?	T4.
Which breast quadrant has the greatest occurrence of cancer, and what type of breast cancer is most common?	Upper outer quadrant (and the axillary tail of Spence). Infiltrating ductal carcinoma is the most common type (70-80%).
Which of the 12 pairs of ribs are considered true ribs?	Pairs 1-7, because they articulate directly with the sternum.
What type of joint is the sternoclavicular joint?	Saddle-type synovial joint with an articular disc.
Which intercostal muscles are most important for inspiration?	External intercostals, because they elevate the ribs and, along with the diaphragm, increase the volume of the thoracic cavity.
Why is the cupula vulnerable to injury?	It is the extension of cervical parietal pleura above the first rib and is vulnerable to trauma associated with the root of the neck (usually penetrating trauma).
What is the inferior extent of the lung and parietal pleura in quiet respiration at the midaxillary line?	The lung extends to the 8th rib, and the pleura to the 10th rib.
The right lung has how many lobes and bronchopulmonary segments?	Three lobes and 10 bronchopulmonary segments.
What is the most common type of lung cancer?	Squamous cell, which usually arises in the main bronchus near the hilum.
Why might a Pancoast tumor present with Horner's syndrome?	The Pancoast tumor is in the apex of the lung and can expand to and impinge on the sympathetic trunk lying posterior to the apex.
What is thoracic outlet syndrome?	Compression of one or more of the structures passing out of the thoracic outlet. The subclavian artery or vein or the lower portion of the brachial plexus is often involved.
As it relates to PE, what is Virchow's triad?	The three major causes of PE, which include venous stasis, trauma, and coagulation disorders.
What is the origin of most PEs?	Deep leg veins, especially those in the calf.

Review Questions

What is COPD, and why is it debilitating?	Chronic obstructive pulmonary disease (chronic bronchitis and emphysema most commonly). Lung compliance is increased, and the elastic recoil of the lungs is decreased, which can collapse the airways during expiration, thus trapping air in the lungs.
Why do most lung abscesses occur in the right lung?	Because the right main bronchus is wider, shorter, and more vertical than the left bronchus, and aspirated infective agents can gain easier access to the right lung.
Where is most reactivation TB localized?	In the apicoposterior segments of the upper lobes of the lungs.
Trace lymph drainage from the hilum of the lung to the paratracheal nodes.	Bronchopulmonary (hilar) nodes to tracheobronchial nodes to paratracheal nodes.
What types of nerve fibers travel in the thoracic cardiac nerves?	Postganglionic sympathetic fibers (to the heart) and visceral afferents from the heart.
Pain from an infection of the pericardium (pericarditis) is conveyed in what nerve(s)?	Phrenic (C3-C5).
Which coronary artery supplies the SA node?	Right, usually via its SA nodal branch.
Trace venous blood from the anterior interventricular septum to the heart.	Tributaries to the great cardiac vein to the coronary sinus to the right atrium.
Why is angina pectoris an example of referred pain?	Visceral afferents from the ischemic heart are conveyed to the upper thoracic spinal cord levels that also receive somatic afferents from the T1 to T4 dermatomes. Both groups of afferents converge in the dorsal horn of the spinal cord, and angina may be perceived as localized to the somatic distribution (T1-T4) rather than identified with the heart.
What are the major causes of MI, and which coronary artery is most often involved?	Major causes of MI include coronary atherosclerosis and thrombosis, and the LAD is the most common site (40-50%).
What are the semilunar valves?	The pulmonary and aortic valves. Each has three semilunar cusps or leaflets (they share a common embryologic origin).
In cardiac auscultation, where is the stethoscope placed to hear the first heart sound ("lub" of the "lub-dub")?	Over the mitral area, in the left fifth intercostal space over the apex of the heart.
What structures are most often involved in IE?	Mitral and aortic valves (85% of patients have heart murmurs).
Why is the left atrium enlarged or dilated in mitral stenosis?	Blood in the left atrium cannot easily pass through the narrowed mitral valve to reach the left ventricle and thus backs up in the left atrium and eventually the lungs.

Review Questions

Trace the conduction pathway through the heart.	SA node to AV node to common AV bundle (of His) to the right and left bundle branches and subendocardial Purkinje system.
What key structures reside in the posterior mediastinum?	Esophagus, aorta, azygos venous system, lymphatics and thoracic duct, and autonomic and spinal nerves.
What veins drain the posterior thoracic wall?	Drainage is largely by tributaries of the azygos system of veins (intercostal veins).
What structure in the embryonic foregut region gives rise to the lung buds?	Laryngotracheal diverticulum.
In the embryo, blood returning from the placenta and yolk sac (via vitelline veins) passes first into which primitive heart chamber?	Sinus venosus.
What does the fourth pair of aortic arches become in the adult?	On the right side, the right subclavian artery; on the left side, the aortic arch.
What is the most common congenital heart defect?	VSD, which usually occurs in the membranous portion of the interventricular septum.
Why can one detect a continuous murmur in a child with a PDA, and where is it auscultated?	The turbulent blood flow from the aorta into the pulmonary trunk via the PDA causes a continuous machine gun murmur over the pulmonary area (upper left sternal border to below the left clavicle). The murmur is continuous because the blood continues to pass through the ductus during systole and diastole from the higher pressure aorta into the lower pressure pulmonary trunk.
What are the hallmarks of tetralogy of Fallot?	Pulmonary stenosis or narrowing of the right ventricular outflow, transposed aorta, right ventricular hypertrophy, and VSD.

6

Abdomen

Introduction The abdomen is the region between the thorax superiorly and the pelvis inferiorly. It is lined externally by muscles that assist in respiration and, by increasing intraabdominal pressure, in micturition, defecation, and childbirth. The abdominal cavity is continuous with the pelvis and contains the gastrointestinal (GI) tract and its associated organs, the urinary system, and the spleen. Knowing which viscera lie in each region or quadrant is key to the correct performance of auscultation, percussion, and palpation of the abdomen, which are part of every physical examination and essential to the process of diagnosing illness.

Surface Anatomy: Key Landmarks

Rectus sheath: sheath containing the rectus abdominis muscle, running from the pubic symphysis and crest to the xiphoid process and fifth to seventh costal cartilages
Linea alba: literally, "white line"; a relatively avascular midline subcutaneous band of fibrous tissue
Semilunar line: lateral border of the rectus abdominis muscle in the rectus sheath
Tendinous intersections: transverse skin grooves that demarcate attachment points of the rectus sheath to the rectus abdominis muscle
Umbilicus: site that marks the T10 dermatome, lying at the level of the intervertebral disc between L3 and L4
Iliac crest: rim of the ilium, lying at about the level of the L4 vertebra
Inguinal ligament: ligament lying deep to a skin crease that marks the division between the lower abdominal wall and thigh

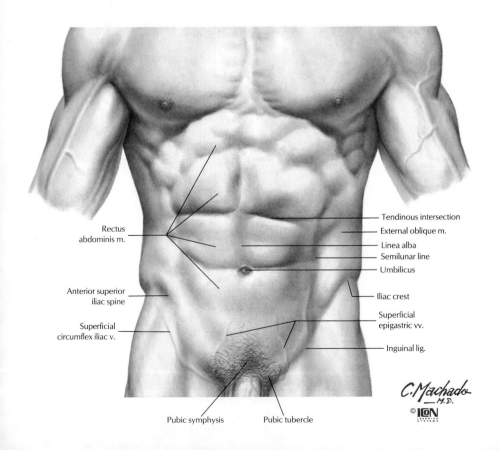

Rectus abdominis m.

Anterior superior iliac spine

Superficial circumflex iliac v.

Tendinous intersection
External oblique m.
Linea alba
Semilunar line
Umbilicus
Iliac crest
Superficial epigastric vv.
Inguinal lig.

C. Machado
—M.D.

©I🜂N

Pubic symphysis   Pubic tubercle

Surface Anatomy: Planes of Reference

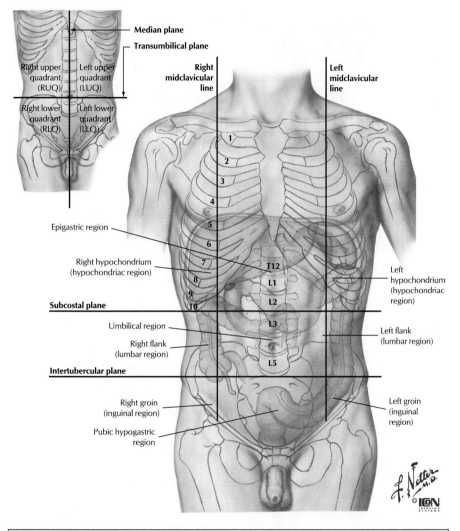

Median plane

Transumbilical plane

Right upper quadrant (RUQ)

Left upper quadrant (LUQ)

Right lower quadrant (RLQ)

Left lower quadrant (LLQ)

Right midclavicular line

Left midclavicular line

Epigastric region

Right hypochondrium (hypochondriac region)

Subcostal plane

Umbilical region

Right flank (lumbar region)

Intertubercular plane

Right groin (inguinal region)

Pubic hypogastric region

Left hypochondrium (hypochondriac region)

Left flank (lumbar region)

Left groin (inguinal region)

T12
L1
L2
L3
L5

1
2
3
4
5
6
7
8
9
10

PLANES OF REFERENCE	DEFINITION
Median	Vertical plane from xiphoid process to pubic symphysis
Transumbilical	Horizontal plane across umbilicus (these two planes divide abdomen into quadrants)
Subcostal	Horizontal plane across inferior margin of the 10th costal cartilage
Intertubercular	Horizontal plane across the tubercles of the ilium and the body of the L5 vertebra
Midclavicular	Two vertical planes through the midpoint of the clavicles (these planes divide the abdomen into nine regions)

These planes of reference are used clinically to highlight the visceral structures found in each quadrant or region and to localize sites of abdominal pain. Knowledge of these quadrants and the nine regions is an essential part of the physical examination of the abdomen.

Abdominal Wall: Superficial Muscles

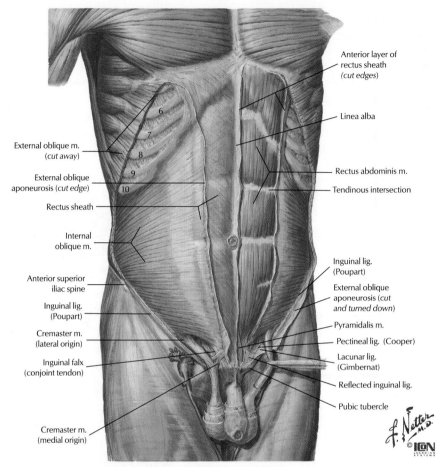

Anterior layer of
rectus sheath
(cut edges)

Linea alba

Rectus abdominis m.

Tendinous intersection

External oblique m.
(cut away)

External oblique
aponeurosis (cut edge)

Rectus sheath

Internal
oblique m.

Anterior superior
iliac spine

Inguinal lig.
(Poupart)

Cremaster m.
(lateral origin)

Inguinal falx
(conjoint tendon)

Cremaster m.
(medial origin)

Inguinal lig.
(Poupart)

External oblique
aponeurosis (cut
and turned down)

Pyramidalis m.

Pectineal lig. (Cooper)

Lacunar lig.
(Gimbernat)

Reflected inguinal lig.

Pubic tubercle

On both sides, most of the external abdominal oblique muscle has been cut away; on the left side, the rectus sheath has been opened to show the rectus abdominis muscle.

MUSCLE	PROXIMAL ATTACHMENT (ORIGIN)	DISTAL ATTACHMENT (INSERTION)	INNERVATION	MAIN ACTIONS
External oblique	External surfaces of 5th to 12th ribs	Linea alba, pubic tubercle, and anterior half of iliac crest	Inferior six thoracic nerves and subcostal nerve	Compresses and supports abdominal viscera; flexes and rotates trunk
Internal oblique	Thoracolumbar fascia, anterior two thirds of iliac crest, and lateral half of inguinal ligament	Inferior borders of 10th to 12th ribs, linea alba, and pubis via conjoint tendon	Ventral rami of inferior six thoracic nerves and first lumbar nerve	Compresses and supports abdominal viscera; flexes and rotates trunk
Transversus abdominis	Internal surfaces of 7-12 costal cartilages, thoracolumbar fascia, iliac crest, and lateral third of inguinal ligament	Linea alba with aponeurosis of internal oblique, pubic crest, and pecten pubis via conjoint tendon	Ventral rami of inferior six thoracic nerves and first lumbar nerve	Compresses and supports abdominal viscera
Rectus abdominis	Pubic symphysis and pubic crest	Xiphoid process and costal cartilages 5-7	Ventral rami of inferior six thoracic nerves	Flexes trunk and compresses abdominal viscera

Abdominal Wall: Deep Muscles

Deep to the rectus abdominis muscle, inferior epigastric vessels (which arise from the external iliac vessels) course superiorly to anastomose with superior epigastric vessels (continuation of internal thoracic vessels). A deeper dissection is shown on the left side.

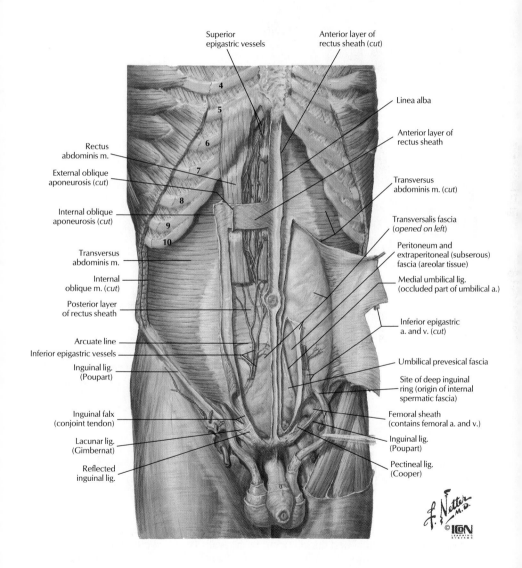

Superior epigastric vessels

Anterior layer of rectus sheath (*cut*)

Linea alba

Anterior layer of rectus sheath

Rectus abdominis m.

External oblique aponeurosis (*cut*)

Internal oblique aponeurosis (*cut*)

Transversus abdominis m.

Internal oblique m. (*cut*)

Posterior layer of rectus sheath

Arcuate line

Inferior epigastric vessels

Inguinal lig. (Poupart)

Inguinal falx (conjoint tendon)

Lacunar lig. (Gimbernat)

Reflected inguinal lig.

Transversus abdominis m. (*cut*)

Transversalis fascia (*opened on left*)

Peritoneum and extraperitoneal (subserous) fascia (areolar tissue)

Medial umbilical lig. (occluded part of umbilical a.)

Inferior epigastric a. and v. (*cut*)

Umbilical prevesical fascia

Site of deep inguinal ring (origin of internal spermatic fascia)

Femoral sheath (contains femoral a. and v.)

Inguinal lig. (Poupart)

Pectineal lig. (Cooper)

Clinical Correlation

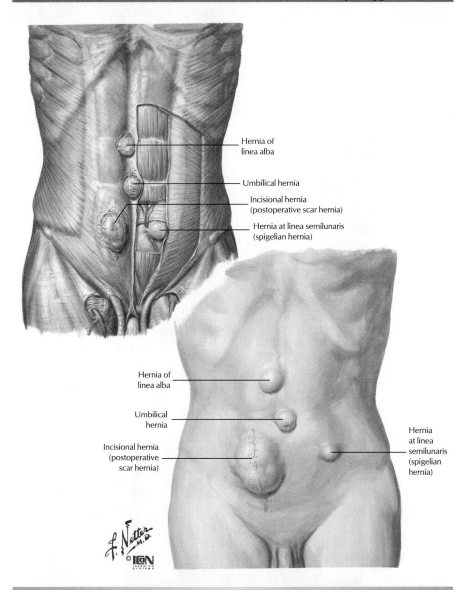

Hernia of
linea alba

Umbilical hernia

Incisional hernia
(postoperative scar hernia)

Hernia at linea semilunaris
(spigelian hernia)

Hernia of
linea alba

Umbilical
hernia

Incisional hernia
(postoperative
scar hernia)

Hernia
at linea
semilunaris
(spigelian
hernia)

To distinguish these hernias from inguinal hernias, they often are called ventral hernias, but like inguinal hernias, all occur in the wall. The most common types are
- **Umbilical**: is usually seen up to the age of 3 years and after the age of 40 years
- **Linea alba**: often occurs in epigastric region; is more common in males than in females; rarely contains viscus
- **Linea semilunaris (spigelian)**: usually occurs in midlife and develops slowly
- **Incisional**: occurs at site of previous laparotomy scar

Abdominal Wall: Veins

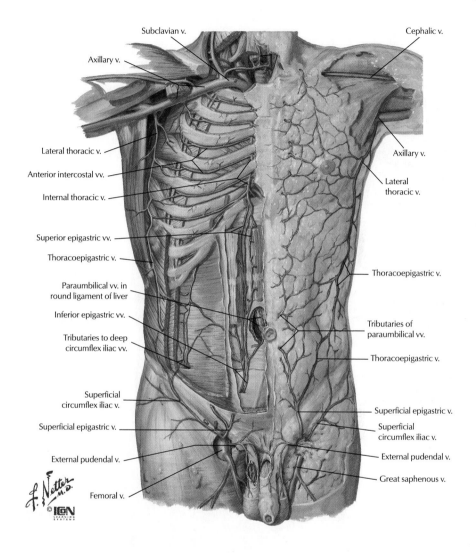

A rich anastomosis of bilateral superficial veins courses over the abdominal wall (the right side shows a deeper dissection).

VEIN	COURSE
Superficial epigastric	Drains into femoral vein
Superficial circumflex iliac	Drains into femoral vein and parallels inguinal ligament
Inferior epigastric	Drains into external iliac vein
Superior epigastric	Drains into internal thoracic vein
Thoracoepigastric	Anastomosis between superficial epigastric and lateral thoracic
Lateral thoracic	Drains into axillary vein

Abdominal Wall: Arteries

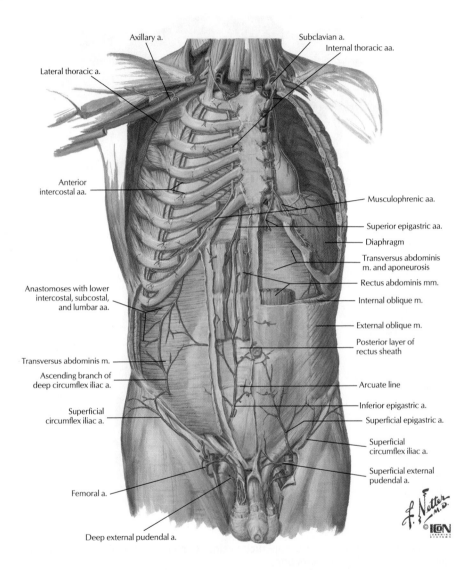

Axillary a.

Subclavian a.

Internal thoracic aa.

Lateral thoracic a.

Anterior intercostal aa.

Musculophrenic aa.

Superior epigastric aa.

Diaphragm

Transversus abdominis m. and aponeurosis

Rectus abdominis mm.

Anastomoses with lower intercostal, subcostal, and lumbar aa.

Internal oblique m.

External oblique m.

Posterior layer of rectus sheath

Transversus abdominis m.

Ascending branch of deep circumflex iliac a.

Arcuate line

Inferior epigastric a.

Superficial circumflex iliac a.

Superficial epigastric a.

Superficial circumflex iliac a.

Superficial external pudendal a.

Femoral a.

Deep external pudendal a.

Right side shows a deeper dissection.

ARTERY	COURSE
Superior epigastric	Arises from internal thoracic and anastomoses with inferior epigastric
Inferior epigastric	Arises from external iliac and anastomoses with superior epigastric
Superficial circumflex iliac	Arises from femoral and anastomoses with deep circumflex iliac
Superficial epigastric	Arises from femoral and runs toward umbilicus
External pudendal	Arises from femoral and runs toward pubis

Abdominal Wall: Rectus Sheath

Section above arcuate line

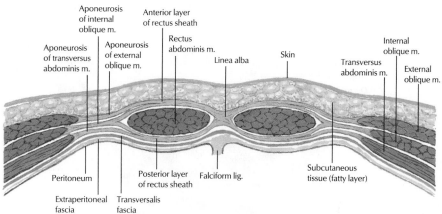

Aponeurosis of internal oblique m.
Anterior layer of rectus sheath
Aponeurosis of transversus abdominis m.
Aponeurosis of external oblique m.
Rectus abdominis m.
Linea alba
Skin
Internal oblique m.
Transversus abdominis m.
External oblique m.
Peritoneum
Posterior layer of rectus sheath
Falciform lig.
Subcutaneous tissue (fatty layer)
Extraperitoneal fascia
Transversalis fascia

Section below arcuate line

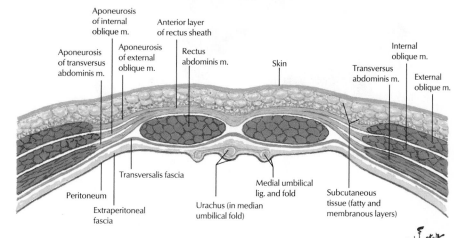

Aponeurosis of internal oblique m.
Anterior layer of rectus sheath
Aponeurosis of transversus abdominis m.
Aponeurosis of external oblique m.
Rectus abdominis m.
Skin
Internal oblique m.
Transversus abdominis m.
External oblique m.
Transversalis fascia
Peritoneum
Medial umbilical lig. and fold
Extraperitoneal fascia
Urachus (in median umbilical fold)
Subcutaneous tissue (fatty and membranous layers)

LAYER	COMMENT
Anterior lamina above arcuate line	Formed by fused aponeuroses of external and internal abdominal oblique muscles
Posterior lamina above arcuate line	Formed by fused aponeuroses of internal abdominal oblique and transversus abdominis muscles
Below arcuate line	All three muscle aponeuroses fuse to form anterior lamina, with rectus abdominis in contact only with transversalis fascia posteriorly

The rectus sheath contains the rectus abdominis muscle (and the inconsistent pyramidalis muscle), superior and inferior epigastric vessels, lymphatics, and ventral rami of T7 to T12 nerves, which penetrate the sheath laterally.

Abdominal Wall: Inguinal Region

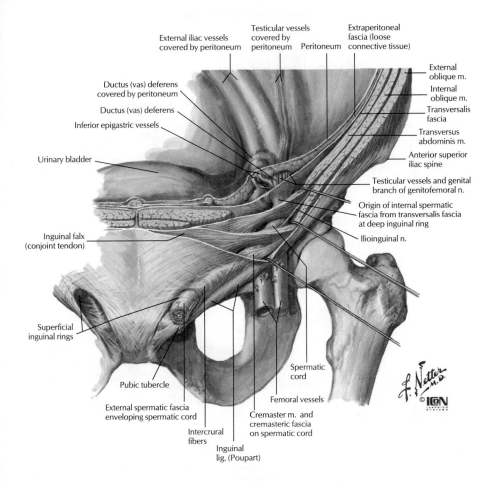

External iliac vessels covered by peritoneum

Testicular vessels covered by peritoneum

Peritoneum

Extraperitoneal fascia (loose connective tissue)

Ductus (vas) deferens covered by peritoneum

Ductus (vas) deferens

Inferior epigastric vessels

Urinary bladder

External oblique m.

Internal oblique m.

Transversalis fascia

Transversus abdominis m.

Anterior superior iliac spine

Testicular vessels and genital branch of genitofemoral n.

Origin of internal spermatic fascia from transversalis fascia at deep inguinal ring

Ilioinguinal n.

Inguinal falx (conjoint tendon)

Superficial inguinal rings

Pubic tubercle

External spermatic fascia enveloping spermatic cord

Intercrural fibers

Inguinal lig. (Poupart)

Cremaster m. and cremasteric fascia on spermatic cord

Femoral vessels

Spermatic cord

FEATURE	COMMENT
Superficial ring	Medial opening in external abdominal oblique aponeurosis
Deep ring	Outpouching in transversalis fascia lateral to inferior epigastric vessels
Inguinal canal	Tunnel extending from deep to superficial ring, paralleling inguinal ligament (transmits spermatic cord or round ligament of uterus)
Anterior wall	Aponeuroses of external and internal abdominal oblique muscles
Posterior wall	Transversalis fascia (medially includes conjoint tendon)
Roof	Arching muscle fibers of internal abdominal oblique and transversus abdominis muscles
Floor	Inguinal ligament (and medially by lacunar ligament, an expanded extension of the ligament)
Inguinal ligament	Ligament extending between anterior superior iliac spine and pubic tubercle (folded inferior border of external abdominal oblique aponeurosis)

Abdominal Wall: Spermatic Cord

The spermatic cord runs in the inguinal canal, exits via the superficial inguinal ring, and passes into the scrotum, where it suspends the testis. As it passes through the inguinal canal, it picks up spermatic fascial layers derived from the abdominal wall as the testis descends in the fetus (see Embryology). The spermatic cord contains the

- Ductus deferens
- Testicular artery, artery of the ductus deferens, and cremasteric artery
- Pampiniform plexus of veins
- Autonomic nerve fibers coursing on arteries and ductus deferens
- Genital branch of the genitofemoral nerve (innervates cremaster muscle)
- Lymphatics

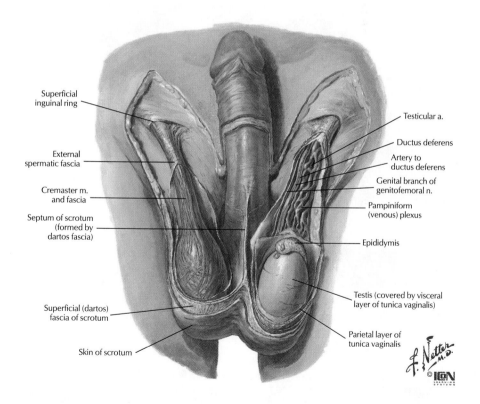

Superficial inguinal ring

External spermatic fascia

Cremaster m. and fascia

Septum of scrotum (formed by dartos fascia)

Superficial (dartos) fascia of scrotum

Skin of scrotum

Testicular a.

Ductus deferens

Artery to ductus deferens

Genital branch of genitofemoral n.

Pampiniform (venous) plexus

Epididymis

Testis (covered by visceral layer of tunica vaginalis)

Parietal layer of tunica vaginalis

Clinical Correlation

Peritoneum
Inguinal lig.
Vas deferens
Obliterated processus vaginalis

Normally obliterated processus vaginalis

Tunica vaginalis

Completely patent processus vaginalis

Partially patent processus vaginalis (small congenital hernia)

Loop of bowel entering hernial sac

Origin of internal spermatic fascia from transversalis fascia at deep inguinal ring

Inferior epigastric vessels

Peritoneum
Extraperitoneal fascia
Transversalis fascia

Superficial inguinal ring

Internal spermatic fascia

External spermatic fascia

Cremaster m. and fascia

Hernial sac

Ductus (vas) deferens and vessels of spermatic cord

Inguinal hernias are distinguished by their relation to the inferior epigastric vessels:
- **Indirect** (75%): occur lateral to inferior epigastric vessels, pass through the deep inguinal ring and inguinal canal in a protrusion of peritoneum along the spermatic cord and within the internal spermatic fascia
- **Direct**: occur medial to inferior epigastric vessels (Hesselbach's triangle) pass through the posterior wall of the inguinal canal, and are separate from the spermatic cord

Indirect hernias often result from incomplete closure of the processus vaginalis (a slip of peritoneum that descends with the testis during development).

Viscera: Peritoneal Cavity

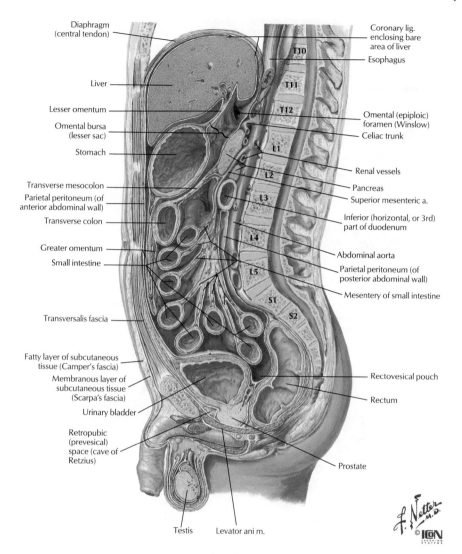

Diaphragm (central tendon)

Coronary lig. enclosing bare area of liver

Esophagus

T10

Liver

T11

Lesser omentum

T12

Omental (epiploic) foramen (Winslow)

Omental bursa (lesser sac)

Celiac trunk

Stomach

L1

Renal vessels

L2

Transverse mesocolon

Pancreas

Parietal peritoneum (of anterior abdominal wall)

L3

Superior mesenteric a.

Transverse colon

Inferior (horizontal, or 3rd) part of duodenum

L4

Greater omentum

Abdominal aorta

Small intestine

Parietal peritoneum (of posterior abdominal wall)

L5

Mesentery of small intestine

S1

S2

Transversalis fascia

Fatty layer of subcutaneous tissue (Camper's fascia)

Membranous layer of subcutaneous tissue (Scarpa's fascia)

Rectovesical pouch

Rectum

Urinary bladder

Retropubic (prevesical) space (cave of Retzius)

Prostate

Testis   Levator ani m.

The peritoneal cavity is a potential space lined with parietal peritoneum (lines the interior aspect of body walls) and visceral peritoneum (covers abdominal organs).

FEATURE	DESCRIPTION
Greater omentum	An "apron" of peritoneum hanging from greater curvature of stomach, folding back on itself to attach to transverse colon
Lesser omentum	Double layer of peritoneum extending from lesser curvature of stomach and proximal duodenum to liver
Mesenteries	Double fold of peritoneum suspending parts of bowel and conveying vessels, lymphatics, and nerves of bowel
Peritoneal ligaments	Double layer of peritoneum attaching viscera to walls or to other viscera

Clinical Correlation

Acute Peritonitis   *Anatomy on pp. 397, 401, 451*

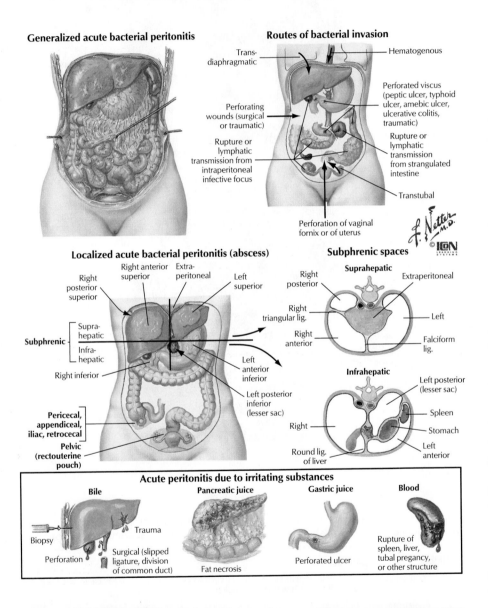

Generalized acute bacterial peritonitis

Routes of bacterial invasion

Trans-diaphragmatic

Hematogenous

Perforating wounds (surgical or traumatic)

Perforated viscus (peptic ulcer, typhoid ulcer, amebic ulcer, ulcerative colitis, traumatic)

Rupture or lymphatic transmission from intraperitoneal infective focus

Rupture or lymphatic transmission from strangulated intestine

Transtubal

Perforation of vaginal fornix or of uterus

Localized acute bacterial peritonitis (abscess)

Right posterior superior

Right anterior superior

Extra-peritoneal

Left superior

Subphrenic — Supra-hepatic / Infra-hepatic

Right inferior

Pericecal, appendiceal, iliac, retrocecal

Pelvic (rectouterine pouch)

Left anterior inferior

Left posterior inferior (lesser sac)

Subphrenic spaces

Suprahepatic

Right posterior

Extraperitoneal

Right triangular lig.

Right anterior

Left

Falciform lig.

Infrahepatic

Left posterior (lesser sac)

Spleen

Right

Stomach

Round lig. of liver

Left anterior

Acute peritonitis due to irritating substances

Bile

Biopsy

Trauma

Perforation

Surgical (slipped ligature, division of common duct)

Pancreatic juice

Fat necrosis

Gastric juice

Perforated ulcer

Blood

Rupture of spleen, liver, tubal pregancy, or other structure

Generalized acute inflammation of the abdomen is called peritonitis. The most common cause is an acute infection. Spread of the infection usually depends on anatomical site and the abdomen's ability to wall off the infected area. Other irritants leading to peritonitis are also illustrated.

Clinical Correlation

Acute Abdomen: Visceral Etiology

Anatomy on pp. 387, 403, 409, 410

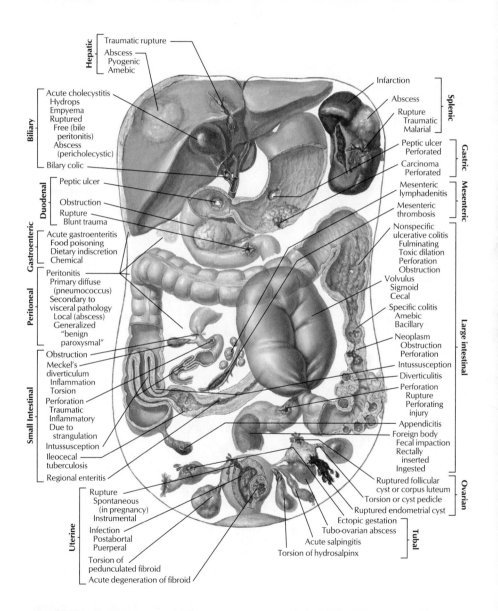

Hepatic
- Traumatic rupture
- Abscess
  - Pyogenic
  - Amebic

Biliary
- Acute cholecystitis
  - Hydrops
  - Empyema
  - Ruptured
  - Free (bile peritonitis)
  - Abscess (pericholecystic)
- Bilary colic

Gastroenteric

Duodenal
- Peptic ulcer
- Obstruction
- Rupture
  - Blunt trauma

Gastroenteric
- Acute gastroenteritis
  - Food poisoning
  - Dietary indiscretion
  - Chemical

Peritoneal
- Peritonitis
  - Primary diffuse (pneumococcus)
  - Secondary to visceral pathology
  - Local (abscess)
  - Generalized "benign paroxysmal"

Small Intestinal
- Obstruction
- Meckel's diverticulum
  - Inflammation
  - Torsion
- Perforation
  - Traumatic
  - Inflammatory
  - Due to strangulation
- Intussusception
- Ileocecal tuberculosis
- Regional enteritis

Uterine
- Rupture
  - Spontaneous (in pregnancy)
  - Instrumental
- Infection
  - Postabortal
  - Puerperal
- Torsion of pedunculated fibroid
- Acute degeneration of fibroid

Splenic
- Infarction
- Abscess
- Rupture
  - Traumatic
  - Malarial

Gastric
- Peptic ulcer
  - Perforated
- Carcinoma
  - Perforated

Mesenteric
- Mesenteric lymphadenitis
- Mesenteric thrombosis

Large intestinal
- Nonspecific ulcerative colitis
  - Fulminating
  - Toxic dilation
  - Perforation
  - Obstruction
- Volvulus
  - Sigmoid
  - Cecal
- Specific colitis
  - Amebic
  - Bacillary
- Neoplasm
  - Obstruction
  - Perforation
- Intussusception
- Diverticulitis
- Perforation
  - Rupture
  - Perforating injury
- Appendicitis
- Foreign body
  - Fecal impaction
  - Rectally inserted
  - Ingested

Ovarian
- Ruptured follicular cyst or corpus luteum
- Torsion or cyst pedicle
- Ruptured endometrial cyst

Tubal
- Ectopic gestation
- Tubo-ovarian abscess
- Acute salpingitis
- Torsion of hydrosalpinx

Abdominal pain (which persists for several hours), tenderness, and evidence of inflammation or visceral dysfunction signal an acute abdomen. The visceral etiology is extensive.

Clinical Correlation

Acute Abdomen: Thoracic, Retroperitoneal, Systemic, Abdominal Wall
Anatomy on pp. 388, 445

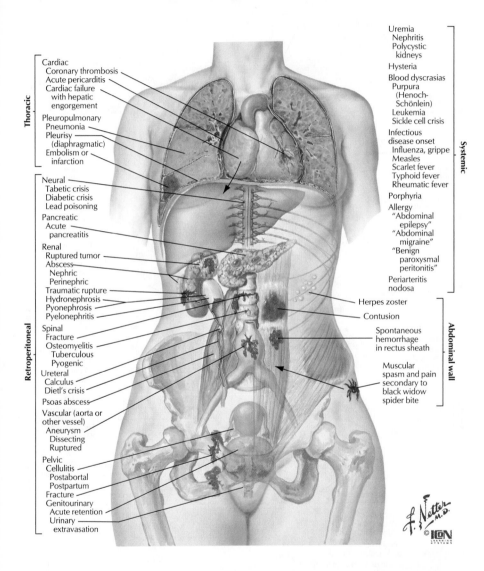

Thoracic

Cardiac
Coronary thrombosis
Acute pericarditis
Cardiac failure
with hepatic
engorgement
Pleuropulmonary
Pneumonia
Pleurisy
(diaphragmatic)
Embolism or
infarction

Retroperitoneal

Neural
Tabetic crisis
Diabetic crisis
Lead poisoning
Pancreatic
Acute
pancreatitis
Renal
Ruptured tumor
Abscess
Nephric
Perinephric
Traumatic rupture
Hydronephrosis
Pyonephrosis
Pyelonephritis
Spinal
Fracture
Osteomyelitis
Tuberculous
Pyogenic
Ureteral
Calculus
Dietl's crisis
Psoas abscess
Vascular (aorta or
other vessel)
Aneurysm
Dissecting
Ruptured
Pelvic
Cellulitis
Postabortal
Postpartum
Fracture
Genitourinary
Acute retention
Urinary
extravasation

Systemic

Uremia
Nephritis
Polycystic
kidneys
Hysteria
Blood dyscrasias
Purpura
(Henoch-
Schönlein)
Leukemia
Sickle cell crisis
Infectious
disease onset
Influenza, grippe
Measles
Scarlet fever
Typhoid fever
Rheumatic fever
Porphyria
Allergy
"Abdominal
epilepsy"
"Abdominal
migraine"
"Benign
paroxysmal
peritonitis"
Periarteritis
nodosa

Abdominal wall

Herpes zoster
Contusion
Spontaneous
hemorrhage
in rectus sheath
Muscular
spasm and pain
secondary to
black widow
spider bite

Thoracic, retroperitoneal, systemic, and abdominal wall etiologies must be considered during assessment of patients with acute abdomen. Referred pain from various visceral structures is common until the disease involves the parietal peritoneum or somatically innervated body wall.

Viscera: Omental Bursa (Lesser Sac)

The omental bursa is an irregular, cul-de-sac space posterior to the stomach and anterior to the retroperitoneal pancreas. It communicates with the greater sac (the rest of the peritoneal cavity) via the epiploic foramen (of Winslow), which lies just posterior to the hepatoduodenal ligament (containing the hepatic artery proper, common bile duct, and portal vein).

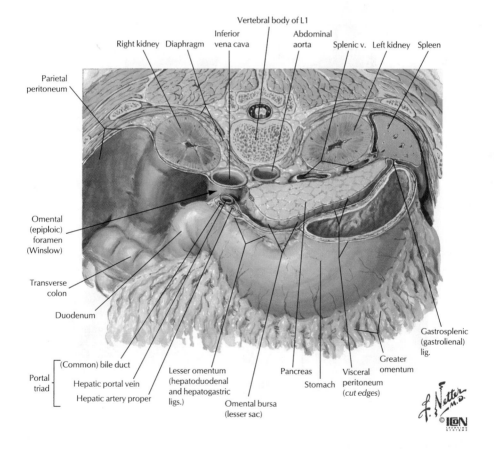

Right kidney Diaphragm Inferior vena cava Vertebral body of L1 Abdominal aorta Splenic v. Left kidney Spleen

Parietal peritoneum

Omental (epiploic) foramen (Winslow)

Transverse colon

Duodenum

Portal triad
- (Common) bile duct
- Hepatic portal vein
- Hepatic artery proper

Lesser omentum (hepatoduodenal and hepatogastric ligs.)

Omental bursa (lesser sac)

Pancreas

Stomach

Visceral peritoneum (cut edges)

Greater omentum

Gastrosplenic (gastrolienal) lig.

Clinical Correlation

Gastroesophageal Reflux Disease *Anatomy on pp. 403, 449*

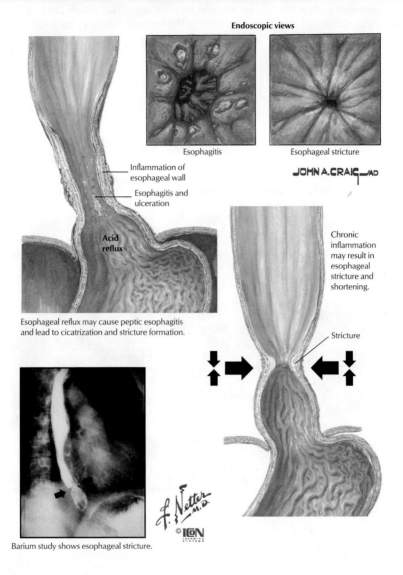

Endoscopic views

Esophagitis

Esophageal stricture

JOHN A. CRAIG AD

Inflammation of esophageal wall

Esophagitis and ulceration

Acid reflux

Chronic inflammation may result in esophageal stricture and shortening.

Esophageal reflux may cause peptic esophagitis and lead to cicatrization and stricture formation.

Stricture

Barium study shows esophageal stricture.

CHARACTERISTIC	DESCRIPTION
Signs and symptoms	Upper abdominal pain, dyspepsia, gas, heartburn, dysphagia (15-20%), bronchospasm or asthma (15-20%)
Prevalence	Common
Age	Reproductive age and older
Causes	Decreased tone of lower esophageal sphincter, sliding hiatal hernia

Viscera: Stomach

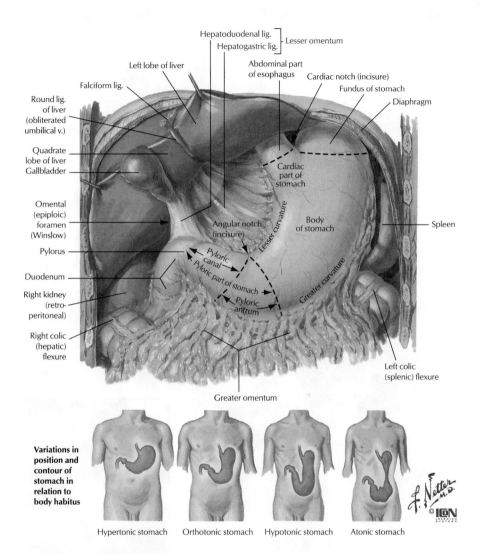

Variations in position and contour of stomach in relation to body habitus

Hypertonic stomach   Orthotonic stomach   Hypotonic stomach   Atonic stomach

FEATURE	DESCRIPTION
Lesser curvature	Right border of stomach; lesser omentum attaches here and extends to liver
Greater curvature	Convex border with greater omentum suspended from its margin
Cardiac part	Area of stomach that communicates with esophagus superiorly
Fundus	Superior part just under left dome of diaphragm
Body	Main part between fundus and pyloric antrum
Pyloric part	Portion that is divided into proximal antrum and distal canal
Pylorus	Site of pyloric sphincter muscle; joins first part of duodenum

Clinical Correlation

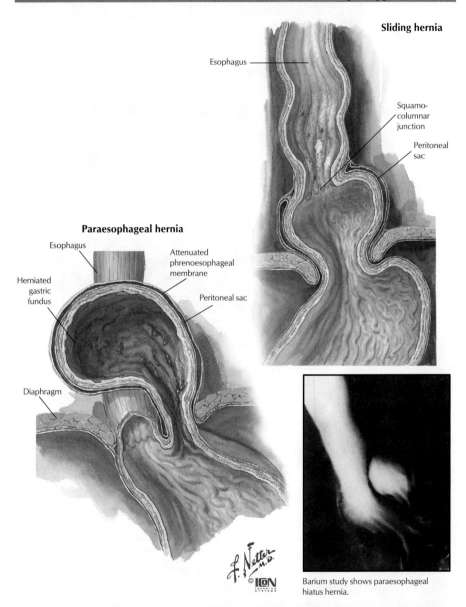

Sliding hernia

Esophagus

Squamo-columnar junction

Peritoneal sac

Paraesophageal hernia

Esophagus

Herniated gastric fundus

Attenuated phrenoesophageal membrane

Peritoneal sac

Diaphragm

Barium study shows paraesophageal hiatus hernia.

Herniation of the diaphragm that involves the stomach is referred to as a hiatal hernia. A widening of the space between the muscular crura forming the esophageal hiatus allows protrusion of part of the stomach. The two anatomical types are
- Sliding, rolling, or axial, hernia (95%): appears as a bell-shaped protrusion
- Paraesophageal, or nonaxial, hernia: usually involves the gastric fundus

Clinical Correlation

Polypoid adenocarcinoma

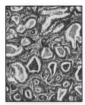

Adenocarcinoma

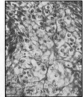

Colloid carcinoma

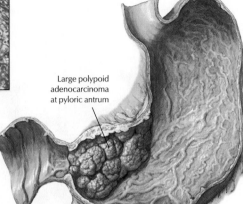

Large polypoid
adenocarcinoma
at pyloric antrum

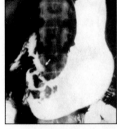

Radiographic appearance of
polypoid adenocarcinoma

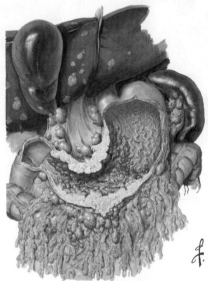

**Carcinoma
of stomach**

Extensive carcinoma
of stomach with
metastases to
lymph nodes, liver,
omentum, tail of
pancreas, and hilus
of spleen; biliary
obstruction

CHARACTERISTIC	DESCRIPTION
Type	95% either intestinal-type adenocarcinomas or diffuse carcinomas
Prevalence	High in Japan, Russia, Colombia, Costa Rica, Hungary; 3% of all cancer deaths in the United States
Age	Intestinal type after 50 years, earlier for diffuse carcinoma
Risk factors	Diet (nitrate, smoked foods, salt intake, few vegetables and fruit), *Helicobacter pylori*, pernicious anemia, blood group A

Viscera: Duodenum

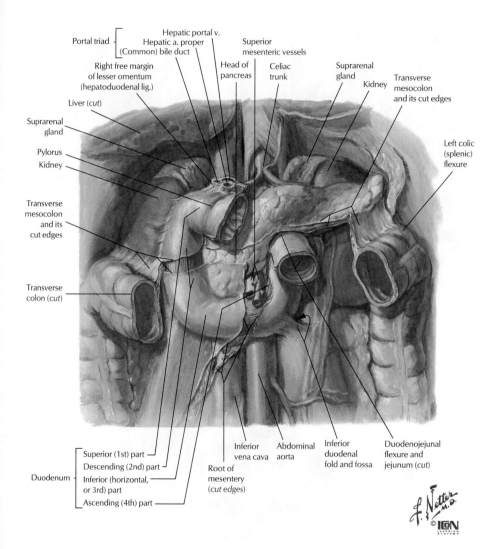

The duodenum is the first part of the small intestine and is principally retroperitoneal.

PART OF DUODENUM	DESCRIPTION
Superior	First part; attachment site for hepatoduodenal ligament of lesser omentum
Descending	Second part; site where bile and pancreatic ducts empty
Inferior	Third part; part that crosses inferior vena cava (IVC) and aorta and is crossed anteriorly by mesenteric vessels
Ascending	Fourth part; portion tethered by suspensory ligament at duodenojejunal flexure

Clinical Correlation

Peptic Ulcer Disease

Anatomy on p. 403

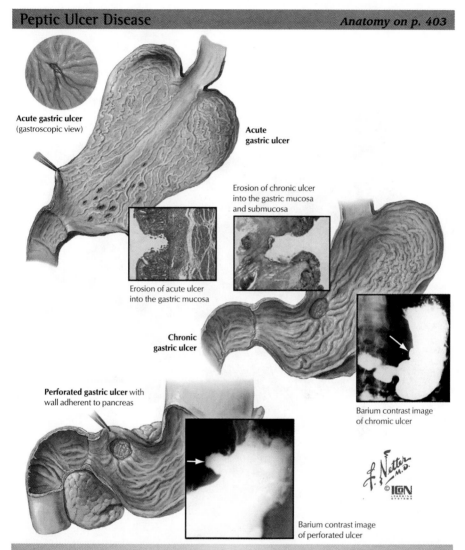

Acute gastric ulcer
(gastroscopic view)

Acute
gastric ulcer

Erosion of chronic ulcer
into the gastric mucosa
and submucosa

Erosion of acute ulcer
into the gastric mucosa

Chronic
gastric ulcer

Perforated gastric ulcer with
wall adherent to pancreas

Barium contrast image
of chromic ulcer

Barium contrast image
of perforated ulcer

Peptic ulcers are GI lesions that may extend through the muscularis mucosae and are remitting, relapsing lesions. Acute lesions are small and shallow, whereas chronic ulcers may erode into the muscularis externa or perforate the serosa.

CHARACTERISTIC	DESCRIPTION
Site	98% in first part of duodenum or stomach, in ratio of approximately 4:1
Prevalence	Worldwide approximately 5%; in United States approximately 2% in males and 1.5% in females
Age	Young adults, increasing with age
Aggravating factors	Mucosal exposure to gastric acid and pepsin; *H. pylori* infection (almost 80% of duodenal ulcers and 70% of gastric ulcers); use of nonsteroidal antiinflammatory drugs, aspirin, or alcohol; smoking

Viscera: Celiac Trunk

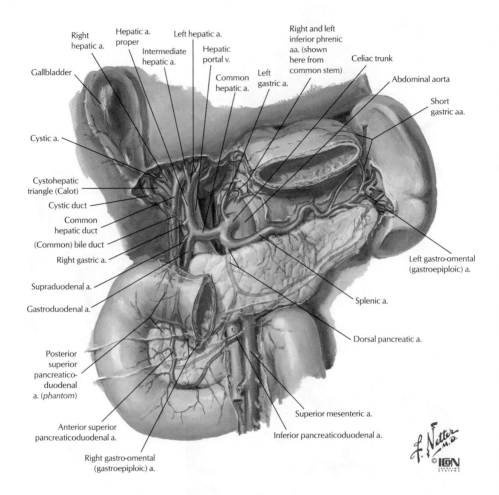

The celiac trunk is one of the three unpaired visceral branches of the aorta that arises just inferior to the aortic hiatus of the diaphragm. It supplies blood to the visceral structures derived from the embryonic foregut and the spleen (not a foregut derivative).

ARTERY	STRUCTURES SUPPLIED
Left gastric	Supplies proximal stomach and distal esophagus
Splenic	Supplies pancreas (dorsal branch), stomach (short gastrics and left gastroepiploic), and spleen
Common hepatic	Divides into proper hepatic and gastroduodenal branches, which supply liver, gallbladder, stomach, duodenum, and pancreas

Viscera: Small Intestine

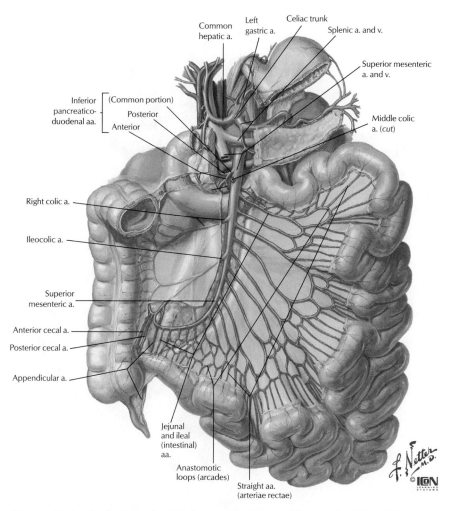

The small intestine includes the duodenum, jejunum, and ileum (distal three fifths). Most of the small intestine and the cecum, ascending colon, and most of the transverse colon are derived from embryonic midgut and are supplied by the superior mesenteric artery (SMA).

ARTERY	STRUCTURES SUPPLIED
SMA	Supplies small intestine and proximal half of colon; arises from aorta posterior to neck of pancreas
Inferior pancreaticoduodenal	Supplies duodenum and pancreas
Middle colic	Supplies transverse colon
Intestinal	Approximately 15 branches supply jejunum and ileum
Ileocolic	Supplies ileum, cecum, and appendix
Right colic	Supplies ascending colon

Viscera: Large Intestine

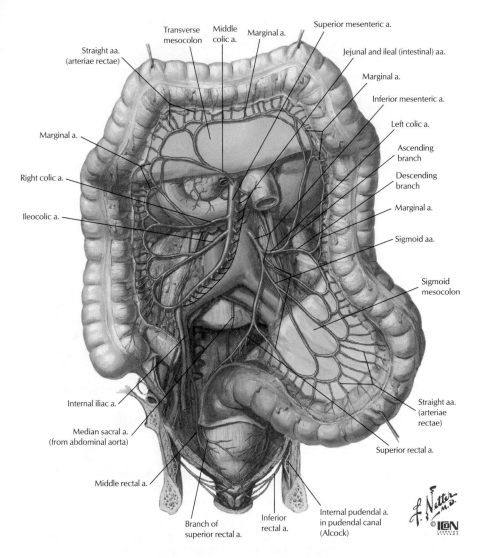

The large intestine includes the cecum (and appendix), ascending colon, transverse colon, descending colon, sigmoid colon, rectum, and anal canal. Embryonic hindgut derivatives include those distal to the distal transverse colon and are supplied by the inferior mesenteric artery (IMA) and its branches.

ARTERY	STRUCTURES SUPPLIED
IMA	Supplies distal colon; arises from aorta approximately 2 cm superior to its bifurcation
Left colic	Supplies distal transverse and descending colon
Sigmoid arteries	Three or four branches supply sigmoid colon
Superior rectal	Supplies proximal rectum (anastomoses with other rectal arteries)

Clinical Correlation

Irritable Bowel Syndrome
Anatomy on p. 410

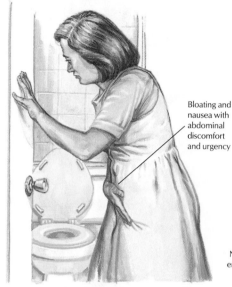

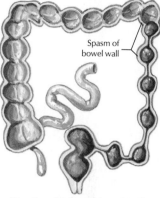

Spasm of bowel wall

Bloating and nausea with abdominal discomfort and urgency

Altered bowel wall sensitivity and motility result in IB symptom complex.

Irritable bowel syndrome is a syndrome of intermittent abdominal pain, diarrhea, and constipation related to altered motility of the gut. Clinical variants include:

1. Spastic colitis characterized by chronic abdominal pain and constipation
2. Intermittent diarrhea that is usually painless
3. Combination of both with alternating diarrhea and constipation

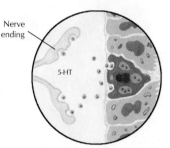

Nerve ending

5-HT

Actions of gut wall 5-hydroxytryptamine (5-HT) may underlie anomalies of motility.

Rome II diagnostic criteria for irritable bowel syndrome	Symptoms suggestive of diagnoses beyond functional bowel disease
12-week history out of past 12 months of abdominal pain and discomfort incorporating two of three features: 1. Relieved by defecation 2. Onset associated with change in stool frequency 3. Onset associated with change in stool form (appearance)	1. Anemia 2. Fever 3. Persistent diarrhea 4. Rectal bleeding 5. Severe constipation 6. Weight loss 7. Nocturnal GI symptoms 8. Family history of GI cancer, inflammatory bowel disease, or celiac disease 9. New onset of symptoms after age 50

JOHN A.CRAIG—AD
©IGN

This syndrome is characterized by intermittent abdominal pain, constipation, or diarrhea caused by altered motility of the bowel. It accounts for approximately 50% of all visits by patients to gastroenterologists.

Clinical Correlation

Crohn's Disease
Anatomy on pp. 409, 410

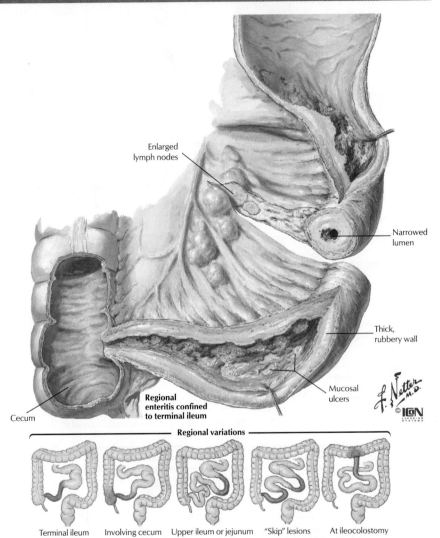

Enlarged lymph nodes

Narrowed lumen

Thick, rubbery wall

Mucosal ulcers

Regional enteritis confined to terminal ileum

Cecum

— Regional variations —

Terminal ileum   Involving cecum   Upper ileum or jejunum   "Skip" lesions   At ileocolostomy

Crohn's disease is an idiopathic inflammatory bowel disease that may affect any segment of the GI tract but usually involves the small intestine and colon.

CHARACTERISTIC	DESCRIPTION
Prevalence	2-10 cases/10,000 population; more common in United States, Britain, Scandinavia
Age	15-30 years
Signs and symptoms	Abdominal pain (paraumbilical and lower right quadrant), diarrhea, fever, dyspareunia, vulvar or perineal fissures or fistulas, urinary tract infection (UTI), arthritis, erythema nodosum

Clinical Correlation

Ulcerative Colitis
Anatomy on p. 410

Intestinal complications

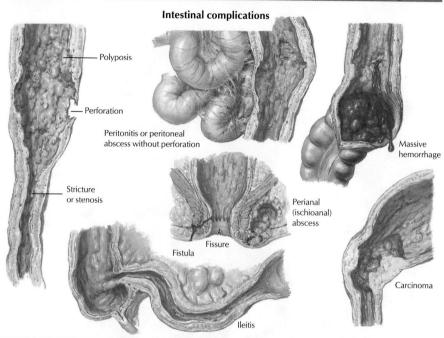

Polyposis

Perforation

Peritonitis or peritoneal abscess without perforation

Stricture or stenosis

Massive hemorrhage

Perianal (ischioanal) abscess

Fissure

Fistula

Carcinoma

Ileitis

Systemic complications

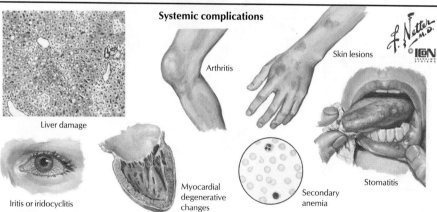

Arthritis

Skin lesions

Liver damage

Iritis or iridocyclitis

Myocardial degenerative changes

Secondary anemia

Stomatitis

Like Crohn's disease, ulcerative colitis is an idiopathic inflammatory bowel disease that begins in the rectum and extends proximally. Usually, the inflammation is limited to the mucosa and submucosa.

CHARACTERISTIC	DESCRIPTION
Prevalence	70-150 cases/100,000 population (80% in rectosigmoid region)
Age	20-50 years; 50% affected are younger than 21 years
Signs and symptoms	Abdominal pain frequently relieved by defecation; diarrhea, fever, arthritis

Clinical Correlation

Colonic Diverticulosis   *Anatomy on p. 410*

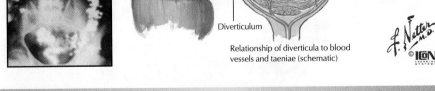

Transverse colon

Descending colon (opened)

Ascending colon

Concretion in diverticulum

Appendix

Peritoneum
Circular muscle
Taenia coli
Epiploic appendix
Concretion in diverticulum
Mucosa
Blood vessel piercing musculature

Diverticulum

Relationship of diverticula to blood vessels and taeniae (schematic)

Most diverticula are acquired (Meckel's, a congenital lesion, is an exception) and are herniations of colonic mucosa through the muscular wall.

CHARACTERISTIC	DESCRIPTION
Site	Most common in distal colon and sigmoid colon
Prevalence	20%, increasing with age to 50% by age 60-80 years
Causes	Exaggerated peristaltic contractions and increased intraluminal pressure and/or intrinsic defect in muscular wall
Risk factors	Low-fiber diet, age (>40 years), history of diverticulitis

Clinical Correlation

Bowel Obstruction: Volvulus

Anatomy on pp. 410, 454

Pathogenesis of sigmoid volvulus

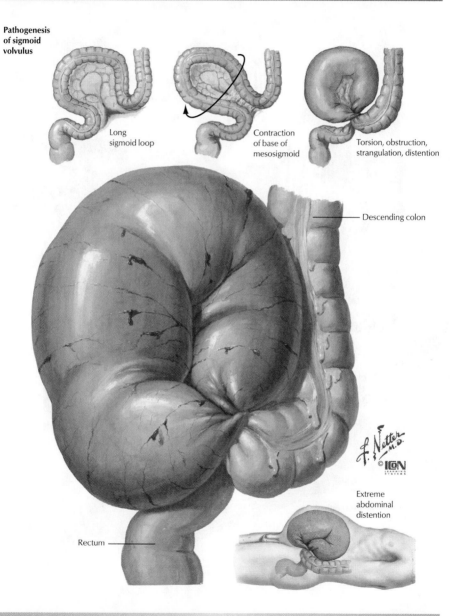

Long sigmoid loop

Contraction of base of mesosigmoid

Torsion, obstruction, strangulation, distention

Descending colon

Rectum

Extreme abdominal distention

Volvulus is a twisting of a bowel loop that may cause bowel obstruction and constriction of the vascular supply, which may lead to infarction. Volvulus affects the small intestine more often than the large, and the sigmoid colon is its most common site in the large bowel. Volvulus is associated with dietary habits, perhaps a bulky vegetable diet that results in an increased fecal load.

Clinical Correlation

Bowel Obstruction: Intussusception

Anatomy on p. 409

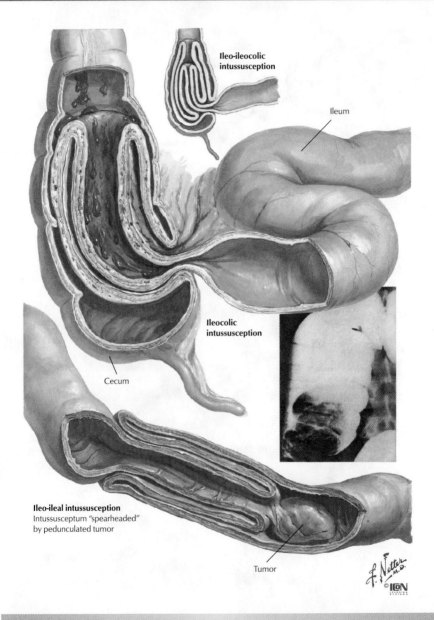

Ileo-ileocolic intussusception

Ileum

Ileocolic intussusception

Cecum

Ileo-ileal intussusception
Intussusceptum "spearheaded" by pedunculated tumor

Tumor

Intussusception is the invagination, or telescoping, of one bowel segment into a contiguous distal segment. In children, the etiology may be linked to excessive peristalsis, whereas in adults, an intraluminal mass, such as a tumor, may become trapped during a peristaltic wave and pull its attachment site forward into the more distal segment. Intestinal obstruction and infarction may occur.

Clinical Correlation

Colorectal Cancer   *Anatomy on p. 410*

Clinical manifestations

Right (ascending) colon

Chronic low-grade bleeding may lead to anemia.

Obstruction uncommon because of large lumen and liquid fecal contents

Lesions of right colon often asymptomatic, or "silent," until disease in advanced stage

Bleeding diluted by fecal stream

Liquid fecal stream passes lesion

Solid stool

Bleeding diluted by feces results in normal-appearing but guaiac-positive stool.

Change in bowel habits may be first symptom of left colon lesions.

Paradoxic diarrhea

Cramping pain

Constipation and obstruction

Left (descending) colon

Tenesmus and urgency

Stool may be blood covered or mixed with blood.

Bleeding

JOHN A. CRAIG—AD
© ICON

Cancer of left colon and rectum frequently causes bleeding and bowel obstruction due to solid feces.

Colorectal cancer is second only to lung cancer in site-specific mortality and accounts for almost 15% of cancer-related deaths in the United States.

CHARACTERISTIC	DESCRIPTION
Site	98% adenocarcinomas: 25% in cecum-ascending colon, 25% in sigmoid colon, 25% in rectum, 25% elsewhere
Prevalence	Highest in United States, Canada, Australia, New Zealand, Denmark, Sweden; males affected 20% more than females
Age	Peak incidence at 60-70 years
Risk factors	Heredity, high-fat diet, increasing age, inflammatory bowel disease, polyps

Clinical Correlation

Surgical Resection of Colon Cancer   *Anatomy on pp. 409, 410*

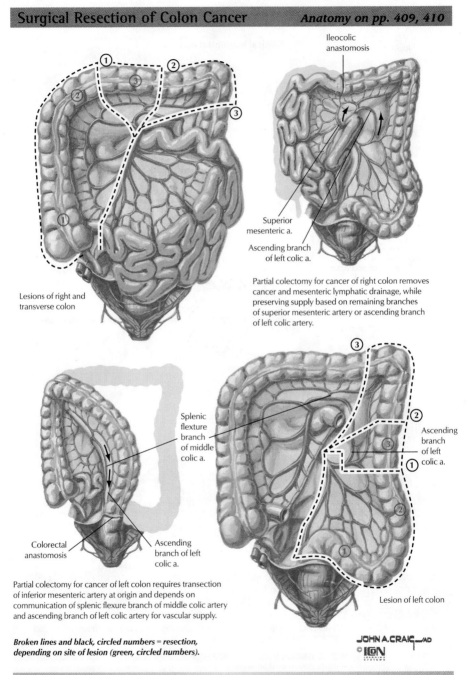

Ileocolic
anastomosis

Lesions of right and
transverse colon

Superior
mesenteric a.

Ascending branch
of left colic a.

Partial colectomy for cancer of right colon removes
cancer and mesenteric lymphatic drainage, while
preserving supply based on remaining branches
of superior mesenteric artery or ascending branch
of left colic artery.

Splenic
flexure
branch
of middle
colic a.

Ascending
branch
of left
colic a.

Colorectal
anastomosis

Ascending
branch of left
colic a.

Partial colectomy for cancer of left colon requires transection
of inferior mesenteric artery at origin and depends on
communication of splenic flexure branch of middle colic artery
and ascending branch of left colic artery for vascular supply.

Lesion of left colon

Broken lines and black, circled numbers = resection,
depending on site of lesion (green, circled numbers).

JOHN A.CRAIG—AD
©ICN

Surgical approaches must preserve the blood supply to the unresected bowel so
that intestinal arterial continuity can be restored by anastomosis after the bowel is
reconnected.

Viscera: Liver

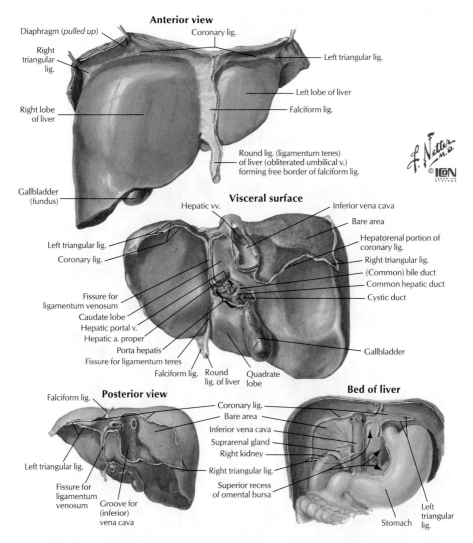

Anterior view

Diaphragm (*pulled up*)
Coronary lig.
Right triangular lig.
Left triangular lig.
Left lobe of liver
Falciform lig.
Right lobe of liver
Round lig. (ligamentum teres) of liver (obliterated umbilical v.) forming free border of falciform lig.
Gallbladder (fundus)

Visceral surface

Hepatic vv.
Inferior vena cava
Bare area
Hepatorenal portion of coronary lig.
Left triangular lig.
Coronary lig.
Right triangular lig.
(Common) bile duct
Common hepatic duct
Cystic duct
Fissure for ligamentum venosum
Caudate lobe
Hepatic portal v.
Hepatic a. proper
Porta hepatis
Fissure for ligamentum teres
Gallbladder
Falciform lig.
Round lig. of liver
Quadrate lobe

Posterior view

Falciform lig.
Coronary lig.
Bare area
Inferior vena cava
Suprarenal gland
Right kidney
Left triangular lig.
Right triangular lig.
Fissure for ligamentum venosum
Groove for (inferior) vena cava
Superior recess of omental bursa

Bed of liver

Stomach
Left triangular lig.

FEATURE	DESCRIPTION
Lobes	Divisions, in functional terms, into right and left lobes, with anatomical subdivisions of right lobe into quadrate and caudate lobes
Round ligament	Ligament that contains obliterated umbilical vein
Falciform ligament	Peritoneal reflection off anterior abdominal wall with round ligament in its margin
Ligamentum venosum	Ligamentous remnant of fetal ductus venosus, allowing fetal blood from placenta to bypass liver
Coronary ligaments	Reflections of peritoneum from liver to diaphragm
Bare area	Area of liver pressed against diaphragm that lacks visceral peritoneum
Porta hepatis	Site at which vessels, ducts, lymphatics, and nerves enter or leave liver

Viscera: Hepatic Portal System and Anastomoses

Venous drainage of the abdominopelvic GI tract occurs via the portal vein (formed by union of the superior mesenteric vein and splenic vein) and its tributaries, which return venous blood to the liver and then via hepatic veins to the IVC and right atrium. Important portocaval anastomoses are illustrated.

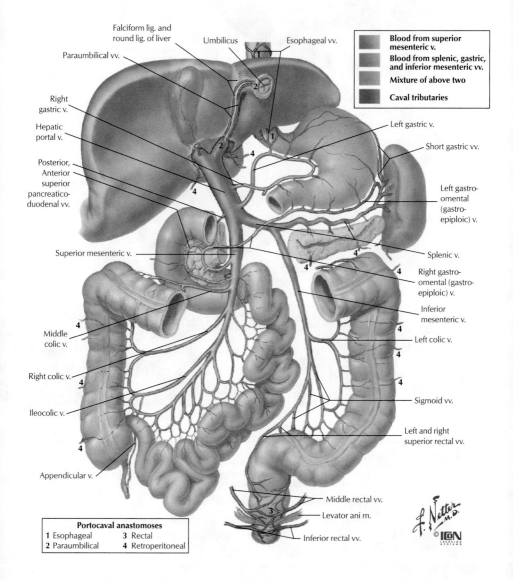

Falciform lig. and round lig. of liver
Umbilicus
Esophageal vv.

Paraumbilical vv.

Blood from superior mesenteric v.
Blood from splenic, gastric, and inferior mesenteric vv.
Mixture of above two
Caval tributaries

Right gastric v.
Hepatic portal v.
Posterior, Anterior superior pancreatico-duodenal vv.

Left gastric v.
Short gastric vv.
Left gastro-omental (gastro-epiploic) v.

Superior mesenteric v.
Splenic v.
Right gastro-omental (gastro-epiploic) v.
Inferior mesenteric v.

Middle colic v.
Right colic v.
Ileocolic v.
Appendicular v.

Left colic v.
Sigmoid vv.
Left and right superior rectal vv.
Middle rectal vv.
Levator ani m.
Inferior rectal vv.

Portocaval anastomoses

1 Esophageal	3 Rectal
2 Paraumbilical	4 Retroperitoneal

Clinical Correlation

Etiology of Cirrhosis
Anatomy on pp. 419, 420

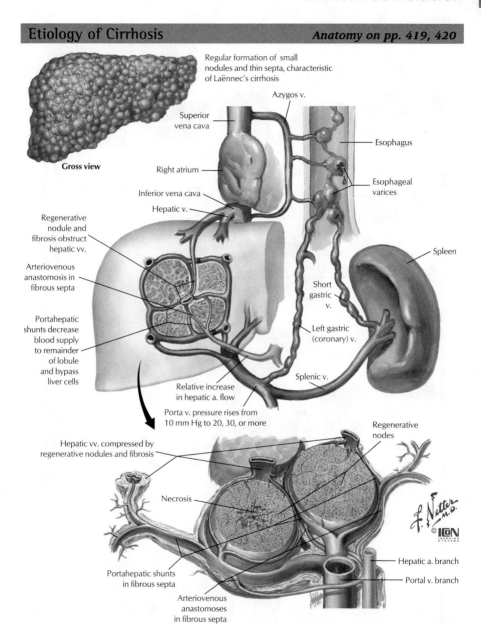

Regular formation of small nodules and thin septa, characteristic of Laënnec's cirrhosis

Gross view

Azygos v.

Superior vena cava

Esophagus

Right atrium

Esophageal varices

Inferior vena cava

Hepatic v.

Regenerative nodule and fibrosis obstruct hepatic vv.

Spleen

Arteriovenous anastomosis in fibrous septa

Short gastric v.

Portahepatic shunts decrease blood supply to remainder of lobule and bypass liver cells

Left gastric (coronary) v.

Relative increase in hepatic a. flow

Splenic v.

Porta v. pressure rises from 10 mm Hg to 20, 30, or more

Regenerative nodes

Hepatic vv. compressed by regenerative nodules and fibrosis

Necrosis

Hepatic a. branch

Portal v. branch

Portahepatic shunts in fibrous septa

Arteriovenous anastomoses in fibrous septa

Cirrhosis, a largely irreversible disease, is characterized by diffuse fibrosis, parenchymal nodular regeneration, and disturbed hepatic architecture. Progressive fibrosis disrupts portal blood flow (portal hypertension), beginning at the level of sinusoids and central veins. Causes include

- Alcoholic liver disease, 60-70%
- Genetic hemochromatosis, 5%
- Viral hepatitis, 10%
- Cryptogenic cirrhosis, 10-15%
- Biliary diseases, 5-10%

Clinical Correlation

Manifestations of Cirrhosis
Anatomy on pp. 419, 420

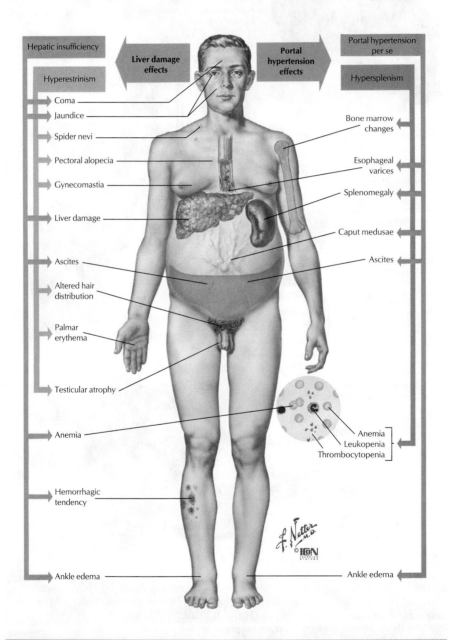

Hepatic insufficiency

Liver damage effects

Portal hypertension effects

Portal hypertension per se

Hyperestrinism

Hypersplenism

Coma

Jaundice

Spider nevi

Pectoral alopecia

Gynecomastia

Liver damage

Ascites

Altered hair distribution

Palmar erythema

Testicular atrophy

Anemia

Hemorrhagic tendency

Ankle edema

Bone marrow changes

Esophageal varices

Splenomegaly

Caput medusae

Ascites

Anemia
Leukopenia
Thrombocytopenia

Ankle edema

With advanced cirrhosis, the clinical manifestations become more obvious. A history of worsening jaundice, dark urine, light stools, and ascites is common.

Clinical Correlation

Ascites
Anatomy on pp. 419, 420

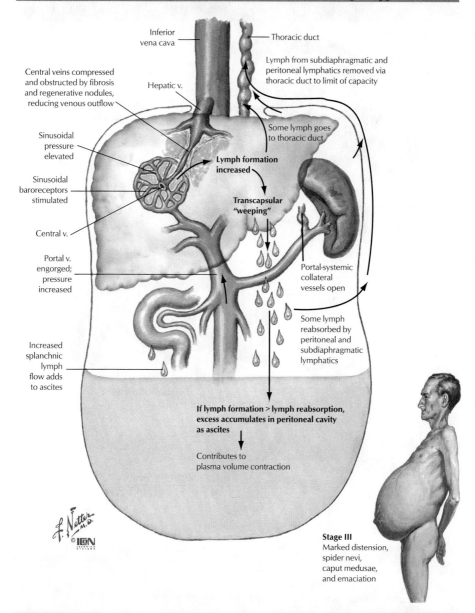

Inferior vena cava

Thoracic duct

Central veins compressed and obstructed by fibrosis and regenerative nodules, reducing venous outflow

Hepatic v.

Lymph from subdiaphragmatic and peritoneal lymphatics removed via thoracic duct to limit of capacity

Sinusoidal pressure elevated

Some lymph goes to thoracic duct

Lymph formation increased

Sinusoidal baroreceptors stimulated

Transcapsular "weeping"

Central v.

Portal v. engorged; pressure increased

Portal-systemic collateral vessels open

Some lymph reabsorbed by peritoneal and subdiaphragmatic lymphatics

Increased splanchnic lymph flow adds to ascites

If lymph formation > lymph reabsorption, excess accumulates in peritoneal cavity as ascites

Contributes to plasma volume contraction

Stage III
Marked distension, spider nevi, caput medusae, and emaciation

Ascites refers to accumulation of excess fluid in the peritoneal cavity (normally a potential space). The pathogenesis, illustrated here for cirrhosis, includes
• Sinusoidal hypertension
• Weeping of hepatic lymph (may approach 10-20 L/day)
• Renal retention of sodium and water

Clinical Correlation

Causes and Consequences of Portal Hypertension

Anatomy on pp. 419, 420

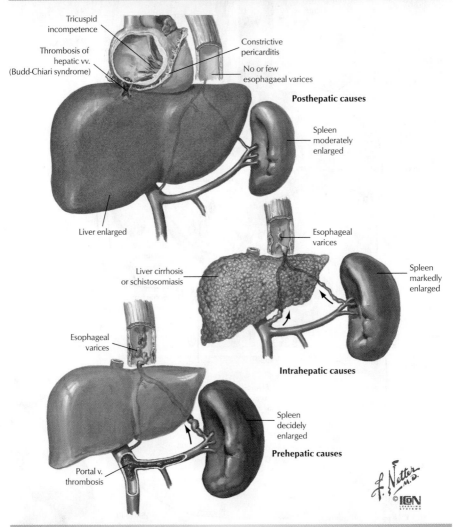

Tricuspid incompetence

Thrombosis of hepatic vv. (Budd-Chiari syndrome)

Constrictive pericarditis

No or few esophagaeal varices

Posthepatic causes

Spleen moderately enlarged

Liver enlarged

Esophageal varices

Liver cirrhosis or schistosomiasis

Spleen markedly enlarged

Esophageal varices

Intrahepatic causes

Spleen decidedly enlarged

Prehepatic causes

Portal v. thrombosis

Resistance to portal blood flow, which causes increased portal venous pressure, can occur via three major mechanisms:
- Prehepatic: obstructed blood flow to the liver
- Posthepatic: obstructed blood flow from the liver to the heart
- Intrahepatic: cirrhosis or other liver diseases

Clinical consequences include
- Ascites (usually detectable when 500 ml fluid accumulates in the abdomen)
- Formation of portocaval venous shunts via natural anastomoses
- Congestive splenomegaly
- Hepatic encephalopathy

Viral Hepatitis
Anatomy on p. 419

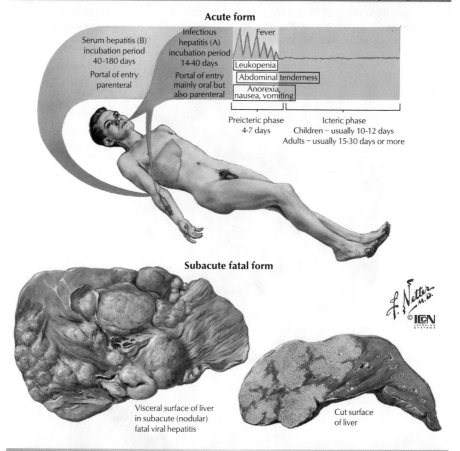

Acute form

Serum hepatitis (B)
incubation period
40-180 days

Portal of entry
parenteral

Infectious
hepatitis (A)
incubation period
14-40 days

Portal of entry
mainly oral but
also parenteral

Fever

Leukopenia

Abdominal tenderness

Anorexia,
nausea, vomiting

Preicteric phase
4-7 days

Icteric phase
Children – usually 10-12 days
Adults – usually 15-30 days or more

Subacute fatal form

Visceral surface of liver
in subacute (nodular)
fatal viral hepatitis

Cut surface
of liver

Viral hepatitis, caused by one of five viruses (hepatitis A to E viruses), affects the liver and involves acute and/or chronic infection with hepatocyte injury, cholestasis, necrosis, portal tract inflammation, and fibrosis. Chronic end-stage infection can lead to cirrhosis with hepatocyte loss, fibrosis, and regenerative nodules. Common signs and symptoms are jaundice, fatigue, abdominal pain, decreased appetite, and nausea, but 80% of patients with HCV infection have no signs or symptoms.

CHARACTERISTIC	HAV	HBV	HCV	HDV	HEV
Type of virus	ssRNA	dsDNA	ssRNA	ssRNA	ssRNA
Transmission route	Fecal-oral	Parenteral, personal contact	Parenteral, personal contact	Parenteral, personal contact	Water-borne
Incubation time (weeks)	2-6	4-26	2-26	4-7	2-8
Presence of chronic hepatitis	No	15-20% of acute infections	>50%	<5% coinfection, 80% superinfection with HBV	No

ss = single stranded; ds = double stranded.

Viscera: Gallbladder and Extrahepatic Ducts

The gallbladder receives, concentrates, and stores bile (capacity of approximately 30-50 ml). The extrahepatic duct system, detailed here, extends from the liver to the gall-bladder and from the gallbladder to the hepatopancreatic ampulla (of Vater), where bile enters the second part of the duodenum. Pancreatic enzymes conveyed by the main pancreatic duct also enter the duodenum at this point.

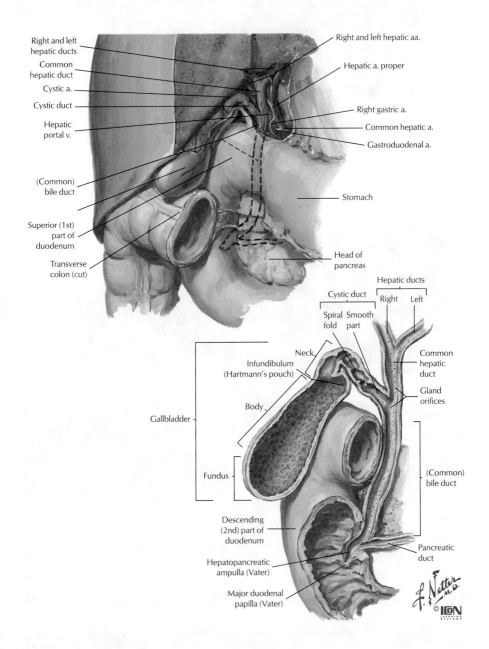

Right and left hepatic ducts

Common hepatic duct

Cystic a.

Cystic duct

Hepatic portal v.

(Common) bile duct

Superior (1st) part of duodenum

Transverse colon (cut)

Right and left hepatic aa.

Hepatic a. proper

Right gastric a.

Common hepatic a.

Gastroduodenal a.

Stomach

Head of pancreas

Hepatic ducts
Right   Left

Cystic duct

Spiral Smooth
fold   part

Neck

Infundibulum
(Hartmann's pouch)

Body

Gallbladder

Fundus

Descending (2nd) part of duodenum

Hepatopancreatic ampulla (Vater)

Major duodenal papilla (Vater)

Common hepatic duct

Gland orifices

(Common) bile duct

Pancreatic duct

Clinical Correlation

Cholelithiasis (Gallstones)   *Anatomy on p. 426*

Mechanisms of biliary pain

Sudden obstruction (biliary colic)

Calculus in Hartmann's pouch

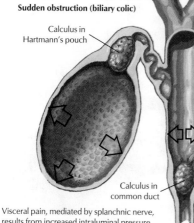

Calculus in common duct

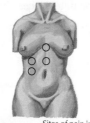

Sites of pain in bilary colic

Visceral pain, mediated by splanchnic nerve, results from increased intraluminal pressure and distention caused by sudden calculous obstruction of cystic or common duct.

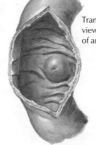

Transduodenal view of bulging of ampulla

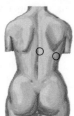

Ampullary stone

Persistent obstruction (acute cholecystitis)

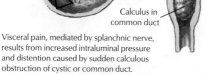

Sites of pain and hyperesthesia in acute cholecystitis

Edema, ischemia, and transmural inflammation

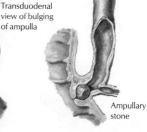

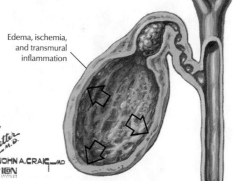

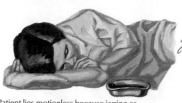

Patient lies motionless because jarring or respiration increases pain. Nausea is common.

Parietal epigastric or right upper quadrant pain results from ischemia and inflammation of gallbladder wall caused by persistent calculous obstruction of cystic duct. Prostaglandins are released.

CHARACTERISTIC	DESCRIPTION
Prevalence	10-20% of adults in developed countries
Types	Cholesterol stones: 80% (crystalline cholesterol monohydrate) Pigment stones: 20% (bilirubin calcium salts)
Risk factors	Increased age, obesity, female, rapid weight loss, estrogenic factors, gallbladder stasis
Complications	Gallbladder inflammation (cholecystitis), obstructive cholestasis or pancreatitis, empyema

Viscera: Pancreas

The pancreas, an exocrine and endocrine organ, lies posterior to the stomach in the floor of the lesser peritoneal sac. It is a retroperitoneal organ, except for the distal tail, which is in contact with the spleen. The head is nestled within the C-shaped curve of the duodenum, with its uncinate process lying posterior to the superior mesenteric vessels.

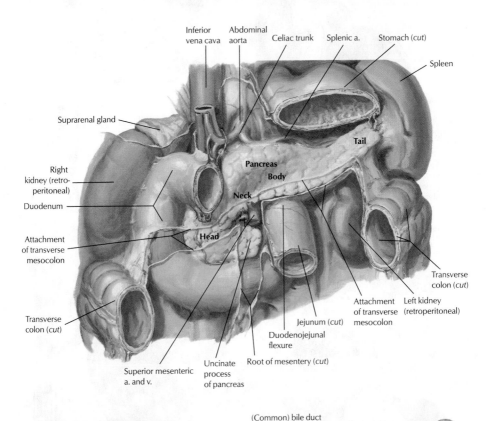

Inferior vena cava — Abdominal aorta — Celiac trunk — Splenic a. — Stomach (cut) — Spleen

Suprarenal gland

Tail

Pancreas
Body

Right kidney (retro-peritoneal)

Neck

Duodenum

Head

Attachment of transverse mesocolon

Transverse colon (cut)

Transverse colon (cut)

Left kidney (retroperitoneal)

Attachment of transverse mesocolon

Jejunum (cut)

Duodenojejunal flexure

Superior mesenteric a. and v.

Uncinate process of pancreas

Root of mesentery (cut)

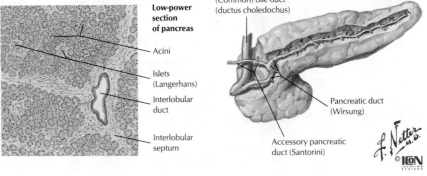

Low-power section of pancreas

(Common) bile duct (ductus choledochus)

Acini

Islets (Langerhans)

Interlobular duct

Interlobular septum

Pancreatic duct (Wirsung)

Accessory pancreatic duct (Santorini)

Clinical Correlation

Zollinger–Ellison Syndrome   *Anatomy on pp. 401, 403, 406, 428*

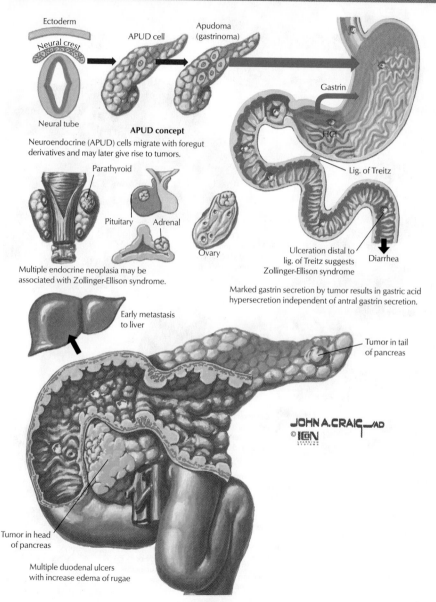

Ectoderm

Neural crest

APUD cell

Apudoma (gastrinoma)

Neural tube

APUD concept

Neuroendocrine (APUD) cells migrate with foregut derivatives and may later give rise to tumors.

Gastrin

HCl

Lig. of Treitz

Parathyroid

Pituitary   Adrenal

Ovary

Multiple endocrine neoplasia may be associated with Zollinger-Ellison syndrome.

Ulceration distal to lig. of Treitz suggests Zollinger-Ellison syndrome

Diarrhea

Marked gastrin secretion by tumor results in gastric acid hypersecretion independent of antral gastrin secretion.

Early metastasis to liver

Tumor in tail of pancreas

JOHN A.CRAIG—AD
©ICON
LEARNING
SYSTEMS

Tumor in head of pancreas

Multiple duodenal ulcers with increase edema of rugae

Zollinger-Ellison syndrome is characterized by gastrin-producing tumors (gastrinomas) that arise in the pancreas, peripancreatic region, or duodenal wall. More than 90% of patients with this syndrome have ulcers, primarily in the duodenum (six times more common than gastric ulcers). Hypergastrinemia leads to a huge increase in gastric acid secretion, which causes peptic ulcers, diarrhea, and gastroesophageal reflux disease.

Clinical Correlation

Carcinoma of the Pancreas

Anatomy on p. 428

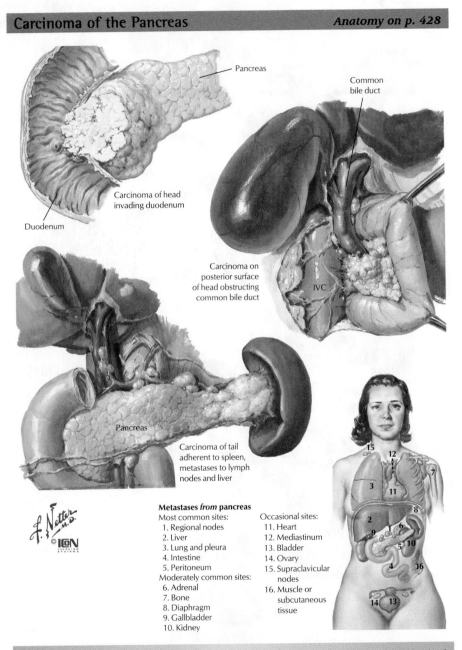

Pancreas

Common bile duct

Carcinoma of head invading duodenum

Duodenum

Carcinoma on posterior surface of head obstructing common bile duct

IVC

Pancreas

Carcinoma of tail adherent to spleen, metastases to lymph nodes and liver

Metastases *from* pancreas

Most common sites:
1. Regional nodes
2. Liver
3. Lung and pleura
4. Intestine
5. Peritoneum

Moderately common sites:
6. Adrenal
7. Bone
8. Diaphragm
9. Gallbladder
10. Kidney

Occasional sites:
11. Heart
12. Mediastinum
13. Bladder
14. Ovary
15. Supraclavicular nodes
16. Muscle or subcutaneous tissue

Carcinoma of the pancreas is the fifth leading cause of cancer deaths in the United States. Pancreatic carcinomas (mostly adenocarcinomas) arise from the exocrine part of the organ; 60% of cancers are found in the pancreatic head (these often cause obstructive jaundice). Islet tumors are less common. Adjacent anatomical sites may be involved; metastases are common.

Viscera: Lymphatics of the Epigastric Region

Lymphatics from the liver (hepatic nodes and vessels), gallbladder (cystic node [Calot]), spleen (splenic nodes), stomach (gastric nodes and vessels), and pancreas (pancreatic nodes) drain mainly to celiac nodes by coursing along arteries derived from the celiac trunk. Lymph is ultimately collected into the cisterna chyli, the dilated proximal end of the thoracic duct (which receives lymph from lumbar and intestinal lymphatics).

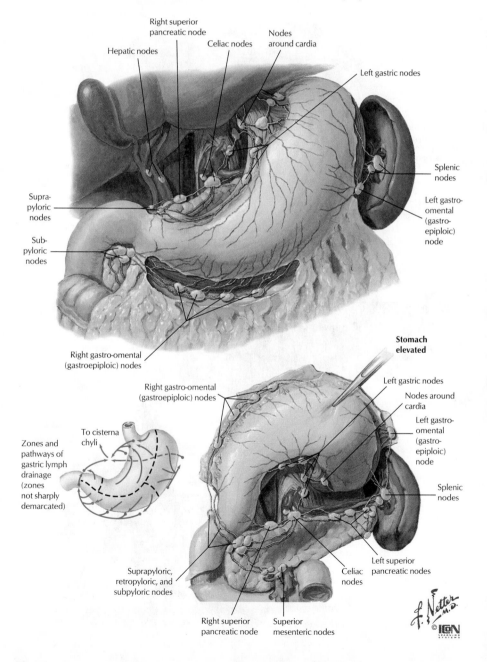

Viscera: Lymphatics of the Colon

Lymph from the small intestine and proximal colon (to about mid–transverse colon) drains into superior mesenteric nodes; lymph from the distal colon and pelvic viscera drains mainly to inferior mesenteric nodes and iliac nodes, respectively. Lymph from some pelvic viscera may also drain to inguinal nodes.

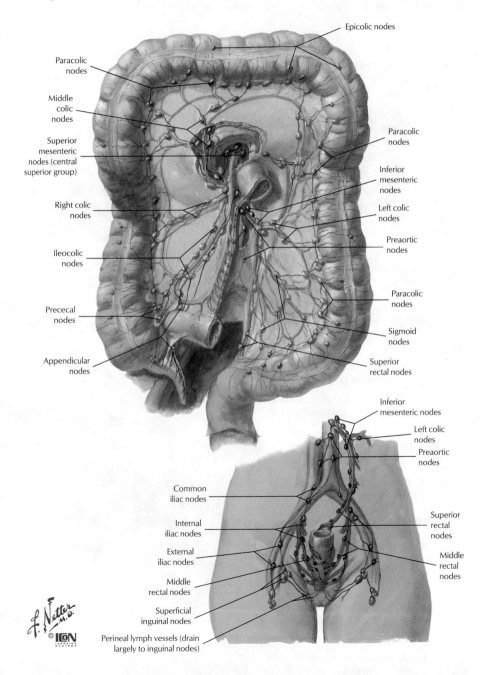

Epicolic nodes

Paracolic nodes

Middle colic nodes

Superior mesenteric nodes (central superior group)

Right colic nodes

Ileocolic nodes

Prececal nodes

Appendicular nodes

Paracolic nodes

Inferior mesenteric nodes

Left colic nodes

Preaortic nodes

Paracolic nodes

Sigmoid nodes

Superior rectal nodes

Inferior mesenteric nodes

Left colic nodes

Preaortic nodes

Common iliac nodes

Internal iliac nodes

External iliac nodes

Middle rectal nodes

Superficial inguinal nodes

Perineal lymph vessels (drain largely to inguinal nodes)

Superior rectal nodes

Middle rectal nodes

Viscera: Kidneys and Suprarenal (Adrenal) Glands

The kidneys and suprarenal glands are retroperitoneal organs, which have a rich vascular supply. The right kidney usually lies somewhat lower than the left, because of the presence of the liver. The right suprarenal gland is often pyramidal, and the left gland is semilunar, as shown here.

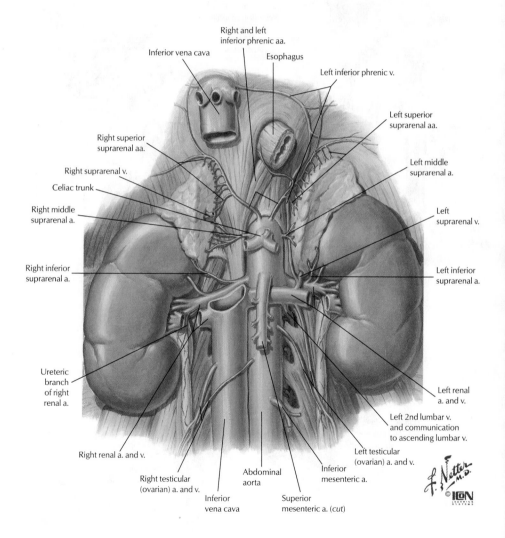

Right and left inferior phrenic aa.

Inferior vena cava

Esophagus

Left inferior phrenic v.

Left superior suprarenal aa.

Right superior suprarenal aa.

Left middle suprarenal a.

Right suprarenal v.

Celiac trunk

Right middle suprarenal a.

Left suprarenal v.

Right inferior suprarenal a.

Left inferior suprarenal a.

Ureteric branch of right renal a.

Left renal a. and v.

Left 2nd lumbar v. and communication to ascending lumbar v.

Right renal a. and v.

Left testicular (ovarian) a. and v.

Right testicular (ovarian) a. and v.

Abdominal aorta

Inferior mesenteric a.

Inferior vena cava

Superior mesenteric a. (cut)

Clinical Correlation

Obstructive Uropathy

Anatomy on pp. 433, 446, 457

Kidney
Anomalies
Prolapse
Calculus
Chronic infection
pyrogenic
granulomatous
Neoplasm
Necrotizing papillitis

Ureter
Anomalies
of number
of termination
Aberrant vessel
Stricture, stenosis
Kinks
Chronic infection
Congenital valve
Retrocaval ureter
Neoplasm
Calculus
Compression
(by nodes, tumor, abscess,
hematoma, bands)
Ureteritis cystica
Ovarian vein syndrome
Periureteral inflammation
(appendicitis, diverticulitis)
Trauma

Kidney
prolapse

Bladder
Ureterocele
Neoplasm
Diverticulum
Calculus
Foreign body
Congenital neck
obstruction
Bilharziasis

Prostate
Benign hypertrophy
Prostatitis, abscess
Cyst
Verumontanitis
Congenital valve
Neoplasm

Female urethra
Neoplasm
Stricture
Diverticulum
Papilloma
Meatal stenosis

Male urethra
Neoplasm
Diverticulum
Stricture
Strangulation
Papilloma
Meatal stenosis
Phimosis

Obstruction to the normal flow of urine, which may occur from the renal calyx to the urethral meatus, can initiate pathologic changes that, when coupled with an infection, can lead to serious uropathies. Various congenital and acquired lesions occur.

Clinical Correlation

Renal Stones (Nephrolithiasis)

Anatomy on pp. 433, 446

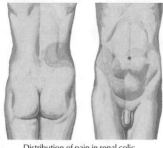

Distribution of pain in renal colic

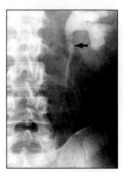

Ureteropelvic obstruction

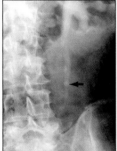

Midureteral obstruction

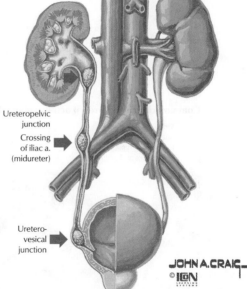

Ureteropelvic junction

Crossing of iliac a. (midureter)

Uretero-vesical junction

JOHN A. CRAIG—AD

© ICN

Distal ureteral obstruction   **Common sites of obstruction**

Renal stones that enter the urinary collecting system may cause renal colic (loin to groin pain) and obstruction at one of the three anatomical sites shown.

CHARACTERISTIC	DESCRIPTION
Type	75% calcium oxalate (phosphate), 15% magnesium ammonium phosphate, 10% uric acid or cystine
Prevalence	Approximately 12% in the United States, highest in Southeast; 2-3 times more common in men than in women; uncommon in African-Americans and Asians
Risk factors	Concentrated urine, heredity, diet, associated diseases (sarcoidosis, inflammatory bowel disease, cancer)

Clinical Correlation

Acute Pyelonephritis   *Anatomy on pp. 433, 446*

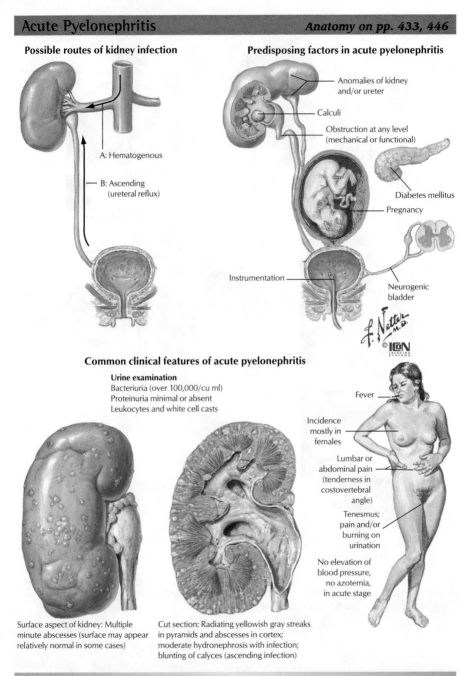

Possible routes of kidney infection

A: Hematogenous

B: Ascending
(ureteral reflux)

Predisposing factors in acute pyelonephritis

Anomalies of kidney
and/or ureter

Calculi

Obstruction at any level
(mechanical or functional)

Diabetes mellitus

Pregnancy

Instrumentation

Neurogenic
bladder

Common clinical features of acute pyelonephritis

Urine examination
Bacteriuria (over 100,000/cu ml)
Proteinuria minimal or absent
Leukocytes and white cell casts

Fever

Incidence
mostly in
females

Lumbar or
abdominal pain
(tenderness in
costovertebral
angle)

Tenesmus;
pain and/or
burning on
urination

No elevation of
blood pressure,
no azotemia,
in acute stage

Surface aspect of kidney: Multiple
minute abscesses (surface may appear
relatively normal in some cases)

Cut section: Radiating yellowish gray streaks
in pyramids and abscesses in cortex;
moderate hydronephrosis with infection;
blunting of calyces (ascending infection)

Acute pyelonephritis, a fairly common inflammation of the kidneys and renal pelvis, results from infection with bacteria (most often *Escherichia coli*) and is a manifestation of UTI. As with UTIs, pyelonephritis occurs more frequently in women than in men.

Clinical Correlation

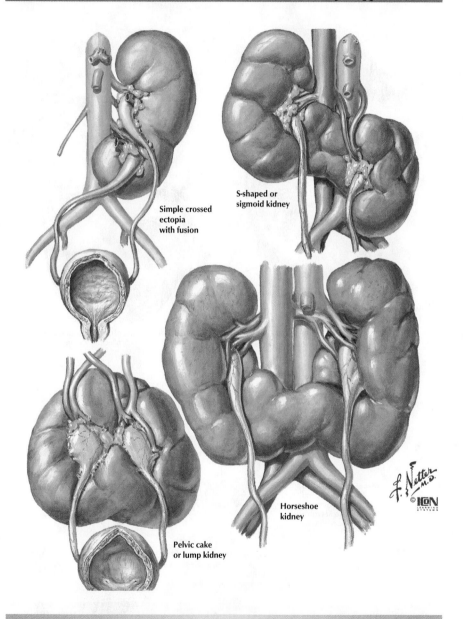

Simple crossed
ectopia
with fusion

S-shaped or
sigmoid kidney

Horseshoe
kidney

Pelvic cake
or lump kidney

   The term renal fusion refers to various common defects in which the two kidneys fuse to become one. The horseshoe kidney, in which developing kidneys fuse (usually lower lobes) anterior to the aorta, often lies low in the abdomen and is the most common kind of fusion. Fused kidneys are close to the midline, have multiple renal arteries, and are malrotated. Obstruction, stone formation, and infection are potential complications.

Clinical Correlation

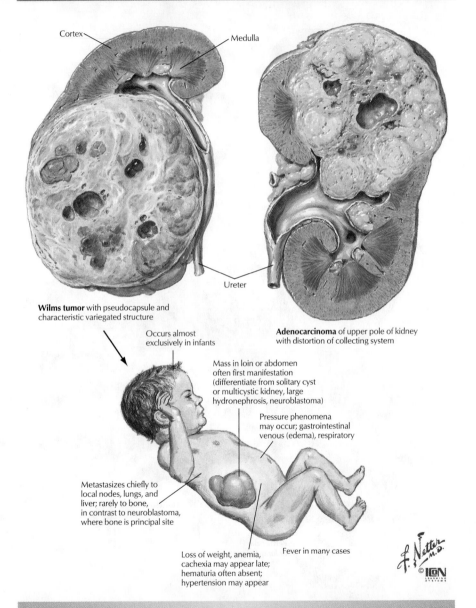

Cortex

Medulla

Wilms tumor with pseudocapsule and
characteristic variegated structure

Ureter

Occurs almost
exclusively in infants

Adenocarcinoma of upper pole of kidney
with distortion of collecting system

Mass in loin or abdomen
often first manifestation
(differentiate from solitary cyst
or multicystic kidney, large
hydronephrosis, neuroblastoma)

Pressure phenomena
may occur; gastrointestinal
venous (edema), respiratory

Metastasizes chiefly to
local nodes, lungs, and
liver; rarely to bone,
in contrast to neuroblastoma,
where bone is principal site

Loss of weight, anemia,
cachexia may appear late;
hematuria often absent;
hypertension may appear

Fever in many cases

Of malignant kidney tumors, 80-90% are adenocarcinomas that arise from tubular epithelium. They account for 2% of all adult cancers, often occur after the age of 50 years, and occur twice as often in men than in women. Wilms tumor is the third most common solid tumor in younger children (aged <10 years) and is associated with congenital malformations related to chromosome 11. Blastemal, stromal, and epithelial cell types can be found in most tumors.

Surgical Approach to the Kidney   *Anatomy on pp. 388, 433, 451*

Lumbar and lateral approaches

Lumbar approach

11th rib resection
Intercostal
12th rib resection
Subcostal

Lateral (flank) approach (extraperitoneal)

Lumbar approach (extraperitoneal)

Patient positioned for flank approach

Paramedian (extraperitoneal or transperitoneal)

Midline or chevron (transperitoneal)

Anterior approaches

Midline
Paramedian
Chevron

JOHN A. CRAIG—AD
©ICON

APPROACH	COMMENT
Lumbar	For removing pelvic and upper urethral stones; involves a nonmuscle-splitting incision that heals quickly
Lateral (flank)	For retrieving renal stones; stresses skeleton and respiratory system because patient is in lateral flexed position
Anterior	Best when flank approach cannot be used; paramedian approach avoids peritoneal cavity
Laparoscopic	Used with instruments introduced through small ipsilateral incisions just lateral to rectus sheath and one near anterior superior iliac spine

Clinical Correlation

Cushing's Syndrome
Anatomy on pp. 45, 433

Causes of Cushing's syndrome

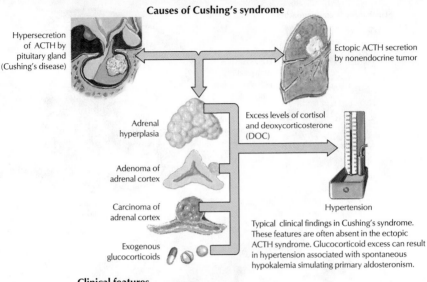

Hypersecretion of ACTH by pituitary gland (Cushing's disease)

Ectopic ACTH secretion by nonendocrine tumor

Adrenal hyperplasia

Excess levels of cortisol and deoxycorticosterone (DOC)

Adenoma of adrenal cortex

Carcinoma of adrenal cortex

Exogenous glucocorticoids

Hypertension

Typical clinical findings in Cushing's syndrome. These features are often absent in the ectopic ACTH syndrome. Glucocorticoid excess can result in hypertension associated with spontaneous hypokalemia simulating primary aldosteronism.

Clinical features

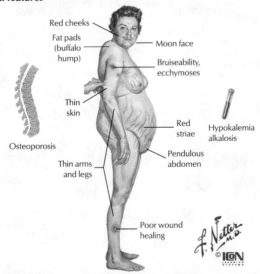

Red cheeks

Fat pads (buffalo hump)

Moon face

Bruiseability, ecchymoses

Thin skin

Osteoporosis

Red striae

Hypokalemia alkalosis

Thin arms and legs

Pendulous abdomen

Poor wound healing

Cushing's syndrome may be caused by any condition that results in increased glucocorticoid levels. Causes include
- Corticotropin dependent
  - Cushing's disease: hypersecretion of corticotropin (70%) (see illustration)
  - Ectopic: corticotropin from nonendocrine tumors, e.g., small cell carcinoma of lung (20%)
- Corticotropin independent
  - Iatrogenic: after administration of exogenous glucocorticoids (75%)
  - Adrenocortical hyperplasia, adenoma, or carcinoma (20%)

Clinical Correlation

**Manifestations of chronic primary adrenal cortical insufficiency
(Addison's disease)**

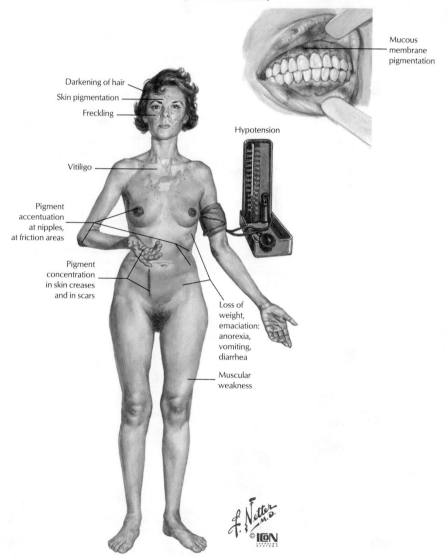

Mucous membrane pigmentation

Darkening of hair

Skin pigmentation

Freckling

Hypotension

Vitiligo

Pigment accentuation at nipples, at friction areas

Pigment concentration in skin creases and in scars

Loss of weight, emaciation: anorexia, vomiting, diarrhea

Muscular weakness

Clinical manifestations of adrenocortical insufficiency do not usually occur until approximately 90% of the adrenal cortex is destroyed. Main causes include
- Autoimmune adrenalitis, 60-70% of cases
- Infectious diseases (tuberculosis, histoplasmosis, HIV infection)
- Metastatic disease (commonly from lung and breast tumors)

Clinical Correlation

Pheochromocytoma

Anatomy on pp. 42, 45, 433

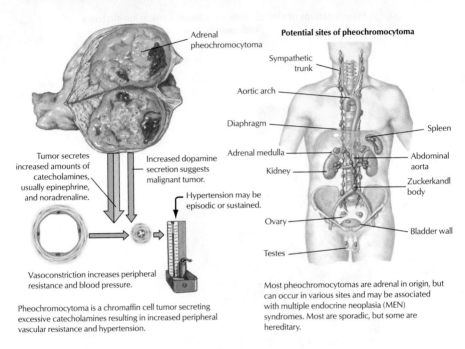

Adrenal pheochromocytoma

Tumor secretes increased amounts of catecholamines, usually epinephrine, and noradrenaline.

Increased dopamine secretion suggests malignant tumor.

Hypertension may be episodic or sustained.

Vasoconstriction increases peripheral resistance and blood pressure.

Pheochromocytoma is a chromaffin cell tumor secreting excessive catecholamines resulting in increased peripheral vascular resistance and hypertension.

Potential sites of pheochromocytoma

Sympathetic trunk

Aortic arch

Diaphragm

Adrenal medulla

Kidney

Ovary

Testes

Spleen

Abdominal aorta

Zuckerkandl body

Bladder wall

Most pheochromocytomas are adrenal in origin, but can occur in various sites and may be associated with multiple endocrine neoplasia (MEN) syndromes. Most are sporadic, but some are hereditary.

Clinical features of pheochromocytoma

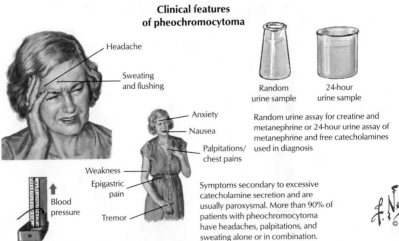

Headache

Sweating and flushing

Anxiety

Nausea

Palpitations/ chest pains

Weakness

Epigastric pain

Blood pressure

Tremor

Random urine sample

24-hour urine sample

Random urine assay for creatine and metanephrine or 24-hour urine assay of metanephrine and free catecholamines used in diagnosis

Symptoms secondary to excessive catecholamine secretion and are usually paroxysmal. More than 90% of patients with pheochromocytoma have headaches, palpitations, and sweating alone or in combination.

Pheochromocytomas are relatively rare neoplasms, composed of chromaffin cells (which synthesize and release catecholamines), that arise from adrenal medullary cells. These tumors may lead to severe hypertension (sustained or paroxysmal) and various clinical features.

Posterior Abdominal Wall: Abdominal Aorta

The abdominal aorta enters the abdomen via the aortic hiatus (T12 vertebral level) and divides into the common iliac arteries anterior to the L4 vertebra. Unpaired GI arteries include the celiac, and superior and inferior mesenteric arteries. Paired arteries to other viscera include the suprarenal, renal, and gonadal arteries. Arteries to musculoskeletal structures include the paired inferior phrenic arteries, the four or five pairs of lumbar arteries, and the unpaired median sacral artery.

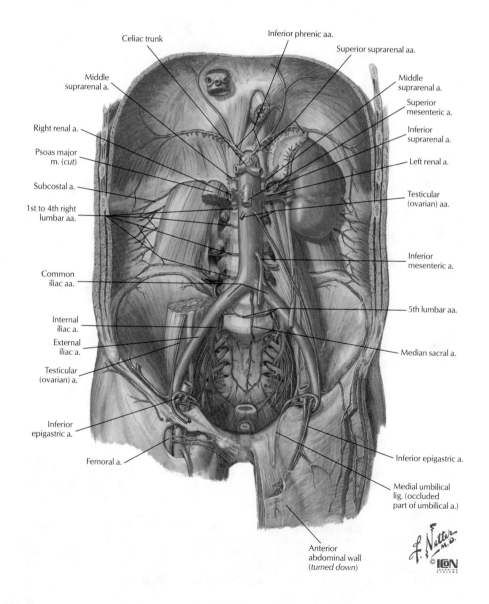

Celiac trunk

Inferior phrenic aa.

Superior suprarenal aa.

Middle suprarenal a.

Middle suprarenal a.

Superior mesenteric a.

Right renal a.

Inferior suprarenal a.

Psoas major m. (cut)

Left renal a.

Subcostal a.

Testicular (ovarian) aa.

1st to 4th right lumbar aa.

Inferior mesenteric a.

Common iliac aa.

5th lumbar aa.

Internal iliac a.

External iliac a.

Median sacral a.

Testicular (ovarian) a.

Inferior epigastric a.

Inferior epigastric a.

Femoral a.

Medial umbilical lig. (occluded part of umbilical a.)

Anterior abdominal wall (turned down)

F. Netter M.D.
©ICN

Clinical Correlation

Surgical Management of Abdominal Aortic Aneurysm

Anatomy on p. 443

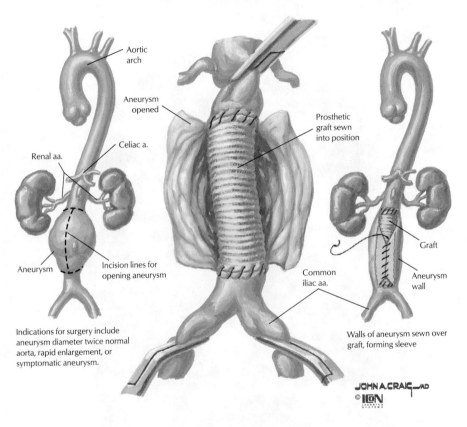

Abdominal aortic aneurysm (infrarenal)

Aortic arch

Aneurysm opened

Celiac a.

Renal aa.

Aneurysm

Incision lines for opening aneurysm

Prosthetic graft sewn into position

Graft

Common iliac aa.

Aneurysm wall

Indications for surgery include aneurysm diameter twice normal aorta, rapid enlargement, or symptomatic aneurysm.

Walls of aneurysm sewn over graft, forming sleeve

JOHN A. CRAIG—AD
© ICON
LEARNING
SYSTEMS

Aneurysms (arterial wall bulges) usually involve large arteries. The multifactorial etiology includes family history, hypertension, breakdown of collagen and/or elastin within a vessel wall that leads to inflammation and weakening of the wall, and atherosclerosis. The abdominal aorta (infrarenal segment) and iliac arteries are most often involved, but the thoracic aorta and femoral and popliteal arteries can also have aneurysms. Symptoms include abdominal and/or back pain, nausea, and early satiety, but up to 75% of patients may be asymptomatic. Surgical repair can be via an open procedure with durable synthetic grafts or an endovascular repair in which a new synthetic lining is inserted, with hooks or stents holding the lining in place.

Posterior Abdominal Wall: Inferior Vena Cava

Structures other than the abdominal GI tract and spleen (which are drained by the hepatic portal system) are drained by tributaries of the IVC, which pierces the diaphragm (at the T8 vertebral level) and enters the right atrium. Primary tributaries from the right side include common iliac, three or four lumbar, gonadal, renal, suprarenal, and inferior phrenic veins; those from the left include common iliac, two or three lumbar, renal (left renal also receives left gonadal and suprarenal veins), and inferior phrenic veins. Two or three hepatic veins also enter the IVC just inferior to the diaphragm.

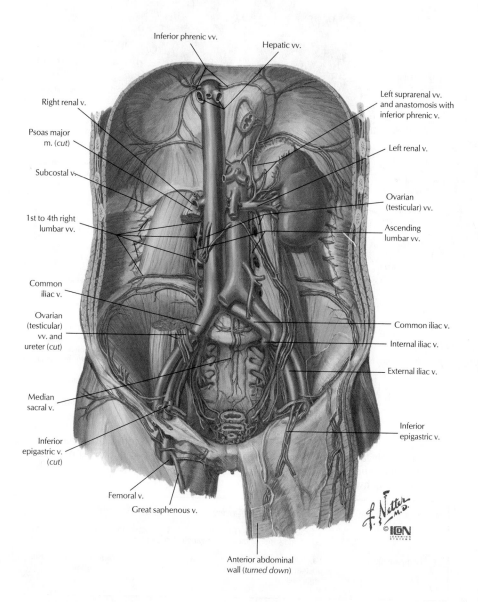

Inferior phrenic vv.

Hepatic vv.

Left suprarenal vv. and anastomosis with inferior phrenic v.

Right renal v.

Psoas major m. (cut)

Left renal v.

Subcostal v.

Ovarian (testicular) vv.

1st to 4th right lumbar vv.

Ascending lumbar vv.

Common iliac v.

Ovarian (testicular) vv. and ureter (cut)

Common iliac v.

Internal iliac v.

External iliac v.

Median sacral v.

Inferior epigastric v.

Inferior epigastric v. (cut)

Femoral v.

Great saphenous v.

Anterior abdominal wall (turned down)

Posterior Abdominal Wall: Autonomic Nerves

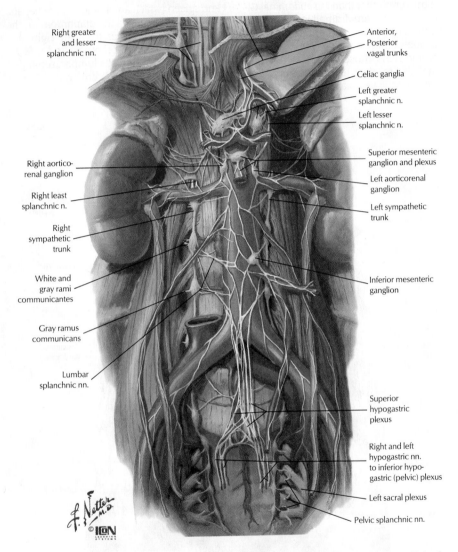

Right greater and lesser splanchnic nn.

Anterior, Posterior vagal trunks

Celiac ganglia

Left greater splanchnic n.

Left lesser splanchnic n.

Superior mesenteric ganglion and plexus

Right aortico-renal ganglion

Left aorticorenal ganglion

Right least splanchnic n.

Left sympathetic trunk

Right sympathetic trunk

Inferior mesenteric ganglion

White and gray rami communicantes

Gray ramus communicans

Lumbar splanchnic nn.

Superior hypogastric plexus

Right and left hypogastric nn. to inferior hypogastric (pelvic) plexus

Left sacral plexus

Pelvic splanchnic nn.

The autonomic pattern of innervation of the abdominal viscera closely parallels the vascular supply laid down during embryonic development (see Chapter 1 [Introduction] for functional aspects). Visceral pain afferents pass to the spinal cord (T5-L2 levels) via sympathetic pathways.

NERVOUS SYSTEM DIVISION	FOREGUT AND MIDGUT DERIVATIVES	HINDGUT DERIVATIVES
Sympathetic	Thoracic splanchnics (T5-T12) to celiac and superior mesenteric ganglia	Lumbar splanchnics (L1-L2) to inferior mesenteric ganglion
Parasympathetic	Vagus nerve (synapse on postganglionic neurons in organ walls)	Pelvic splanchnics (S2-S4) to inferior mesenteric and hypogastric ganglia or plexuses

Clinical Correlation

Visceral Referred Pain

Anatomy on pp. 387, 446, 453

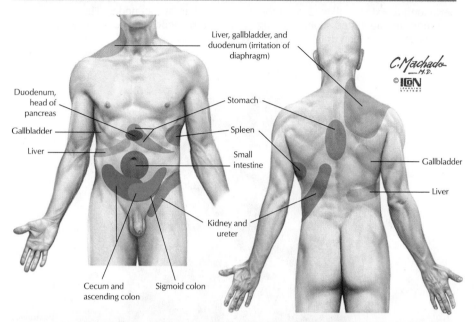

Liver, gallbladder, and duodenum (irritation of diaphragm)

Duodenum, head of pancreas

Gallbladder

Liver

Stomach

Spleen

Small intestine

Gallbladder

Liver

Kidney and ureter

Cecum and ascending colon

Sigmoid colon

Pain afferents pass from abdominal viscera to the spinal cord largely by following thoracic and lumbar splanchnic sympathetic nerves (T5-L2). Thus, visceral pain may be perceived as somatic pain over these dermatomes; this type of pain is known clinically as referred pain. Pain afferents from pelvic viscera largely follow pelvic parasympathetic splanchnic nerves (S2-S4) into the cord, so this pain is felt over these dermatomes. Common sites of referred visceral pain are illustrated; spinal cord levels vary from person to person.

ORGAN	SPINAL CORD LEVEL	ANTERIOR ABDOMINAL REGION OR QUADRANT
Stomach	T5-T9	Epigastric or left hypochondrium
Spleen	T6-T8	Left hypochondrium
Duodenum	T5-T8	Epigastric or right hypochondrium
Pancreas	T7-T9	Inferior part of epigastric
Liver or gallbladder*	T6-T9	Epigastric or right hypochondrium
Jejunum	T6-T10	Umbilical
Ileum	T7-T10	Umbilical
Cecum	T10-T11	Umbilical or right lumbar or right lower quadrant
Appendix	T10-T11	Umbilical or right inguinal or right lower quadrant
Ascending colon	T10-T12	Umbilical or right lumbar
Sigmoid colon	L1-L2	Left lumbar or left lower quadrant
Kidney	T10-L1	Lower hypochondrium or lumbar
Ureter	T11-L1	Lumbar to inguinal (loin to groin)

Irritation of the diaphragm leads to pain referred to the back (inferior scapula) and shoulder region.

Posterior Abdominal Wall: Lymphatics

Lymph from viscera and interior body walls ultimately collects in lymph nodes associated with major vascular channels. The flow pattern is inguinal nodes (lower extremity and perineum) to external iliac to common iliac to lumbar (aortic) nodes. The viscera drain to inferior (hindgut) and superior (midgut) mesenteric nodes and celiac nodes (foregut). The cisterna chyli then drains all lymph to the thoracic duct.

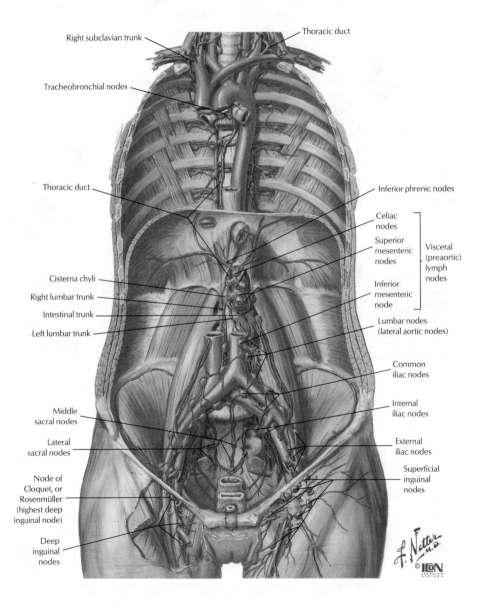

Posterior Abdominal Wall: Muscles

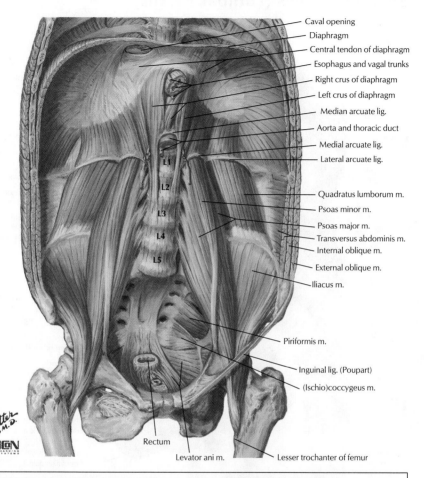

Caval opening
Diaphragm
Central tendon of diaphragm
Esophagus and vagal trunks
Right crus of diaphragm
Left crus of diaphragm
Median arcuate lig.
Aorta and thoracic duct
Medial arcuate lig.
Lateral arcuate lig.
Quadratus lumborum m.
Psoas minor m.
Psoas major m.
Transversus abdominis m.
Internal oblique m.
External oblique m.
Iliacus m.
Piriformis m.
Inguinal lig. (Poupart)
(Ischio)coccygeus m.
Lesser trochanter of femur
Levator ani m.
Rectum

L1
L2
L3
L4
L5

MUSCLE	SUPERIOR ATTACHMENT (ORIGIN)	INFERIOR ATTACH-MENT (INSERTION)	INNERVATION	ACTIONS
Psoas major	Transverse processes of lumbar vertebrae; sides of bodies of T12-L5 vertebrae, and intervening intervertebral discs	Lesser trochanter of femur	Lumbar plexus via ventral branches of L2-L4 nerves	Acting superiorly with iliacus, flexes hip; acting inferiorly, flexes vertebral column laterally; used to balance trunk in sitting position; acting inferiorly with iliacus, flexes trunk
Iliacus	Superior two thirds of iliac fossa, ala of sacrum, and anterior sacroiliac ligaments	Lesser trochanter of femur and shaft inferior to it, and to psoas major tendon	Femoral nerve	Flexes hip and stabilizes hip joint; acts with psoas major
Quadratus lumborum	Medial half of inferior border of 12th rib and tips of lumbar transverse processes	Iliolumbar ligament and internal lip of iliac crest	Ventral branches of T12 and L1-L4 nerves	Extends and laterally flexes vertebral column; fixes 12th rib during inspiration
Diaphragm	Thoracic outlet: xiphoid, lower six costal cartilages, L1-L3 vertebrae	Converge into central tendon	Phrenic nerve	Draws central tendon down and forward during inspiration

Posterior Abdominal Wall: Somatic Nerves (Lumbar Plexus)

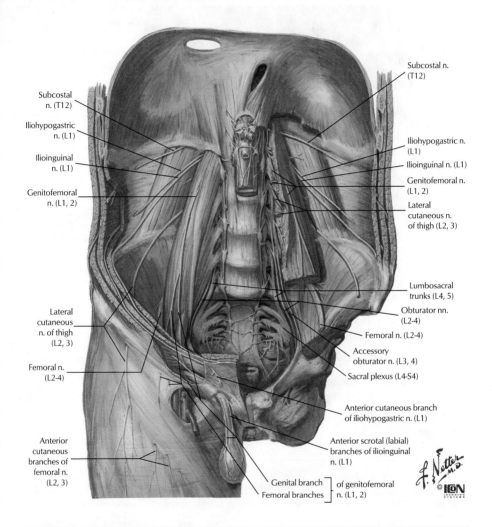

Subcostal n. (T12)

Subcostal n. (T12)

Iliohypogastric n. (L1)

Ilioinguinal n. (L1)

Genitofemoral n. (L1, 2)

Iliohypogastric n. (L1)

Ilioinguinal n. (L1)

Genitofemoral n. (L1, 2)

Lateral cutaneous n. of thigh (L2, 3)

Lumbosacral trunks (L4, 5)

Obturator nn. (L2-4)

Femoral n. (L2-4)

Lateral cutaneous n. of thigh (L2, 3)

Accessory obturator n. (L3, 4)

Femoral n. (L2-4)

Sacral plexus (L4-S4)

Anterior cutaneous branch of iliohypogastric n. (L1)

Anterior cutaneous branches of femoral n. (L2, 3)

Anterior scrotal (labial) branches of ilioinguinal n. (L1)

Genital branch ⎫ of genitofemoral
Femoral branches ⎭ n. (L1, 2)

NERVE	FUNCTION AND INNERVATION
Subcostal	Last thoracic nerve; courses inferior to 12th rib
Iliohypogastric	Motor and sensory (above pubis and posterolateral buttocks)
Ilioinguinal	Motor and sensory (sensory to inguinal region)
Genitofemoral	Genital branch to cremaster muscle, femoral branch to femoral triangle
Lateral cutaneous nerve of thigh	Sensory to anterolateral thigh
Femoral	Motor in pelvis (to iliacus) and anterior thigh muscles, sensory to thigh and medial leg
Obturator	Motor to adductor muscles in thigh, sensory to medial thigh
Accessory obturator	Inconstant (10%); motor to pectineus muscle

Abdominal Cross Section: T12 Vertebral Level

The T12 vertebral level corresponds to the level at which the aorta pierces the diaphragm. Liver, stomach, spleen, kidneys, and suprarenal glands can be seen. The lesser and greater (peritoneal) sacs and lesser omentum are shown to good advantage. Access to the lesser sac (omental bursa) is gained by way of the epiploic foramen (of Winslow), situated posterior to the hepatoduodenal ligament and anterior to the IVC.

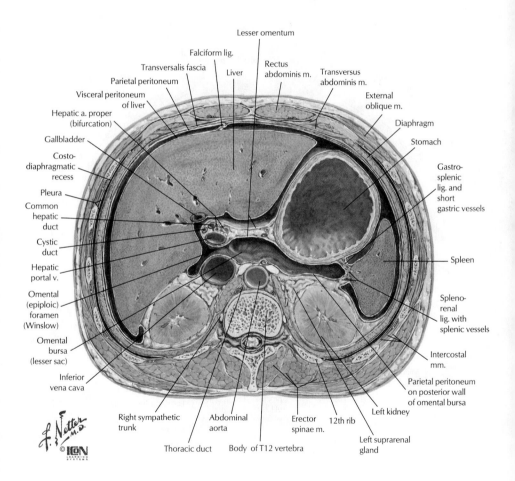

Labels (clockwise from top):
Lesser omentum
Falciform lig.
Transversalis fascia
Liver
Rectus abdominis m.
Transversus abdominis m.
Parietal peritoneum
Visceral peritoneum of liver
External oblique m.
Hepatic a. proper (bifurcation)
Diaphragm
Gallbladder
Stomach
Costo-diaphragmatic recess
Gastro-splenic lig. and short gastric vessels
Pleura
Common hepatic duct
Cystic duct
Spleen
Hepatic portal v.
Omental (epiploic) foramen (Winslow)
Spleno-renal lig. with splenic vessels
Omental bursa (lesser sac)
Intercostal mm.
Inferior vena cava
Parietal peritoneum on posterior wall of omental bursa
Right sympathetic trunk
Abdominal aorta
Erector spinae m.
12th rib
Left kidney
Thoracic duct
Body of T12 vertebra
Left suprarenal gland

Abdominal Cross Section: L3–4 Vertebral Level

At this level (intervertebral disc between L3 and L4), note the loops of mesenteric small intestine, retroperitoneal (secondarily) ascending and descending colon, and transverse colon (tethered by the transverse mesocolon). Posterior, lateral, and anterior abdominal wall muscles are clearly seen. Note how the greater omentum drapes over the abdominal viscera like an apron, keeping the visceral peritoneum from contacting the parietal peritoneum lining the inner aspect of the abdominal wall. Similarly, it can "wall off" infections to protect other viscera.

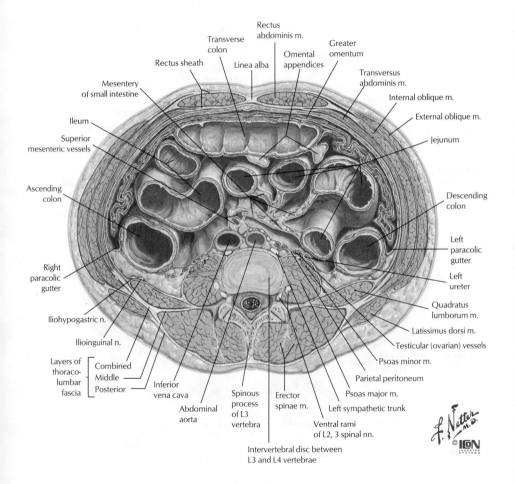

Rectus abdominis m.
Transverse colon
Rectus sheath
Linea alba
Omental appendices
Greater omentum
Transversus abdominis m.
Mesentery of small intestine
Internal oblique m.
External oblique m.
Ileum
Jejunum
Superior mesenteric vessels
Ascending colon
Descending colon
Left paracolic gutter
Right paracolic gutter
Left ureter
Iliohypogastric n.
Quadratus lumborum m.
Latissimus dorsi m.
Ilioinguinal n.
Testicular (ovarian) vessels
Psoas minor m.
Layers of thoracolumbar fascia — Combined / Middle / Posterior
Inferior vena cava
Parietal peritoneum
Psoas major m.
Abdominal aorta
Spinous process of L3 vertebra
Erector spinae m.
Left sympathetic trunk
Ventral rami of L2, 3 spinal nn.
Intervertebral disc between L3 and L4 vertebrae

Embryology: Summary of Gut Development

5 weeks

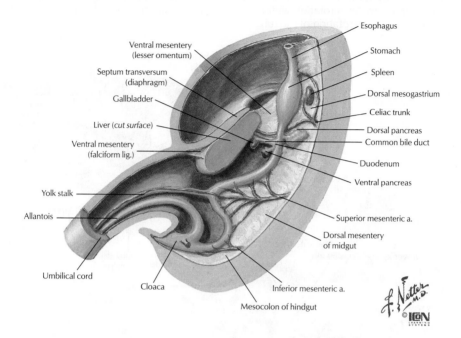

The embryonic gut begins as a midline tube that is divided into foregut, midgut, and hindgut regions, each with its own visceral blood supply and autonomic innervation.

	FOREGUT	MIDGUT	HINDGUT
Organs	Stomach Liver Gallbladder Pancreas Spleen 1st half duodenum	2nd half duodenum Jejunum Ileum Cecum Ascending colon 2/3 of transverse colon	Left 1/3 of transverse colon Descending colon Sigmoid colon Rectum
Arteries	Celiac trunk: Splenic artery Left gastric Common hepatic	Superior mesenteric: Ileocolic Right colic Middle colic	Inferior mesenteric: Left colic Sigmoid branches Superior rectal
Ventral mesentery	Lesser omentum Falciform ligament Coronary/triangular ligaments	None	None
Dorsal mesentery	Gastrosplenic ligament Splenorenal ligament Gastrocolic ligament Greater omentum	Mesointestine Mesoappendix Transverse mesocolon	Sigmoid mesocolon
Nerve supply Parasympathetic	Vagus	Vagus	Pelvic splanchnic nerves (S2-S4)
Sympathetic	Thoracic splanchnics (T5-T11)	Thoracic splanchnics (T11-T12)	Lumbar splanchnics (L1-L2)

Embryology: Gut Tube Rotation

The midgut region is suspended by the dorsal mesogastrium, partially extends into the umbilical cord, initially makes an 180° loop around the axis of the SMA, and undergoes rapid growth (forms the small bowel). By week 10, the bowel returns to the abdominal cavity and completes rotation with a 90° swing to the left lower quadrant (arrow), thus ending a full 270° rotation of the tube.

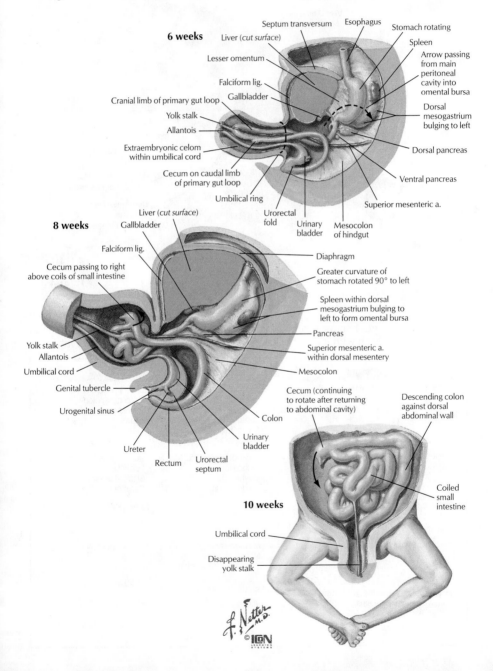

6 weeks

Septum transversum
Esophagus
Stomach rotating
Liver (*cut surface*)
Spleen
Arrow passing from main peritoneal cavity into omental bursa
Lesser omentum
Falciform lig.
Dorsal mesogastrium bulging to left
Cranial limb of primary gut loop
Gallbladder
Yolk stalk
Allantois
Extraembryonic celom within umbilical cord
Dorsal pancreas
Cecum on caudal limb of primary gut loop
Ventral pancreas
Umbilical ring
Superior mesenteric a.
Dorsal pancreas

8 weeks

Liver (*cut surface*)
Gallbladder
Falciform lig.
Cecum passing to right above coils of small intestine
Yolk stalk
Allantois
Umbilical cord
Genital tubercle
Urogenital sinus
Ureter
Rectum
Urorectal septum
Urorectal fold
Urinary bladder
Mesocolon of hindgut
Diaphragm
Greater curvature of stomach rotated 90° to left
Spleen within dorsal mesogastrium bulging to left to form omental bursa
Pancreas
Superior mesenteric a. within dorsal mesentery
Mesocolon
Cecum (continuing to rotate after returning to abdominal cavity)
Colon
Urinary bladder

10 weeks

Descending colon against dorsal abdominal wall
Coiled small intestine
Umbilical cord
Disappearing yolk stalk

Embryology: Foregut Organ Development

Growing from the abdominal foregut are endodermal buds that give rise to the liver, gallbladder, and pancreas (parenchyma of these organs is formed largely by mesoderm). As the foregut grows, the stomach swings to the left and the duodenum folds to the right in a C shape, so the ventral pancreatic bud (forms part of pancreatic head and uncinate process) is flipped to the left, where it fuses with the dorsal bud. Likewise, the common bile duct assumes a posterior relationship with the duodenum and fuses with the main pancreatic duct (of Wirsung).

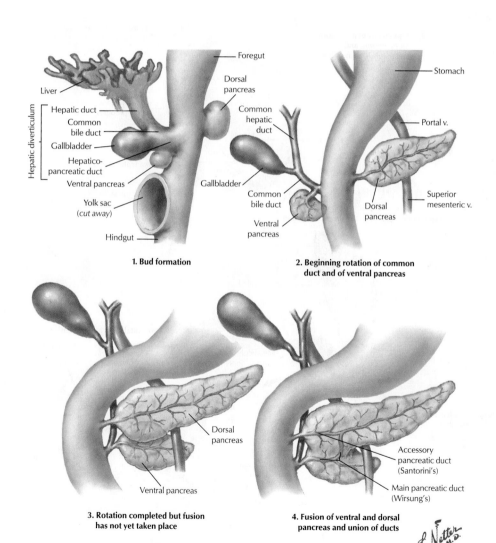

Foregut

Dorsal pancreas

Liver

Hepatic duct

Common bile duct

Gallbladder

Hepatico-pancreatic duct

Ventral pancreas

Yolk sac (*cut away*)

Hindgut

Hepatic diverticulum

Common hepatic duct

1. Bud formation

Stomach

Portal v.

Gallbladder

Common bile duct

Ventral pancreas

Dorsal pancreas

Superior mesenteric v.

2. Beginning rotation of common duct and of ventral pancreas

Dorsal pancreas

Ventral pancreas

3. Rotation completed but fusion has not yet taken place

Accessory pancreatic duct (Santorini's)

Main pancreatic duct (Wirsung's)

4. Fusion of ventral and dorsal pancreas and union of ducts

Embryology: Development of the Urinary System

Initially, intermediate mesoderm differentiates into nephrogenic (kidney) tissue and forms a pronephros (that degenerates) and mesonephros (that functions briefly) retroperitoneally in the posterior abdominal wall. The definitive kidney develops from metanephric tissue into which the ureteric bud grows and differentiates into the renal pelvis, calyces, and collecting ducts. The cloaca (Latin, "sewer") develops into an anterior urogenital sinus and posterior rectum.

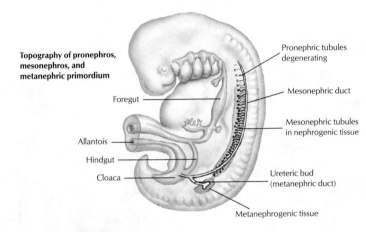

Topography of pronephros, mesonephros, and metanephric primordium

Pronephric tubules degenerating

Foregut

Mesonephric duct

Mesonephric tubules in nephrogenic tissue

Allantois

Hindgut

Cloaca

Ureteric bud (metanephric duct)

Metanephrogenic tissue

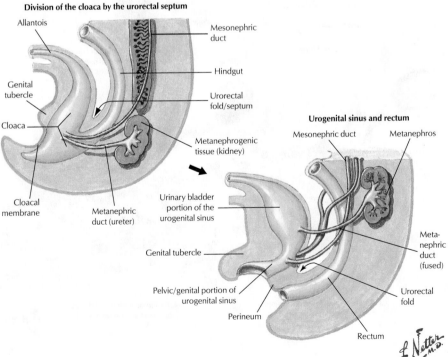

Division of the cloaca by the urorectal septum

Allantois

Mesonephric duct

Hindgut

Genital tubercle

Urorectal fold/septum

Cloaca

Metanephrogenic tissue (kidney)

Cloacal membrane

Metanephric duct (ureter)

Urogenital sinus and rectum

Mesonephric duct

Metanephros

Urinary bladder portion of the urogenital sinus

Genital tubercle

Meta-nephric duct (fused)

Pelvic/genital portion of urogenital sinus

Urorectal fold

Perineum

Rectum

Embryology: Kidney Ascent and Rotation

Via differential growth and migration, the kidneys ascend from deep in the pelvis to the posterior abdominal wall (always retroperitoneal). The hilum of the kidney first faces anteriorly, but kidneys normally rotate 90° so that the renal pelvis faces medially and renal vessels connect at the hilum.

Apparent "ascent and rotation" of the kidneys in embryologic development

Frontal view   Cross section

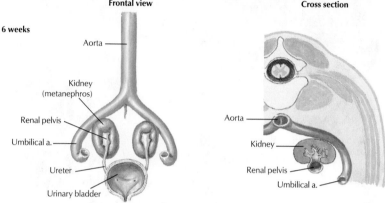

6 weeks

Aorta

Kidney (metanephros)

Renal pelvis

Umbilical a.

Ureter

Urinary bladder

Aorta

Kidney

Renal pelvis

Umbilical a.

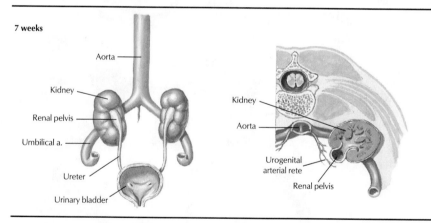

7 weeks

Aorta

Kidney

Renal pelvis

Umbilical a.

Ureter

Urinary bladder

Kidney

Aorta

Urogenital arterial rete

Renal pelvis

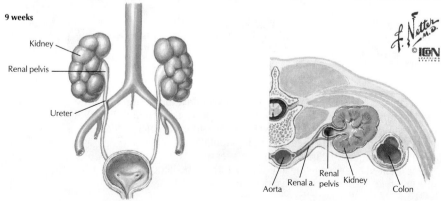

9 weeks

Kidney

Renal pelvis

Ureter

Aorta   Renal a.   Renal pelvis   Kidney   Colon

Clinical Correlation

Anatomy on pp. 453, 454

Meckel's Diverticulum

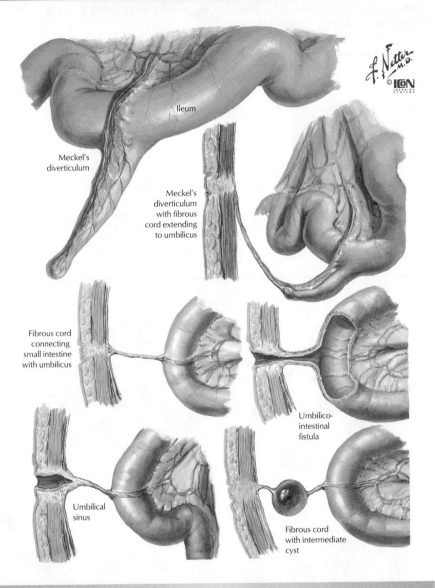

Ileum

Meckel's diverticulum

Meckel's diverticulum with fibrous cord extending to umbilicus

Fibrous cord connecting small intestine with umbilicus

Umbilico-intestinal fistula

Umbilical sinus

Fibrous cord with intermediate cyst

Meckel's diverticulum is the most common developmental anomaly of the bowel and occurs as a result of failure of involution of the vitelline (omphalomesenteric, yolk stalk) duct. It often is referred to as the syndrome of 2s because it
- Occurs in approximately 2% of the population
- Is approximately 2 inches long, on average
- Is located approximately 2 feet proximal to the ileocecal junction
- Often contains at least 2 types of mucosa

Clinical Correlation

Congenital Megacolon (Hirschsprung's Disease)

Anatomy on pp. 44, 446

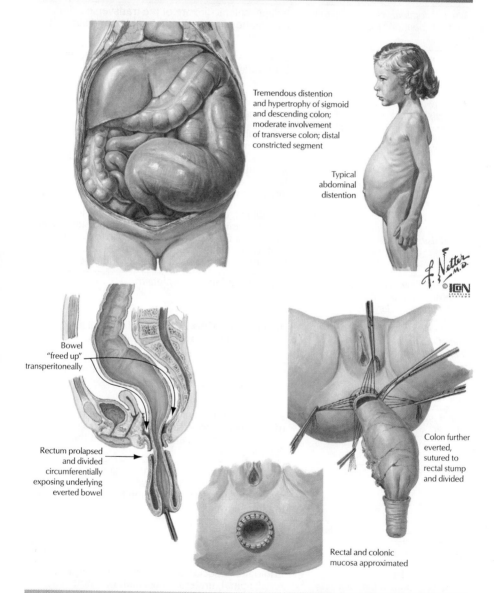

Tremendous distention and hypertrophy of sigmoid and descending colon; moderate involvement of transverse colon; distal constricted segment

Typical abdominal distention

Bowel "freed up" transperitoneally

Rectum prolapsed and divided circumferentially exposing underlying everted bowel

Colon further everted, sutured to rectal stump and divided

Rectal and colonic mucosa approximated

Congenital megacolon results from failure of neural crest cells to migrate distally along the colon (usually sigmoid colon and rectum), which leads to an aganglionic segment that lacks both Meissner's submucosal and Auerbach's myenteric plexuses. Distention proximal to the aganglionic region may occur shortly after birth or may cause symptoms only later, in early childhood. Surgical repair involves prolapse and eversion of the segment.

Review Questions

What are the linea alba and semi-lunar lines?	The linea alba is a relatively avascular midline band of subcutaneous fibrous tissue; semilunar lines demarcate the lateral borders of the rectus sheath.
What abdominal viscera lie in the left hypochondriac region?	Spleen, splenic flexure of the transverse colon, pancreatic tail, stomach (variable), and part of the left kidney.
What are the three muscle layers of the abdominal wall lateral to the rectus sheath?	External and internal abdominal obliques and transversus abdominis.
Name two abdominal wall (ventral) hernias.	Umbilical, linea alba, linea semilunaris, and incisional.
What are the layers of the abdominal wall?	Skin, subcutaneous tissue (fatty Camper's fascia and membranous Scarpa's fascia in lower abdomen); external oblique, internal oblique, and transversus abdominis muscles; transversalis fascia; extraperitoneal fascia (preperitoneal fat); and peritoneum.
Identify two superficial routes that venous blood returning to the heart could use.	Inferior epigastrics to superior epigastrics to internal thoracic veins to subclavian veins, and superficial circumflex iliac to thoracoepigastric to lateral thoracic to axillary veins (subclavian and axillary then join major veins at the root of the neck).
What anastomotic arteries lie posterior to the rectus abdominis muscle?	Superior and inferior epigastric.
What layers form the anterior lamina of the rectus sheath below the arcuate line?	Aponeuroses of the external and internal abdominal oblique and the transversus abdominis.
What nerve is in the spermatic cord, and what does it innervate?	Genital branch of the genitofemoral nerve. It innervates the cremaster muscle.
What is an indirect inguinal hernia?	A hernia that occurs lateral to the inferior epigastric vessels, passes through the deep inguinal ring and inguinal canal, and may appear at the superficial inguinal ring.
What is the inguinal (Hesselbach's) triangle?	Area bounded by the inguinal ligament, inferior epigastric vessels, and lateral border of the rectus sheath. Hernias through this area are direct inguinal hernias.
What structure can limit spread of a suprahepatic abscess across the midline?	Falciform ligament.
Identify at least five causes of acute abdomen that may originate from retroperitoneal structures.	Etiologies associated with neural, pancreatic, renal, spinal, ureteral, muscular, or vascular structures, or skeletal fractures.
What are peritoneal signs of an acute abdomen?	Tenderness, percussion and rebound tenderness, guarding, and pain with motion.

Review Questions

What is the access point to the lesser sac?	The epiploic foramen (of Winslow), just posterior to the hepatoduodenal ligament and anterior to the IVC.
What ventral mesentery derivative connects the stomach to the liver?	Hepatogastric ligament portion of the lesser omentum.
What is the most common type of hiatal hernia?	Sliding (rolling or axial) hernia (95%).
In advanced gastric carcinoma, metastases may involve what adjacent structures?	Liver, omentum, pancreas, spleen, and lymph nodes.
What intraabdominal organ is most often injured in blunt trauma?	Spleen.
Where does the hepatopancreatic ampulla terminate?	In the lumen of the second, or descending, part of the duodenum.
Where do most peptic ulcers occur?	First part of the duodenum.
If a peptic ulcer of the first part of the duodenum starts bleeding, which artery is most likely responsible?	Gastroduodenal.
What are the three major branches of the celiac artery (trunk), and what do they supply?	Left gastric, common hepatic, and splenic. They supply the spleen and the foregut derivatives of the GI tract.
What structures are supplied blood by the SMA?	Midgut derivatives of the GI tract.
Why is the superior rectal artery an important anastomotic vessel?	It has anastomoses with the middle and inferior rectal arteries arising from the internal iliac and pudendal arteries, respectively.
Where is McBurney's point?	One third along the line connecting the anterior superior iliac spine to the umbilicus. It is a good landmark for locating an inflamed appendix (point of tenderness).
According to the Rome II diagnostic criteria, what features must one look for in a diagnosis of irritable bowel syndrome?	A 12-week history in the past year plus two of the following three features: relief by defecation, onset associated with change in stool frequency, and onset associated with change in stool appearance.
Where is the pain of Crohn's disease localized?	Paraumbilical region and lower right quadrant.
Most cases of ulcerative colitis are limited to what regions of the bowel?	Rectum and sigmoid colon (80%).
What is the most common site for the occurrence of diverticula?	Distal transverse colon, descending colon, and sigmoid colon.

Review Questions

What is volvulus?	A twisting of a bowel loop that may cause obstruction, compromise the bowel vascular supply, and lead to infarction.
Distinguish between symptoms of cancer of the ascending colon versus those of cancer of the descending colon.	Right colon cancer is often asymptomatic (silent) until the disease reaches an advanced stage; left colon cancer often leads to changes in bowel habits (constipation or diarrhea).
Partial colectomy of the descending colon requires transection of the IMA. How will the colorectal anastomosis get its blood supply?	Via the splenic flexure (marginal) branch of the middle colic artery (from SMA) and the ascending portion of the left colic branch, along with anastomoses from the rectal arteries (from the internal iliac/pudendal).
What is the bare area of the liver?	The portion that is pressed against the diaphragm and is not covered with visceral peritoneum (appears dull).
What are the four important sites of portocaval anastomoses?	Esophageal, paraumbilical, rectal, and retroperitoneal.
Why does cirrhosis lead to portal hypertension?	Diffuse fibrosis and nodular regeneration of damaged parenchyma significantly alter the liver's architecture and disrupt the central veins and sinusoids, which makes perfusion of the liver via the portal vein difficult.
What clinical signs are commonly seen with advancing cirrhosis?	Deepening jaundice, dark urine, light stools, and ascites.
Besides cirrhosis or other liver diseases, how can portal hypertension occur?	Prehepatic: obstructed blood flow to the liver (portal vein thrombosis); or posthepatic: obstructed blood flow from the liver to the heart (hepatic vein thrombosis).
Account for the referred pain of biliary colic.	Gallbladder distention initiates visceral pain mediated by the greater splanchnic nerve (most likely the T6-T9 dermatome levels) that causes pain in the epigastric and right hypochondriac region (may refer to the scapular region, and right shoulder if diaphragm is irritated).
What is the cystohepatic (Calot's) triangle?	Area bounded by the cystic duct, common hepatic duct, and cystic artery. It is important to identify each of these structures, especially the cystic artery, during gallbladder surgery.
Why can many pancreatic cancers be difficult to diagnose?	If they occur in the pancreatic head, they may obstruct the flow of bile and present with jaundice. However, cancers of the body and tail do not; these may remain silent until the cancer erodes into the posterior body wall and affects other structures, including the nerves, by which time metastases have often occurred.
Where does the thoracic lymphatic duct begin?	In the abdomen at the cisterna chyli, which is the dilated beginning of the duct that receives lymph from lumbar and interstitial lymphatics.

Review Questions

Which adrenal (suprarenal) gland usually has a semilunar shape?	Left. The right one is often pyramidal.
Identify three common anatomical sites where a renal calculus (stone) may become lodged and obstruct urine flow.	Ureteropelvic junction, where the ureter crosses the external iliac vessels, and the ureterovesical junction.
What is the most common type of renal fusion?	Horseshoe kidney, in which two kidneys fuse congenitally, usually at the lower poles.
What are the clinical features of Wilms tumor?	Loin or abdominal mass, often in an infant; fever; loss of weight; anemia; and cachexia.
Which approach to the kidney avoids entering the peritoneal cavity?	Lumbar, lateral (flank), and paramedian anterior.
What are some clinical features of Cushing's disease (hypersecretion of corticotropin)?	Fat pads (buffalo hump on upper back), hypertension, flushed cheeks, moon face, ecchymoses, red striae across abdomen, thin skin, pendulous abdomen, and poor wound healing.
What are some clinical features of pheochromocytoma and potential sites of this tumor?	Headache, sweating and flushing, anxiety, nausea, palpitations and chest pain, severe hypertension, weakness, epigastric pain, and tremor. These tumors arise from chromaffin cells of neural crest origin and are found most often in the adrenal medulla or along the sympathetic trunk and autonomic ganglia.
Into which veins do the gonadal veins empty?	The right vein empties into the IVC, and the left vein empties into the left renal vein.
How are thoracic splanchnic nerves distributed to the abdominal GI tract?	They distribute to the foregut and midgut derivatives of the GI tract by synapsing in the celiac and superior mesenteric ganglia and sending postganglionic fibers to the viscera on the vessels of the celiac artery and SMA.
What is the area of referred pain from the jejunum?	Umbilical region.
What is the area of referred pain for appendicitis?	Umbilical region early, then the lower right quadrant.
What is the insertion of the iliopsoas muscle, and what is its function?	It inserts into the lesser trochanter of the femur and is the major flexor of the thigh at the hip joint.
Which nerves of the lumbar plexus arise from L2 to L4 ventral rami, and what do they innervate?	Femoral, which innervates anterior compartment muscles of the thigh (largely knee extensors), and obturator, which innervates medial compartment muscles of the thigh (largely hip adductors).
What are the derivatives of the embryonic ventral mesentery?	Lesser omentum, falciform ligament, and coronary ligaments of the liver.
What is the parasympathetic innervation to the abdominal GI tract?	Foregut and midgut derivatives are innervated by the vagus nerve; the hindgut is innervated by the pelvic splanchnics (S2-S4).

Review Questions

What is the axis around which the gut tube rotates during development?	The SMA.
Which pancreatic bud gives rise to the main pancreatic duct (of Wirsung)?	The proximal portion of the main duct is derived from the ventral pancreatic bud; the distal half comes originally from the dorsal pancreatic bud.
What is the metanephros?	The mesoderm into which the ureteric bud grows and differentiates to form the definitive human kidney.
What is the most common developmental anomaly of the bowel?	Meckel's diverticulum. It results from failure of involution of the vitelline duct.
What is Hirschsprung's disease, and what is its cause?	Congenital megacolon, resulting from failure of neural crest cells to migrate distally along the colon (usually affects sigmoid colon and rectum), leads to an aganglionic segment that lacks both Meissner's and Auerbach's plexuses.

7

Pelvis and Perineum

CHAPTER OUTLINE

Introduction The bowl-shaped pelvic cavity is continuous superiorly with the abdomen and bounded inferiorly by the perineum, which lies between the thighs. The pelvis contains the terminal gastrointestinal tract and urinary system and the reproductive organs. The perineum provides support to the pelvic viscera and contains the external genitalia.

Surface Anatomy: Key Landmarks

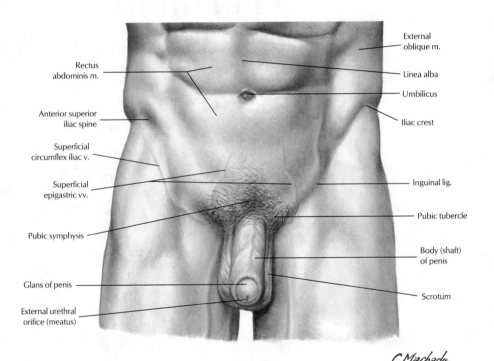

Surface Anatomy: Key Landmarks (continued)

Umbilicus: site that marks the T10 dermatome, lying at the level of the intervertebral disc between L3 and L4

Iliac crest: rim of the ilium, lying at approximately the level of the L4 vertebra

Anterior superior iliac spine: superior attachment point for the inguinal ligament

Pubic tubercle: inferior attachment point for the inguinal ligament

Posterior superior iliac spine: site often demarcated by dimpling of overlying skin

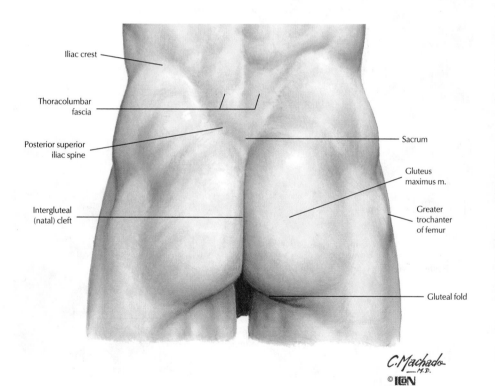

Pelvis: Bony Pelvis and Ligaments

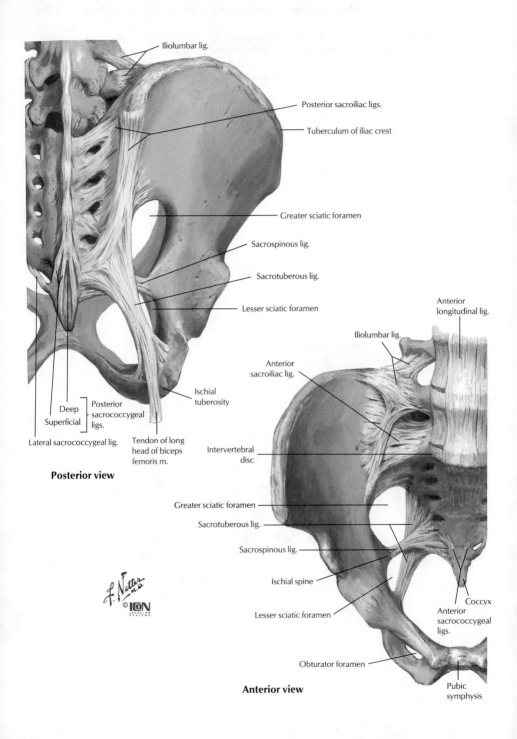

Iliolumbar lig.

Posterior sacroiliac ligs.

Tuberculum of iliac crest

Greater sciatic foramen

Sacrospinous lig.

Sacrotuberous lig.

Lesser sciatic foramen

Ischial
tuberosity

Deep
Superficial
Posterior
sacrococcygeal
ligs.

Lateral sacrococcygeal lig.

Tendon of long
head of biceps
femoris m.

Posterior view

Anterior
longitudinal lig.

Iliolumbar lig.

Anterior
sacroiliac lig.

Intervertebral
disc

Greater sciatic foramen

Sacrotuberous lig.

Sacrospinous lig.

Ischial spine

Lesser sciatic foramen

Coccyx

Anterior
sacrococcygeal
ligs.

Obturator foramen

Pubic
symphysis

Anterior view

Pelvis: Bony Pelvis and Ligaments (continued)

The bony pelvis was reviewed in Chapter 4 (Lower Limb).

LIGAMENT	ATTACHMENT	COMMENT
Lumbosacral Joint*		
Intervertebral (IV) disc	Between L5 and sacrum	Allows little movement
Iliolumbar	Transverse process of L5 to crest of ilium	Can be involved in avulsion fracture
Sacroiliac (Plane Synovial) Joint		
Sacroiliac	Sacrum to ilium	Allows little movement; consists of posterior (strong), anterior (provides rotational stability), and interosseous (strongest) ligaments
Sacrococcygeal (Symphysis) Joint		
Sacrococcygeal	Between coccyx and sacrum	Allows some movement; consists of anterior, posterior, and lateral ligaments; contains an IV disc between S5 and C1
Pubic Symphysis		
Pubic	Between pubic bones	Allows some movement, fibrocartilage disc
Accessory Ligaments		
Sacrotuberous	Iliac spines and sacrum to ischial tuberosity	Provides vertical stability
Sacrospinous	Ischial spine to sacrum and coccyx	Divides sciatic notch into greater and lesser sciatic foramina

Other ligaments include those binding any two vertebrae and facet joints (see Chapter 2 [Back]).

Pelvis: Muscles of the Pelvic Floor

Superior view

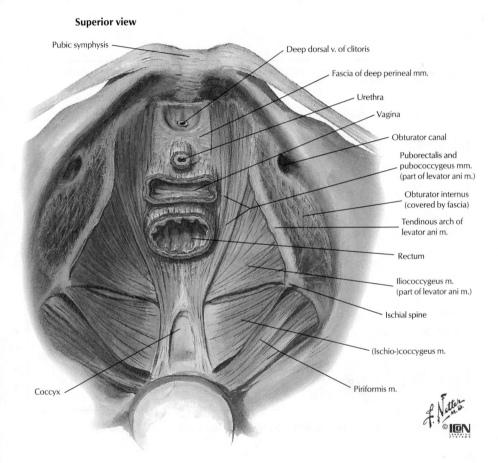

Pubic symphysis

Deep dorsal v. of clitoris

Fascia of deep perineal mm.

Urethra

Vagina

Obturator canal

Puborectalis and pubococcygeus mm. (part of levator ani m.)

Obturator internus (covered by fascia)

Tendinous arch of levator ani m.

Rectum

Iliococcygeus m. (part of levator ani m.)

Ischial spine

(Ischio-)coccygeus m.

Piriformis m.

Coccyx

Pelvis: Muscles of the Pelvic Floor (continued)

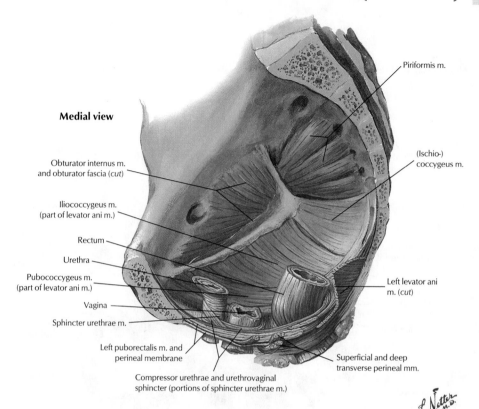

Medial view

Piriformis m.

(Ischio-) coccygeus m.

Obturator internus m. and obturator fascia (*cut*)

Iliococcygeus m. (part of levator ani m.)

Rectum

Urethra

Pubococcygeus m. (part of levator ani m.)

Vagina

Sphincter urethrae m.

Left puborectalis m. and perineal membrane

Compressor urethrae and urethrovaginal sphincter (portions of sphincter urethrae m.)

Left levator ani m. (*cut*)

Superficial and deep transverse perineal mm.

The levator ani and coccygeus muscles comprise the pelvic diaphragm, an important supporting structure of the pelvic floor.

MUSCLE	PROXIMAL ATTACHMENT (ORIGIN)	DISTAL ATTACHMENT (INSERTION)	INNERVATION	MAIN ACTIONS
Obturator internus	Pelvic aspect of obturator membrane and pelvic bones	Greater trochanter of femur	Nerve to obturator internus	Rotates external thigh laterally; abducts flexed thigh at hip
Piriformis	Anterior surface of second to fourth sacral segments and sacrotuberous ligament	Greater trochanter of femur	Ventral rami of S1-2	Rotates external thigh laterally; abducts flexed thigh; stabilizes hip joint
Levator ani	Body of pubis, tendinous arch of obturator fascia, and ischial spine	Perineal body, coccyx, anococcygeal raphe, walls of prostate or vagina, rectum, and anal canal	Ventral rami of S3-4, perineal nerve	Supports pelvic viscera; raises pelvic floor
Coccygeus (ischiococcygeus)	Ischial spine and sacrospinous ligament	Inferior sacrum and coccyx	Ventral rami of S4-5	Supports pelvic viscera; draws coccyx forward

Pelvic Cavity: Reproductive Viscera in the Female

Median (sagittal) section

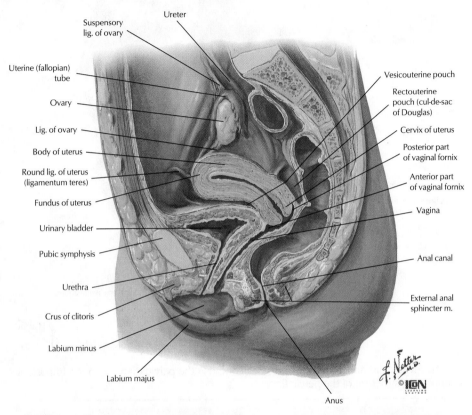

FEATURE	CHARACTERISTICS
Ovary	Is suspended between suspensory ligament of ovary (contains ovarian vessels, nerves, lymphatics) and ovarian ligament (tethered to uterus)
Uterine tube (fallopian tube, oviduct)	Runs in mesosalpinx of broad ligament
Uterus	Consists of body (fundus and isthmus) and cervix; is supported by pelvic diaphragm and ligaments
Vagina	Includes fornix—recess around protruding uterine cervix

Compared with the male pelvis, the female pelvis generally has smaller bones, an oval rather than heart-shaped inlet, a larger pelvic outlet, a wider pelvic cavity with flared iliac fossae, a larger subpubic angle, and a shorter, wider sacrum—all adaptations for childbirth.

Pelvic Cavity: Peritoneal Relationships of Female Pelvic Viscera

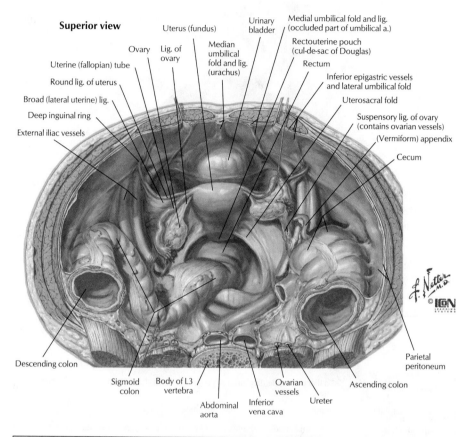

Superior view

Uterus (fundus)

Ovary Lig. of ovary

Uterine (fallopian) tube

Round lig. of uterus

Broad (lateral uterine) lig.

Deep inguinal ring

External iliac vessels

Median umbilical fold and lig. (urachus)

Urinary bladder

Medial umbilical fold and lig. (occluded part of umbilical a.)

Rectouterine pouch (cul-de-sac of Douglas)

Rectum

Inferior epigastric vessels and lateral umbilical fold

Uterosacral fold

Suspensory lig. of ovary (contains ovarian vessels)

(Vermiform) appendix

Cecum

Parietal peritoneum

Descending colon

Sigmoid colon

Body of L3 vertebra

Abdominal aorta

Inferior vena cava

Ovarian vessels

Ureter

Ascending colon

FEATURE	CHARACTERISTICS
Ascending colon	Retroperitoneal
Descending colon	Retroperitoneal
Sigmoid colon	Part of colon tethered by sigmoid mesocolon
Rectum	Part of large intestine that becomes retroperitoneal as it descends into pelvis
Urinary bladder	Organ covered by peritoneum
Vesicouterine pouch	Peritoneal recess between bladder and uterus
Rectouterine pouch (of Douglas)	Peritoneal recess between rectum and uterus, lowest point in female pelvis (accessed with needle via posterior vaginal fornix)
Uterus	Organ covered with peritoneum
Ureteric fold	Peritoneum covering ureter as it courses to bladder
Broad ligament	Peritoneal fold that "suspends" uterus and uterine tubes
Round ligament of uterus	Ligament that reflects off uterus and keeps it anteverted and anteflexed; passes into inguinal canal and ends in labia majora

Pelvic Cavity: Pelvic Arteries in the Female

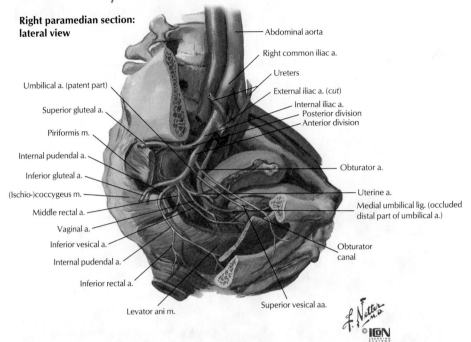

Right paramedian section: lateral view

- Umbilical a. (patent part)
- Superior gluteal a.
- Piriformis m.
- Internal pudendal a.
- Inferior gluteal a.
- (Ischio-)coccygeus m.
- Middle rectal a.
- Vaginal a.
- Inferior vesical a.
- Internal pudendal a.
- Inferior rectal a.
- Levator ani m.

- Abdominal aorta
- Right common iliac a.
- Ureters
- External iliac a. (*cut*)
- Internal iliac a.
  - Posterior division
  - Anterior division
- Obturator a.
- Uterine a.
- Medial umbilical lig. (occluded distal part of umbilical a.)
- Obturator canal
- Superior vesical aa.

f. Netter m.d.
©ICON

ARTERY (DIVISION)	COURSE AND STRUCTURES SUPPLIED
Common iliac	Divides into external (to thigh) and internal (to pelvis) iliac
Internal iliac	Divides into posterior division (P) and anterior division (A)
Iliolumbar (P)	To iliacus muscle (iliac artery), psoas, quadratus lumborum, and spine (lumbar artery)
Lateral sacral (P)	Piriformis muscle and sacrum (meninges and nerves)
Superior gluteal (P)	Between lumbosacral trunk and S1 nerves, through greater sciatic foramen and into gluteal region
Inferior gluteal (A)	Between S1 or S2 and S2 or S3 to gluteal region
Internal pudendal (A)	To perineal structures
Umbilical (A)	Gives rise to superior vesical artery to bladder and becomes medial umbilical ligament when it reaches anterior abdominal wall
Obturator (A)	Passes into medial thigh via obturator foramen (with nerve)
Uterine (A)	Runs over levator ani and ureter to reach uterus
Vaginal (A)	From internal iliac or uterine, passes to vagina
Middle rectal (A)	To lower rectum and superior part of anal canal
Ovarian	From abdominal aorta, runs in suspensory ligament of ovary
Superior rectal	Continuation of inferior mesenteric artery (IMA) to rectum
Median sacral	From aortic bifurcation, unpaired artery to sacrum and coccyx

Arteries in the male are similar, except that uterine, vaginal, and ovarian branches are replaced by arteries to the ductus deferens (from a vesical branch), prostate (from inferior vesical), and testis (from aorta). Significant variability exists for these arteries, so they are best named for the structure supplied. Corresponding veins (usually multiple veins) to these arteries drain into the internal iliac vein directly or into other larger veins.

Pelvic Cavity: Uterus and Adnexa

Posterior view

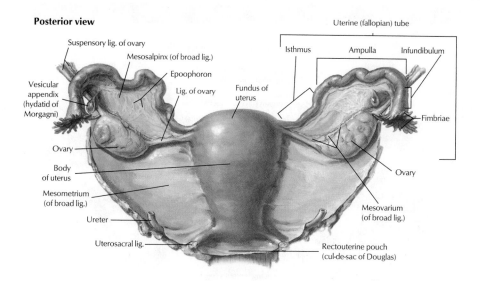

Suspensory lig. of ovary

Mesosalpinx (of broad lig.)

Epoophoron

Vesicular appendix (hydatid of Morgagni)

Lig. of ovary

Fundus of uterus

Uterine (fallopian) tube

Isthmus   Ampulla   Infundibulum

Fimbriae

Ovary

Body of uterus

Mesometrium (of broad lig.)

Ureter

Uterosacral lig.

Ovary

Mesovarium (of broad lig.)

Rectouterine pouch (cul-de-sac of Douglas)

Frontal section

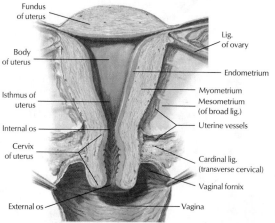

Fundus of uterus

Body of uterus

Isthmus of uterus

Internal os

Cervix of uterus

External os

Lig. of ovary

Endometrium

Myometrium

Mesometrium (of broad lig.)

Uterine vessels

Cardinal lig. (transverse cervical)

Vaginal fornix

Vagina

FEATURE	CHARACTERISTICS
Broad ligament of uterus	Includes mesovarium (enfolds ovary), mesosalpinx (enfolds uterine tube), and mesometrium (remainder of ligament)
Ovaries	Are suspended by suspensory ligament of ovary from lateral pelvic wall and tethered to uterus by ovarian ligament
Uterine tubes	Consist of fimbriated end (collects ova), infundibulum, ampulla, isthmus, and uterine parts
Transverse cervical (cardinal or Mackenrodt's) ligaments	Are fibromuscular condensations of pelvic fascia that support uterus
Uterosacral ligaments	Extend from sides of cervix to sacrum, support uterus, and lie beneath peritoneum (uterosacral fold)

Clinical Correlation

Urinary Tract Infections: Cystitis   *Anatomy on pp. 472, 473, 494*

Factors in Etiology of Cystitis

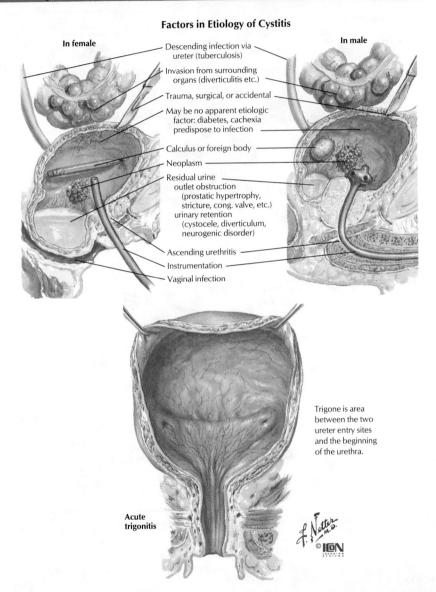

In female

In male

- Descending infection via ureter (tuberculosis)
- Invasion from surrounding organs (diverticulitis etc.)
- Trauma, surgical, or accidental
- May be no apparent etiologic factor: diabetes, cachexia predispose to infection
- Calculus or foreign body
- Neoplasm
- Residual urine outlet obstruction (prostatic hypertrophy, stricture, cong. valve, etc.) urinary retention (cystocele, diverticulum, neurogenic disorder)
- Ascending urethritis
- Instrumentation
- Vaginal infection

Trigone is area between the two ureter entry sites and the beginning of the urethra.

Acute trigonitis

Urinary tract infection (UTI) is more common in women—because they have shorter urethras, urinary tract trauma, and exposure to pathogens during sexual activity—although, as illustrated, a number of other risk factors may also precipitate infection. *Escherichia coli* is the usual pathogen. UTI may lead to urethritis, cystitis (bladder inflammation, including trigonitis), and pyelonephritis. Symptoms of cystitis include dysuria, frequency, urgency, suprapubic discomfort and tenderness, and hematuria (infrequent).

Clinical Correlation

Stress Incontinence in Women

Anatomy on pp. 470-475

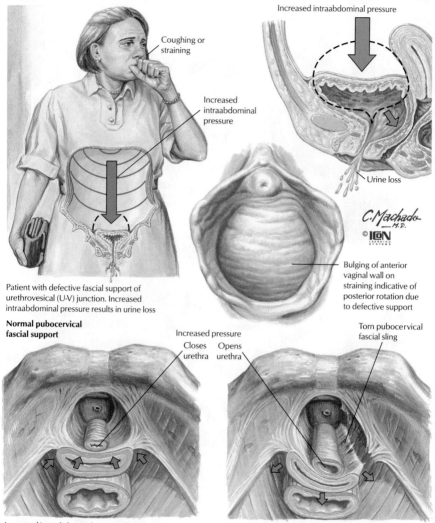

Increased intraabdominal pressure

Coughing or straining

Increased intraabdominal pressure

Urine loss

C. Machado —M.D.

© ICON

Patient with defective fascial support of urethrovesical (U-V) junction. Increased intraabdominal pressure results in urine loss

Bulging of anterior vaginal wall on straining indicative of posterior rotation due to defective support

Normal pubocervical fascial support

Increased pressure
Closes   Opens
urethra   urethra

Torn pubocervical fascial sling

Increased intraabdominal pressure forces urethra against intact pubocervical fascia, closing urethra and maintaining continence.

Defective fascial support allows posterior rotation of U-V junction due to increased pressure, opening urethra and causing urine loss.

Involuntary loss of urine after an increase in intraabdominal pressure is often associated with weakening of supporting structures including
- Medial and lateral pubovesical ligaments
- Vesicocervical fascia (pubovesical fascia at the urethrovesical junction) that blends with the perineal membrane and perineal body
- Levator ani (provides some support for urethrovesical junction)
- Functional integrity of the urethral sphincter

Common predisposing factors include multiparity, obesity, chronic cough, and lifting.

Clinical Correlation

Urethrocele and Cystocele   *Anatomy on pp. 472, 473, 475*

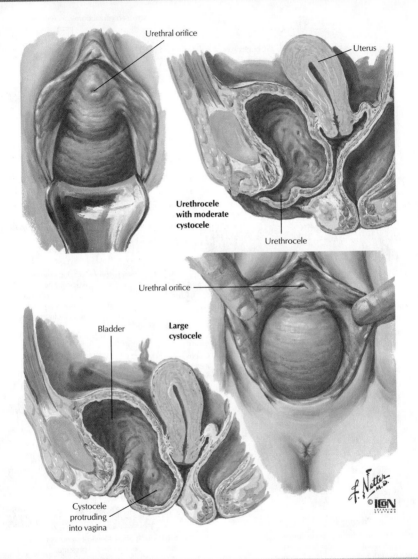

Urethral orifice

Uterus

Urethrocele
with moderate
cystocele

Urethrocele

Urethral orifice

Bladder   **Large
cystocele**

Cystocele
protruding
into vagina

A urethrocele is a prolapse of the urethra; a cystocele is a prolapse of the bladder that is caused by loss of support of the anterior vagina by attenuation of pubovesical and vesicocervical fasciae.

CHARACTERISTIC	DESCRIPTION
Prevalence	10-15% of women
Age	≥40 years
Risk factors	Multiparity, obesity, chronic cough, heavy lifting

Clinical Correlation

Uterine Prolapse

Anatomy on pp. 472, 473, 475

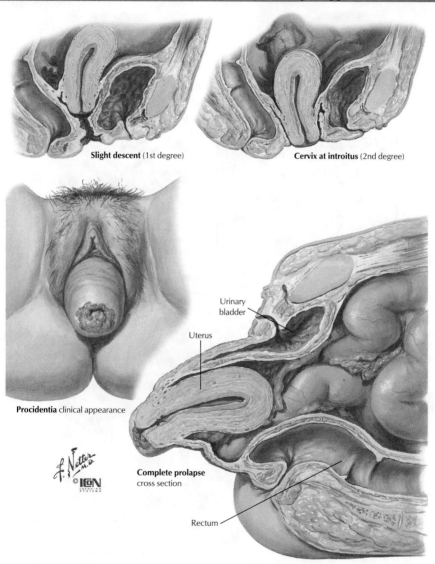

Slight descent (1st degree)

Cervix at introitus (2nd degree)

Procidentia clinical appearance

Urinary bladder

Uterus

Complete prolapse cross section

Rectum

Uterine prolapse involves loss of support by cardinal or uterosacral ligaments and by levator ani.

CHARACTERISTIC	DESCRIPTION
Prevalence	Some descent common in parous women
Age	Late reproductive and older age groups
Risk factors	Birth trauma, obesity, chronic cough, lifting, weak ligaments

Clinical Correlation

Cervical Carcinoma   *Anatomy on pp. 472, 473, 475*

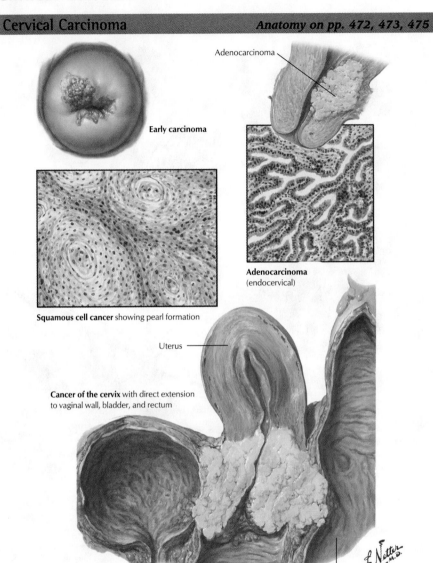

Adenocarcinoma

Early carcinoma

Adenocarcinoma
(endocervical)

Squamous cell cancer showing pearl formation

Uterus

Cancer of the cervix with direct extension
to vaginal wall, bladder, and rectum

Rectum

Approximately 85-90% of cervical carcinomas are squamous carcinomas; approximately 10-15% are adenocarcinomas.

CHARACTERISTIC	DESCRIPTION
Risk factors	Early sexual activity, multiple sex partners, human papillomavirus (HPV) infection, African-American, smoking
Prevalence	15,000 cases/year, with 6000 deaths/year
Age	40-60 years

Clinical Correlation

Cervical Cell Pathology   *Anatomy on p. 475*

**Cervical cell pathology
in squamous tissue**

Grades and cell types

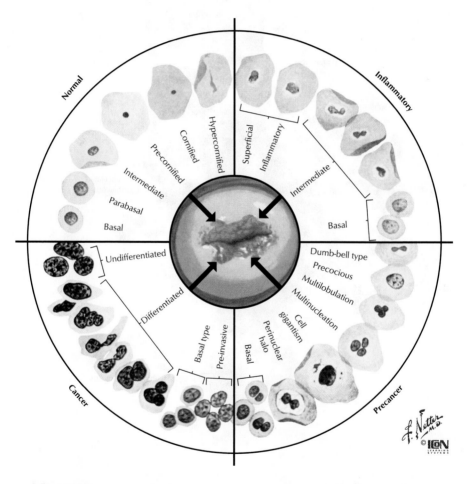

The Papanicolaou test, or Pap smear, revolutionized early diagnosis and treatment of cervical carcinoma. Colposcopy (examination with a colposcope, a low-magnification optical instrument) allows direct visualization of the cervix, vagina, and vulva to reveal the cervical transition (transformation) zone, where cervical epithelium changes from simple columnar to stratified squamous epithelium.

Clinical Correlation

Uterine Leiomyomas (Fibroids)   *Anatomy on pp. 472, 473, 475*

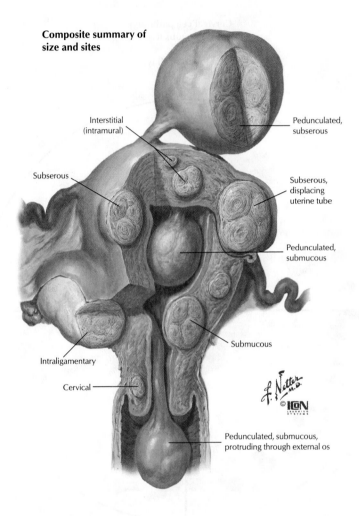

Composite summary of size and sites

Interstitial (intramural)

Subserous

Intraligamentary

Cervical

Pedunculated, subserous

Subserous, displacing uterine tube

Pedunculated, submucous

Submucous

Pedunculated, submucous, protruding through external os

Leiomyomas are benign tumors of smooth muscle cells of the myometrium. Because they are firm, they are commonly referred to as fibroids.

CHARACTERISTIC	DESCRIPTION
Prevalence	30% of all women; 40-50% of women older than 50 years; most common benign tumor in women
Risk factors	Nulliparity, early menarche, African-American (4- to 10-fold increase)
Growth	Stimulated by estrogen, oral contraceptives, epidermal growth factor

Clinical Correlation

Endometriosis   *Anatomy on pp. 472, 473, 475*

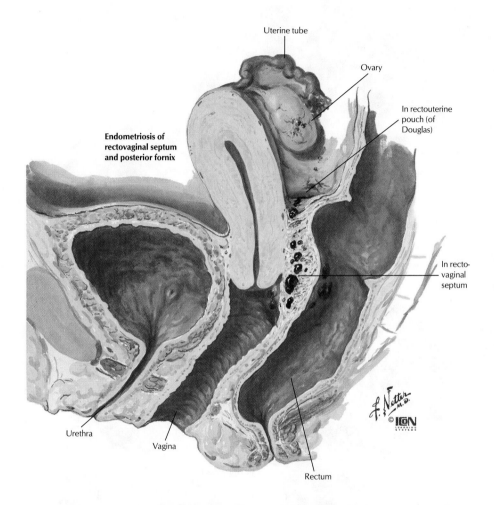

Uterine tube

Ovary

In rectouterine pouch (of Douglas)

Endometriosis of rectovaginal septum and posterior fornix

In rectovaginal septum

Urethra

Vagina

Rectum

Endometriosis is a progressive, benign condition characterized by ectopic foci of endometrial tissue in the pelvis (ovary, rectouterine pouch, uterine ligaments, tubes) or peritoneal cavity.

CHARACTERISTIC	DESCRIPTION
Prevalence	5-10% of all women; 30-50% of infertility patients
Age	30-50 years
Causes	Genetic, menstrual backflow through tubes, lymphatic or vascular spread, metaplasia of coelomic epithelium
Risk factors	Obstructive anomalies (cervical or vaginal outflow pathway)

Clinical Correlation

Uterine Endometrial Carcinoma   *Anatomy on p. 475*

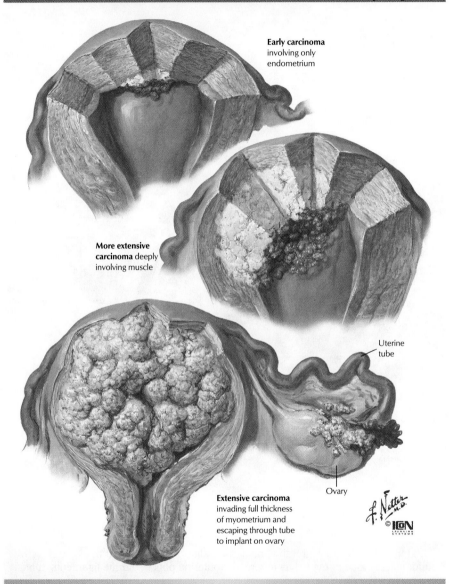

Early carcinoma involving only endometrium

More extensive carcinoma deeply involving muscle

Uterine tube

Extensive carcinoma invading full thickness of myometrium and escaping through tube to implant on ovary

Ovary

Endometrial carcinoma is the most common malignancy of the female reproductive tract. It often occurs between the ages of 55 and 65 years. Risk factors include
- Obesity (increased estrogen synthesis)
- Estrogen replacement therapy without concomitant progestin
- Breast or colon cancer
- Early menarche or late menopause (prolonged estrogen stimulation)
- Chronic anovulation
- Diabetes

Clinical Correlation

Chronic Pelvic Inflammatory Disease
Anatomy on p. 475

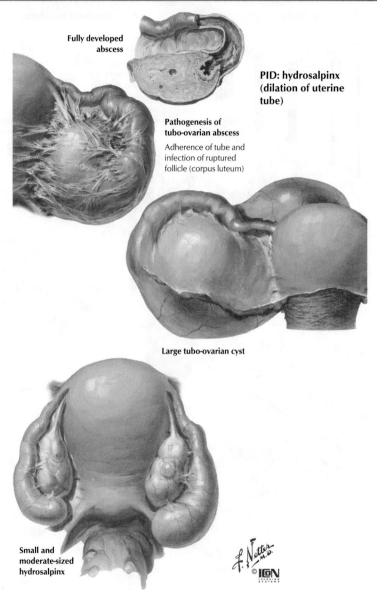

Fully developed abscess

PID: hydrosalpinx (dilation of uterine tube)

Pathogenesis of tubo-ovarian abscess

Adherence of tube and infection of ruptured follicle (corpus luteum)

Large tubo-ovarian cyst

Small and moderate-sized hydrosalpinx

Recurrent or chronic infections of the uterine tubes or other adnexa (uterine appendages), which result in cystic dilation (hydrosalpinx), can account for approximately 40% of female infertility. The most affected ages are 15-25 years; risk factors include early sexual activity, multiple partners, sexually transmitted diseases (STDs), and pelvic inflammatory disease (PID). Unilateral or bilateral adnexal masses (usually sausage shaped) may be palpable.

Clinical Correlation

Dysfunctional Uterine Bleeding

Anatomy on p. 475

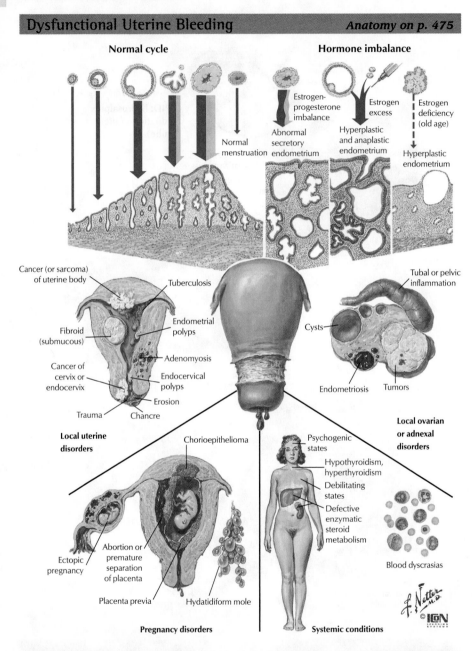

Normal cycle

Hormone imbalance

Estrogen-progesterone imbalance

Estrogen excess

Estrogen deficiency (old age)

Normal menstruation

Abnormal secretory endometrium

Hyperplastic and anaplastic endometrium

Hyperplastic endometrium

Cancer (or sarcoma) of uterine body

Tuberculosis

Tubal or pelvic inflammation

Fibroid (submucous)

Endometrial polyps

Cysts

Cancer of cervix or endocervix

Adenomyosis

Endocervical polyps

Trauma

Chancre

Erosion

Endometriosis

Tumors

Local uterine disorders

Chorioepithelioma

Psychogenic states

Local ovarian or adnexal disorders

Hypothyroidism, hyperthyroidism

Debilitating states

Defective enzymatic steroid metabolism

Ectopic pregnancy

Abortion or premature separation of placenta

Blood dyscrasias

Placenta previa

Hydatidiform mole

Pregnancy disorders

Systemic conditions

Dysfunctional uterine bleeding involves an irregular cycle or intermenstrual bleeding (painless) with no clinically identifiable cause; it accounts for approximately 10-15% of all gynecologic office visits. The etiology and pathogenesis are extensive and include local uterine or ovarian and adnexal disorders, as well as systemic and pregnancy-related disorders.

Clinical Correlation

Ectopic Pregnancy
Anatomy on pp. 52, 475

Sites of ectopic implantation

Interstitial

Tubal (isthmic)

Tubal (ampullar)

Abdominal

Infundibular (ostial)

Ovarian

Cervical

Unruptured tubal pregnancy

Villi invading tubular wall

Chorion

Amnion

Hemorrhage in tubal wall

Lumen of tube

Section through tubal pregnancy

Ectopic pregnancy is implantation of a blastocyst outside the endometrial cavity.

CHARACTERISTIC	DESCRIPTION
Prevalence	10-15/1000 pregnancies (highest rates in Jamaica and Vietnam)
Age	>40% in 25- to 34-year-old group
Causes	Uterine tube damage or poor tubal motility
Risk factors	Tubal damage (infections), previous history, age (>35 years), nonwhite, smoking, intrauterine contraceptive device use, endometriosis

Clinical Correlation

Ovarian Cysts   *Anatomy on pp. 473, 475*

Differential Diagnosis

Low-lying
cecum

Distended
bladder

Simple serous cyst
(Serous cystoma)

Appendiceal abscess

Redundant
sigmoid
colon

Pregnancy, hydramnios,
hydatid mole,
hematometra, pyometra

Ovarian cysts usually arise from epithelial ovarian components (follicular cysts, luteal cysts, capsule) and are asymptomatic, normally small, and often benign (>90%). However, timely diagnosis is important and difficult. As illustrated, the differential diagnosis includes conditions that may present as lower abdominopelvic masses.

Clinical Correlation

Ovarian Cysts (continued)

Anatomy on pp. 473, 475

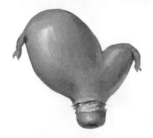

Bicornuate uterus
(with pregnancy in
one horn, or interstitial
pregnancy)

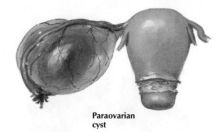

**Paraovarian
cyst**

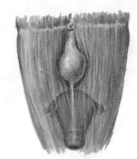

**Desmoid;
urachal cyst**

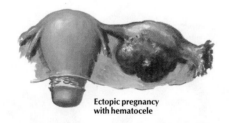

**Ectopic pregnancy
with hematocele**

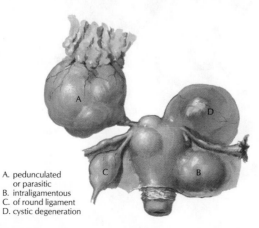

A. pedunculated
   or parasitic
B. intraligamentous
C. of round ligament
D. cystic degeneration

Clinical Correlation

Ovarian Tumors   *Anatomy on pp. 473, 475*

Papillary serous cystadenocarcinoma

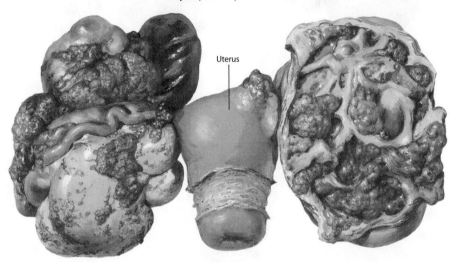

Uterus

Clear cell carcinoma of ovary

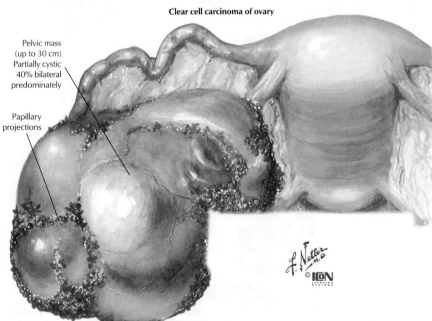

Pelvic mass
(up to 30 cm)
Partially cystic
40% bilateral
predominately

Papillary
projections

Clinical Correlation

Epithelial stromal ovarian tumors

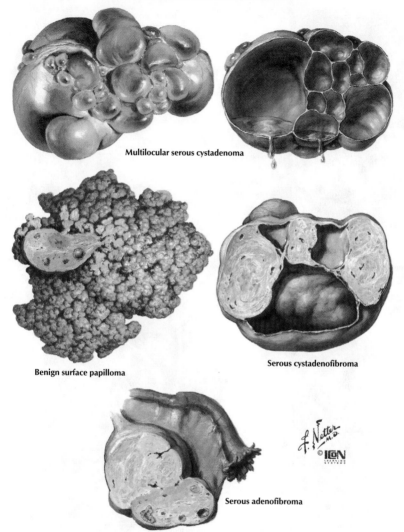

Multilocular serous cystadenoma

Benign surface papilloma

Serous cystadenofibroma

Serous adenofibroma

CHARACTERISTIC	DESCRIPTION
Derivation	Surface epithelial-stromal: 65-70% (85-90% of all malignancies); germ cell: 15-20%; sex-cord stroma: 5-10%
Types of epithelial-stromal tumors	Serous, mucinous, endometrioid, clear cell, Brenner, cystadenofibroma
Age	Benign tumors: women aged 20-29 years; malignant tumors: 50% in women older than 50 years
Risk factors	Family history, high-fat diet, age, nulliparity, early menarche, late menopause, white race, higher socioeconomic status

Clinical Correlation

Metastases of Ovarian Carcinoma *Anatomy on pp. 472, 473, 504, 508*

Routes of metastases

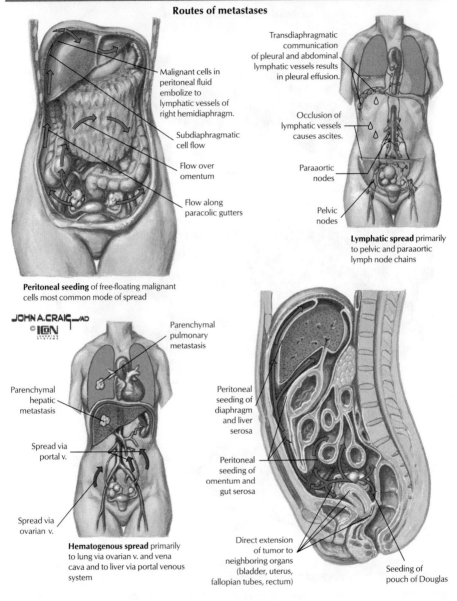

Malignant cells in peritoneal fluid embolize to lymphatic vessels of right hemidiaphragm.

Subdiaphragmatic cell flow

Flow over omentum

Flow along paracolic gutters

Peritoneal seeding of free-floating malignant cells most common mode of spread

JOHN A. CRAIG—AD
©ICON
LEARNING SYSTEMS

Transdiaphragmatic communication of pleural and abdominal lymphatic vessels results in pleural effusion.

Occlusion of lymphatic vessels causes ascites.

Paraaortic nodes

Pelvic nodes

Lymphatic spread primarily to pelvic and paraaortic lymph node chains

Parenchymal pulmonary metastasis

Parenchymal hepatic metastasis

Spread via portal v.

Spread via ovarian v.

Hematogenous spread primarily to lung via ovarian v. and vena cava and to liver via portal venous system

Peritoneal seeding of diaphragm and liver serosa

Peritoneal seeding of omentum and gut serosa

Direct extension of tumor to neighboring organs (bladder, uterus, fallopian tubes, rectum)

Seeding of pouch of Douglas

Ovarian neoplasms are a clinical challenge because they are asymptomatic until late in the course of disease. They often present with symptoms related to metastases to distant sites. Symptoms include weight loss, increasing abdominal girth, ascites, and lower abdominal discomfort. Various routes of metastasis are illustrated.

Clinical Correlation

Assisted Reproduction

Anatomy on p. 475

In vitro fertilization

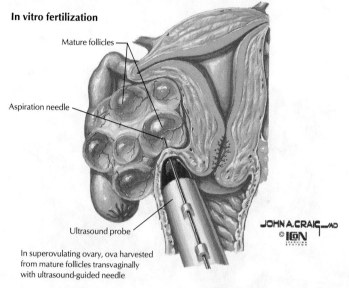

Mature follicles

Aspiration needle

Ultrasound probe

In superovulating ovary, ova harvested from mature follicles transvaginally with ultrasound-guided needle

JOHN A. CRAIG—MD

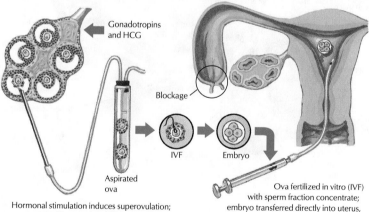

Gonadotropins and HCG

Blockage

IVF

Embryo

Aspirated ova

Hormonal stimulation induces superovulation; ova aspirated from mature follicles

Ova fertilized in vitro (IVF) with sperm fraction concentrate; embryo transferred directly into uterus, bypassing tubal occlusion

Approximately 10-15% of infertile couples may benefit from various assisted reproductive strategies.

TECHNIQUE	DEFINITION
Artificial insemination	Use of donor sperm
GIFT	Gamete intrafallopian transfer
IUI	Intrauterine insemination (partner's or donor's sperm)
IVF/ET	In vitro fertilization with embryo transfer to uterine cavity (illustrated)
ZIFT	In vitro fertilization with zygote transfer to fallopian tube

Pelvic Cavity: Reproductive Viscera in the Male

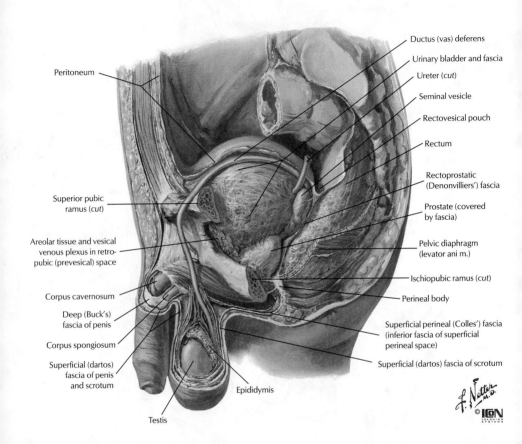

Peritoneum

Superior pubic ramus (*cut*)

Areolar tissue and vesical venous plexus in retro-pubic (prevesical) space

Corpus cavernosum

Deep (Buck's) fascia of penis

Corpus spongiosum

Superficial (dartos) fascia of penis and scrotum

Testis

Epididymis

Ductus (vas) deferens

Urinary bladder and fascia

Ureter (*cut*)

Seminal vesicle

Rectovesical pouch

Rectum

Rectoprostatic (Denonvilliers') fascia

Prostate (covered by fascia)

Pelvic diaphragm (levator ani m.)

Ischiopubic ramus (*cut*)

Perineal body

Superficial perineal (Colles') fascia (inferior fascia of superficial perineal space)

Superficial (dartos) fascia of scrotum

FEATURE	CHARACTERISTICS
Testes	Develop in retroperitoneal abdominal wall and descend into scrotum
Epididymis	Consists of head, body, and tail; functions in maturation and storage of sperm
Ductus (vas) deferens	Passes in spermatic cord through inguinal canal to join duct of seminal vesicle (ejaculatory duct)
Seminal vesicles	Secrete alkaline seminal fluid
Prostate gland	Surrounds prostatic urethra and secretes prostatic fluid

Note that the pelvic ductus deferens, seminal vesicles, and prostate gland lie deep to the peritoneum, which reflects off of the pelvic walls, bladder, and rectum.

Clinical Correlation

Vasectomy
Anatomy on p. 494

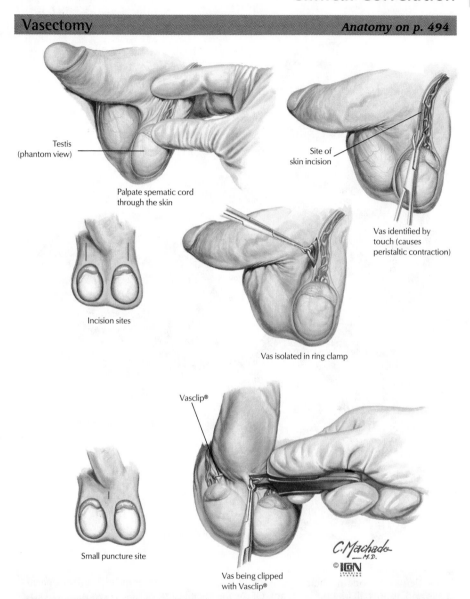

Testis
(phantom view)

Palpate spematic cord
through the skin

Site of
skin incision

Vas identified by
touch (causes
peristaltic contraction)

Incision sites

Vas isolated in ring clamp

Vasclip®

Small puncture site

Vas being clipped
with Vasclip®

   Vasectomy offers birth control with a failure rate below that of the pill, condom, intrauterine device, and tubal ligation. It can be performed as an office procedure with local anesthetic (approximately 500,000/year in the United States). One approach uses a small incision on each side of the scrotum to isolate the vas deferens; another uses a small puncture (no incision) in the scrotal skin to isolate both right and left vas. The muscular vas is identified, and a small segment is isolated between two small metal clips or sutures. The isolated segment is resected, the clipped ends of the vas are cauterized, and the incision is closed (or, in the nonincisional approach, the puncture wound is left unsutured).

Clinical Correlation

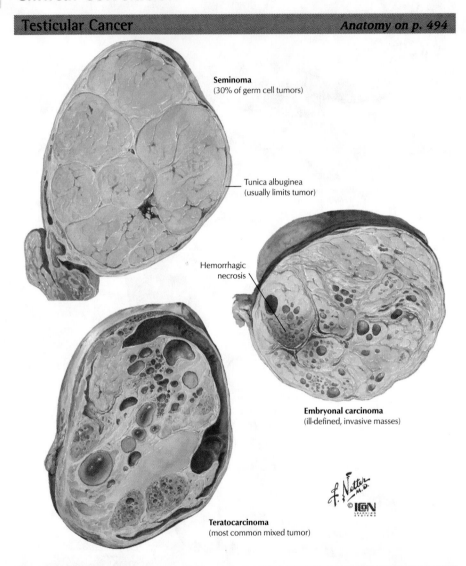

Seminoma
(30% of germ cell tumors)

Tunica albuginea
(usually limits tumor)

Hemorrhagic
necrosis

Embryonal carcinoma
(ill-defined, invasive masses)

Teratocarcinoma
(most common mixed tumor)

Testicular tumors are heterogeneous neoplasms, 95% of them arising from germ cells and almost all being malignant. Of the germ cell tumors, 60% show mixed histologic features, and 40% show a single histologic pattern.

CHARACTERISTIC	DESCRIPTION
Prevalence	2/100,000 males
Peak incidence age	15- to 34-year-old group
Presentation	Firm, painless enlargement of testis
Sertoli or Leydig cell tumors	Uncommon and more often benign than germ cell tumors

Clinical Correlation

Hydrocele and Varicocele
Anatomy on p. 494

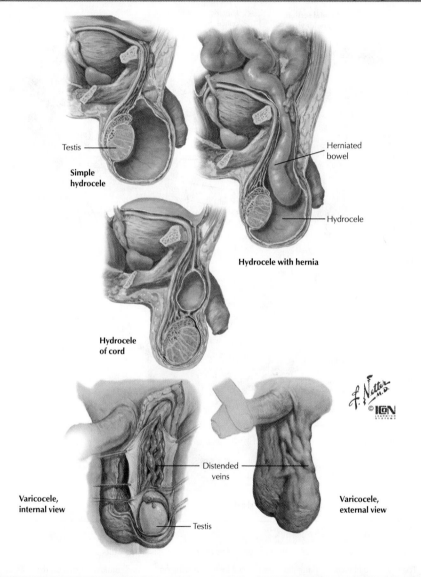

Testis

Simple hydrocele

Herniated bowel

Hydrocele

Hydrocele with hernia

Hydrocele of cord

Varicocele, internal view

Distended veins

Testis

Varicocele, external view

The most common cause of scrotal enlargement is hydrocele—excessive accumulation of serous fluid within the tunica vaginalis (usually a potential space). An infection (in the testis or epididymis), trauma, or tumor may lead to hydrocele, or it may be idiopathic. Varicocele is abnormal dilation and tortuosity of the pampiniform venous plexus. Almost all varicoceles are on the left side, perhaps because the left testicular vein drains into the left renal vein rather than the larger inferior vena cava, as the right testicular vein does. A varicocele is evident at physical examination when a patient stands but usually resolves when the patient is recumbent.

Pelvic Cavity: Bladder, Prostate, and Seminal Vesicles

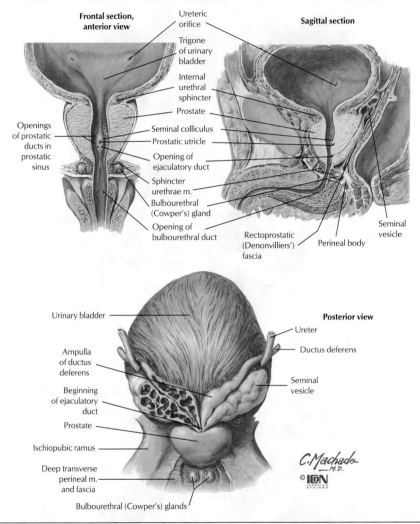

Frontal section, anterior view

Ureteric orifice

Sagittal section

Trigone of urinary bladder

Internal urethral sphincter

Prostate

Openings of prostatic ducts in prostatic sinus

Seminal colliculus

Prostatic utricle

Opening of ejaculatory duct

Sphincter urethrae m.

Bulbourethral (Cowper's) gland

Opening of bulbourethral duct

Rectoprostatic (Denonvilliers') fascia

Perineal body

Seminal vesicle

Urinary bladder

Posterior view

Ureter

Ductus deferens

Ampulla of ductus deferens

Beginning of ejaculatory duct

Prostate

Ischiopubic ramus

Deep transverse perineal m. and fascia

Seminal vesicle

Bulbourethral (Cowper's) glands

C. Machado
—M.D.
©ICN
LEARNING SYSTEMS

CHARACTERISTIC	DESCRIPTION
Urinary bladder	Organ with detrusor muscle (smooth muscle) lining walls
Trigone of the bladder	Triangular area marked by two ureteric orifices and urinary internal urethral orifice (at eminence called uvula)
Prostate gland	Walnut-sized gland with five lobes (anterior, middle, posterior, right and left lateral); middle prone to benign hypertrophy
Seminal vesicles	Lobulated glands whose ducts join ductus deferens to form ejaculatory duct
Bulbourethral (Cowper's) glands	Glands that lie adjacent to external urethral sphincter muscle and secrete mucus-rich fluid that lubricates urethra
Urethra	Three-part structure: prostatic, membranous (surrounded by external urethral sphincter muscle), and spongy (penile)

Clinical Correlation

Transurethral Resection of the Prostate

Anatomy on p. 498

JOHN A. CRAIG—AD
© ICN
LEARNING
SYSTEMS

Tissue chips

Hypertrophic prostate

Prostatic fossa

Bladder neck mm.

Intravesical view of hypertrophy

Postoperative view

Explosion

Air

Gas

Bladder perforation

Capsular perforation

Removal of hypertrophied inner zone by resection

Surgical complications

Postoperative urethral stricture

Benign prostatic hypertrophy is fairly common (20% of males by the age of 40 years) and its occurrence increases with age (in 90% of men older than 80 years). It is really nodular hyperplasia, not hypertrophy, that results from proliferation of epithelial and stromal tissues, often in the periurethral area. This growth can lead to symptoms that may include urinary urgency, decreased stream force, frequency, and nocturia. Symptoms may necessitate transurethral resection of the prostate in which the obstructing periurethral part of the gland is removed via resectoscope. Although relatively rare, several surgical complications are illustrated.

Clinical Correlation

Prostatic Carcinoma   *Anatomy on pp. 494, 498*

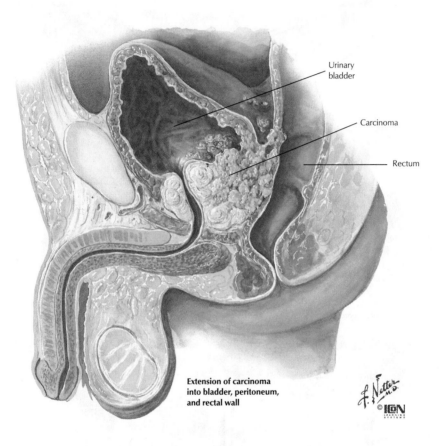

Urinary
bladder

Carcinoma

Rectum

**Extension of carcinoma
into bladder, peritoneum,
and rectal wall**

Prostatic carcinoma is the most common visceral cancer in males and the second leading cause of death in men older than 50 years (lung cancer is the first).

CHARACTERISTIC	DESCRIPTION
Site	70% arise in outer glands (adenocarcinomas) and are palpable by digital rectal examination
Metastases	Regional pelvic lymph nodes, bone, seminal vesicles, bladder, and periurethral zones
Etiology	Hormonal (androgens), genetic, environmental factors
Prevalence	Increased in African-Americans and Scandinavians, few in Japan

Clinical Correlation

Prostate Cancer: Metastases   *Anatomy on p. 498*

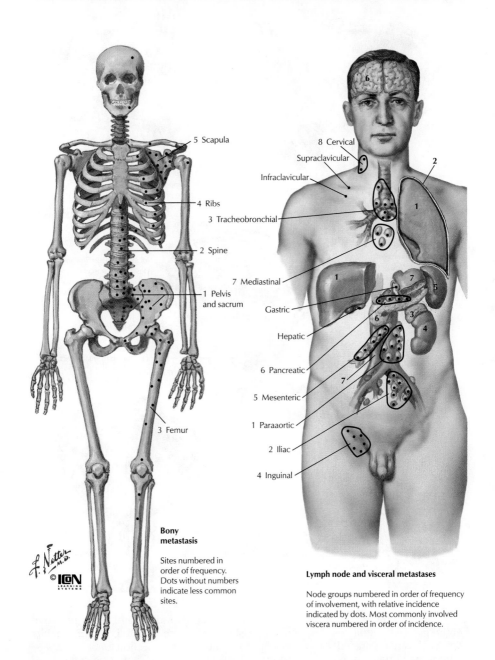

5 Scapula

4 Ribs

3 Tracheobronchial

2 Spine

7 Mediastinal

1 Pelvis and sacrum

Gastric

Hepatic

6 Pancreatic

5 Mesenteric

1 Paraaortic

2 Iliac

4 Inguinal

3 Femur

8 Cervical

Supraclavicular

Infraclavicular

Bony metastasis

Sites numbered in order of frequency. Dots without numbers indicate less common sites.

Lymph node and visceral metastases

Node groups numbered in order of frequency of involvement, with relative incidence indicated by dots. Most commonly involved viscera numbered in order of incidence.

Clinical Correlation

Radical Prostatectomy
Anatomy on pp. 494, 498, 507

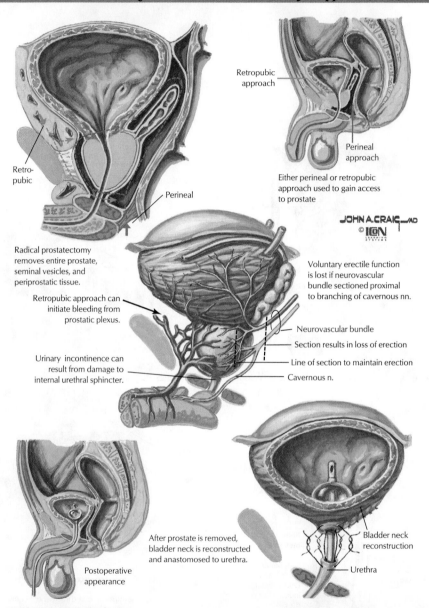

Retropubic approach

Perineal approach

Either perineal or retropubic approach used to gain access to prostate

JOHN A. CRAIG—AD
© ICN

Retro-pubic

Perineal

Radical prostatectomy removes entire prostate, seminal vesicles, and periprostatic tissue.

Voluntary erectile function is lost if neurovascular bundle sectioned proximal to branching of cavernous nn.

Retropubic approach can initiate bleeding from prostatic plexus.

Neurovascular bundle

Section results in loss of erection

Line of section to maintain erection

Cavernous n.

Urinary incontinence can result from damage to internal urethral sphincter.

After prostate is removed, bladder neck is reconstructed and anastomosed to urethra.

Bladder neck reconstruction

Urethra

Postoperative appearance

A common treatment of localized prostate cancer is radical prostatectomy—the entire gland, seminal vesicles, and periprostatic tissue are resected. The retropubic approach is often preceded by regional pelvic lymph node dissection for cancer staging. In the perianal approach (used less often), lymph nodes cannot be simultaneously sampled. Side effects of the treatment include erectile dysfunction, urinary incontinence, or both.

Pelvic Cavity: Rectum and Ischioanal Fossae

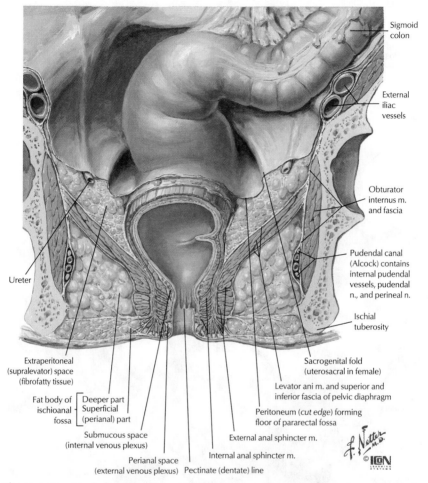

Sigmoid colon

External iliac vessels

Obturator internus m. and fascia

Pudendal canal (Alcock) contains internal pudendal vessels, pudendal n., and perineal n.

Ischial tuberosity

Ureter

Extraperitoneal (supralevator) space (fibrofatty tissue)

Fat body of ischioanal fossa { Deeper part / Superficial (perianal) part }

Submucous space (internal venous plexus)

Perianal space (external venous plexus) Pectinate (dentate) line

Sacrogenital fold (uterosacral in female)

Levator ani m. and superior and inferior fascia of pelvic diaphragm

Peritoneum (*cut edge*) forming floor of pararectal fossa

External anal sphincter m.

Internal anal sphincter m.

The rectum extends from the sigmoid colon to the anal canal. The anal canal lies below the pelvic diaphragm and ends at the anus (external anal sphincter muscle).

FEATURE	CHARACTERISTICS
Pelvic diaphragm	Consists of levator ani and coccygeus muscles; supports pelvic viscera
Pudendal (Alcock's) canal	Conveys vessels and nerves to perineal region
Rectal ampulla	Is dilation just superior to pelvic diaphragm; stores feces
Ischioanal fossa	Consist of fibrous and fatty tissue surrounding anal canal
Anal valves	Are mucosal folds with anal columns extending superiorly
Internal sphincter	Smooth muscle anal sphincter
Pectinate line	Demarcates visceral (above) from somatic (below) portions of anal canal by type of epithelium, innervation, and embryology
External sphincter	Skeletal muscle sphincter (subcutaneous, superficial and deep)

Pelvic Cavity: Arteries of the Rectum and Anal Canal

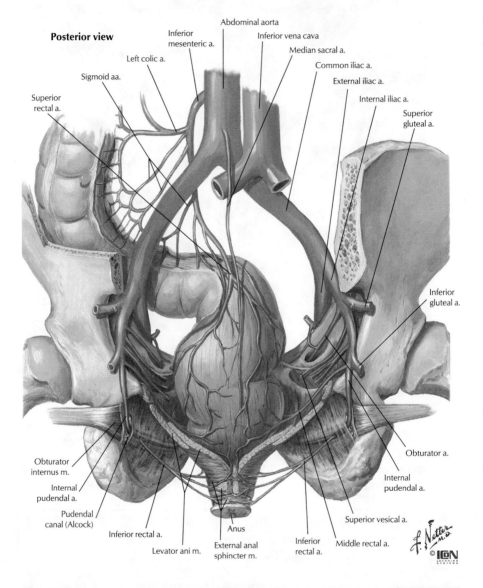

Posterior view

Inferior mesenteric a.

Abdominal aorta

Inferior vena cava

Median sacral a.

Left colic a.

Common iliac a.

External iliac a.

Sigmoid aa.

Internal iliac a.

Superior rectal a.

Superior gluteal a.

Inferior gluteal a.

Obturator a.

Obturator internus m.

Internal pudendal a.

Internal pudendal a.

Pudendal canal (Alcock)

Inferior rectal a.

Levator ani m.

Anus

External anal sphincter m.

Inferior rectal a.

Middle rectal a.

Superior vesical a.

ARTERY	COURSE AND STRUCTURES SUPPLIED
Superior rectal	Continuation of inferior mesenteric artery
Middle rectal	From internal iliac, vesical, or uterine (female) artery, supplies pelvic diaphragm, rectum, and proximal anal canal
Inferior rectal	From internal pudendal artery, supplies external anal sphincter
Median sacral	From aorta, supplies sacrum and coccyx, and rectum

Pelvic Cavity: Veins of the Rectum and Anal Canal

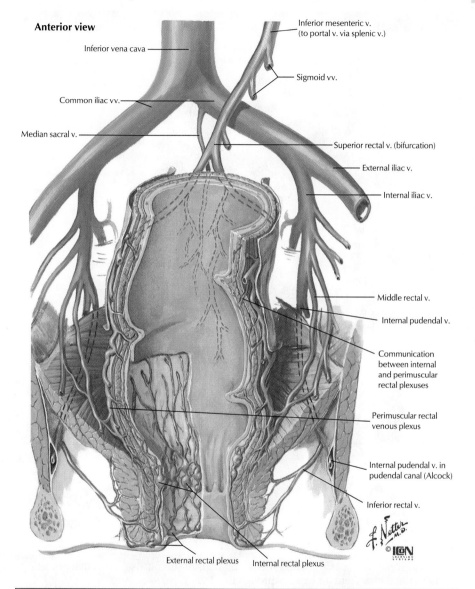

Anterior view

Inferior mesenteric v. (to portal v. via splenic v.)

Inferior vena cava

Sigmoid vv.

Common iliac vv.

Median sacral v.

Superior rectal v. (bifurcation)

External iliac v.

Internal iliac v.

Middle rectal v.

Internal pudendal v.

Communication between internal and perimuscular rectal plexuses

Perimuscular rectal venous plexus

Internal pudendal v. in pudendal canal (Alcock)

Inferior rectal v.

External rectal plexus   Internal rectal plexus

VEIN	CONNECTION
Superior rectal	Drains into inferior mesenteric vein (portal system)
Middle rectal	Drain into internal iliac vein (caval system)
Inferior rectal	Drain into internal pudendal and then internal iliac vein
Median sacral	Drains into left common iliac vein

Rectal venous drainage provides an important portocaval anastomosis between the superior rectal vein (portal system) and the other three venous tributaries (caval system).

Clinical Correlation

Hemorrhoids   *Anatomy on p. 505*

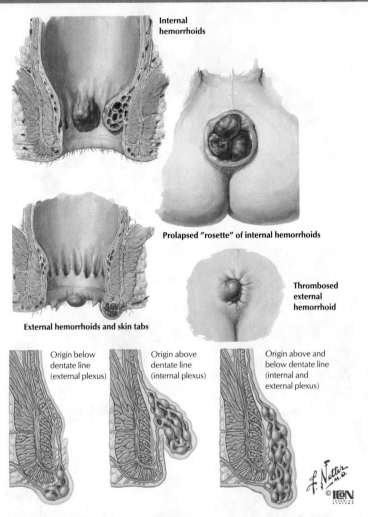

Internal hemorrhoids

Prolapsed "rosette" of internal hemorrhoids

Thrombosed external hemorrhoid

External hemorrhoids and skin tabs

Origin below dentate line (external plexus)

Origin above dentate line (internal plexus)

Origin above and below dentate line (internal and external plexus)

Hemorrhoids are symptomatic varicose dilations of submucosal veins that protrude into the anal canal and/or extend through the anus.

CHARACTERISTIC	DESCRIPTION
Types	Internal: dilations of veins of internal rectal plexus External: dilations of veins of external rectal plexus Mixed: combination of internal and external
Prevalence	50-80% of all Americans; more common after pregnancy
Signs and symptoms	Perianal swelling, itching, pain, rectal bleeding, constipation, hematochezia, inflammation
Risk factors	Pregnancy, obesity, chronic cough, constipation, heavy lifting, sedentary work or lifestyle, hepatic disease, colon malignancy, portal hypertension, anal intercourse

Pelvic Cavity: Nerves

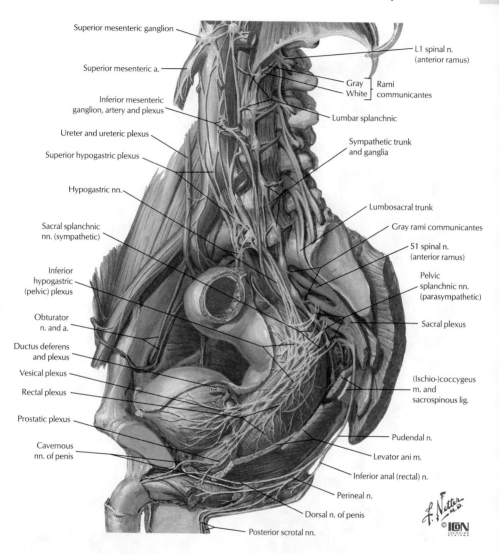

Superior mesenteric ganglion

Superior mesenteric a.

Inferior mesenteric ganglion, artery and plexus

Ureter and ureteric plexus

Superior hypogastric plexus

Hypogastric nn.

Sacral splanchnic nn. (sympathetic)

Inferior hypogastric (pelvic) plexus

Obturator n. and a.

Ductus deferens and plexus

Vesical plexus

Rectal plexus

Prostatic plexus

Cavernous nn. of penis

L1 spinal n. (anterior ramus)

Gray ⎫ Rami
White ⎭ communicantes

Lumbar splanchnic

Sympathetic trunk and ganglia

Lumbosacral trunk

Gray rami communicantes

S1 spinal n. (anterior ramus)

Pelvic splanchnic nn. (parasympathetic)

Sacral plexus

(Ischio-)coccygeus m. and sacrospinous lig.

Pudendal n.

Levator ani m.

Inferior anal (rectal) n.

Perineal n.

Dorsal n. of penis

Posterior scrotal nn.

NERVE	INNERVATION
Lumbar splanchnics	From L1 to L2 or L3; sympathetics to hypogastric plexus (superior and inferior) to innervate hindgut derivatives and pelvic reproductive viscera
Sacral splanchnics	From L1 to L2 or L3: sympathetics to inferior hypogastric plexus that first travel down the sympathetic chain before synapsing in the plexus
Pelvic splanchnics	From S2 to S4: parasympathetics to inferior hypogastric plexus to innervate hindgut derivatives and pelvic reproductive viscera
Inferior hypogastric plexus	Plexus of nerves (splanchnics) and ganglia where sympathetic and parasympathetic preganglionic fibers synapse
Pudendal nerve	From S2 to S4: somatic nerve that innervates skin and skeletal muscle of pelvic diaphragm and perineum (from sacral plexus)

Pelvic Cavity: Lymphatics

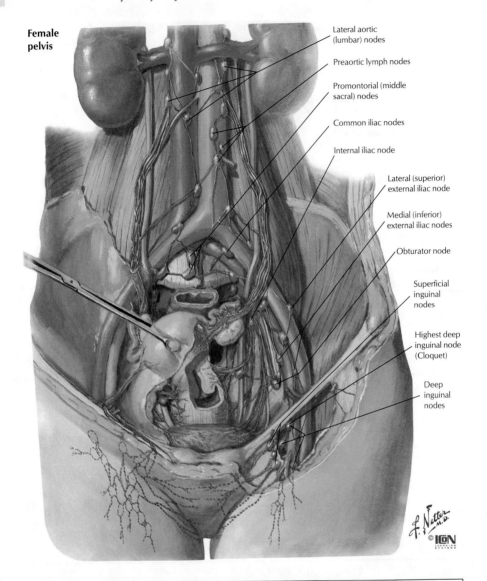

Female pelvis

Lateral aortic (lumbar) nodes

Preaortic lymph nodes

Promontorial (middle sacral) nodes

Common iliac nodes

Internal iliac node

Lateral (superior) external iliac node

Medial (inferior) external iliac nodes

Obturator node

Superficial inguinal nodes

Highest deep inguinal node (Cloquet)

Deep inguinal nodes

LYMPH NODE	DRAINAGE
Superficial inguinal	Receive lymph from perineum (and lower limb and abdomen) and deep pelvic viscera and drain it to external iliac nodes
Deep inguinal	Receive lymph from perineum (and lower limb) and drain it to external iliac nodes
Internal iliac	Receive lymph from pelvic viscera and drain it along iliac nodes, ultimately to reach aortic (lumbar) nodes
External iliac	Convey lymph along iliac nodes to reach aortic (lumbar) nodes
Gonadal lymphatics	Drain lymph from gonads directly to aortic (lumbar) nodes

Perineum: Male

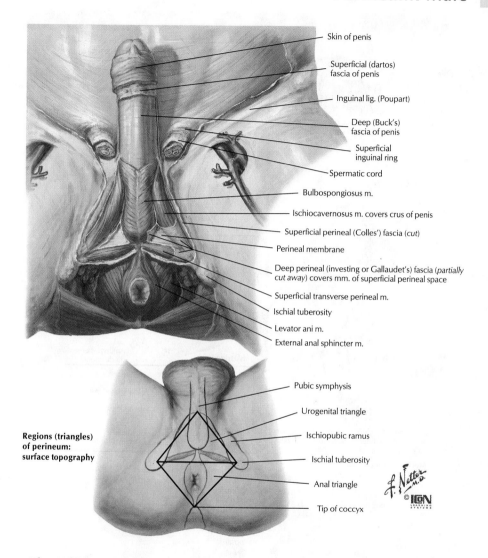

Skin of penis

Superficial (dartos) fascia of penis

Inguinal lig. (Poupart)

Deep (Buck's) fascia of penis

Superficial inguinal ring

Spermatic cord

Bulbospongiosus m.

Ischiocavernosus m. covers crus of penis

Superficial perineal (Colles') fascia (*cut*)

Perineal membrane

Deep perineal (investing or Gallaudet's) fascia (*partially cut away*) covers mm. of superficial perineal space

Superficial transverse perineal m.

Ischial tuberosity

Levator ani m.

External anal sphincter m.

Pubic symphysis

Urogenital triangle

Ischiopubic ramus

Ischial tuberosity

Anal triangle

Tip of coccyx

Regions (triangles) of perineum: surface topography

The perineum, a diamond-shaped region between the thighs, can be divided into an anterior urogenital triangle and a posterior anal triangle. Perineal boundaries include the

Pubic symphysis anteriorly
Ischial tuberosities laterally
Coccyx posteriorly

Muscles of the superficial perineal space are the skeletal type and include

Ischiocavernosus: surround the corpus cavernosum (penile crus; erectile tissue)
Bulbospongiosus: surround the bulb of the penis (erectile tissue)
Superficial transverse perineal (STP): stabilizes the central tendon of the perineum

The perineal central tendon is an important anchoring structure for the perineum, and the bulbospongiosus, STP, levator ani, and external anal sphincter all arise from it. Fat and fibrous tissue fill the ischioanal fossa.

Clinical Correlation

Erectile Dysfunction   *Anatomy on pp. 507, 511*

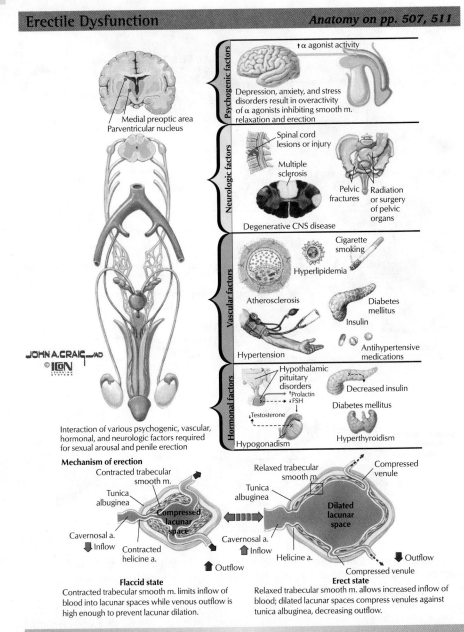

↑α agonist activity

Psychogenic factors
Depression, anxiety, and stress disorders result in overactivity of α agonists inhibiting smooth m. relaxation and erection

Medial preoptic area
Parventricular nucleus

Neurologic factors
Spinal cord lesions or injury

Multiple sclerosis

Pelvic fractures

Radiation or surgery of pelvic organs

Degenerative CNS disease

Vascular factors
Cigarette smoking

Hyperlipidemia

Atherosclerosis

Diabetes mellitus

Insulin

Hypertension

Antihypertensive medications

JOHN A. CRAIG—AD
©ICON LEARNING SYSTEMS

Hormonal factors
Hypothalamic pituitary disorders
↑Prolactin
↓FSH
Decreased insulin

↓Testosterone

Diabetes mellitus

Hypogonadism

Hyperthyroidism

Interaction of various psychogenic, vascular, hormonal, and neurologic factors required for sexual arousal and penile erection

Mechanism of erection

Contracted trabecular smooth m.

Tunica albuginea

Compressed lacunar space

Cavernosal a.
⬇ Inflow

Contracted helicine a.

⬆ Outflow

Relaxed trabecular smooth m.

Tunica albuginea

Compressed venule

Dilated lacunar space

Cavernosal a.
⬆ Inflow

Helicine a.

⬇ Outflow

Compressed venule

Flaccid state
Contracted trabecular smooth m. limits inflow of blood into lacunar spaces while venous outflow is high enough to prevent lacunar dilation.

Erect state
Relaxed trabecular smooth m. allows increased inflow of blood; dilated lacunar spaces compress venules against tunica albuginea, decreasing outflow.

Erectile dysfunction (ED) is an inability to achieve and/or maintain penile erection sufficient for sexual intercourse. Its occurrence increases with age; its probable causes are illustrated. Normal erectile function occurs when a sexual stimulus causes release of nitric oxide from nerve endings and endothelial cells of the corpus cavernosum, thus relaxing smooth muscle tone and increasing blood flow, which compresses veins in the tunica albuginea and engorges erectile tissues. Available drugs aid corpus smooth muscle relaxation.

Perineum: Deeper Structures of the Male Perineum

The deep perineal space lies superior to the superficial space, its contents including the external urethral sphincter, the often indistinct deep transverse perineal muscle, and the fascial layers covering these skeletal muscles (old term: urogenital diaphragm). Most important, the external urethral sphincter is under voluntary control and is innervated by the perineal nerve, a branch of the pudendal nerve.

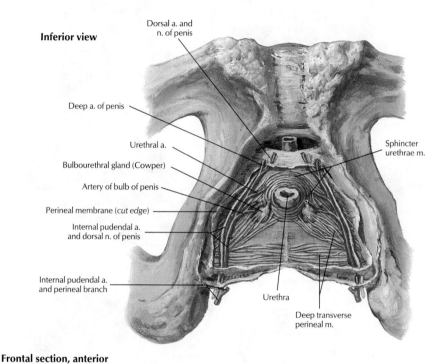

Inferior view

Dorsal a. and n. of penis

Deep a. of penis

Urethral a.

Bulbourethral gland (Cowper)

Artery of bulb of penis

Perineal membrane (*cut edge*)

Internal pudendal a. and dorsal n. of penis

Internal pudendal a. and perineal branch

Sphincter urethrae m.

Urethra

Deep transverse perineal m.

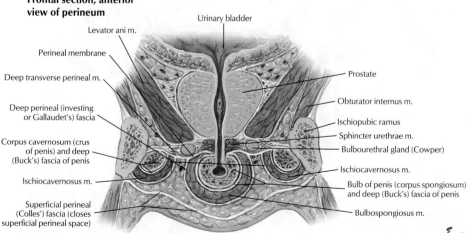

Frontal section, anterior view of perineum

Levator ani m.

Perineal membrane

Deep transverse perineal m.

Deep perineal (investing or Gallaudet's) fascia

Corpus cavernosum (crus of penis) and deep (Buck's) fascia of penis

Ischiocavernosus m.

Superficial perineal (Colles') fascia (closes superficial perineal space)

Urinary bladder

Prostate

Obturator internus m.

Ischiopubic ramus

Sphincter urethrae m.

Bulbourethral gland (Cowper)

Ischiocavernosus m.

Bulb of penis (corpus spongiosum) and deep (Buck's) fascia of penis

Bulbospongiosus m.

Clinical Correlation

Urethral Trauma in the Male   *Anatomy on pp. 498, 509, 511*

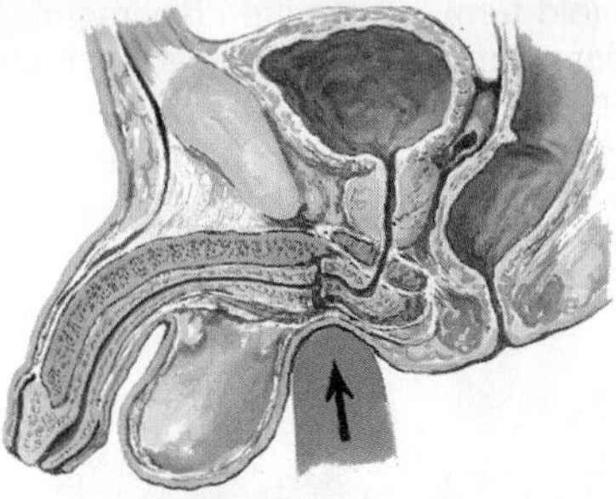

Straddle Injury

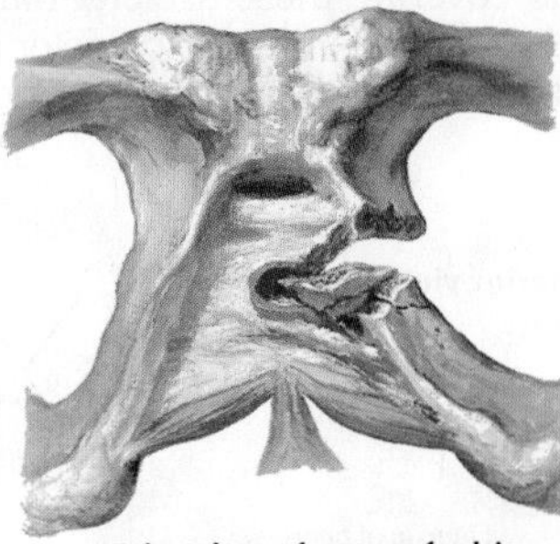

Injury due to fracture of pelvis

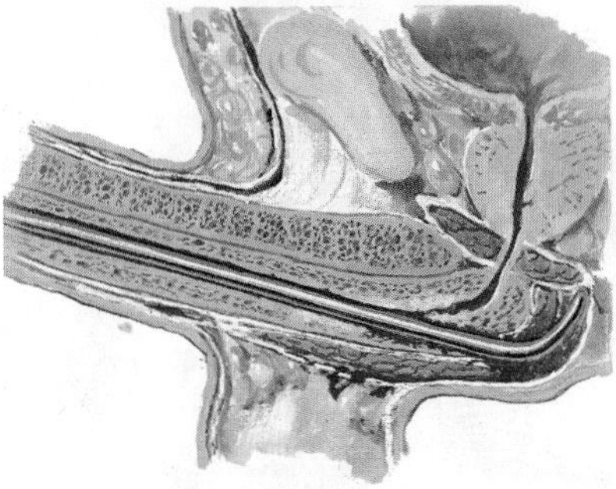

Injury from within (false passage)

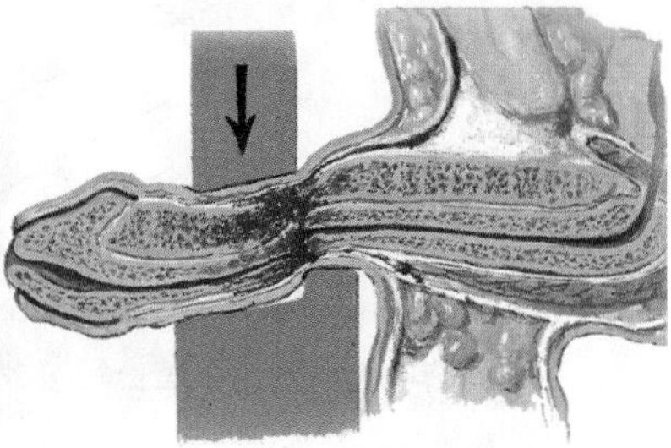

Direct external trauma

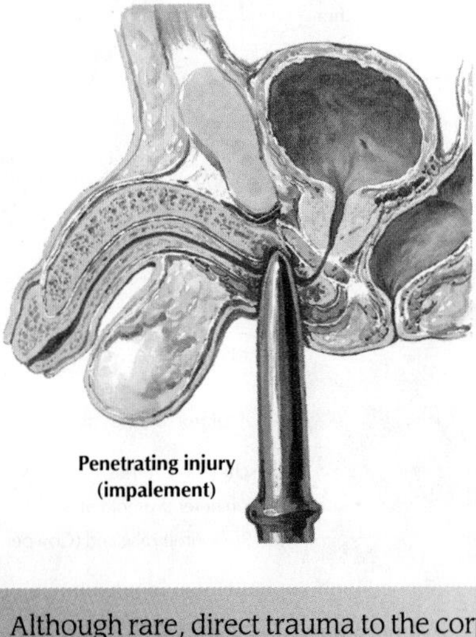

Penetrating injury
(impalement)

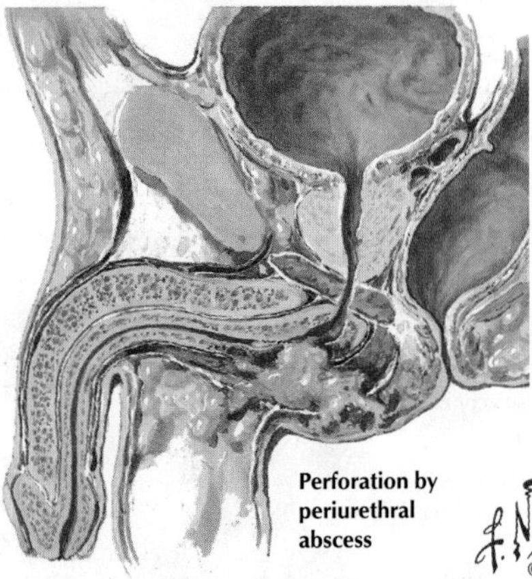

Perforation by
periurethral
abscess

Although rare, direct trauma to the corpora cavernosa can occur. Rupture of the thick tunica albuginea usually involves Buck's fascia (deep fascia of penis), and blood extravasates quickly, which causes penile swelling. Urethral rupture is more common and involves one of three mechanisms:
- External trauma or penetrating injury
- Internal injury (by catheter, instrument, or foreign body)
- Spontaneous rupture (increased intraurethral pressure or periurethral inflammation)

Clinical Correlation

Urine Extravasation
Anatomy on pp. 494, 498, 511

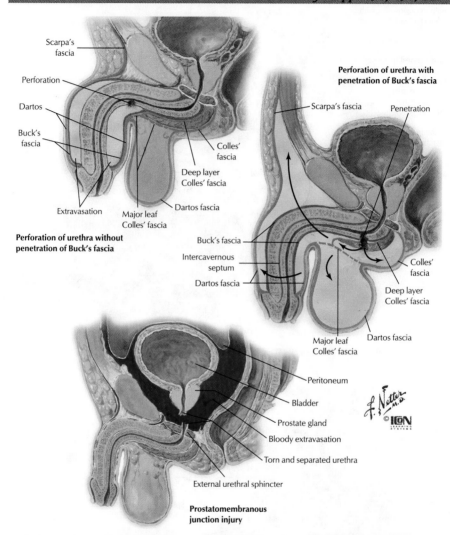

Scarpa's fascia

Perforation

Dartos

Buck's fascia

Extravasation

Major leaf Colles' fascia

Dartos fascia

Major leaf Colles' fascia

Deep layer Colles' fascia

Colles' fascia

Perforation of urethra without penetration of Buck's fascia

Perforation of urethra with penetration of Buck's fascia

Scarpa's fascia

Penetration

Buck's fascia

Intercavernous septum

Dartos fascia

Colles' fascia

Deep layer Colles' fascia

Dartos fascia

Major leaf Colles' fascia

Peritoneum

Bladder

Prostate gland

Bloody extravasation

Torn and separated urethra

External urethral sphincter

Prostatomembranous junction injury

Rupture of the male urethra can lead to urine extravasation into various pelvic or perineal spaces that are largely limited by fascial planes.

INJURY SITE	CONSEQUENCES
Penile urethra, Buck's fascia intact	Localized swelling confined to penis
Penile urethra, Buck's fascia ruptured	Eventual collection of urine deep to Colles' fascia (superficial perineal fascia); perineum: superficial pouch; penis; scrotum: deep to dartos (superficial) fascia; lower abdominal wall: deep to Scarpa's fascia
Prostatomembranous junction	Potential injury with anterior pelvic fractures, which may lead to retroperitoneal hematoma and urine extravasation

Perineum: Female

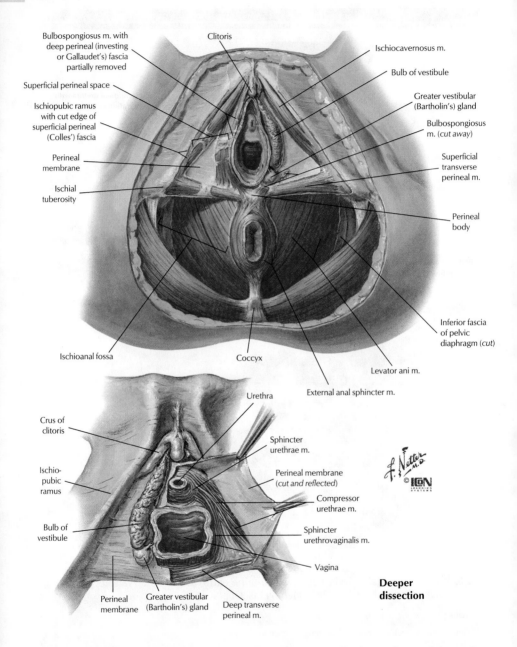

Bulbospongiosus m. with deep perineal (investing or Gallaudet's) fascia partially removed

Superficial perineal space

Ischiopubic ramus with cut edge of superficial perineal (Colles') fascia

Perineal membrane

Ischial tuberosity

Clitoris

Ischiocavernosus m.

Bulb of vestibule

Greater vestibular (Bartholin's) gland

Bulbospongiosus m. (*cut away*)

Superficial transverse perineal m.

Perineal body

Inferior fascia of pelvic diaphragm (*cut*)

Ischioanal fossa

Coccyx

Levator ani m.

External anal sphincter m.

Crus of clitoris

Ischio-pubic ramus

Bulb of vestibule

Urethra

Sphincter urethrae m.

Perineal membrane (*cut and reflected*)

Compressor urethrae m.

Sphincter urethrovaginalis m.

Vagina

Perineal membrane

Greater vestibular (Bartholin's) gland

Deep transverse perineal m.

Deeper dissection

The muscles and structures of the female perineum are similar to those of the male except that the vagina bisects the bulbospongiosus muscle and bulb, which results in a split muscle and bulb of the vestibule (erectile tissue) surrounding the vulva (region defined by labia minora). The ischiocavernosus muscle surrounds the crus of the clitoris (erectile tissue). The central tendon is especially important in the female because it maintains the integrity of the perineum.

Perineum: Nerves

Innervation of the perineum is by the pudendal nerve (S2-S4) and its branches (inferior rectal and perineal nerves); it enters the perineum via the pudendal canal. The perineal nerve divides into superficial and deep branches. The pudendal nerve, which terminates as the dorsal nerve of the clitoris (or penis), is a somatic nerve (innervates skin and skeletal muscle). Coursing with these nerves are branches from the internal pudendal artery: inferior rectal, perineal, labial (scrotal), vestibule (bulb), and deep and dorsal arteries of the clitoris (penis).

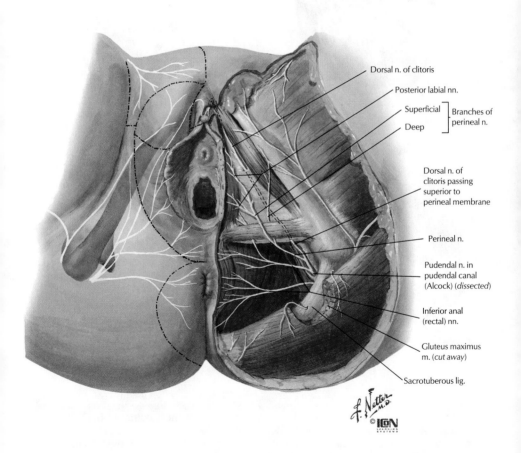

Dorsal n. of clitoris

Posterior labial nn.

Superficial ⎤ Branches of
Deep   ⎦ perineal n.

Dorsal n. of clitoris passing superior to perineal membrane

Perineal n.

Pudendal n. in pudendal canal (Alcock) (*dissected*)

Inferior anal (rectal) nn.

Gluteus maximus m. (*cut away*)

Sacrotuberous lig.

Clinical Correlation

Sexually Transmitted Diseases   *Anatomy on pp. 509, 514*

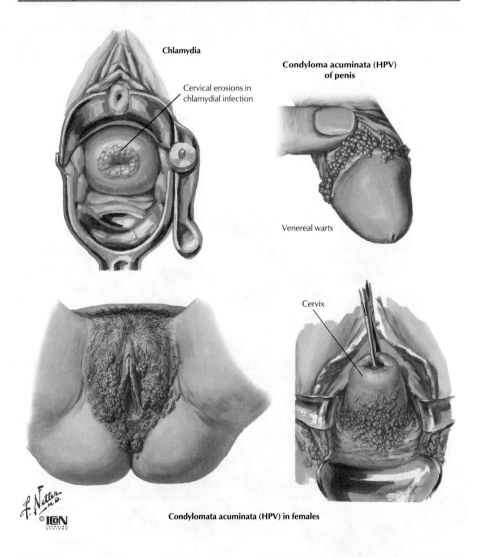

Chlamydia

Cervical erosions in chlamydial infection

Condyloma acuminata (HPV) of penis

Venereal warts

Cervix

Condylomata acuminata (HPV) in females

HPV and *Chlamydia trachomatis* infections are the two most common STDs in the United States. HPV infections (>90% of which are benign) are characterized in both sexes by warty lesions caused most often by serotypes 6 and 11. The virus is commonly spread by skin-to-skin contact; the incubation period is 3 weeks to 8 months. HPV is highly associated with cervical cancer in women. Chlamydia is the most common bacterial STD, with antibodies present in up to 40% of all sexually active women (which suggests previous infection). Infected structures include the urethra, cervix, greater vestibular glands, and uterine tubes in women and the urethra, epididymis, and prostate in men. A common risk factor for both STDs is having multiple sexual partners.

Clinical Correlation

Sexually Transmitted HIV

Anatomy on pp. 509, 514

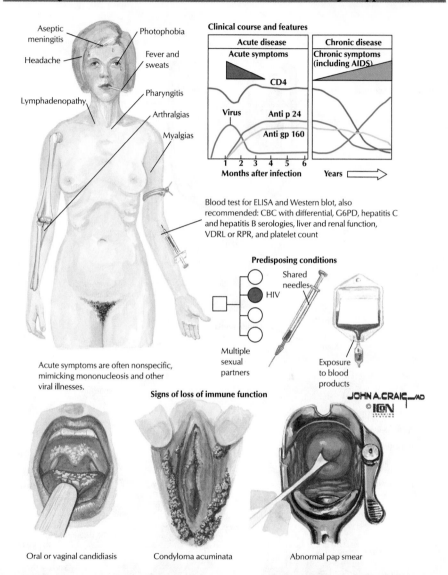

Aseptic meningitis

Photophobia

Headache

Fever and sweats

Lymphadenopathy

Pharyngitis

Arthralgias

Myalgias

Clinical course and features

Acute disease	Chronic disease
Acute symptoms	Chronic symptoms (including AIDS)

CD4

Virus   Anti p 24

Anti gp 160

1 2 3 4 5 6
Months after infection   Years ⟹

Blood test for ELISA and Western blot, also recommended: CBC with differential, G6PD, hepatitis C and hepatitis B serologies, liver and renal function, VDRL or RPR, and platelet count

Predisposing conditions

Shared needles

HIV

Multiple sexual partners

Exposure to blood products

Acute symptoms are often nonspecific, mimicking mononucleosis and other viral illnesses.

JOHN A. CRAIG—AD
© ICN

Signs of loss of immune function

Oral or vaginal candidiasis

Condyloma acuminata

Abnormal pap smear

HIV-1 and HIV-2, which infect CD4⁺ white cells, cause acquired immunodeficiency syndrome (AIDS), although AIDS does not develop in everyone who is HIV positive. Sexual contact with an HIV-infected person is a common mode of transmission; blood, blood-derived products, and transfer from infected mothers to fetuses and infants also spread the disease. The initial presentation often mimics mononucleosis or flulike symptoms, including fever, fatigue, rash, headache, lymphadenopathy (cervical, axillary, and inguinal nodes), pharyngitis, diarrhea, and vomiting. More than 39 million people worldwide have HIV infection or AIDS.

Embryology: Urogenital Derivatives

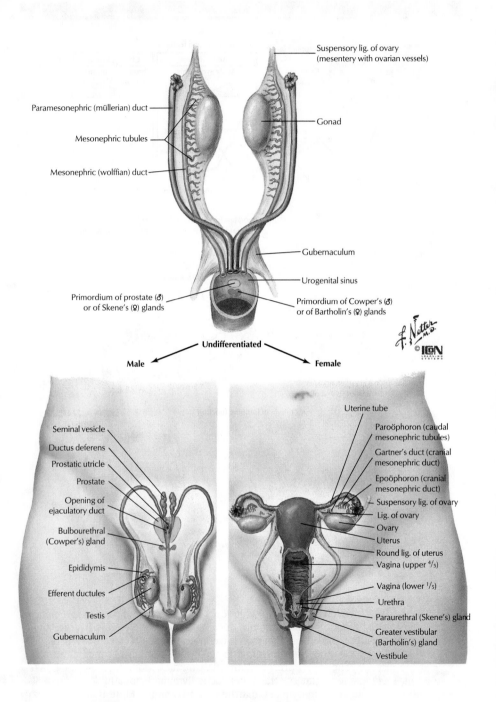

Suspensory lig. of ovary
(mesentery with ovarian vessels)

Paramesonephric (müllerian) duct

Gonad

Mesonephric tubules

Mesonephric (wolffian) duct

Gubernaculum

Urogenital sinus

Primordium of prostate (♂)
or of Skene's (♀) glands

Primordium of Cowper's (♂)
or of Bartholin's (♀) glands

Undifferentiated

Male

Female

Seminal vesicle

Ductus deferens

Prostatic utricle

Prostate

Opening of
ejaculatory duct

Bulbourethral
(Cowper's) gland

Epididymis

Efferent ductules

Testis

Gubernaculum

Uterine tube

Paroöphoron (caudal
mesonephric tubules)

Gartner's duct (cranial
mesonephric duct)

Epoöphoron (cranial
mesonephric duct)

Suspensory lig. of ovary

Lig. of ovary

Ovary

Uterus

Round lig. of uterus

Vagina (upper 4/5)

Vagina (lower 1/5)

Urethra

Paraurethral (Skene's) gland

Greater vestibular
(Bartholin's) gland

Vestibule

Embryology: Urogenital Derivatives (continued)

MALE	FEMALE
From the Urogenital Sinus	
Urinary bladder Urethra (except navicular fossa) Prostate gland Bulbourethral glands	Urinary bladder Urethra Lower vagina (and vaginal epithelium) Vestibule Greater vestibular/urethral glands
From the Mesonephric Duct and Tubules	
Efferent ductules Duct of epididymis Ductus deferens Ejaculatory duct Seminal vesicles	Degenerates (Ureter, renal pelvis, calices, and collecting tubules in both sexes)
From the Paramesonephric Duct	
Degenerates	Uterine tubes, uterus, upper vagina

Embryology: Homologues of External Genital Organs

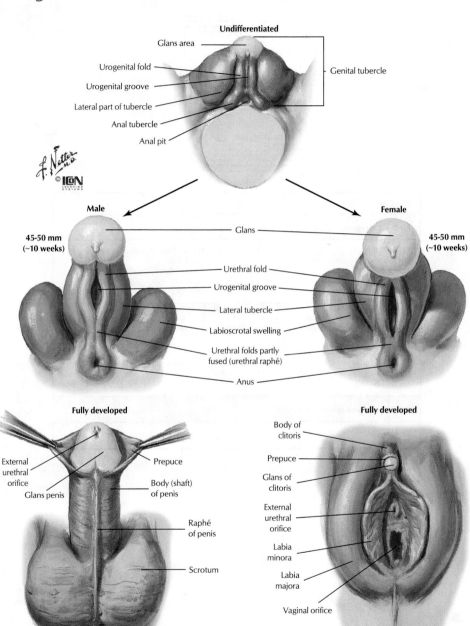

Undifferentiated

Glans area

Urogenital fold

Urogenital groove

Lateral part of tubercle

Anal tubercle

Anal pit

Genital tubercle

Male

45-50 mm (~10 weeks)

Female

45-50 mm (~10 weeks)

Glans

Urethral fold

Urogenital groove

Lateral tubercle

Labioscrotal swelling

Urethral folds partly fused (urethral raphé)

Anus

Fully developed

External urethral orifice

Glans penis

Prepuce

Body (shaft) of penis

Raphé of penis

Scrotum

Fully developed

Body of clitoris

Prepuce

Glans of clitoris

External urethral orifice

Labia minora

Labia majora

Vaginal orifice

Perineal raphé

Perianal tissues

Embryology: Homologues of External Genital Organs (continued)

MALE	FEMALE
From the Genital Tubercle/Phallus	
Penis:	*Clitoris:*
Glans penis	Glans clitoridis
Corpora cavernosum penis	Corpora cavernosa clitoridis
Corpus spongiosum penis	Bulb of vestibule
From the Urogenital Folds	
Ventral aspect of penis	Labia minora
Most of the penile urethra	Perineal raphé
Perineal raphé	Perianal tissue (and external anal
Perianal tissue (and external sphincter)	sphincter)
From the Labioscrotal Folds	
Scrotum	Labia majora
From the Gubernaculum	
Gubernaculum testis	Ovarian ligament
	Round ligament of uterus

Clinical Correlation

Hypospadias and Epispadias

Anatomy on p. 520

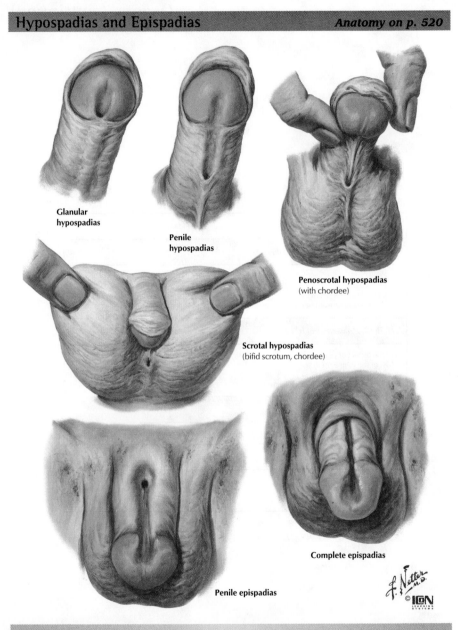

Glanular
hypospadias

Penile
hypospadias

Penoscrotal hypospadias
(with chordee)

Scrotal hypospadias
(bifid scrotum, chordee)

Complete epispadias

Penile epispadias

Hypospadias and epispadias are congenital anomalies of the penis. Hypospadias is far more common (1 in 300 male births) and is characterized by failure of fusion of the urogenital folds, which normally seal the penile (spongy) urethra within the penis. The defect occurs on the ventral aspect of the penis (corpus spongiosum). Hypospadias may be associated with inguinal hernias and undescended testes. Epispadias (rare: 1 in 30,000 male births) is characterized by a urethral orifice on the dorsal aspect of the penis.

Clinical Correlation

Uterine Anomalies
Anatomy on pp. 518, 519

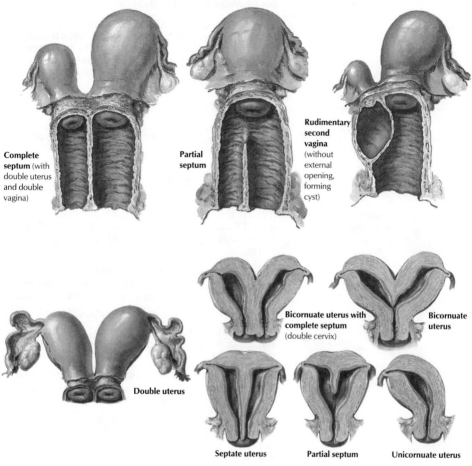

Complete septum (with double uterus and double vagina)

Partial septum

Rudimentary second vagina (without external opening, forming cyst)

Double uterus

Bicornuate uterus with complete septum (double cervix)

Bicornuate uterus

Septate uterus

Partial septum

Unicornuate uterus

Incomplete fusion of the distal paramesonephric (müllerian) ducts can lead to septation of the uterus or partial or complete duplication of the uterus (bicornuate uterus). The prevalence is up to 3% for septate uterine anomalies but only approximately 0.1% for bicornuate anomalies. If only one paramesonephric duct persists and develops, a unicornuate uterus results. These conditions seem to be transmitted by a polygenic or multifactorial pattern and have a higher risk for recurrent spontaneous abortions (15-25%), premature labor, uterine pain, breech or transverse deliveries, and dysmenorrhea.

Review Questions

What dermatome level is demarcated by the umbilicus?	T10.
What kind of joint is the sacroiliac joint?	Plane synovial joint that allows for little movement but provides rotational stability.
What important spaces are created by the sacrospinous ligament?	The greater and lesser sciatic foramina. These foramina provide an avenue for structures passing from the pelvis into the gluteal region and posterior thigh, and an avenue for the pudendal vessels and nerves to enter the pudendal canal and pass to the perineum.
What muscles make up the pelvic diaphragm?	Levator ani and coccygeus.
What is the origin (proximal attachment) of the levator ani muscle?	Pubis, tendinous arch of the obturator fascia, and ischial spine.
What are the descriptive subdivisions of the uterus?	Body (fundus and isthmus) and cervix.
Why is the rectouterine pouch (of Douglas) important?	It is the lowest point in the female pelvis (peritoneal fluids may collect here), and access to drain these fluids is possible via the posterior vaginal fornix.
What are the descriptive subdivisions of the broad ligament?	Mesovarium (surrounds and suspends the ovary), mesosalpinx (surrounds and suspends the uterine tubes), and mesometrium (surrounds and supports the uterus).
Why are UTIs more common in women than in men?	The urethra is shorter in women and opens into the vulva, which provides a moist, warm environment for bacteria to colonize.
What is stress incontinence?	Involuntary loss of urine associated with increased intraabdominal pressure, as occurs when lifting, coughing, or sneezing.
What structures may be involved in stress incontinence in women?	Stress incontinence may result from a loss of functional integrity of the pubovesical ligaments, vesicocervical fascia, levator ani, and/or urethral sphincter.
Uterine prolapse may occur with the loss of support of which important structures?	Cardinal and uterosacral ligaments and the levator ani muscle.
What is the origin of cervical cancer?	A neoplasm of the squamous epithelium (85-90%) at the transitional zone. HPV is a common risk factor.
What is the most common type of cancer of the female reproductive tract?	Endometrial carcinoma.
What is the most common type of ovarian carcinoma, and what are common routes of metastatic spread?	Surface epithelial-stromal tumors are most common (85-90% of all malignancies). Peritoneal seeding is the usual route of spread, but hematogenous spread to lungs and liver and lymphatic spread to the pelvic and aortic nodes may also occur.

Review Questions

Which branches of the internal iliac artery arise from its posterior division?	Iliolumbar, lateral sacral, and superior gluteal arteries.
Why might a varicocele resolve with the patient recumbent?	Most varicoceles occur on the left side, and when the patient is recumbent, the venous return to the left renal vein via the left testicular vein is facilitated by not having to move against gravity, thus relieving the pressure in the dilated pampiniform plexus of veins. If an abdominal mass compresses the left testicular or renal vein, causing varicocele, the condition may not resolve in the recumbent position.
How does the urinary bladder empty itself?	Appropriate central nervous system reflexes initiate voiding via stimulation of pelvic splanchnic nerves to the bladder, which cause contraction of the detrusor smooth muscle of the bladder wall. Voluntary relaxation of external sphincter urethrae muscle tone occurs in conjunction with the detrusor contraction but is mediated by the somatic nervous system. In males, sympathetic relaxation of the internal sphincter (females lack an internal sphincter) also occurs with detrusor muscle contraction.
What are descriptive subdivisions of the male urethra?	Prostatic, membranous, and spongy (penile).
What are the three most common sites of bony metastases of prostatic carcinoma?	Pelvis-sacrum, spine, and femur.
What is the innervation of the external anal sphincter?	Inferior anal (rectal) nerves from the pudendal nerve (S2-S4).
Which rectal veins are involved in portocaval anastomoses?	The inferior and middle rectal veins (tributaries of the internal iliac vein—caval system) anastomose with the superior rectal vein from the inferior mesenteric vein, a tributary of the portal venous system.
What are common causes of hemorrhoids?	Constipation and straining (increased intraabdominal pressure), portal hypertension, and pregnancy.
What is the parasympathetic innervation of the pelvic viscera?	Parasympathetic preganglionic fibers arise from S2 to S4 via pelvic splanchnics that course to the inferior hypogastric plexus (pelvic), synapse there, and then innervate pelvic viscera (smooth muscle and glands).
Lymphatic spread of cancer cells from a malignant ovarian tumor may involve the aortic (lumbar) lymph nodes directly. Why?	The lymphatic vessels of the ovary follow the ovarian artery directly back to the abdominal aorta and infiltrate aortic nodes in this region.
Why is the central tendon of the perineum important?	It anchors the perineum because it provides for the attachment of many skeletal muscles of the perineum as well as fascial layers.

Review Questions

What is a common cause of erectile dysfunction in males?	Loss of functionality in the nerves that relax the smooth muscle tone of the corpus cavernosum, which thus impedes blood flow into cavernous erectile tissue. Current medications facilitate smooth muscle relaxation and increase blood flow.
What are the two most common STDs in the United States?	HPV and chlamydia. HPV is also associated with cervical cancer.
What is hypospadias?	A congenital anomaly of the penis characterized by the failure of the urogenital folds to fuse. Consequently, a portion of the spongy urethra may be exposed on the ventral aspect of the body of the penis.
What is the fate of the paramesonephric duct in males and females?	In males, it essentially degenerates but in females forms the uterine tubes, uterus, and upper vagina.

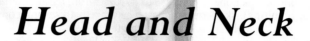

Head and Neck

8

Introduction The head protects the brain, participates in communication and expresses our emotions, and houses the special senses. It consists of the cranium, orbits, ears, nasal cavities, and oral cavity. It is largely innervated by the cranial nerves. The neck connects the head to the thorax and is the conduit for visceral structures, which pass cranially or caudally within the tightly partitioned fascial sleeves of the neck.

Surface Anatomy: Key Landmarks

Glabella: smooth prominence on frontal bone above root of the nose
Zygomatic bone: cheek bone, vulnerable to fractures from facial trauma
Ear (auricle, or pinna): skin-covered elastic cartilage with several consistent features including the helix, antihelix, tragus, and antitragus
Philtrum: midline infranasal depression of the upper lip; distorted with cleft lip
Nasolabial sulcus: line between nose and corner of lip; less prominent with paralysis of facial muscles, e.g., Bell's palsy
Thyroid cartilage: laryngeal prominence, or "Adam's apple," vulnerable to trauma
Jugular (suprasternal) notch: midline depression between the two sternal heads of the sternocleidomastoid muscle (SCM)

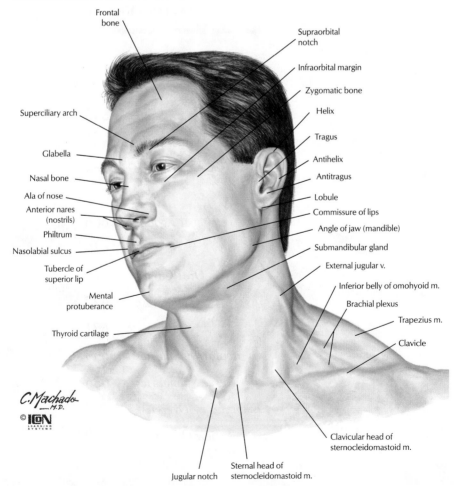

Frontal bone
Supraorbital notch
Infraorbital margin
Zygomatic bone
Helix
Superciliary arch
Tragus
Glabella
Antihelix
Nasal bone
Antitragus
Ala of nose
Lobule
Anterior nares (nostrils)
Commissure of lips
Philtrum
Angle of jaw (mandible)
Nasolabial sulcus
Submandibular gland
Tubercle of superior lip
External jugular v.
Mental protuberance
Inferior belly of omohyoid m.
Brachial plexus
Thyroid cartilage
Trapezius m.
Clavicle
Clavicular head of sternocleidomastoid m.
Sternal head of sternocleidomastoid m.
Jugular notch

C. Machado
—M.D.
© ICN LEARNING SYSTEMS

Neck: Cervical Plexus

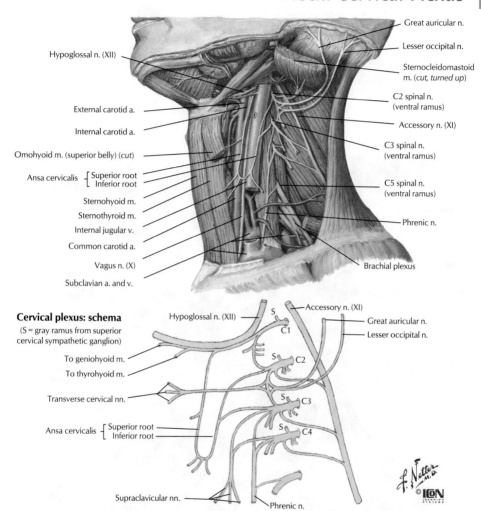

Great auricular n.

Lesser occipital n.

Hypoglossal n. (XII)

Sternocleidomastoid m. (cut, turned up)

C2 spinal n. (ventral ramus)

External carotid a.

Accessory n. (XI)

Internal carotid a.

C3 spinal n. (ventral ramus)

Omohyoid m. (superior belly) (cut)

Ansa cervicalis { Superior root / Inferior root

C5 spinal n. (ventral ramus)

Sternohyoid m.

Sternothyroid m.

Internal jugular v.

Phrenic n.

Common carotid a.

Vagus n. (X)

Brachial plexus

Subclavian a. and v.

Cervical plexus: schema
(S = gray ramus from superior cervical sympathetic ganglion)

Accessory n. (XI)

Hypoglossal n. (XII)

S / C1

Great auricular n.

Lesser occipital n.

To geniohyoid m.

To thyrohyoid m.

S / C2

Transverse cervical nn.

S / C3

Ansa cervicalis { Superior root / Inferior root

S / C4

Supraclavicular nn.

Phrenic n.

The cervical nerve plexus is derived from ventral rami of C1 to C4 spinal nerves.

NERVE	INNERVATION
C1	Travels with CN XII to innervate geniohyoid and thyrohyoid muscles
Ansa cervicalis	Is C1-C3 loop that sends motor branches to infrahyoid muscles
Lesser occipital	From C2, is sensory to neck and scalp posterior to ear
Great auricular	From C2 to C3, is sensory over parotid gland and posterior ear
Transverse cervical	From C2 to C3, is sensory to anterior triangle of neck
Supraclavicular	From C3 to C4, are anterior, middle, and posterior sensory branches to skin over clavicle and shoulder region
Phrenic	From C3 to C5, is motor and sensory nerve to diaphragm
Motor branches	Are small twigs that supply scalene muscles, levator scapulae, and prevertebral muscles

Neck: Muscles

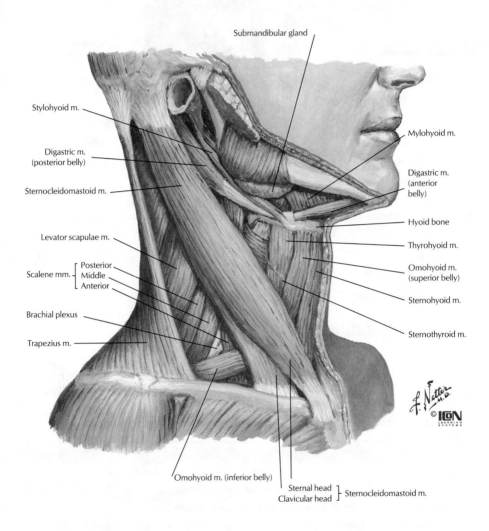

Submandibular gland

Stylohyoid m.

Digastric m. (posterior belly)

Sternocleidomastoid m.

Levator scapulae m.

Scalene mm. { Posterior Middle Anterior

Brachial plexus

Trapezius m.

Mylohyoid m.

Digastric m. (anterior belly)

Hyoid bone

Thyrohyoid m.

Omohyoid m. (superior belly)

Sternohyoid m.

Sternothyroid m.

Omohyoid m. (inferior belly)

Sternal head ⎤
Clavicular head ⎦ Sternocleidomastoid m.

Neck: Muscles (continued)

Muscles of the neck divide it into several triangles for descriptive purposes. The posterior triangle is bounded by the trapezius, SCM, and middle third of the clavicle. The anterior triangle is bounded by median line of the neck, anterior border of the SCM, and inferior border of the mandible. These major triangles can be further subdivided.

MUSCLE	ORIGIN	INSERTION	INNERVATION	MAIN ACTIONS
Sternocleido-mastoid	*Sternal head*: anterior surface of manubrium *Clavicular head*: medial third of clavicle	Mastoid process and lateral half of superior nuchal line	Spinal root of cranial nerve (CN) XI and C2-C3	Tilts head to one side, i.e., laterally flexes and rotates head so face is turned superiorly toward opposite side; acting together, muscles flex neck
Posterior scalene	Posterior tubercles of transverse processes of C4-C6	External border of second rib	C6-C8	Flexes neck laterally; elevates second rib
Middle scalene	Posterior tubercles of transverse processes of C2-C7	Superior surface of first rib	C3-C8	Flexes neck laterally; elevates first rib
Anterior scalene	Anterior tubercles of transverse processes of C3-C6	First rib	C5-C7	Flexes neck laterally; elevates first rib
Digastric	*Anterior belly*: digastric fossa of mandible *Posterior belly*: mastoid notch	Intermediate tendon to hyoid bone	*Anterior belly*: mylohyoid nerve, a branch of inferior alveolar nerve *Posterior belly*: facial nerve	Depresses mandible; raises hyoid bone and steadies it during swallowing and speaking
Sternohyoid	Manubrium of sternum and medial end of clavicle	Body of hyoid bone	C1-C3 from ansa cervicalis	Depresses hyoid bone after swallowing
Sternothyroid	Posterior surface of manubrium	Oblique line of thyroid cartilage	C2 and C3 from ansa cervicalis	Depresses larynx after swallowing
Thyrohyoid	Oblique line of thyroid cartilage	Body and greater horn of hyoid bone	C1 via hypoglossal nerve	Depresses hyoid bone and elevates larynx
Omohyoid	Superior border of scapula near suprascapular notch	Inferior border of hyoid bone	C1-C3 from ansa cervicalis	Depresses, retracts, and steadies hyoid bone
Mylohyoid	Mylohyoid line of mandible	Raphe and body of hyoid bone	Mylohyoid nerve, a branch of inferior alveolar nerve	Elevates hyoid bone, floor of mouth, and tongue during swallowing and speaking
Stylohyoid	Styloid process of temporal bone	Body of hyoid bone	Facial nerve	Elevates and retracts hyoid bone, thus elongating floor of mouth

Neck: Subclavian Artery

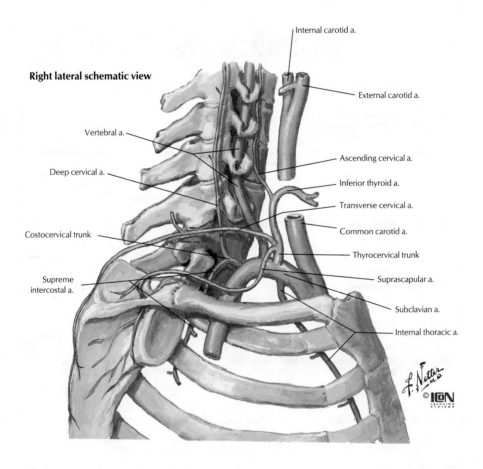

Right lateral schematic view

Internal carotid a.

External carotid a.

Vertebral a.

Ascending cervical a.

Deep cervical a.

Inferior thyroid a.

Transverse cervical a.

Common carotid a.

Costocervical trunk

Thyrocervical trunk

Supreme
intercostal a.

Suprascapular a.

Subclavian a.

Internal thoracic a.

Neck: Subclavian Artery (continued)

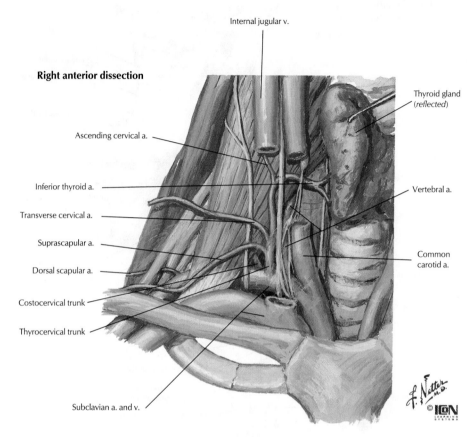

Internal jugular v.

Right anterior dissection

Thyroid gland
(reflected)

Ascending cervical a.

Inferior thyroid a.

Vertebral a.

Transverse cervical a.

Suprascapular a.

Dorsal scapular a.

Common
carotid a.

Costocervical trunk

Thyrocervical trunk

Subclavian a. and v.

The subclavian artery is divided for descriptive purposes into three parts by the anterior scalene muscle. Part 1 lies medial, part 2 lies posterior, and part 3 lies lateral to the anterior scalene muscle.

BRANCH	COURSE
Part 1	
Vertebral	Ascends through C6 to C1 transverse foramina and enters foramen magnum
Internal thoracic	Descend parasternally to anastomose with superior epigastric artery
Thyrocervical trunk	Gives rise to inferior thyroid, transverse cervical, and suprascapular arteries
Part 2	
Costocervical trunk	Gives rise to deep cervical and supreme intercostal arteries
Part 3	
Dorsal scapular	Is inconstant; may also arise from transverse cervical artery

Neck: Carotid Artery

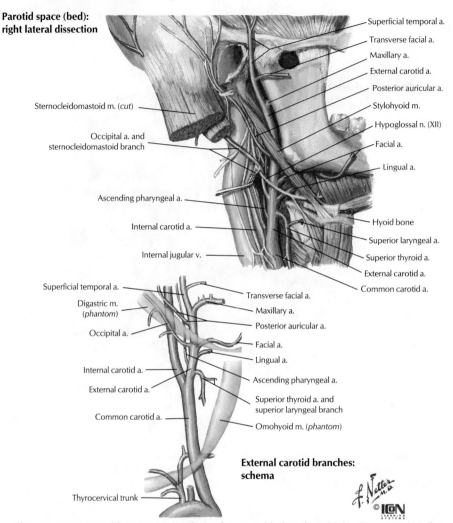

Parotid space (bed): right lateral dissection

Superficial temporal a.
Transverse facial a.
Maxillary a.
External carotid a.
Posterior auricular a.
Stylohyoid m.
Hypoglossal n. (XII)
Facial a.
Lingual a.

Sternocleidomastoid m. (cut)
Occipital a. and sternocleidomastoid branch

Ascending pharyngeal a.
Internal carotid a.
Internal jugular v.

Hyoid bone
Superior laryngeal a.
Superior thyroid a.
External carotid a.
Common carotid a.

Superficial temporal a.
Digastric m. (phantom)
Occipital a.
Internal carotid a.
External carotid a.
Common carotid a.

Transverse facial a.
Maxillary a.
Posterior auricular a.
Facial a.
Lingual a.
Ascending pharyngeal a.
Superior thyroid a. and superior laryngeal branch
Omohyoid m. (phantom)

External carotid branches: schema

Thyrocervical trunk

The common carotid artery ascends in the carotid sheath (which also contains the internal jugular vein and vagus nerve) and divides into the internal carotid (IC) artery (no branches in the neck) and external carotid artery (branches described in the table).

BRANCH	COURSE AND STRUCTURES SUPPLIED
Superior thyroid	Supplies thyroid gland, larynx, and infrahyoid muscles
Ascending pharyngeal	Supplies pharyngeal region, middle ear, meninges, and prevertebral muscles
Lingual	Passes deep to hyoglossus muscle to supply the tongue
Facial	Courses over the mandible and supplies the face
Occipital	Supplies SCM and anastomoses with costocervical trunk
Posterior auricular	Supplies region posterior to ear
Maxillary	Passes into infratemporal fossa (described later)
Superficial temporal	Supplies face, temporalis muscle, and lateral scalp

Neck: Fascial Layers

Cross section

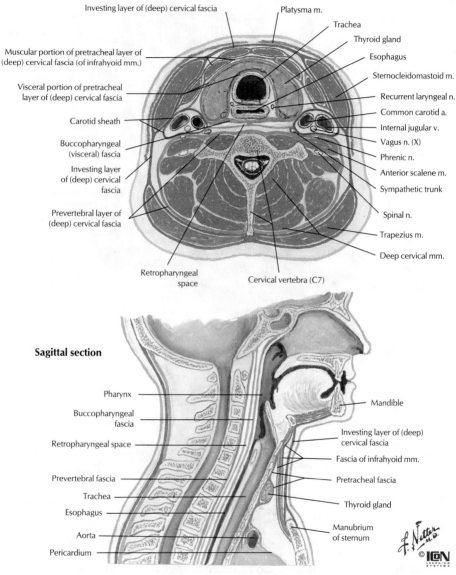

Investing layer of (deep) cervical fascia

Platysma m.

Trachea

Thyroid gland

Esophagus

Muscular portion of pretracheal layer of (deep) cervical fascia (of infrahyoid mm.)

Sternocleidomastoid m.

Visceral portion of pretracheal layer of (deep) cervical fascia

Recurrent laryngeal n.

Common carotid a.

Carotid sheath

Internal jugular v.

Buccopharyngeal (visceral) fascia

Vagus n. (X)

Phrenic n.

Investing layer of (deep) cervical fascia

Anterior scalene m.

Sympathetic trunk

Prevertebral layer of (deep) cervical fascia

Spinal n.

Trapezius m.

Deep cervical mm.

Retropharyngeal space

Cervical vertebra (C7)

Sagittal section

Pharynx

Mandible

Buccopharyngeal fascia

Investing layer of (deep) cervical fascia

Retropharyngeal space

Fascia of infrahyoid mm.

Prevertebral fascia

Pretracheal fascia

Trachea

Thyroid gland

Esophagus

Manubrium of sternum

Aorta

Pericardium

The deep cervical fascia of the neck tightly invests the neck structures (and thus edema in the neck can be painful), provides natural avenues for the spread of infections, and is divided into three layers:

Investing: it surrounds the neck and invests the trapezius and SCM muscles
Pretracheal (visceral): limited to the anterior neck, it invests the infrahyoid muscles, thyroid gland, trachea, and esophagus
Prevertebral: a tubular sheath, it invests prevertebral muscles and vertebral column

The carotid sheath blends with these fascial layers but is distinct and contains the common carotid artery, internal jugular vein, and vagus nerve.

Neck: Thyroid Gland

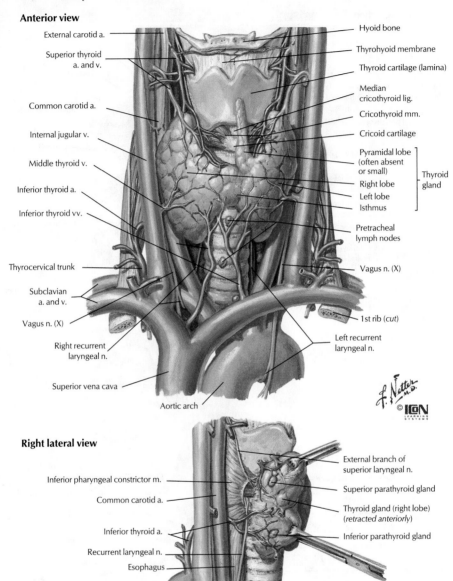

Anterior view

External carotid a.

Superior thyroid a. and v.

Common carotid a.

Internal jugular v.

Middle thyroid v.

Inferior thyroid a.

Inferior thyroid vv.

Thyrocervical trunk

Subclavian a. and v.

Vagus n. (X)

Right recurrent laryngeal n.

Superior vena cava

Aortic arch

Hyoid bone

Thyrohyoid membrane

Thyroid cartilage (lamina)

Median cricothyroid lig.

Cricothyroid mm.

Cricoid cartilage

Pyramidal lobe (often absent or small)

Right lobe

Left lobe

Isthmus

} Thyroid gland

Pretracheal lymph nodes

Vagus n. (X)

1st rib (cut)

Left recurrent laryngeal n.

Right lateral view

Inferior pharyngeal constrictor m.

Common carotid a.

Inferior thyroid a.

Recurrent laryngeal n.

Esophagus

External branch of superior laryngeal n.

Superior parathyroid gland

Thyroid gland (right lobe) (retracted anteriorly)

Inferior parathyroid gland

The thyroid gland lies at the C5 to T1 vertebral level, anterior to the trachea, and has two pairs (variable) of parathyroid glands embedded on its posterior surface. The thyroid secretes thyroxine and thyrocalcitonin.

FEATURE	CHARACTERISTICS
Lobes	Right and left, with a thin isthmus joining them
Blood supply	Superior and inferior thyroid arteries
Venous drainage	Superior, middle, and inferior thyroid veins
Pyramidal lobe	Variable (50% of time) superior extension of thyroid tissue

Clinical Correlation

Hyperthroidism with Diffuse Goiter (Graves' Disease)

Anatomy on pp. 535, 536

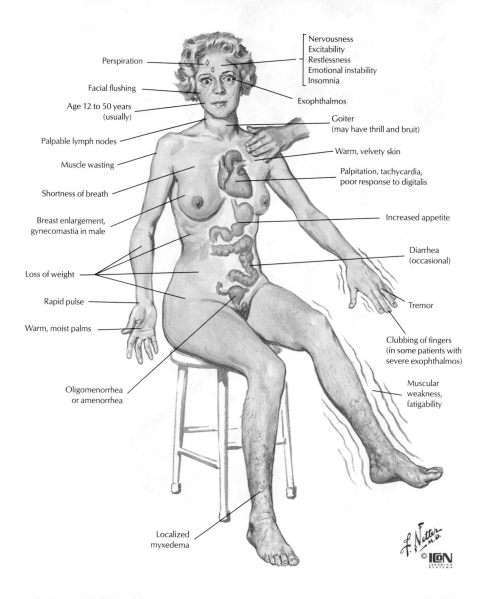

Perspiration

Facial flushing

Age 12 to 50 years (usually)

Palpable lymph nodes

Muscle wasting

Shortness of breath

Breast enlargement, gynecomastia in male

Loss of weight

Rapid pulse

Warm, moist palms

Oligomenorrhea or amenorrhea

Localized myxedema

Nervousness
Excitability
Restlessness
Emotional instability
Insomnia

Exophthalmos

Goiter
(may have thrill and bruit)

Warm, velvety skin

Palpitation, tachycardia, poor response to digitalis

Increased appetite

Diarrhea
(occasional)

Tremor

Clubbing of fingers
(in some patients with severe exophthalmos)

Muscular
weakness,
fatigability

Graves' disease is the most common cause of hyperthyroidism in patients younger than 40 years. Excess synthesis and release of thyroid hormone (T_3 and T_4) result in thyrotoxicosis, which up-regulates tissue metabolism and leads to symptoms indicating increased metabolism.

Clinical Correlation

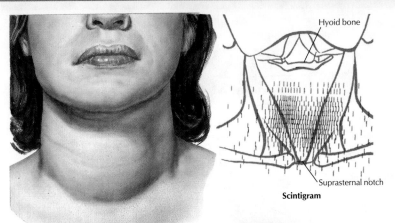

Hyoid bone

Suprasternal notch

Scintigram

**Diffuse goiter of
moderate size**

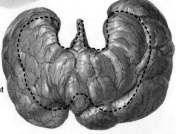

**Diffuse
enlargement
and engorgement
of thyroid gland**
(broken line
indicates normal
size of gland)

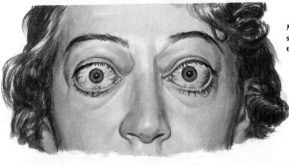

**Moderately
severe
exophthalmos**

CHARACTERISTIC	DESCRIPTION
Etiology	Autoimmune disease with antibodies directed against thyroid-stimulating hormone (TSH) receptor, stimulating release of hormone or increasing thyroid epithelial cell activity; familial predisposition
Prevalence	Seven times more common in women than in men; peak incidence between 20 and 40 years of age
Signs	Thyrotoxicosis (hyperfunctional state), lid lag, exophthalmos (infiltrative increase in retrobulbar connective tissue and extraocular muscles), pretibial myxedema (thickened skin on leg); most common cause of endogenous hyperthyroidism

Clinical Correlation

Hypothyroidism

Anatomy on pp. 535, 536, 645

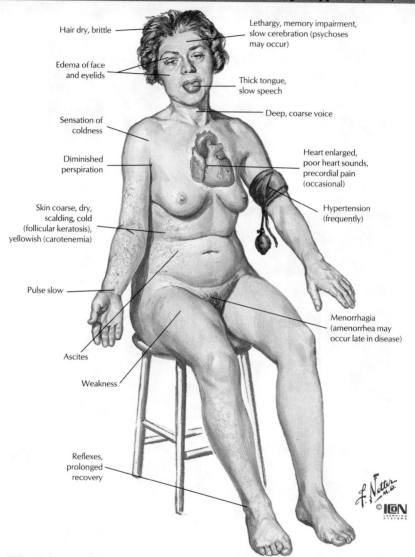

Hair dry, brittle

Edema of face and eyelids

Sensation of coldness

Diminished perspiration

Skin coarse, dry, scalding, cold (follicular keratosis), yellowish (carotenemia)

Pulse slow

Ascites

Weakness

Reflexes, prolonged recovery

Lethargy, memory impairment, slow cerebration (psychoses may occur)

Thick tongue, slow speech

Deep, coarse voice

Heart enlarged, poor heart sounds, precordial pain (occasional)

Hypertension (frequently)

Menorrhagia (amenorrhea may occur late in disease)

Primary hypothyroidism is a disease in which the thyroid gland produces inadequate amounts of thyroid hormone to meet the body's needs (TSH levels are increased).

CHARACTERISTIC	DESCRIPTION
Etiology	Surgical ablation (thyroidectomy), radiation damage, Hashimoto's thyroiditis (autoimmune inflammatory disorder), idiopathic causes
Prevalence	More common in women than in men; can occur in any age group; congenital cases approximately 1 in 5000 births
Signs and symptoms	Myxedema (clinical manifestations illustrated)

Clinical Correlation

Manifestations of Primary Hyperparathyroidism

Anatomy on pp. 536, 645

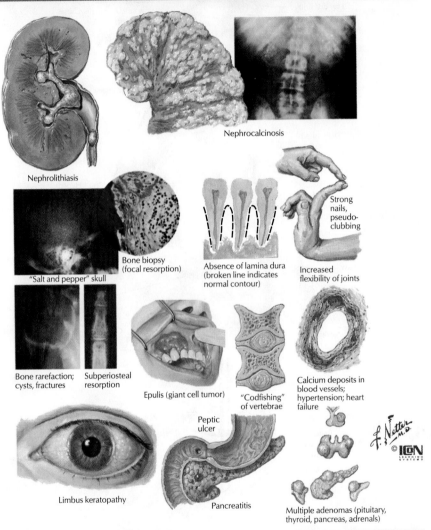

Nephrolithiasis

Nephrocalcinosis

"Salt and pepper" skull

Bone biopsy (focal resorption)

Absence of lamina dura (broken line indicates normal contour)

Strong nails, pseudo-clubbing

Increased flexibility of joints

Bone rarefaction; cysts, fractures

Subperiosteal resorption

Epulis (giant cell tumor)

"Codfishing" of vertebrae

Calcium deposits in blood vessels; hypertension; heart failure

Peptic ulcer

Limbus keratopathy

Pancreatitis

Multiple adenomas (pituitary, thyroid, pancreas, adrenals)

CHARACTERISTIC	DESCRIPTION
Etiology	Hypertrophy of parathyroid glands (>85% are solitary benign adenomas), which leads to secretion of excess parathyroid hormone that causes increased calcium levels
Presentation	Mild or nonspecific symptoms including fatigue, constipation, polyuria, polydipsia, depression, skeletal pain, and nausea
Prevalence	Approximately 100,000 new cases/year in the United States; 2:1 prevalence in women, which increases with age
Management	Surgical removal of parathyroid glands

Neck: Laryngeal Cartilages

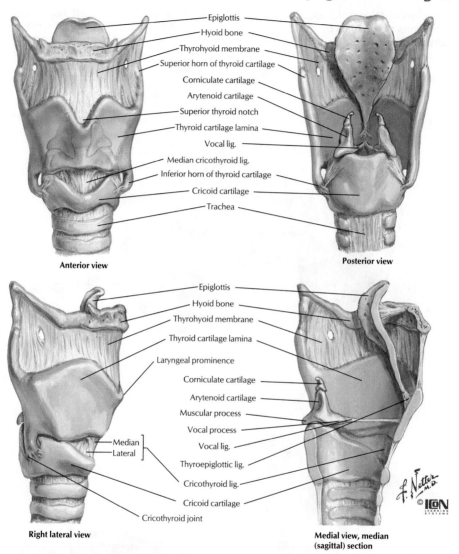

Anterior view

- Epiglottis
- Hyoid bone
- Thyrohyoid membrane
- Superior horn of thyroid cartilage
- Corniculate cartilage
- Arytenoid cartilage
- Superior thyroid notch
- Thyroid cartilage lamina
- Vocal lig.
- Median cricothyroid lig.
- Inferior horn of thyroid cartilage
- Cricoid cartilage
- Trachea

Posterior view

Right lateral view

- Epiglottis
- Hyoid bone
- Thyrohyoid membrane
- Thyroid cartilage lamina
- Laryngeal prominence
- Corniculate cartilage
- Arytenoid cartilage
- Muscular process
- Vocal process
- Median
- Lateral
- Vocal lig.
- Thyroepiglottic lig.
- Cricothyroid lig.
- Cricoid cartilage
- Cricothyroid joint

Medial view, median (sagittal) section

The larynx lies at the C3 to C6 vertebral level, just superior to the trachea, and consists of nine cartilages joined by ligaments and membranes.

CARTILAGE	DESCRIPTION
Thyroid	Two hyaline laminae and the laryngeal prominence (Adam's apple)
Cricoid	Signet ring-shaped hyaline cartilage just inferior to thyroid
Epiglottis	Spoon-shaped fibrocartilage plate attached to thyroid
Arytenoid	Paired pyramidal cartilages that rotate on cricoid cartilage
Corniculate	Paired cartilages that lie on apex of arytenoid cartilages
Cuneiform	Paired cartilages in aryepiglottic folds that have no articulations

Neck: Muscles of the Larynx

The vocal folds (true vocal cords) control phonation much like a reed instrument. Vibrations of the folds produce sounds as air passes through the rima glottidis (space between the folds). The posterior cricoarytenoid muscles are important: they are the only laryngeal muscles that abduct the vocal folds (all others are adductors). The vestibular (false vocal) folds have a protective function.

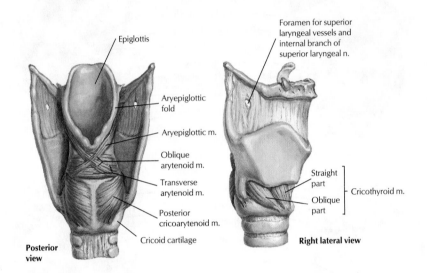

Epiglottis

Aryepiglottic fold

Aryepiglottic m.

Oblique arytenoid m.

Transverse arytenoid m.

Posterior cricoarytenoid m.

Cricoid cartilage

Posterior view

Foramen for superior laryngeal vessels and internal branch of superior laryngeal n.

Straight part
Oblique part
Cricothyroid m.

Right lateral view

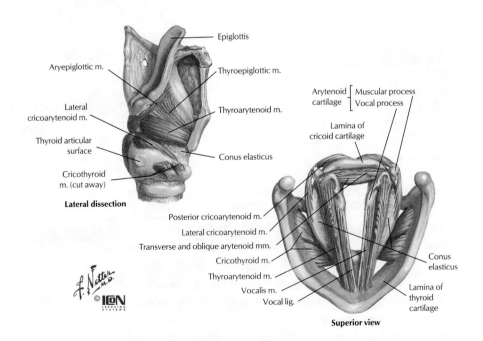

Aryepiglottic m.

Lateral cricoarytenoid m.

Thyroid articular surface

Cricothyroid m. (cut away)

Lateral dissection

Epiglottis

Thyroepiglottic m.

Thyroarytenoid m.

Conus elasticus

Arytenoid cartilage
Muscular process
Vocal process

Lamina of cricoid cartilage

Posterior cricoarytenoid m.
Lateral cricoarytenoid m.
Transverse and oblique arytenoid mm.
Cricothyroid m.
Thyroarytenoid m.
Vocalis m.
Vocal lig.

Conus elasticus

Lamina of thyroid cartilage

Superior view

Clinical Correlation

Hoarseness
Anatomy on pp. 542, 631

Inflammation of the larynx

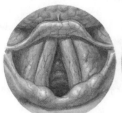
Acute laryngitis

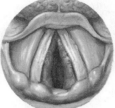
Subglottic inflammation and swelling in inflammatory croup

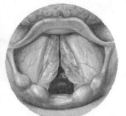
Edematous vocal cords in chronic laryngitis

Lesions of the vocal cords

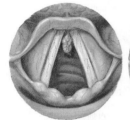
Pedunculated papilloma at anterior commissure

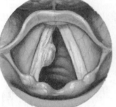
Sessile polyp

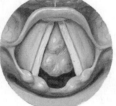
Subglottic polyp

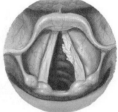
Hyperkeratosis of right cord

Cancer of the larynx

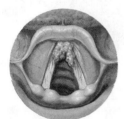
Carcinoma involving anterior commissure

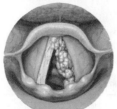
Extensive carcinoma of right vocal cord involving arytenoid region

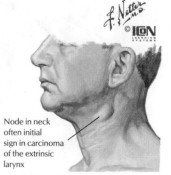
Node in neck often initial sign in carcinoma of the extrinsic larynx

---

Hoarseness can be due to any condition that results in improper vibration or coaptation of the vocal folds.

CONDITION	DESCRIPTION
Acute laryngitis	Inflammation and edema caused by smoking, gastroesophageal reflux disease, chronic rhinosinusitis, cough, voice overuse, myxedema, infection
Stiffness	Caused by surgical scarring or inflammation
Mass lesion	Caused by nodule, cyst, granuloma, neoplasm, fungal infection
Paralysis or paresis	Occurs after viral infection, recurrent laryngeal nerve lesion, or stroke; can have congenital causes or be iatrogenic

Neck: Prevertebral Muscles

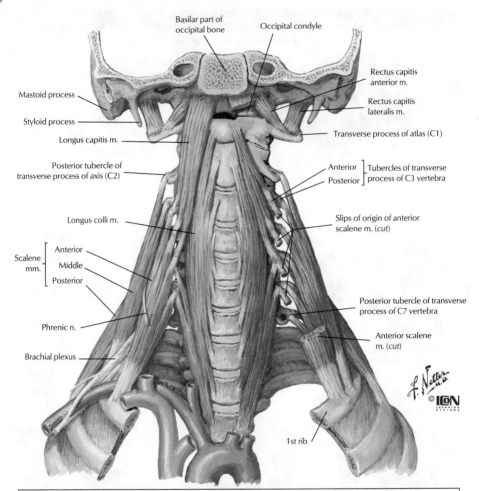

MUSCLE	INFERIOR ATTACHMENT (ORIGIN)	SUPERIOR ATTACHMENT (INSERTION)	INNERVATION	MAIN ACTIONS
Longus colli	Body of T1-T3 with attachments to bodies of C4-C7 and transverse processes of C3-C6	Anterior tubercle of C1 (atlas)	C2-C6 spinal nerves	Flexes cervical vertebrae; allows slight rotation
Longus capitis	Anterior tubercles of C3-C6 transverse processes	Basilar part of occipital bone	C2-C3 spinal nerves	Flexes head
Rectus capitis anterior	Lateral mass of C1 (atlas)	Base of skull, anterior to occipital condyle	C1-C2 spinal nerves	Flexes head
Rectus capitis lateralis	Transverse process of C1 (atlas)	Jugular process of occipital bone	C1-C2 spinal nerves	Flexes and helps to stabilize head

Skull: Anterior and Lateral Aspects

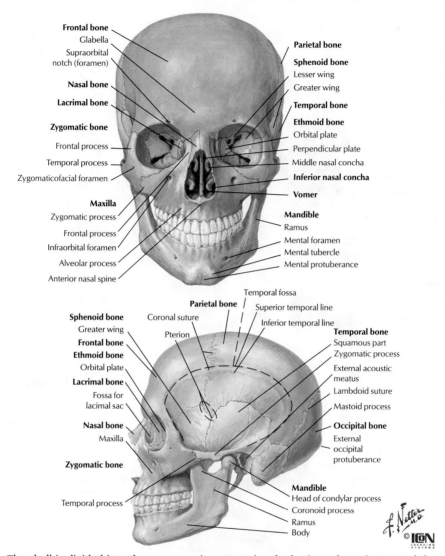

Frontal bone
Glabella
Supraorbital notch (foramen)
Nasal bone
Lacrimal bone
Zygomatic bone
Frontal process
Temporal process
Zygomaticofacial foramen
Maxilla
Zygomatic process
Frontal process
Infraorbital foramen
Alveolar process
Anterior nasal spine

Parietal bone
Sphenoid bone
Lesser wing
Greater wing
Temporal bone
Ethmoid bone
Orbital plate
Perpendicular plate
Middle nasal concha
Inferior nasal concha
Vomer
Mandible
Ramus
Mental foramen
Mental tubercle
Mental protuberance

Temporal fossa
Parietal bone
Coronal suture
Superior temporal line
Inferior temporal line
Pterion
Sphenoid bone
Greater wing
Frontal bone
Ethmoid bone
Orbital plate
Lacrimal bone
Fossa for lacimal sac
Nasal bone
Maxilla
Zygomatic bone
Temporal process

Temporal bone
Squamous part
Zygomatic process
External acoustic meatus
Lambdoid suture
Mastoid process
Occipital bone
External occipital protuberance
Mandible
Head of condylar process
Coronoid process
Ramus
Body

The skull is divided into the neurocranium (contains the brain and meninges) and the viscerocranium (facial skeleton). Sutures are immobile fibrous joints between skull bones.

FEATURE	DESCRIPTION
Frontal	Forms forehead, is thicker anteriorly, and contains frontal sinuses
Orbit	Is composed of contributions from seven different bones
Maxilla	Forms part of cheek; contains 16 maxillary teeth and sinuses
Zygomatic	Forms cheek and lateral orbital walls
Temporal	Contains middle and inner ear and vestibular system for balance
Mandible	Forms lower jaw that contains 16 mandibular teeth

Skull: Sagittal Aspect

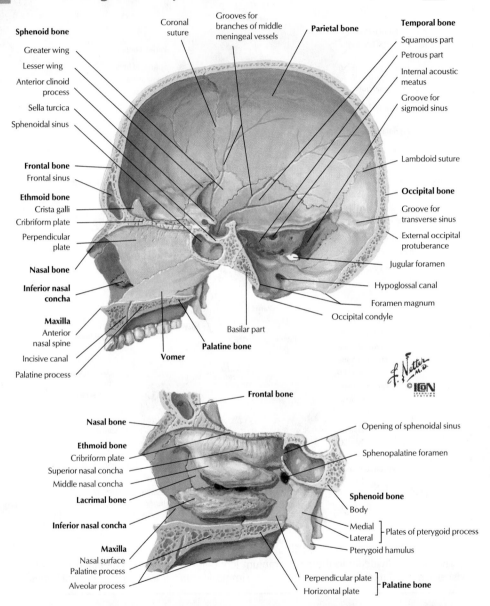

Sphenoid bone
- Greater wing
- Lesser wing
- Anterior clinoid process
- Sella turcica
- Sphenoidal sinus

Frontal bone
- Frontal sinus

Ethmoid bone
- Crista galli
- Cribriform plate
- Perpendicular plate

Nasal bone

Inferior nasal concha

Maxilla
- Anterior nasal spine
- Incisive canal
- Palatine process

Coronal suture

Grooves for branches of middle meningeal vessels

Parietal bone

Temporal bone
- Squamous part
- Petrous part
- Internal acoustic meatus
- Groove for sigmoid sinus

Lambdoid suture

Occipital bone
- Groove for transverse sinus
- External occipital protuberance
- Jugular foramen
- Hypoglossal canal
- Foramen magnum
- Occipital condyle

Basilar part

Palatine bone

Vomer

Frontal bone

Nasal bone

Ethmoid bone
- Cribriform plate
- Superior nasal concha
- Middle nasal concha

Lacrimal bone

Inferior nasal concha

Maxilla
- Nasal surface
- Palatine process
- Alveolar process

Opening of sphenoidal sinus

Sphenopalatine foramen

Sphenoid bone
- Body
- Medial
- Lateral } Plates of pterygoid process
- Pterygoid hamulus

Perpendicular plate
Horizontal plate } Palatine bone

FEATURE	CHARACTERISTICS
Nasal septum	Formed by perpendicular plate of ethmoid, vomer, and palatine bones and septal cartilages
Lateral nasal wall	Formed by superior and middle conchae of ethmoid, inferior concha, nasal bone, maxilla, and lacrimal, palatine, and sphenoid bones
Temporal	Contains middle and inner ear and vestibular system

Skull: Superior Aspect of Cranial Base

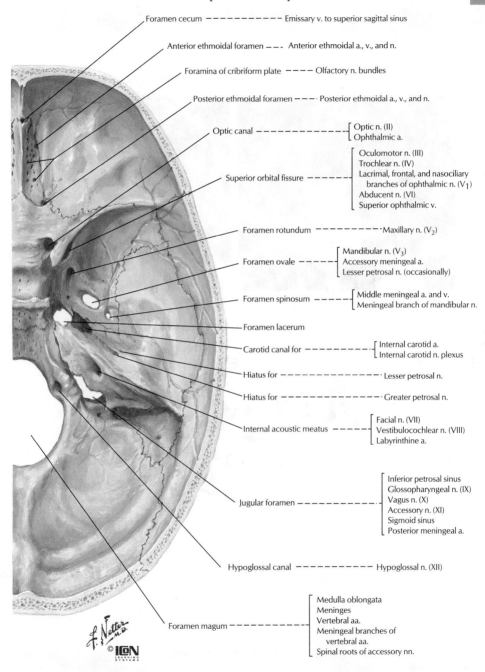

Foramen cecum — — — — — — — — Emissary v. to superior sagittal sinus

Anterior ethmoidal foramen — — — Anterior ethmoidal a., v., and n.

Foramina of cribriform plate — — — — Olfactory n. bundles

Posterior ethmoidal foramen — — — Posterior ethmoidal a., v., and n.

Optic canal — — — — — — — — — — [Optic n. (II)
[Ophthalmic a.

Superior orbital fissure — — — — — [Oculomotor n. (III)
Trochlear n. (IV)
Lacrimal, frontal, and nasociliary
    branches of ophthalmic n. (V_1)
Abducent n. (VI)
Superior ophthalmic v.

Foramen rotundum — — — — — — — — Maxillary n. (V_2)

Foramen ovale — — — — — [Mandibular n. (V_3)
Accessory meningeal a.
Lesser petrosal n. (occasionally)

Foramen spinosum — — — — — [Middle meningeal a. and v.
[Meningeal branch of mandibular n.

Foramen lacerum

Carotid canal for — — — — — — — — [Internal carotid a.
[Internal carotid n. plexus

Hiatus for — — — — — — — — — — — Lesser petrosal n.

Hiatus for — — — — — — — — — — — Greater petrosal n.

Internal acoustic meatus — — — — [Facial n. (VII)
Vestibulocochlear n. (VIII)
Labyrinthine a.

Jugular foramen — — — — — — — [Inferior petrosal sinus
Glossopharyngeal n. (IX)
Vagus n. (X)
Accessory n. (XI)
Sigmoid sinus
Posterior meningeal a.

Hypoglossal canal — — — — — — — — Hypoglossal n. (XII)

Foramen magum — — — — — — — [Medulla oblongata
Meninges
Vertebral aa.
Meningeal branches of
    vertebral aa.
Spinal roots of accessory nn.

The interior aspect of the skull shows the three cranial fossae—anterior (contains orbital roof and frontal lobes), middle (temporal lobes), and posterior (cerebellum, pons, medulla oblongata)—and the key foramina and structures passing through them.

Clinical Correlation

Compound Depressed Skull Fractures   *Anatomy on pp. 546, 558, 564*

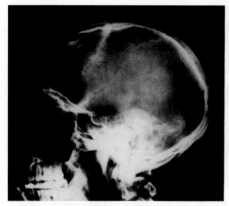

Left frontal depressed skull fracture

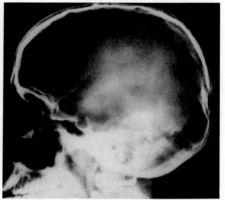

Occipital depressed skull fracture

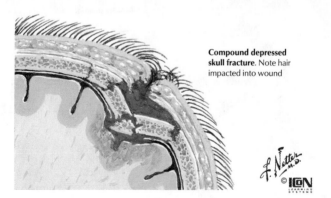

Compound depressed skull fracture. Note hair impacted into wound

Skull fractures may be classified as
- **Linear**: with a distinct fracture line
- **Comminuted**: with multiple fragments (depressed if driven inward, to compress or tear the dura mater)
- **Diastasis**: fracture along a suture line
- **Basilar**: fracture of the base of the skull

Any fracture that communicates with a lacerated scalp, paranasal sinuses, or middle ear is termed compound. Compound depressed fractures must be treated surgically.

Clinical Correlation

Zygomatic Fractures
Anatomy on pp. 545, 546, 594

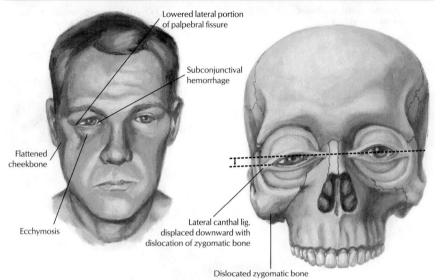

Lowered lateral portion of palpebral fissure

Subconjunctival hemorrhage

Flattened cheekbone

Ecchymosis

Lateral canthal lig. displaced downward with dislocation of zygomatic bone

Dislocated zygomatic bone

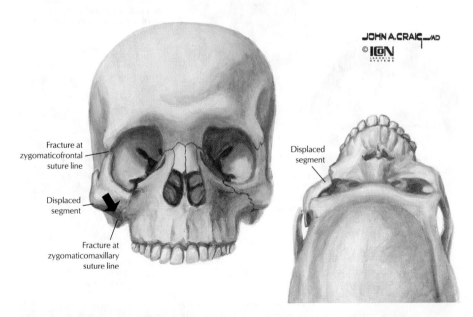

JOHN A. CRAIG, MD
© ICON
LEARNING SYSTEMS

Fracture at zygomaticofrontal suture line

Displaced segment

Fracture at zygomaticomaxillary suture line

Displaced segment

Trauma to the zygomatic bone (cheekbone) can disrupt the zygomatic complex and its articulations with the frontal, maxillary, temporal, sphenoid, and palatine bones. Often, fractures involve suture lines with the frontal and maxillary bones, with displacement inferiorly, medially, and posteriorly. Typical clinical presentation is illustrated. Ipsilateral ocular and visual changes may include diplopia (upper outer gaze) and hyphema, with immediate attention required.

Clinical Correlation

Midface Fractures   *Anatomy on pp. 545, 546, 628, 631*

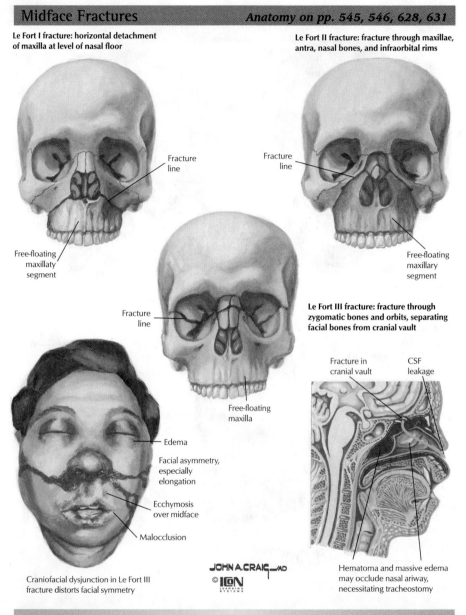

Le Fort I fracture: horizontal detachment of maxilla at level of nasal floor

Fracture line

Free-floating maxillaty segment

Le Fort II fracture: fracture through maxillae, antra, nasal bones, and infraorbital rims

Fracture line

Free-floating maxillary segment

Fracture line

Le Fort III fracture: fracture through zygomatic bones and orbits, separating facial bones from cranial vault

Free-floating maxilla

Fracture in cranial vault   CSF leakage

Edema

Facial asymmetry, especially elongation

Ecchymosis over midface

Malocclusion

Craniofacial dysjunction in Le Fort III fracture distorts facial symmetry

JOHN A. CRAIG—MD
© ICON
LEARNING SYSTEMS

Hematoma and massive edema may occlude nasal airiway, necessitating tracheostomy

Midface fractures (of maxillae, naso-orbital complex, zygomatic bones) were classified by Le Fort as follows:
- **Le Fort I**: horizontal detachment of maxilla at the level of the nasal floor
- **Le Fort II**: pyramidal fracture that includes both maxillae and nasal bones, medial portions of both antra, infraorbital rims, orbits, and orbital floors
- **Le Fort III**: includes Le Fort II and fracture of both zygomatic bones; may cause airway problems, nasolacrimal apparatus obstruction, and cerebrospinal fluid (CSF) leakage

Skull: Mandible

**Mandible of adult:
anterolateral superior view**

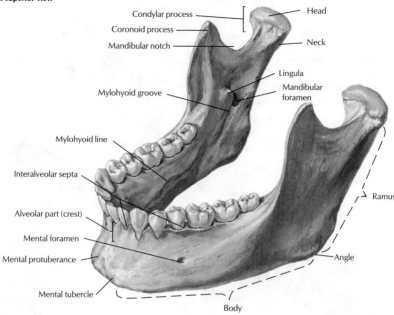

Condylar process — Head
Coronoid process
Mandibular notch — Neck
Lingula
Mylohyoid groove — Mandibular foramen
Mylohyoid line
Interalveolar septa
Alveolar part (crest)
Mental foramen
Mental protuberance — Angle
Mental tubercle — Ramus
Body

**Mandible of adult:
left posterior view**

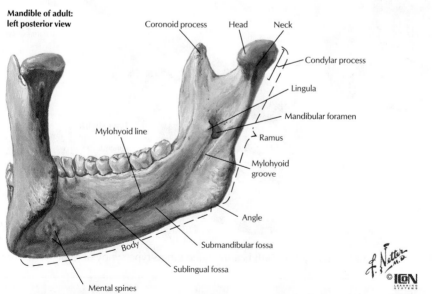

Coronoid process   Head   Neck
Condylar process
Lingula
Mandibular foramen
Mylohyoid line
Ramus
Mylohyoid groove
Angle
Body
Submandibular fossa
Sublingual fossa
Mental spines

FEATURE	CHARACTERISTICS
Mandibular head	Articulates with mandibular fossa of temporal bone
Mandibular foramen	Inferior alveolar nerve, artery, and vein enter mandible at this opening
Teeth	16 teeth: 4 incisors, 2 canines, 4 premolars (bicuspid), 6 molars (third molars called wisdom teeth)

Skull: Temporomandibular Joint

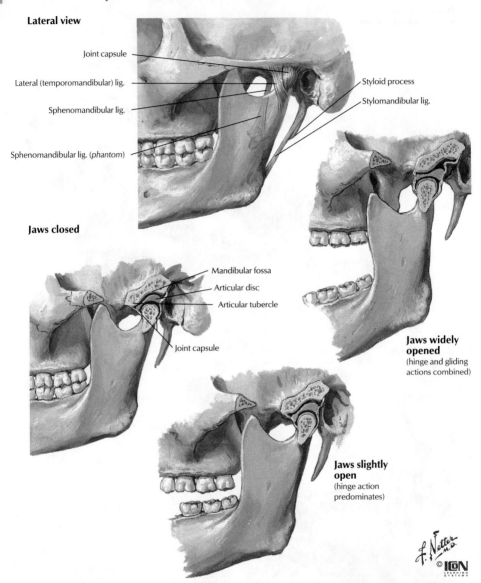

Lateral view

Joint capsule

Lateral (temporomandibular) lig.

Sphenomandibular lig.

Sphenomandibular lig. (*phantom*)

Styloid process

Stylomandibular lig.

Jaws closed

Mandibular fossa

Articular disc

Articular tubercle

Joint capsule

Jaws widely opened
(hinge and gliding actions combined)

Jaws slightly open
(hinge action predominates)

The temporomandibular joint (TMJ) is a modified hinge-type synovial joint.

LIGAMENT	ATTACHMENT	COMMENT
Capsule	Temporal fossa and tubercle to mandibular head	Permits side-to-side motion, protrusion, and retrusion
Lateral (TMJ)	Temporal to mandible	Thickened fibrous band of capsule
Articular disc	Between temporal bone and mandible	Divides joint into two synovial compartments

Clinical Correlation

Mandibular Fractures *Anatomy on pp. 552, 619*

Anatomy of mandible predisposes it to multiple fractures.

Condyle

Subcondylar area can fracture from blow to chin.

Third molar area may be weakened by partially erupted molar.

Distorted soft-tissue contours

Malocclusion

Ecchymosis or laceration of chin (in children)

Cuspid area is weakened by long tooth.

Displaced segment

Step defects

Displaced segment

Step defect

Mylohyoid m.

Bleeding caused by fracture is trapped by fanlike attachment of mylohoid musculature to mandible, and presents clinically as ecchymosis in floor of mouth.

JOHN A. CRAIG—AD
© ICN LEARNING SYSTEMS

Because of its vulnerable location, the mandible is the second most commonly fractured facial bone (nasal bone is the first). The mandible's U shape renders it liable to multiple fractures (>50%); the most common sites are the cuspid (canine tooth) area and the third molar area. Oozing blood from the mandible collects in loose tissues of the mouth floor (ecchymosis) and is virtually pathognomonic of a fracture.

Face and Scalp: Parotid Gland and Facial Nerve

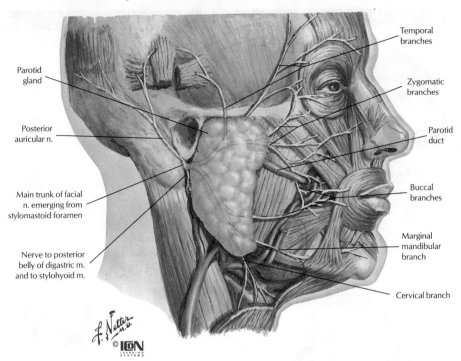

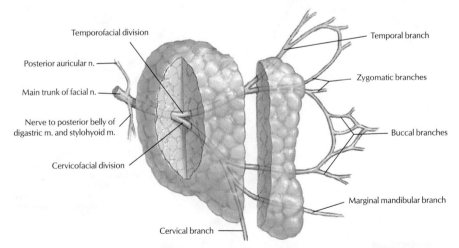

The parotid gland is the largest of the three pairs of salivary glands and is encased within the parotid sheath, a tough extension of the deep cervical fascia. The terminal portion of the facial nerve courses through the gland and distributes to the face in five groups of branches that innervate the muscles of facial expression:

- Temporal
- Zygomatic
- Buccal
- Marginal mandibular
- Cervical

Clinical Correlation

Facial Nerve (Bell's) Palsy   *Anatomy on pp. 554, 556, 639*

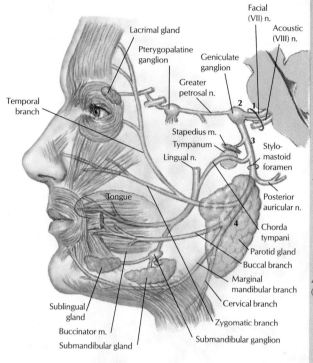

Lacrimal gland

Pterygopalatine ganglion

Geniculate ganglion

Greater petrosal n.

Facial (VII) n.

Acoustic (VIII) n.

Temporal branch

Stapedius m.

Tympanum

Lingual n.

Stylo-mastoid foramen

Tongue

Posterior auricular n.

Chorda tympani

Parotid gland

Buccal branch

Marginal mandibular branch

Cervical branch

Zygomatic branch

Submandibular ganglion

Sublingual gland

Buccinator m.

Submandibular gland

Sites of lesions and their manifestations

1. Intracranial and/or internal auditory meatus
   All symptoms of 2, 3, and 4, plus deafness due to involvement of eighth cranial nerve.

2. Geniculate ganglion
   All symptoms of 3 and 4, plus pain behind ear. Herpes of tympanum and of external auditory meatus may occur.

3. Facial canal
   All symptoms of 4, plus loss of taste in anterior tongue and decreased salivation on affected side due to chorda tympani involvement. Hyperacusis due to effect on nerve branch to stapedius muscle.

4. Below stylomastoid foramen (parotid gland tumor, trauma)
   Facial paralysis (mouth draws to opposite side; on affected side, patient unable to close eye or wrinkle forehead; food collects between teeth and cheek due to paralysis of buccinator muscle).

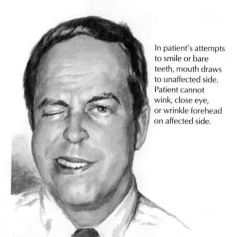

In patient's attempts to smile or bare teeth, mouth draws to unaffected side. Patient cannot wink, close eye, or wrinkle forehead on affected side.

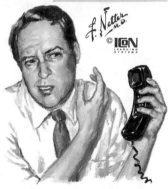

Hyperacusis: Patient holds phone away from ear.

Acute, unilateral facial palsy is the most common cause of facial muscle weakness and cranial neuropathy and may often be caused by herpes simplex virus (HSV) infection. Manifestations associated with lesions at points along the path of CN VII are illustrated.

Face and Scalp: Muscles of Facial Expression

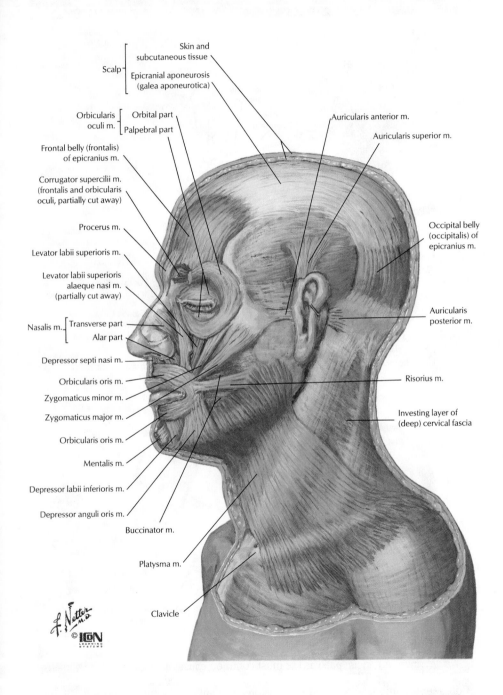

Scalp {
Skin and subcutaneous tissue
Epicranial aponeurosis (galea aponeurotica)

Orbicularis oculi m. {
Orbital part
Palpebral part

Frontal belly (frontalis) of epicranius m.

Corrugator supercilii m. (frontalis and orbicularis oculi, partially cut away)

Procerus m.

Levator labii superioris m.

Levator labii superioris alaeque nasi m. (partially cut away)

Nasalis m. {
Transverse part
Alar part

Depressor septi nasi m.

Orbicularis oris m.

Zygomaticus minor m.

Zygomaticus major m.

Orbicularis oris m.

Mentalis m.

Depressor labii inferioris m.

Depressor anguli oris m.

Buccinator m.

Platysma m.

Clavicle

Auricularis anterior m.

Auricularis superior m.

Occipital belly (occipitalis) of epicranius m.

Auricularis posterior m.

Risorius m.

Investing layer of (deep) cervical fascia

Face and Scalp: Muscles of Facial Expression (continued)

All of these muscles are supplied by the facial nerve (CN VII). Not all of the muscles of facial expression are listed in the table.

MUSCLE	ORIGIN	INSERTION	MAIN ACTIONS
Frontalis	Skin of forehead	Epicranial aponeurosis	Elevates eyebrows and forehead
Orbicularis oculi	Medial orbital margin, medial palpebral ligament, and lacrimal bone	Skin around margin of orbit; tarsal plate	Closes eyelids
Nasalis	Superior part of canine ridge of maxilla	Nasal cartilages	Draws ala of nose toward septum
Orbicularis oris	Median plane of maxilla superiorly and mandible inferiorly; other fibers from deep surface of skin	Mucous membrane of lips	Closes and protrudes lips (e.g., purses them during whistling and sucking)
Levator labii superioris	Frontal process of maxilla and infraorbital region	Skin of upper lip and alar cartilage	Elevates lip, dilates nostril, raises angle of mouth
Platysma	Superficial fascia of deltoid and pectoral regions	Mandible, skin of cheek, angle of mouth, and orbicularis oris	Depresses mandible and tenses skin of lower face and neck
Mentalis	Incisive fossa of mandible	Skin of chin	Elevates and protrudes lower lip
Buccinator	Mandible, pterygomandibular raphe, and alveolar processes of maxilla and mandible	Angle of mouth	Presses cheek against molar teeth, thereby aiding chewing

Face and Scalp: Arteries and Veins

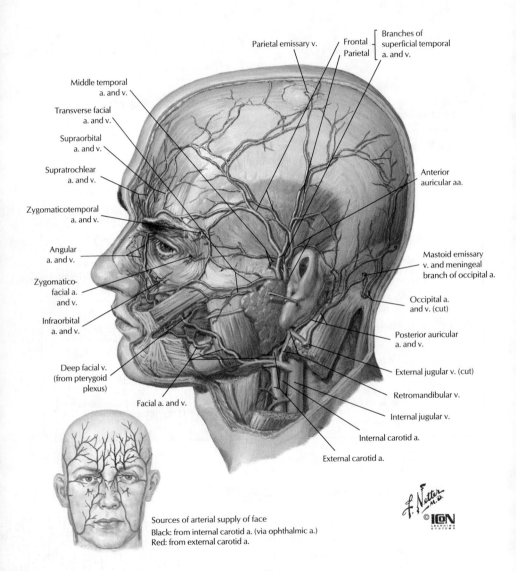

Parietal emissary v.

Frontal · Parietal — Branches of superficial temporal a. and v.

Middle temporal a. and v.

Transverse facial a. and v.

Supraorbital a. and v.

Supratrochlear a. and v.

Zygomaticotemporal a. and v.

Angular a. and v.

Zygomatico- facial a. and v.

Infraorbital a. and v.

Deep facial v. (from pterygoid plexus)

Facial a. and v.

Anterior auricular aa.

Mastoid emissary v. and meningeal branch of occipital a.

Occipital a. and v. (cut)

Posterior auricular a. and v.

External jugular v. (cut)

Retromandibular v.

Internal jugular v.

Internal carotid a.

External carotid a.

Sources of arterial supply of face
Black: from internal carotid a. (via ophthalmic a.)
Red: from external carotid a.

The vascular supply to the face and scalp is rich. Scalp wounds bleed profusely because arteries in this area have extensive anastomoses and, when lacerated, are held open by the dense fibrous tissue of the scalp, which prevents retraction into subcutaneous tissue.

Face and Scalp: Cutaneous Nerves

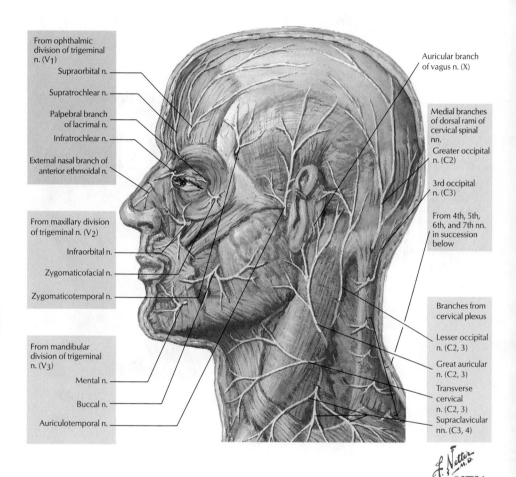

From ophthalmic division of trigeminal n. (V₁)
- Supraorbital n.
- Supratrochlear n.
- Palpebral branch of lacrimal n.
- Infratrochlear n.
- External nasal branch of anterior ethmoidal n.

From maxillary division of trigeminal n. (V₂)
- Infraorbital n.
- Zygomaticofacial n.
- Zygomaticotemporal n.

From mandibular division of trigeminal n. (V₃)
- Mental n.
- Buccal n.
- Auriculotemporal n.

Auricular branch of vagus n. (X)

Medial branches of dorsal rami of cervical spinal nn.
- Greater occipital n. (C2)
- 3rd occipital n. (C3)
- From 4th, 5th, 6th, and 7th nn. in succession below

Branches from cervical plexus
- Lesser occipital n. (C2, 3)
- Great auricular n. (C2, 3)
- Transverse cervical n. (C2, 3)
- Supraclavicular nn. (C3, 4)

Cutaneous nerves of the face and scalp arise primarily from the trigeminal nerve, with some contributions from the cervical plexus. The trigeminal nerve has three divisions:

Ophthalmic (CN V₁): sensory
Maxillary (CN V₂): sensory
Mandibular (CN V₃): sensory and motor

Sensory nerve cell bodies reside in the trigeminal (also known as semilunar or gasserian) ganglion.

Clinical Correlation

Trigeminal Neuralgia
Anatomy on pp. 559, 638

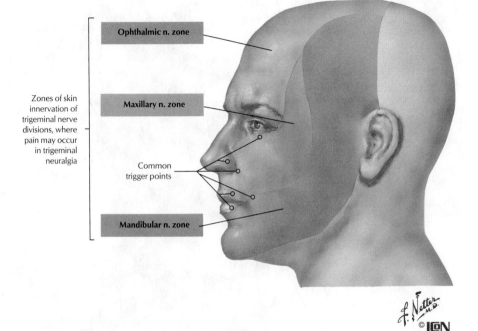

Zones of skin innervation of trigeminal nerve divisions, where pain may occur in trigeminal neuralgia

Ophthalmic n. zone

Maxillary n. zone

Common trigger points

Mandibular n. zone

Trigeminal neuralgia (or tic douloureux) is a neurologic condition characterized by episodes of brief, intense facial pain over one of the three areas of distribution of CN V. The pain is so intense that the patient winces, which produces a facial muscle tic.

CHARACTERISTIC	DESCRIPTION
Etiology	Uncertain; possibly vascular compression of trigeminal sensory ganglion by superior cerebellar artery
Presentation	Recurrent, lancinating, burning pain, usually affecting V_2 or V_3 unilaterally (<6% involve V_1), usually in a person older than 50 years
Triggers	Touch; draft of cool air

Clinical Correlation

Herpes Zoster (Shingles)

Anatomy on pp. 559, 638

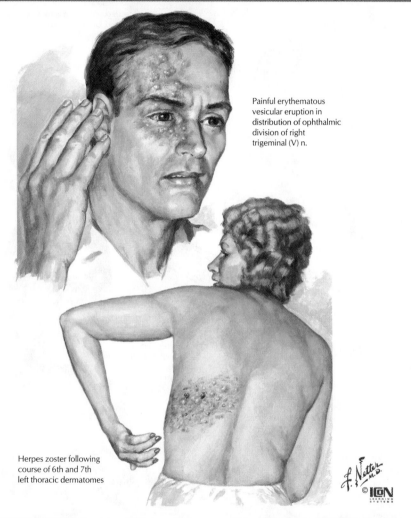

Painful erythematous vesicular eruption in distribution of ophthalmic division of right trigeminal (V) n.

Herpes zoster following course of 6th and 7th left thoracic dermatomes

Herpes zoster, or shingles, is the most common infection of the peripheral nervous system (PNS). It is an acute neuralgia confined to the dermatome distribution of a specific spinal or cranial sensory nerve root.

CHARACTERISTIC	DESCRIPTION
Etiology	Reactivation of previous infection of dorsal root or sensory ganglion by varicella-zoster virus (which causes chickenpox)
Prevalence	Approximately 0.5% of population
Presentation	Vesicular rash confined to a radicular or cranial nerve sensory distribution; initial intense burning localized pain with vesicles appearing 72-96 hours later
Sites affected	Usually one or several contiguous unilateral dermatomes (T5-L2), CN V (semilunar ganglion), or CN VII (geniculate ganglion)

Clinical Correlation

Organisms enter through large, small, or even unrecognized wound. Deep, infected punctures are most susceptible, because organisms thrive best anaerobically.

Clostridium tetani: gram-positive, spore-bearing rods

Toxin produced locally passes via bloodstream or along nerves to CNS.

Motor neurons of spinal cord (anterior horn) and of brainstem become hyperactive because toxin specifically attacks inhibitory (Renshaw) cells.

Spasm of jaw, facial, and neck muscles (trismus [lockjaw], risus sardonicus) and dysphagia are often early symptoms.

Complete tetanic spasm in advanced disease. Patient rigid in moderate opisthotonos, with arms extended, abdomen boardlike. Respiratory arrest may occur.

The PNS motor unit is vulnerable to three bacteria-produced toxins: tetanospasmin (motor neuron), diphtheria toxin (peripheral nerve), and botulin (neuromuscular junction). The hearty spore of *Clostridium tetani* is commonly found in soil, dust, and feces and can enter the body through wounds, blisters, burns, skin ulcers, insect bites, and surgical procedures. Symptoms include restlessness, low-grade fever, and stiffness or soreness. Eventually, nuchal rigidity, trismus (lockjaw), dysphagia, laryngospasm, and acute, massive muscle spasms can occur. Prophylaxis (immunization) is the best management.

Clinical Correlation

Alopecia

Anatomy on pp. 6, 561

Hair loss

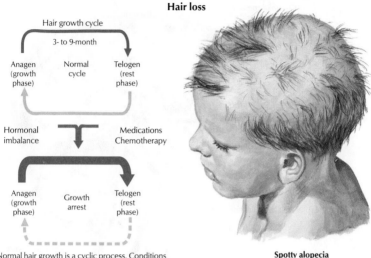

Hair growth cycle

3- to 9-month

Anagen (growth phase) → Normal cycle → Telogen (rest phase)

Hormonal imbalance / Medications Chemotherapy

Anagen (growth phase) → Growth arrest → Telogen (rest phase)

Normal hair growth is a cyclic process. Conditions that upset the grow-rest cycling may delay replacement of normal hair loss, resulting in alopecia. Such conditions are usually reversible.

Spotty alopecia

Conditions associated with increased risk of hair loss

Pregnancy and delivery

Oral contraceptive use

Polycystic ovaries

Medications and chemotherapy

Pituitary hyperplasia

Family history of balding

Postmenopausal without hormone replacement

Estrogen

Adrenal hyperplasia

Diabetes mellitus

Hair loss can occur for various reasons, but alopecia areata is a specific disease whose etiology is uncertain. Alopecia areata shows a genetic predisposition and has been linked to a number of autoimmune disorders. It occurs primarily in children and young adults and is characterized by sudden loss of oval patches of hair.

Brain: Meninges and Cerebrospinal Fluid

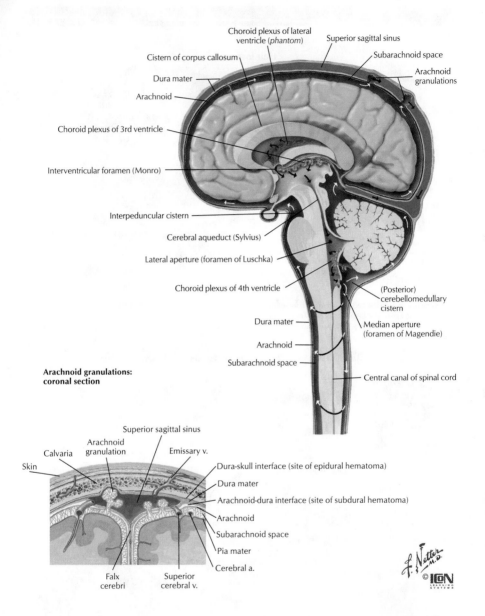

Choroid plexus of lateral ventricle (*phantom*)
Superior sagittal sinus
Subarachnoid space
Arachnoid granulations
Cistern of corpus callosum
Dura mater
Arachnoid
Choroid plexus of 3rd ventricle
Interventricular foramen (Monro)
Interpeduncular cistern
Cerebral aqueduct (Sylvius)
Lateral aperture (foramen of Luschka)
Choroid plexus of 4th ventricle
(Posterior) cerebellomedullary cistern
Dura mater
Median aperture (foramen of Magendie)
Arachnoid
Subarachnoid space
Central canal of spinal cord

Arachnoid granulations: coronal section

Superior sagittal sinus
Arachnoid granulation
Emissary v.
Calvaria
Skin
Dura-skull interface (site of epidural hematoma)
Dura mater
Arachnoid-dura interface (site of subdural hematoma)
Arachnoid
Subarachnoid space
Pia mater
Cerebral a.
Falx cerebri
Superior cerebral v.

The subarachnoid space (between the arachnoid and pia mater) contains CSF, which
- Supports and cushions the spinal cord and brain
- Fulfills some functions normally provided by the lymphatic system
- Occupies a volume of approximately 150 ml in the subarachnoid space
- Is produced by choroid plexuses in the brain's ventricles
- Is produced at a rate of approximately 500 ml/day
- Is reabsorbed largely by arachnoid granulations and by small central nervous system (CNS) capillaries

Clinical Correlation

Meningitis   *Anatomy on p. 564*

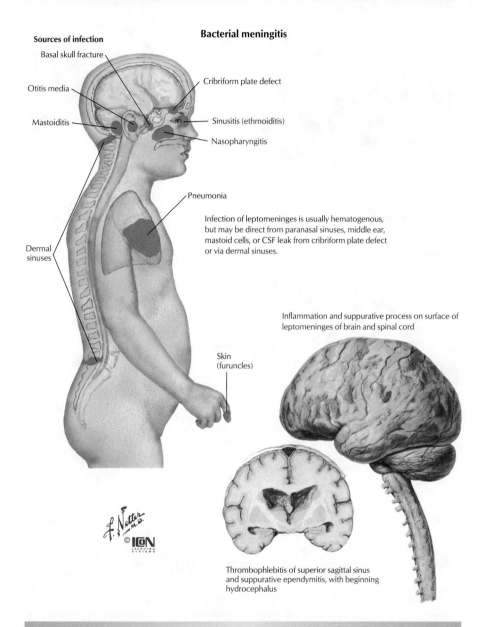

Sources of infection

Bacterial meningitis

Basal skull fracture

Cribriform plate defect

Otitis media

Mastoiditis

Sinusitis (ethmoiditis)

Nasopharyngitis

Pneumonia

Infection of leptomeninges is usually hematogenous, but may be direct from paranasal sinuses, middle ear, mastoid cells, or CSF leak from cribriform plate defect or via dermal sinuses.

Dermal sinuses

Inflammation and suppurative process on surface of leptomeninges of brain and spinal cord

Skin (furuncles)

Thrombophlebitis of superior sagittal sinus and suppurative ependymitis, with beginning hydrocephalus

Meningitis is a serious condition defined as inflammation of the arachnoid and pia mater meningeal layers. It results most often from bacterial or aseptic causes—the latter include viral infections, drug reactions, and systemic diseases. Patients with meningitis usually present with headache, fever, and a painful, stiff neck. Diagnosis is made by lumbar puncture and examination of CSF.

Clinical Correlation

Hydrocephalus

Anatomy on p. 564

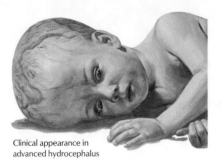

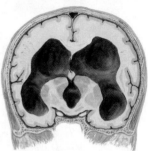

Section through brain showing marked dilatation of lateral and 3rd ventricles

Clinical appearance in advanced hydrocephalus

Potential lesion sites in obstructive hydrocephalus

1. Interventricular foramina (of Monro)
2. Cerebral aqueduct (of Sylvius)
3. Lateral apertures (of Luschka)
4. Median aperture (of Magendie)

Shunt procedure for hydrocephalus

Reservoir at end of cannula implanted beneath galea permits transcutaneous needle puncture for withdrawal of CSF, introduction of antibiotics, or dye to test patency of shunt.

Cannula inserted into lateral ventricle

One-way valve to prevent reflux of blood or peritoneal fluid and control CSF pressure

Drainage tube may be introduced into internal jugular v. and thence into right atrium via neck incision, or may be continued subcutaneously to abdomen.

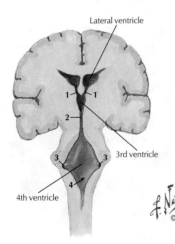

Lateral ventricle

3rd ventricle

4th ventricle

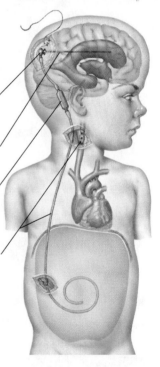

Accumulation of excess CSF (via overproduction or decreased absorption) within the brain's ventricular system is called hydrocephalus.

TYPE	DEFINITION
Obstructive	Congenital stenosis of cerebral aqueduct (of Sylvius), or obstruction at other sites (illustrated) by tumors
Communicating	Obstruction outside the ventricular system, e.g., subarachnoid space (hemorrhage) or at arachnoid granulations
Normal pressure	Adult syndrome of progressive dementia, gait disorders, and urinary incontinence; computed tomography shows ventricular dilation and brain atrophy

Brain: Dural Venous Sinuses

Dural sinuses and their relationship to the cranial nerves, falx cerebri and falx cerebelli, and tentorium cerebelli are shown. Most venous drainage occurs posteriorly
(although these veins lack valves, and blood may flow in either direction). Blood ultimately collects in the sigmoid sinus and then drains into the origin of the internal jugular vein.

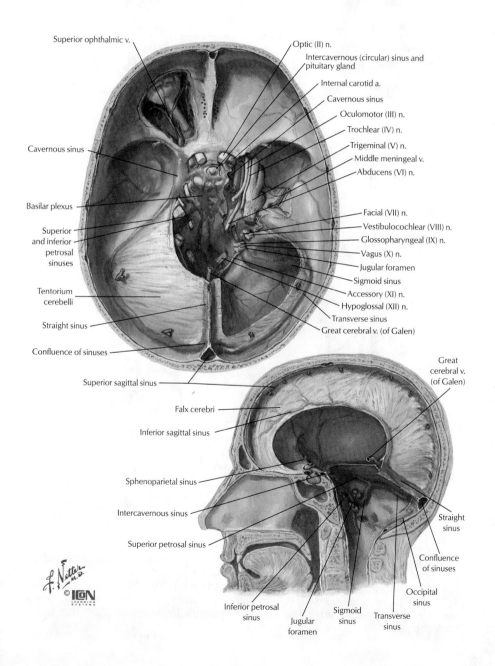

Superior ophthalmic v.
Optic (II) n.
Intercavernous (circular) sinus and pituitary gland
Internal carotid a.
Cavernous sinus
Oculomotor (III) n.
Trochlear (IV) n.
Trigeminal (V) n.
Middle meningeal v.
Abducens (VI) n.
Cavernous sinus
Basilar plexus
Superior and inferior petrosal sinuses
Facial (VII) n.
Vestibulocochlear (VIII) n.
Glossopharyngeal (IX) n.
Vagus (X) n.
Jugular foramen
Sigmoid sinus
Tentorium cerebelli
Accessory (XI) n.
Hypoglossal (XII) n.
Transverse sinus
Straight sinus
Great cerebral v. (of Galen)
Confluence of sinuses
Superior sagittal sinus
Great cerebral v. (of Galen)
Falx cerebri
Inferior sagittal sinus
Sphenoparietal sinus
Straight sinus
Intercavernous sinus
Confluence of sinuses
Superior petrosal sinus
Occipital sinus
Inferior petrosal sinus
Jugular foramen
Sigmoid sinus
Transverse sinus

Clinical Correlation

Anterior Pituitary Deficiency　　　*Anatomy on pp. 45, 567, 572, 627*

Pituitary anterior lobe deficiency in the adult

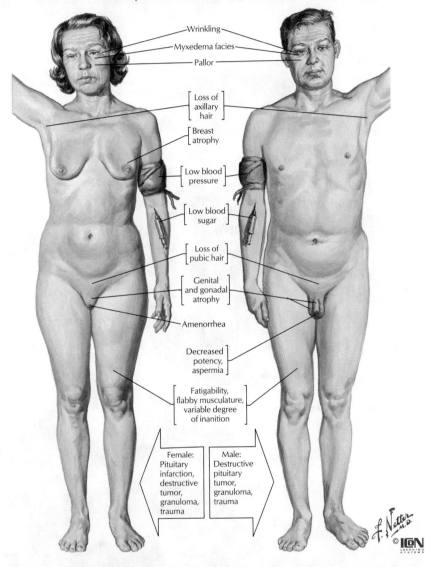

Wrinkling
Myxedema facies
Pallor

Loss of axillary hair

Breast atrophy

Low blood pressure

Low blood sugar

Loss of pubic hair

Genital and gonadal atrophy

Amenorrhea

Decreased potency, aspermia

Fatigability, flabby musculature, variable degree of inanition

Female: Pituitary infarction, destructive tumor, granuloma, trauma

Male: Destructive pituitary tumor, granuloma, trauma

The anterior pituitary produces six polypeptide hormones that regulate other endocrine glands via negative feedback. Most dysfunction of this gland is caused by tumors, usually benign, that disrupt normal hormone release. The first hormone lost as a result of large mass lesions of the gland is usually growth hormone (GH), followed by luteinizing hormone (LH) and follicle-stimulating hormone (FSH), then corticotropin and TSH, and, last, prolactin.

Clinical Correlation

Pituitary Adenomas   *Anatomy on pp. 567, 572, 627*

Acidophil adenoma

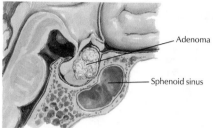

Adenoma

Sphenoid sinus

Relatively small, slow-growing adenoma, causing endocrine symptoms (acromegaly) with little mechanical disturbance

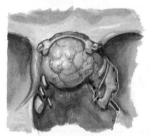

Invasive (malignant) adenoma; extension into right cavernous sinus

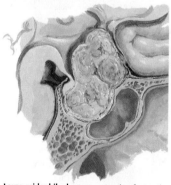

Large acidophil adenoma; extensive destruction of pituitary substance, compression of optic chiasm, invasion of third ventricle and floor of sella

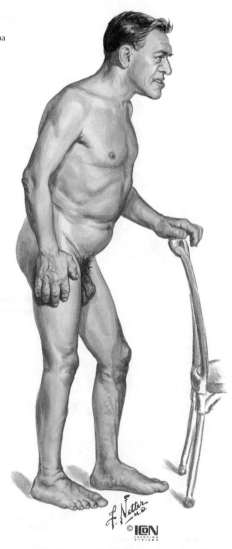

Anterior pituitary gland adenomas may lead to hypersecretion of pituitary hormones. Prolactin hypersecretion is most common, followed by GH and corticotropin (TSH and gonadotropin hypersecretion is rare). GH overproduction, which results in gigantism in children and acromegaly in adults, leads to enlargement of soft tissues (tongue, skin, organs) and bones, sweating, fatigue, weakness, and arthralgias. Such adenomas can expand into the cavernous sinus (to cause deficits of CNs III, IV, V_1, V_2, and/or VI) or compress the optic chiasm (to cause bitemporal hemianopia).

Clinical Correlation

Pituitary Tumor Resection   *Anatomy on pp. 45, 546, 572, 631*

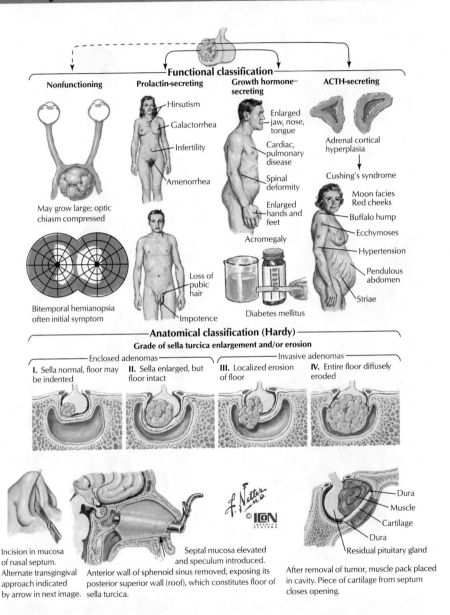

Functional classification

Nonfunctioning

May grow large; optic chiasm compressed

Bitemporal hemianopsia often initial symptom

Prolactin-secreting

- Hirsutism
- Galactorrhea
- Infertility
- Amenorrhea
- Loss of pubic hair
- Impotence

Growth hormone–secreting

- Enlarged jaw, nose, tongue
- Cardiac, pulmonary disease
- Spinal deformity
- Enlarged hands and feet

Acromegaly

Diabetes mellitus

ACTH-secreting

Adrenal cortical hyperplasia

Cushing's syndrome

- Moon facies Red cheeks
- Buffalo hump
- Ecchymoses
- Hypertension
- Pendulous abdomen
- Striae

Anatomical classification (Hardy)
Grade of sella turcica enlargement and/or erosion

Enclosed adenomas

I. Sella normal, floor may be indented

II. Sella enlarged, but floor intact

Invasive adenomas

III. Localized erosion of floor

IV. Entire floor diffusely eroded

Incision in mucosa of nasal septum. Alternate transgingival approach indicated by arrow in next image.

Septal mucosa elevated and speculum introduced. Anterior wall of sphenoid sinus removed, exposing its posterior superior wall (roof), which constitutes floor of sella turcica.

- Dura
- Muscle
- Cartilage
- Dura
- Residual pituitary gland

After removal of tumor, muscle pack placed in cavity. Piece of cartilage from septum closes opening.

Most pituitary tumors are adenomas of the anterior pituitary (gliomas of the posterior lobe are rare). Fortunately, development of the transsphenoidal surgical approach to the sella turcica permits resection of the tumor and preservation of normal glandular tissue.

Brain: Surface Anatomy and Functional Regions

Several circumscribed regions on the cerebral cortex are associated with specific functions. Key surface landmarks, typical of the human brain, are used to divide the brain into lobes.

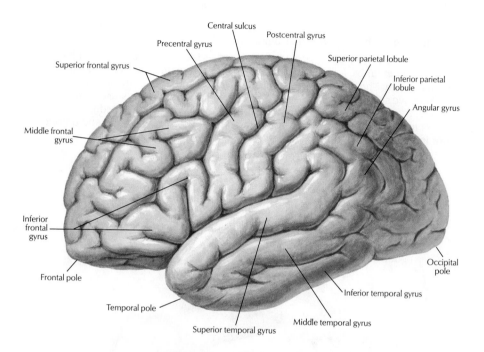

Central sulcus
Precentral gyrus
Postcentral gyrus
Superior frontal gyrus
Superior parietal lobule
Inferior parietal lobule
Angular gyrus
Middle frontal gyrus
Inferior frontal gyrus
Frontal pole
Occipital pole
Inferior temporal gyrus
Temporal pole
Middle temporal gyrus
Superior temporal gyrus

Functional areas of the brain

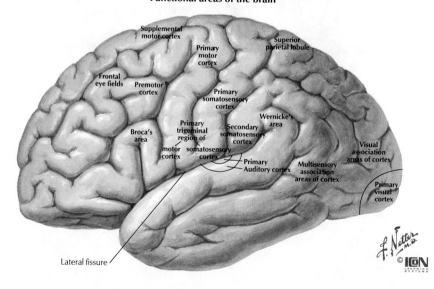

Supplemental motor cortex
Primary motor cortex
Superior parietal lobule
Frontal eye fields
Premotor cortex
Primary somatosensory cortex
Broca's area
Primary trigeminal region of motor cortex
Secondary somatosensory cortex
Wernicke's area
somatosensory cortex
Primary Auditory cortex
Multisensory association areas of cortex
Visual association areas of cortex
Primary visual cortex
Lateral fissure

Brain: Surface Anatomy and Functional Regions (continued)

The cerebral cortex is divided into lobes:

Frontal
Parietal
Occipital
Temporal (not shown in this midsagittal view)

The cingulate cortex is highlighted and labeled as the limbic lobe to reflect its association with other limbic forebrain structures and hypothalamic control of the autonomic nervous system. The thalamus is the gateway to the cortex, simplistically functioning as the "executive secretary" to the cortex. The cerebellum coordinates smooth motor activities and processes muscle position. The brainstem (midbrain, pons, medulla oblongata) conveys motor and sensory input from the body and conveys somatic and autonomic motor information to peripheral targets.

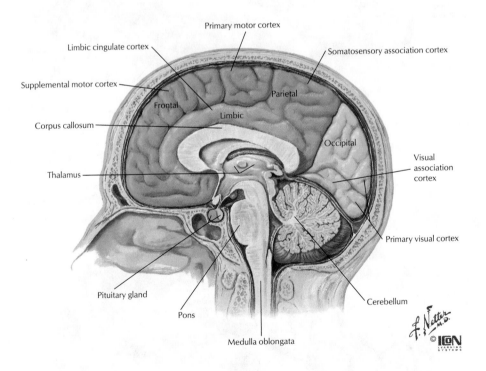

Brain: Arterial Supply

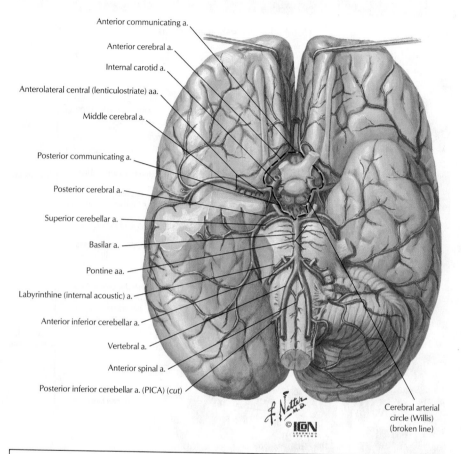

Anterior communicating a.

Anterior cerebral a.

Internal carotid a.

Anterolateral central (lenticulostriate) aa.

Middle cerebral a.

Posterior communicating a.

Posterior cerebral a.

Superior cerebellar a.

Basilar a.

Pontine aa.

Labyrinthine (internal acoustic) a.

Anterior inferior cerebellar a.

Vertebral a.

Anterior spinal a.

Posterior inferior cerebellar a. (PICA) (cut)

Cerebral arterial circle (Willis) (broken line)

ARTERY	COURSE AND STRUCTURES SUPPLIED
Vertebral	From subclavian artery, supplies cerebellum
Posterior inferior cerebellar	From vertebral artery, goes to posteroinferior cerebellum
Basilar	From both vertebrals, goes to brainstem, cerebellum, cerebrum
Anterior inferior cerebellar	From basilar, supplies inferior cerebellum
Superior cerebellar	From basilar, supplies superior cerebellum
Posterior cerebral	From basilar, supplies inferior cerebrum, occipital lobe
Posterior communicating	Cerebral arterial circle (of Willis)
Internal carotid (IC)	From common carotid, supplies cerebral lobes and eye
Middle cerebral	From IC, goes to lateral aspect of cerebral hemispheres
Anterior communicating	Cerebral arterial circle (of Willis)
Anterior cerebral	From IC, goes to cerebral hemispheres (except occipital lobe)

Clinical Correlation

Congenital Cerebral Aneurysms   *Anatomy on p. 573*

Distribution of cerebral aneurysms

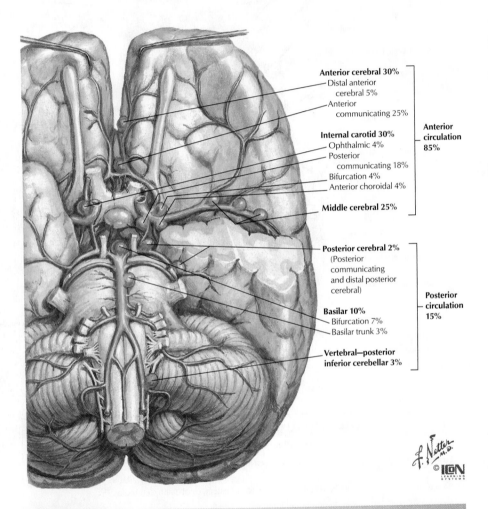

Anterior cerebral 30%
— Distal anterior cerebral 5%
— Anterior communicating 25%

Internal carotid 30%
— Ophthalmic 4%
— Posterior communicating 18%
— Bifurcation 4%
— Anterior choroidal 4%

Middle cerebral 25%

} Anterior circulation 85%

Posterior cerebral 2%
(Posterior communicating and distal posterior cerebral)

Basilar 10%
— Bifurcation 7%
— Basilar trunk 3%

Vertebral–posterior inferior cerebellar 3%

} Posterior circulation 15%

The most common cause of subarachnoid hemorrhage is the rupture of a saccular, or berry, aneurysm.

CHARACTERISTIC	DESCRIPTION
Etiology	Congenital defect in tunica media of arteries at branch points
Prevalence	1%, but a higher association with certain diseases (polycystic kidney, fibromuscular dysplasia, coarctation of aorta); women slightly more affected than men; age 30-65 years
Presentation	Sudden, severe headache; vomiting; alterations in consciousness; meningeal signs include neck rigidity and pain spreading from occipital region to neck, back, and lower limbs

Clinical Correlation

Epidural Hematomas   *Anatomy on pp. 564, 573, 609*

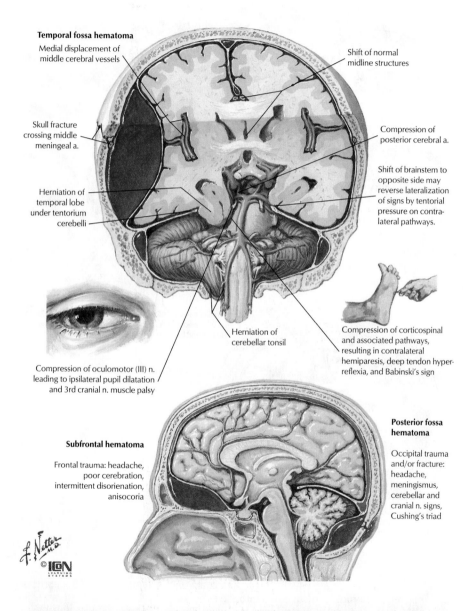

Temporal fossa hematoma
Medial displacement of middle cerebral vessels

Shift of normal midline structures

Skull fracture crossing middle meningeal a.

Compression of posterior cerebral a.

Shift of brainstem to opposite side may reverse lateralization of signs by tentorial pressure on contralateral pathways.

Herniation of temporal lobe under tentorium cerebelli

Compression of oculomotor (III) n. leading to ipsilateral pupil dilatation and 3rd cranial n. muscle palsy

Herniation of cerebellar tonsil

Compression of corticospinal and associated pathways, resulting in contralateral hemiparesis, deep tendon hyperreflexia, and Babinski's sign

Subfrontal hematoma

Frontal trauma: headache, poor cerebration, intermittent disorienation, anisocoria

Posterior fossa hematoma

Occipital trauma and/or fracture: headache, meningismus, cerebellar and cranial n. signs, Cushing's triad

Epidural hematomas result most often from vehicular accidents, falls, and sports injuries. The source of the bleeding is usually arterial (85%); common locations include the frontal, temporal (middle meningeal artery is very susceptible), and occipital regions.

Clinical Correlation

Subdural Hematomas
Anatomy on pp. 564, 567

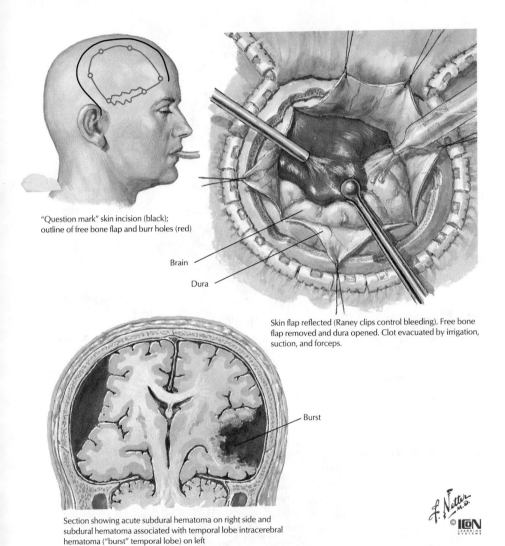

"Question mark" skin incision (black); outline of free bone flap and burr holes (red)

Brain

Dura

Skin flap reflected (Raney clips control bleeding). Free bone flap removed and dura opened. Clot evacuated by irrigation, suction, and forceps.

Burst

Section showing acute subdural hematoma on right side and subdural hematoma associated with temporal lobe intracerebral hematoma ("burst" temporal lobe) on left

Subdural hematomas are usually due to an acute venous hemorrhage of the cortical bridging veins draining cortical blood into the superior sagittal sinus. Half are associated with skull fractures. Clinical signs include a decreasing level of consciousness, ipsilateral pupillary dilation, and contralateral hemiparesis. These hematomas develop within 1 week after injury but often present within hours. Chronic subdural hematomas are most common in the elderly and long-term alcoholics who have some brain atrophy, which increases the space traversed by the bridging veins.

Clinical Correlation

Carotid–Cavernous Sinus Fistula
Anatomy on pp. 567, 634

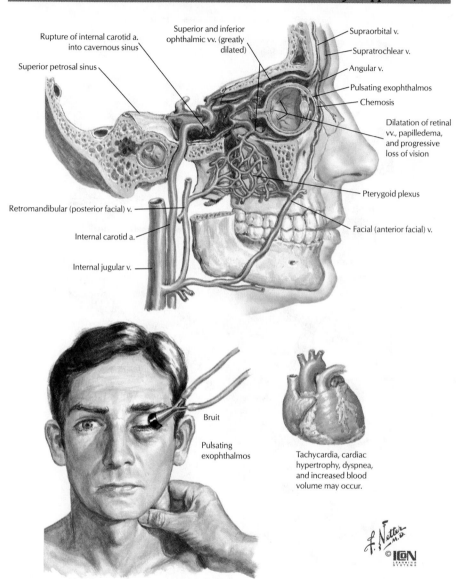

Rupture of internal carotid a. into cavernous sinus

Superior and inferior ophthalmic vv. (greatly dilated)

Superior petrosal sinus

Supraorbital v.

Supratrochlear v.

Angular v.

Pulsating exophthalmos

Chemosis

Dilatation of retinal vv., papilledema, and progressive loss of vision

Retromandibular (posterior facial) v.

Internal carotid a.

Internal jugular v.

Pterygoid plexus

Facial (anterior facial) v.

Bruit

Pulsating exophthalmos

Tachycardia, cardiac hypertrophy, dyspnea, and increased blood volume may occur.

Bruit obliterated by carotid compression

More common than symptomatic intracavernous sinus aneurysms but less common than subarachnoid saccular (berry) aneurysms, carotid-cavernous sinus fistulas often result from trauma and are more common in men than in women. They are high-pressure (arterial) low-flow lesions characterized by an orbital bruit, exophthalmos, chemosis, and extraocular muscle palsies (CNs III, IV, and VI). Blood collecting in the cavernous sinus drains via several venous pathways, as illustrated.

Clinical Correlation

Stroke

Anatomy on pp. 564, 573

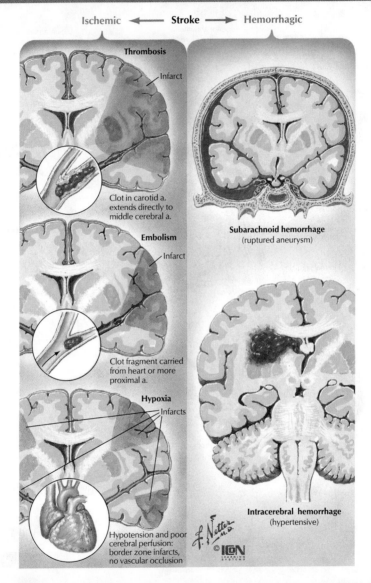

Ischemic ← **Stroke** → Hemorrhagic

Thrombosis

Infarct

Clot in carotid a. extends directly to middle cerebral a.

Embolism

Infarct

Clot fragment carried from heart or more proximal a.

Hypoxia

Infarcts

Hypotension and poor cerebral perfusion: border zone infarcts, no vascular occlusion

Subarachnoid hemorrhage (ruptured aneurysm)

Intracerebral hemorrhage (hypertensive)

Stroke is a localized brain injury caused by a vascular episode that lasts more than 24 hours (whereas transient ischemic attacks [TIAs] are focal ischemic episodes that last less than 24 hours). Stroke is classified into two types:

- **Ischemic** (80%): thrombotic or embolic, resulting from atherosclerosis of extracranial (usually carotid) and/or intracranial arteries or from underlying heart disease
- **Hemorrhagic**: occurs when a cerebral vessel weakens and ruptures, which causes intracranial bleeding, usually affecting a larger brain area

Clinical Correlation

Other Etiologic Mechanisms of Stroke   *Anatomy on pp. 564, 573*

Cardiac emboli

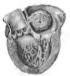
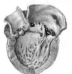

Cardiomyopathy with thrombi

Mitral valve prolapse with clots

Atrial myxomatous tumor emboli

Marantic emboli

Probe-patent foramen ovale transmitting venous clots

Carotid or intracerebral arterial disorders

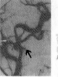

Migraine

Angiogram showing dissection of carotid artery, with high-grade stenosis and pseudo-aneurysm

Intracerebral aneurysm. Spasm in distal vessel

Giant cell arteritis

Drug-induced mechanisms

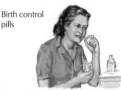

Birth control pills

Drug addiction ("mainliner")

Monoamine oxidase (MAO) inhibitors (potentiated by wine and cheese)

Hematologic disorders

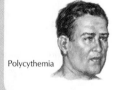
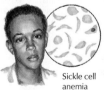
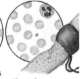

Polycythemia

Sickle cell anemia

Thrombocytosis

Thrombocytopenia

Infectious diseases

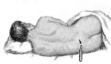

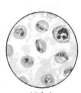

Herpes zoster (ophthalmic)

CNS syphilis

Meningitis

Malaria

Clinical Correlation

Ischemia in the Internal Carotid Artery Territory

Anatomy on pp. 573, 598

Clinical manifestations

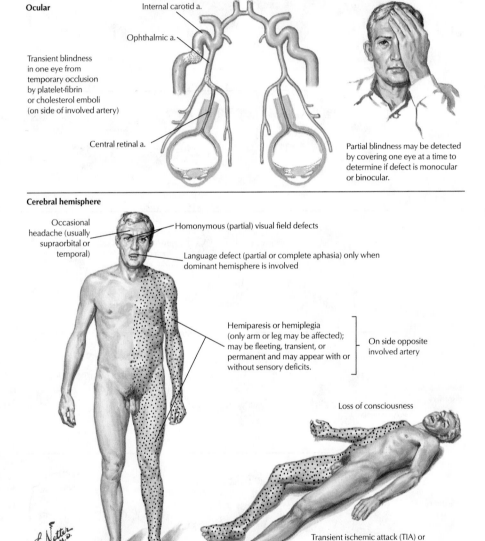

Ocular

Internal carotid a.

Ophthalmic a.

Transient blindness in one eye from temporary occlusion by platelet-fibrin or cholesterol emboli (on side of involved artery)

Central retinal a.

Partial blindness may be detected by covering one eye at a time to determine if defect is monocular or binocular.

Cerebral hemisphere

Occasional headache (usually supraorbital or temporal)

Homonymous (partial) visual field defects

Language defect (partial or complete aphasia) only when dominant hemisphere is involved

Hemiparesis or hemiplegia (only arm or leg may be affected); may be fleeting, transient, or permanent and may appear with or without sensory deficits.

On side opposite involved artery

Loss of consciousness

Transient ischemic attack (TIA) or full stroke (CVA) hemiplegia or hemiparesis contralateral to lesion

A TIA or true stroke involving the IC artery territory can lead to ipsilateral visual disturbances with or without contralateral motor and sensory changes. A defect in the dominant hemisphere may lead to aphasia.

Clinical Correlation

Collateral Circulation after Internal
Carotid Artery Occlusion   *Anatomy on pp. 534, 573, 609, 633*

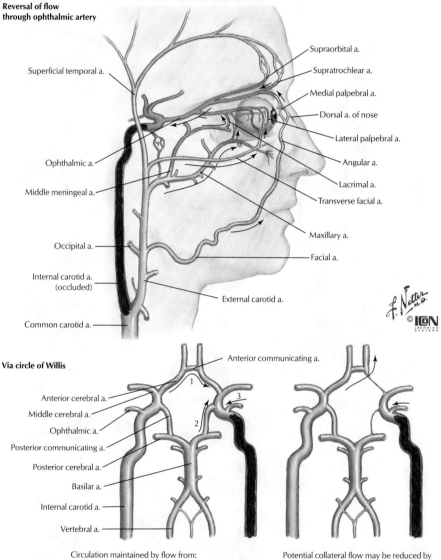

Reversal of flow through ophthalmic artery

Superficial temporal a.

Ophthalmic a.

Middle meningeal a.

Occipital a.

Internal carotid a. (occluded)

Common carotid a.

Supraorbital a.

Supratrochlear a.

Medial palpebral a.

Dorsal a. of nose

Lateral palpebral a.

Angular a.

Lacrimal a.

Transverse facial a.

Maxillary a.

Facial a.

External carotid a.

F. Netter M.D.
© ICON LEARNING SYSTEMS

Via circle of Willis

Anterior communicating a.

Anterior cerebral a.

Middle cerebral a.

Ophthalmic a.

Posterior communicating a.

Posterior cerebral a.

Basilar a.

Internal carotid a.

Vertebral a.

Circulation maintained by flow from:
1. Opposite internal carotid a. (anterior circulation)
2. Vertebrobasilar system (posterior circulation)
3. Ophthalmic a.

Potential collateral flow may be reduced by anomalous insufficiency of segments of circle of Willis.

If a major artery, such as the IC artery, becomes occluded, extracranial and intracranial (circle of Willis) anastomoses may provide collateral routes of circulation. These routes are more likely to develop when occlusion is gradual (as in atherosclerosis) rather than acute (as in embolic obstruction).

Clinical Correlation

Ischemia in the Vertebrobasilar Artery Territory

Anatomy on pp. 573, 637, 638

Clinical manifestations

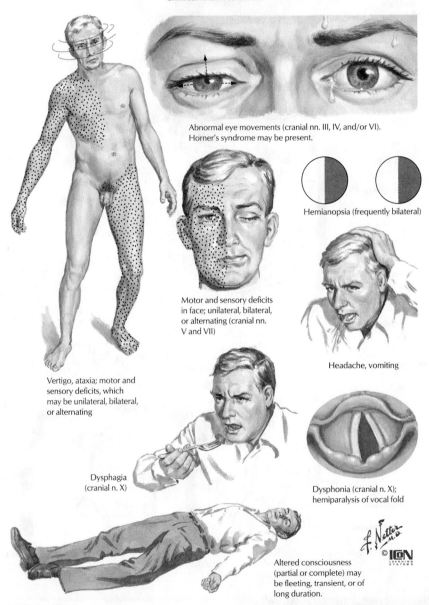

Abnormal eye movements (cranial nn. III, IV, and/or VI). Horner's syndrome may be present.

Hemianopsia (frequently bilateral)

Motor and sensory deficits in face; unilateral, bilateral, or alternating (cranial nn. V and VII)

Headache, vomiting

Vertigo, ataxia; motor and sensory deficits, which may be unilateral, bilateral, or alternating

Dysphagia (cranial n. X)

Dysphonia (cranial n. X); hemiparalysis of vocal fold

Altered consciousness (partial or complete) may be fleeting, transient, or of long duration.

Of all strokes, 20% occur in the vertebrobasilar territory. Dysfunction may involve the brainstem, cerebellar hemispheres, or occipital lobes. Clinical manifestations vary because the basilar artery is a midline vessel with branches to both sides of the brain.

Clinical Correlation

Giant Cell Arteritis and Polymyalgia Rheumatica

Anatomy on pp. 558, 598

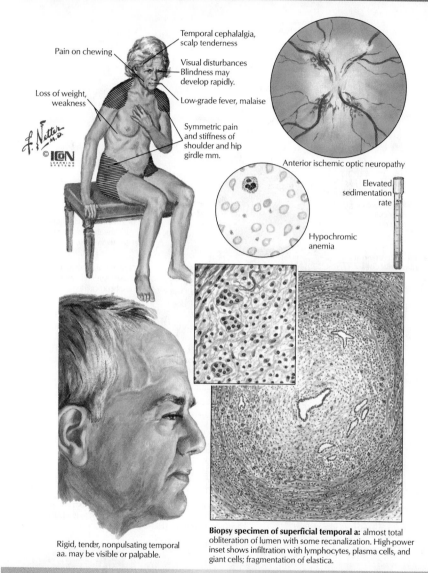

Temporal cephalalgia, scalp tenderness

Pain on chewing

Visual disturbances Blindness may develop rapidly.

Loss of weight, weakness

Low-grade fever, malaise

Symmetric pain and stiffness of shoulder and hip girdle mm.

Anterior ischemic optic neuropathy

Elevated sedimentation rate

Hypochromic anemia

Rigid, tender, nonpulsating temporal aa. may be visible or palpable.

Biopsy specimen of superficial temporal a: almost total obliteration of lumen with some recanalization. High-power inset shows infiltration with lymphocytes, plasma cells, and giant cells; fragmentation of elastica.

These two conditions are linked and coexist or develop sequentially. They are associated with increased erythrocyte sedimentation rate, interleukin 6, and human leukocyte antigen-DR4. The etiology is uncertain but may include infections and local degenerative, genetic, and autoimmune processes. Both conditions usually affect people older than 50 years, women more than men, and those of north European descent. Giant cell arteritis is a medical emergency because it can lead to unilateral blindness (arteries most affected are the temporal, which can be biopsied, and the ophthalmic). Both diseases respond to systemic steroid treatment.

Clinical Correlation

Vascular (Multiinfarct) Dementia   *Anatomy on p. 573*

Clinical characteristics of vascular (multiinfarct) dementia

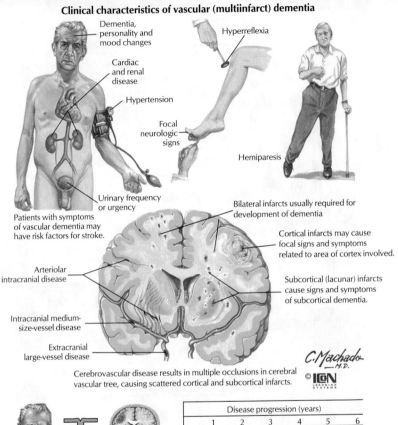

Dementia, personality and mood changes

Hyperreflexia

Cardiac and renal disease

Hypertension

Focal neurologic signs

Hemiparesis

Urinary frequency or urgency

Patients with symptoms of vascular dementia may have risk factors for stroke.

Bilateral infarcts usually required for development of dementia

Cortical infarcts may cause focal signs and symptoms related to area of cortex involved.

Arteriolar intracranial disease

Subcortical (lacunar) infarcts cause signs and symptoms of subcortical dementia.

Intracranial medium-size-vessel disease

Extracranial large-vessel disease

Cerebrovascular disease results in multiple occlusions in cerebral vascular tree, causing scattered cortical and subcortical infarcts.

C. Machado M.D.

© ICON LEARNING SYSTEMS

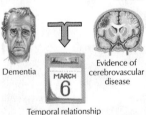

Dementia

MARCH 6

Evidence of cerebrovascular disease

Temporal relationship

Triad of characteristics that suggests vascular etiology

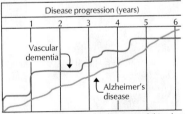

Disease progression (years)

Vascular dementia

Alzheimer's disease

Clinical progression. Vascular dementia exhibits abrupt onset and stepwise progression in contrast to gradual onset and progression of Alzheimer's disease.

Dementia is an acquired neurologic syndrome that presents with multiple cognitive deficits. By definition, it includes one or more of the following: short-term memory impairment, behavioral disturbance, and difficulties with daily functioning and independence. It can be classed as degenerative, vascular, alcoholic, or HIV related. The most common cause of degenerative dementia is Alzheimer's disease. Vascular dementias, resulting from anoxic damage from small infarcts, account for approximately 15-20% of dementia cases. Multiinfarct dementia is associated with heart disease, diabetes mellitus (DM), hypertension, and inflammatory diseases.

Clinical Correlation

Extrapyramidal Disorders (Parkinson's Disease)

Anatomy on pp. 571, 572

Parkinson's disease

Dementia

Masklike facies

Rigidity and flexed posturing

Tremor

Short shuffling gait

Dopamine projections to corpus striatum from substantia nigra

Loss of dopamine projections to frontal cortex from ventral tegmentum may result in dementia

Lewy body

Substantia nigra shows marked loss of neurons and pigment. Residual neurons may exhibit Lewy bodies.

Dopamine

Normal

Dopamine

Parkinson's disease

C. Machado —M.D.

© ICON
LEARNING
SYSTEMS

Parkinson's disease is an extrapyramidal disorder characterized by motor impairment, specifically
- Rigidity
- Expressionless face
- Stooped posture
- Shuffling gait
- Pill-rolling tremor

The disease results from progressive loss of dopamine (DA)-secreting neurons of the substantia nigra, which project to the corpus striatum (accounts for motor impairment) and frontal cortex (cause of dementia). Dementia is increasingly recognized in advanced disease, in up to 25% of cases.

Clinical Correlation

Manifestations of Brain Tumors
Anatomy on pp. 571, 598

Intracranial pressure triad

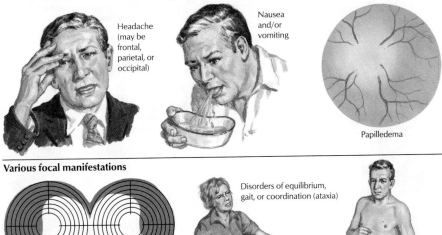

Headache (may be frontal, parietal, or occipital)

Nausea and/or vomiting

Papilledema

Various focal manifestations

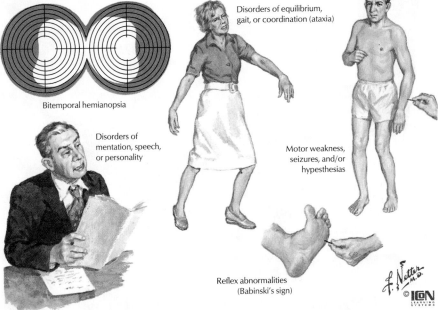

Bitemporal hemianopsia

Disorders of equilibrium, gait, or coordination (ataxia)

Disorders of mentation, speech, or personality

Motor weakness, seizures, and/or hypesthesias

Reflex abnormalities (Babinski's sign)

Clinical signs and symptoms of brain tumors depend on the location and the degree to which intracranial pressure (ICP) is increased. Slow-growing tumors in relatively silent areas (e.g., frontal lobes) may go undetected and can become quite large before symptoms occur. Small tumors in key brain areas can lead to seizures, hemiparesis, or aphasia. Increased ICP can initiate broader damage by compressing critical brain structures. Early symptoms of ICP include malaise, headache, nausea, papilledema, and, less often, abducent nerve palsy and Parinaud's syndrome (classic signs of hydrocephalus: loss of upward gaze, downward ocular deviation ["setting sun" syndrome], lid retraction, light-near dissociation of pupils). Types of primary tumors include gliomas (50% of tumors), meningiomas (20%), pituitary tumors (15%), and neuromas (7%).

Clinical Correlation

Gliomas

Anatomy on pp. 33, 571

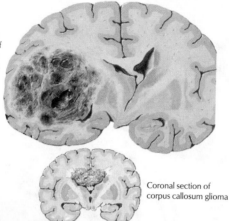

Large, hemispheric glioblastoma multiforme with central areas of necrosis. Brain distorted to opposite side.

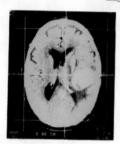

Coronal section of corpus callosum glioma

CT-guided stereotactic brain biopsy

CT scan taken with basic frame on patient's head. Biopsy needle directed at target by coordinates dialed directly on stereotactic frame.

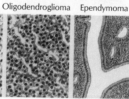
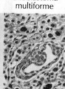
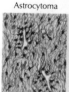

Patient, head draped, on operating table. Biopsy specimen taken via burr hole under local anesthesia.

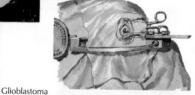

| Astrocytoma | Glioblastoma multiforme | Oligodendroglioma | Ependymoma |

Approximately 50% of primary brain tumors are gliomas (incidence in children is even higher), which arise from supporting cells (glia) of the brain.

TYPE	CHARACTERISTICS
Astrocytoma	Fibrillary (infiltrating) and pilocytic (more common in children)
Oligodendroglioma	More common in adults; usually occurs in cerebral hemispheres
Ependymoma	Usually arises in a brain ventricle or spinal cord central canal; causes increased ICP and hydrocephalus

Clinical Correlation

Meningiomas

Anatomy on pp. 564, 571

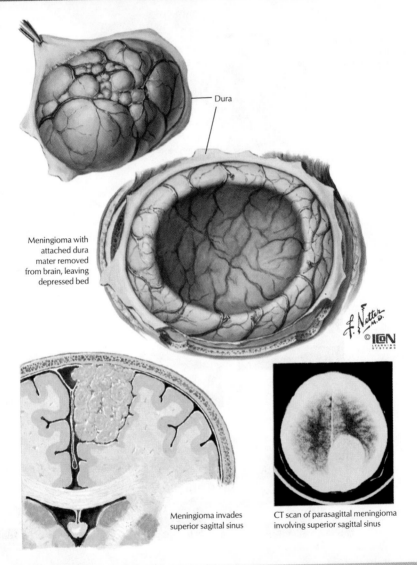

Dura

Meningioma with attached dura mater removed from brain, leaving depressed bed

Meningioma invades superior sagittal sinus

CT scan of parasagittal meningioma involving superior sagittal sinus

Meningiomas, slow-growing benign tumors, arise from meningothelial cells of the arachnoid mater.

CHARACTERISTIC	DESCRIPTION
Prevalence	5-20% of all brain tumors; two times more common in women than in men; increasing prevalence with age
Location	Most outside brain parenchyma; arise in cranial vault and spinal cord
Presentation	Usually increased ICP; occasionally seizures and neurologic deficits

Clinical Correlation

Metastatic Brain Tumors   *Anatomy on pp. 109, 571*

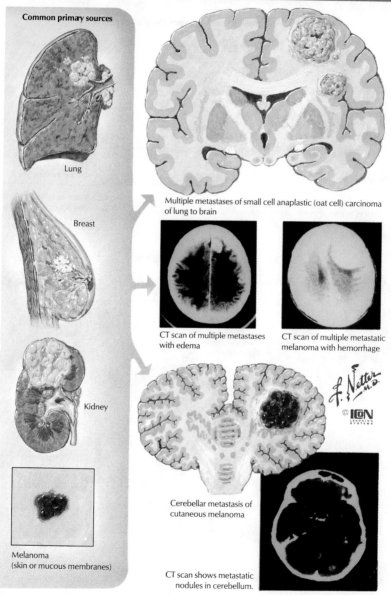

Common primary sources

Lung

Breast

Kidney

Melanoma
(skin or mucous membranes)

Multiple metastases of small cell anaplastic (oat cell) carcinoma of lung to brain

CT scan of multiple metastases with edema

CT scan of multiple metastatic melanoma with hemorrhage

Cerebellar metastasis of cutaneous melanoma

CT scan shows metastatic nodules in cerebellum.

Metastatic tumors are more common than primary brain tumors. Most spread via the bloodstream, with cells seeded between white and gray matter. Some tumors metastasize directly from head and neck cancers or by means of Batson's vertebral venous plexus. Presentation includes increased ICP and often headache (50%) and seizures (25%).

Clinical Correlation

Viral Encephalitis

Anatomy on pp. 597, 638

Possible route of transmission in herpes simplex encephalitis

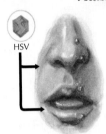
HSV

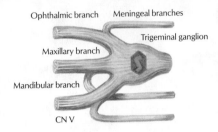
Ophthalmic branch   Meningeal branches
Trigeminal ganglion
Maxillary branch
Mandibular branch
CN V

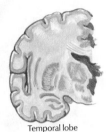
Temporal lobe

Primary infection	Latent phase	Reactivation (lytic phase)
Virus enters via cutaneous or mucosal surfaces to infect sensory or autonomic n. endings with transport to cell bodies in ganglia.	Virus replicates in ganglia before establishing latent phase.	Reactivation of HSV in trigeminal ganglion can result in spread to brain (temporal lobe) via meningeal branches of CN V.

Clinical features of HSV encephalitis

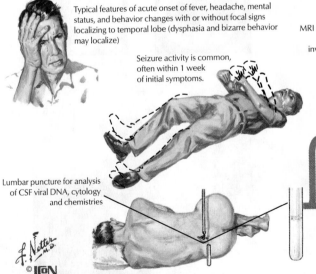

Typical features of acute onset of fever, headache, mental status, and behavior changes with or without focal signs localizing to temporal lobe (dysphasia and bizarre behavior may localize)

Seizure activity is common, often within 1 week of initial symptoms.

Lumbar puncture for analysis of CSF viral DNA, cytology and chemistries

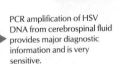
MRI demonstrating temporal lobe involvement is a diagnostic cornerstone

PCR amplification of HSV DNA from cerebrospinal fluid provides major diagnostic information and is very sensitive.

HSV encephalitis CSF cytology and chemical studies typically show:
WBC: moderate
RBC: +/−
Protein: moderate
Glucose: normal

CHARACTERISTIC	DESCRIPTION
Etiology	HSV-1, arboviruses, and enteroviruses more common causes than cytomegalovirus, Epstein-Barr virus, HIV, varicella-zoster virus, and others
Pathophysiology	Infection of brain parenchyma, with perivascular infiltrates, microglial nodules, and inclusion bodies
Prevalence	2-4 cases/million; occurs in all ages but more common in adolescents or young adults and those older than 50 years
Presentation	Hallmark: cognitive deficits

Clinical Correlation

Unipolar Depression

Anatomy on p. 571

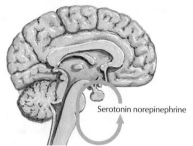

Serotonin norepinephrine

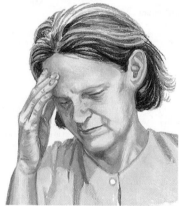

Depression is a biochemically mediated state most likely based on abnormalities in metabolism of serotonin and norepinephrine.

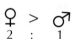

♀ > ♂
2 : 1

Female gender predominates.

Clinical syndrome characterized by withdrawal, anger, frustration, and loss of pleasure

Associated symptoms and comorbidities

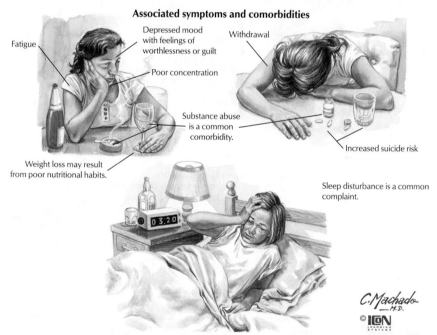

Fatigue

Depressed mood with feelings of worthlessness or guilt

Withdrawal

Poor concentration

Substance abuse is a common comorbidity.

Increased suicide risk

Weight loss may result from poor nutritional habits.

Sleep disturbance is a common complaint.

C. Machado —M.D.

© ICON
LEARNING
SYSTEMS

Occasionally feeling depressed is a nonpathologic process, whereas depression, the illness, interferes with patients' usual functioning. Depression is associated with an imbalance in neurotransmission of monoamines (serotonin, norepinephrine, DA). Major depression occurs in 4% of the general population. Clinical signs and symptoms include depressed mood, anxiety, guilt, and suicidal thoughts, among others. Risk factors include female sex, family history, personal history of previous depression, postpartum status, lack of social supports, and substance abuse.

Clinical Correlation

Migraine Headache   *Anatomy on pp. 529, 571, 638*

Mechanisms in migraine

Central mechanisms

Pain perception

Peripheral mechanisms

Migraine may be initiated by afferent stimulation from central centers in cortex, thalamus, and hypothalamus or by peripheral afferent stimulation via trigeminal n. or cervical roots C1-3.

Periaqueductal gray matter

Nucleus raphe dorsalis

Locus ceruleus

Local defect in endogenous pain control system prevents inhibition of pain stimulation (disinhibition) in spinal nucleus of trigeminal n.

Trigeminal n. pain pathway

Unopposed pain stimulation in spinal nucleus of trigeminal n.

V₁   Peripheral inflow

V₂

Central pain pathway

V₃

Trigeminal (V) n.

Trigeminal vascular reflex
Afferent stimulation of pain centers in spinal nucleus of trigeminal n. increased and perpetuated by cycle of parasympathetic dilation of internal and external carotid aa. mediated via facial n., resulting in stimulation of pain centers by trigeminal n. afferents

Nucleus raphe magnus

Facial (VII) n.

Parasympathetic (vasodilation) outflow

Second-order neuron

Impaired inhibition in endogenous pain control system

Pain stimulation in spinal nucleus of trigeminal n. via afferent input from higher sources and via cervical roots C1-3

C1-3 pain pathway

C. Machado
— M.D.

© ICON
LEARNING

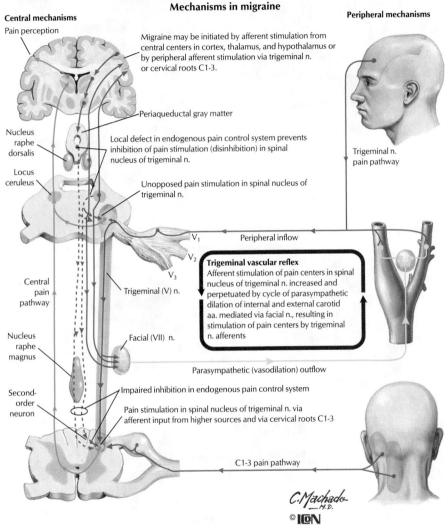

CHARACTERISTIC	DESCRIPTION
Etiology	Role suggested for serotonin and DA receptor activation and/or trigeminal stimulation and neurogenic inflammation of blood vessels; 70-80% family history
Prevalence	18% female, 6% male in United States; 80% have first attack by age 30 years
Presentation	Dizziness, tinnitus, scotomas, photophobia, weakness, aphasia, vomiting, visual scintillations (zigzag lines)
Triggers	Intense light, sound, or odors; certain foods (e.g., MSG); stress; fatigue; irregular sleep; hormonal fluctuations; weather changes

Clinical Correlation

Respiratory Function in Head Injury *Anatomy on pp. 571, 573*

Causes of impaired O_2 and CO_2 exchange

Hypoxia and acidosis of neurons

Hemispheric and/or basal ganglia lesions
may cause Cheyne-Stokes respiration

Indirect injury to brainstem
from intracranial clot may cause uncal herniation

$O_2 \downarrow CO_2 \uparrow$
$NaHCO_3 \rightarrow HHCO$

Hypoxia and acidosis result in rapidly deteriorating neuronal function.

Injury to upper brainstem
may result in rapid, shallow breathing (central neurogenic hyperventilation)

Pneumotaxic center

Apneustic center

Injury to medulla
often results in very irregular respiration (ataxic)

Medullary center

Impaired blood supply to brain
due to shock (hypovolemic or neurogenic) or arterial injury

Airway obstruction
by blood, mucus, vomitus, foreign body (false teeth), or impacted tongue impairs respiratory exchange

Increased intracranial pressure

Phrenic n.

Chest injury
(fractured ribs, flail chest, sucking wounds, pneumothorax, hemothorax) impairs breathing

Intercostal nn.

Hypercapnia increases cerebral blood volume, leading to additional increase in intracranial pressure, which further embarrasses respiration: a vicious cycle of deterioration.

Delayed complications
(pulmonary embolus, fat embolus, disseminated intravascular coagulation)
or
Metabolic factors
may further alter respiration (ketoacidosis, uremia, salicylism, hepatic encephalopathy, poisoning)

Management of patients with head injury must include careful assessment and monitoring of respiration, because the brain depends on aerobic metabolism in most situations and requires a significant blood supply (15-20% of cardiac output) and oxygen supply (20% of the body's utilization).

Orbit: Eyelids and Lacrimal Apparatus

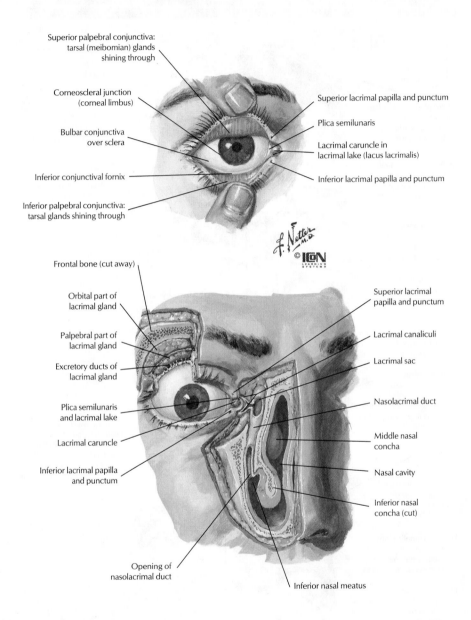

Superior palpebral conjunctiva: tarsal (meibomian) glands shining through

Corneoscleral junction (corneal limbus)

Bulbar conjunctiva over sclera

Inferior conjunctival fornix

Inferior palpebral conjunctiva: tarsal glands shining through

Superior lacrimal papilla and punctum

Plica semilunaris

Lacrimal caruncle in lacrimal lake (lacus lacrimalis)

Inferior lacrimal papilla and punctum

Frontal bone (cut away)

Orbital part of lacrimal gland

Palpebral part of lacrimal gland

Excretory ducts of lacrimal gland

Plica semilunaris and lacrimal lake

Lacrimal caruncle

Inferior lacrimal papilla and punctum

Opening of nasolacrimal duct

Inferior nasal meatus

Superior lacrimal papilla and punctum

Lacrimal canaliculi

Lacrimal sac

Nasolacrimal duct

Middle nasal concha

Nasal cavity

Inferior nasal concha (cut)

The eyelids protect the eyeballs and keep the corneas moist. The lacrimal apparatus includes the

Lacrimal glands: secrete tears; innervated by facial nerve parasympathetics
Lacrimal ducts: excretory ducts of the glands
Lacrimal canaliculi: collect tears and convey them to lacrimal sacs
Nasolacrimal ducts: convey tears from lacrimal sacs to the nasal cavity (inferior meatus)

Orbit: Muscles

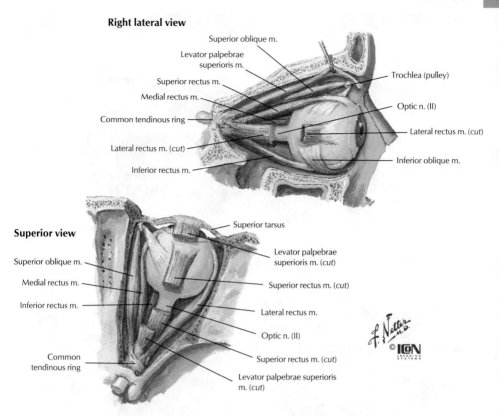

Right lateral view

Superior oblique m.

Levator palpebrae
superioris m.

Superior rectus m.

Medial rectus m.

Common tendinous ring

Lateral rectus m. (*cut*)

Inferior rectus m.

Trochlea (pulley)

Optic n. (II)

Lateral rectus m. (*cut*)

Inferior oblique m.

Superior view

Superior oblique m.

Medial rectus m.

Inferior rectus m.

Common
tendinous ring

Superior tarsus

Levator palpebrae
superioris m. (*cut*)

Superior rectus m. (*cut*)

Lateral rectus m.

Optic n. (II)

Superior rectus m. (*cut*)

Levator palpebrae superioris
m. (*cut*)

MUSCLE	ORIGIN	INSERTION	INNERVATION	MAIN ACTIONS
Levator palpebrae superioris	Sphenoid bone, anterosuperior optic canal	Tarsal plate and skin of upper eyelid	Oculomotor nerve (superior tarsal muscle supplied by sympathetic fibers)	Elevates upper eyelid
Superior rectus (SR)	Common tendinous ring (anulus of Zinn)	Sclera just posterior to cornea	Oculomotor nerve	Elevates, adducts, and rotates eyeball medially
Inferior rectus (IR)	Common tendinous ring (anulus of Zinn)	Sclera just posterior to cornea	Oculomotor nerve	Depresses, adducts, and rotates eyeball medially
Medial rectus	Common tendinous ring (anulus of Zinn)	Sclera just posterior to cornea	Oculomotor nerve	Adducts eyeball
Lateral rectus	Common tendinous ring (anulus of Zinn)	Sclera just posterior to cornea	Abducent nerve	Abducts eyeball
Superior oblique (SO)	Body of sphenoid bone	Passes through a trochlea and inserts into sclera	Trochlear nerve	Medially rotates, depresses, and abducts eyeball
Inferior oblique (IO)	Floor of orbit	Sclera deep to lateral rectus muscle	Oculomotor nerve	Laterally rotates and elevates and abducts eyeball

Clinical Correlation

General Testing of Extraocular Muscles   *Anatomy on pp. 595, 637*

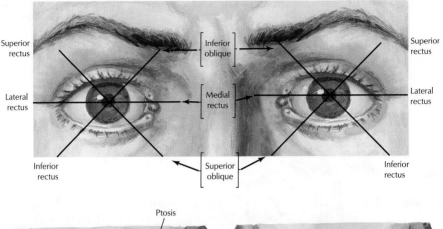

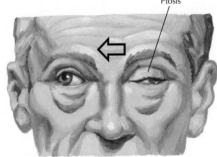

Attempted right gaze in patient with
left third nerve palsy

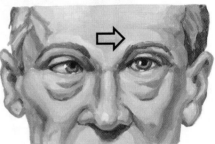

Attempted left gaze in patient with
left sixth nerve palsy

Because extraocular muscles act as synergists and antagonists and may be responsible for multiple movements, it is difficult to test each muscle individually. However, the generalist can obtain an idea of extraocular muscle (or nerve) impairment by checking the ability of individual muscles to elevate or depress the globe with the eye abducted or adducted, thereby aligning the globe with the pull (line of contraction) of the muscle. One can use an H pattern to assess how each eye tracks movement of an object (the tester's finger). For example, when the finger is held up and to the right of the patient's eyes, the patient must primarily use the SR of the right eye and the IO of the left eye to focus on the finger. Pure abduction is done by the lateral rectus; pure adduction is done by the medial rectus. In all other cases, two muscles elevate the eye (SR and IO, with minimal intorsion or extorsion) and two muscles depress the eye (IR and SO, with minimal intorsion or extorsion) in abduction and adduction, respectively. At the end of this test, the examiner can bring the finger directly to the midline to test convergence (medial rectus muscles). If an eye movement disorder is detected via this method, a specialist may be consulted for further evaluation.

Orbit: Nerves

Superior view

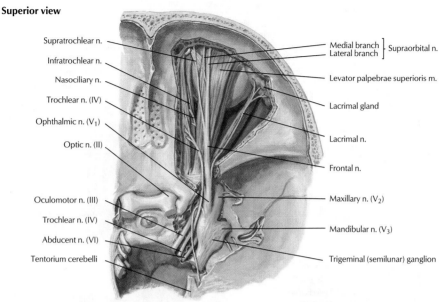

Supratrochlear n.

Infratrochlear n.

Nasociliary n.

Trochlear n. (IV)

Ophthalmic n. (V₁)

Optic n. (II)

Oculomotor n. (III)

Trochlear n. (IV)

Abducent n. (VI)

Tentorium cerebelli

Medial branch ⎤ Supraorbital n.
Lateral branch ⎦

Levator palpebrae superioris m.

Lacrimal gland

Lacrimal n.

Frontal n.

Maxillary n. (V₂)

Mandibular n. (V₃)

Trigeminal (semilunar) ganglion

Levator palpebrae superioris, superior rectus, and superior oblique mm. partially cut away

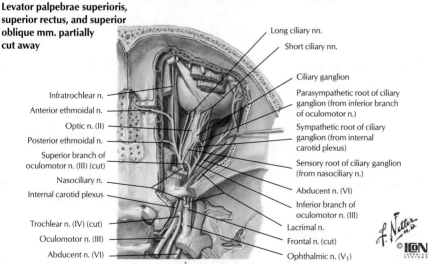

Infratrochlear n.

Anterior ethmoidal n.

Optic n. (II)

Posterior ethmoidal n.

Superior branch of oculomotor n. (III) (cut)

Nasociliary n.

Internal carotid plexus

Trochlear n. (IV) (cut)

Oculomotor n. (III)

Abducent n. (VI)

Long ciliary nn.

Short ciliary nn.

Ciliary ganglion

Parasympathetic root of ciliary ganglion (from inferior branch of oculomotor n.)

Sympathetic root of ciliary ganglion (from internal carotid plexus)

Sensory root of ciliary ganglion (from nasociliary n.)

Abducent n. (VI)

Inferior branch of oculomotor n. (III)

Lacrimal n.

Frontal n. (cut)

Ophthalmic n. (V₁)

NERVE (CN)	INNERVATION
Optic (II)	Leaves via optic canal and carries sensory axons to brain
Oculomotor (III)	Motor to five muscles; conveys parasympathetics to ciliary body and ciliary muscle (for accommodation) and sphincter pupillae muscle
Trochlear (IV)	Motor to SO muscle
Abducent (VI)	Motor to lateral rectus muscle
Ophthalmic (V₁)	Sensory to orbit and eye (frontal, lacrimal, nasociliary nerves)

Orbit: Eyeball (Globe)

Horizontal section

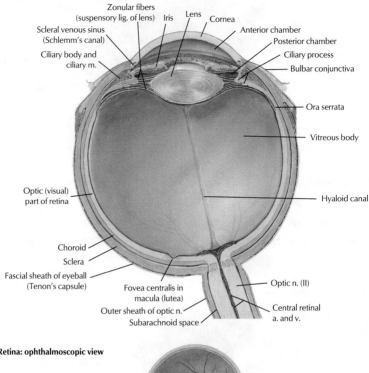

Retina: ophthalmoscopic view

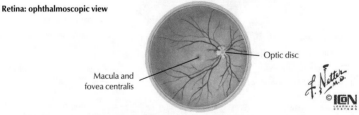

FEATURE	DEFINITION
Sclera	Outer fibrous layer of eyeball
Cornea	Transparent part of outer layer; very sensitive to pain
Choroid	Vascular middle layer of eyeball
Ciliary body	Vascular and muscular extension of choroid anteriorly
Ciliary process	Radiating pigmented folds on ciliary body that secret aqueous humor that fills posterior and anterior chambers
Iris	Contractile diaphragm with central aperture (pupil)
Lens	Transparent lens supported in capsule by zonular fibers
Retina	Optically receptive part of optic nerve (optic retina)
Macula lutea	Retinal area of most acute vision
Optic disc	Nonreceptive area where optic nerve axons leave retina for brain

Clinical Correlation

Eyelid Infection and Conjunctival Disorders

Anatomy on pp. 594, 598

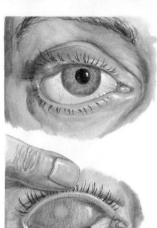

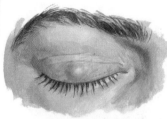
Acute meibomianitis

Chalazion

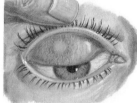
Chalazion; lid everted

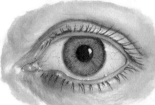
Hordeolum (sty) of lower lid

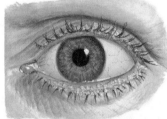
Blepharitis

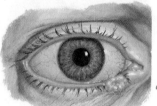

Carcinoma of lower lid

CONDITION	DESCRIPTION
Meibomianitis	Inflammation of meibomian (tarsal) glands
Chalazion	Cyst formation in meibomian gland
Hordeolum (sty)	Infection of sebaceous gland at base of eyelash follicle
Blepharitis	Inflammation of eyelash margin (scaly or ulcerated)
Conjunctival hyperemia (bloodshot eye)	Dilated, congested conjunctival vessels caused by local irritants (e.g., dust, smoke) (not illustrated)
Conjunctivitis (pink eye)	Common inflammation; result of injection of conjunctival vessels caused by allergy, infection, or external irritant
Subconjunctival hemorrhage	Painless, homogeneous red area; result of rupture of subconjunctival capillaries

Clinical Correlation

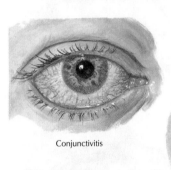

Conjunctivitis

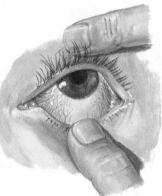

Finger pressure test

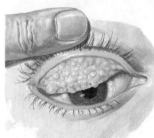

Vernal conjunctivitis

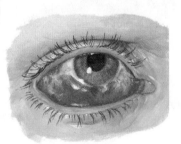

Subconjunctival hemorrhage

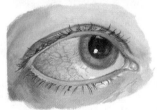

Episcleritis

Clinical Correlation

Ocular Refractive Disorders (Ametropias)   *Anatomy on p. 598*

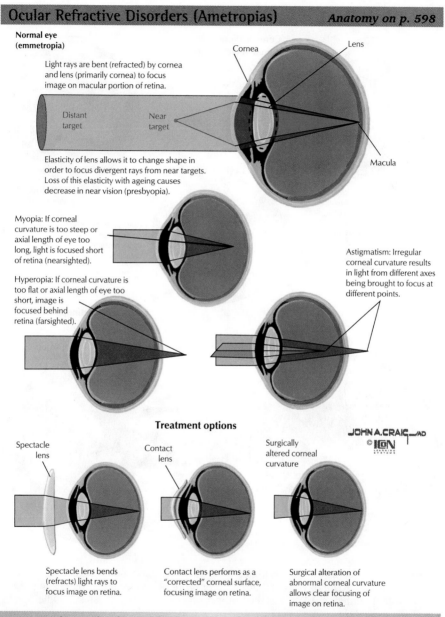

Normal eye (emmetropia)

Light rays are bent (refracted) by cornea and lens (primarily cornea) to focus image on macular portion of retina.

Cornea

Lens

Distant target

Near target

Elasticity of lens allows it to change shape in order to focus divergent rays from near targets. Loss of this elasticity with ageing causes decrease in near vision (presbyopia).

Macula

Myopia: If corneal curvature is too steep or axial length of eye too long, light is focused short of retina (nearsighted).

Hyperopia: If corneal curvature is too flat or axial length of eye too short, image is focused behind retina (farsighted).

Astigmatism: Irregular corneal curvature results in light from different axes being brought to focus at different points.

Treatment options

JOHN A.CRAIG—MD
©ICN

Spectacle lens

Contact lens

Surgically altered corneal curvature

Spectacle lens bends (refracts) light rays to focus image on retina.

Contact lens performs as a "corrected" corneal surface, focusing image on retina.

Surgical alteration of abnormal corneal curvature allows clear focusing of image on retina.

Ametropias are the aberrant focusing of light rays on a site other than the optimal site on the retina (macula). Optically, the cornea, lens, and axial length of the eyeball must be in precise balance to achieve sharp focus on the macula. Common disorders include

- **Myopia** (nearsightedness): 80% of ametropias
- **Hyperopia** (farsightedness): age-related occurrence
- **Astigmatism**: nonspherical cornea causes focusing at multiple locations instead of at a single point; affects 25-40% of the population
- **Presbyopia**: age-related progressive loss of accommodative ability (lens is less flexible)

Clinical Correlation

Diabetic Retinopathy
Anatomy on p. 598

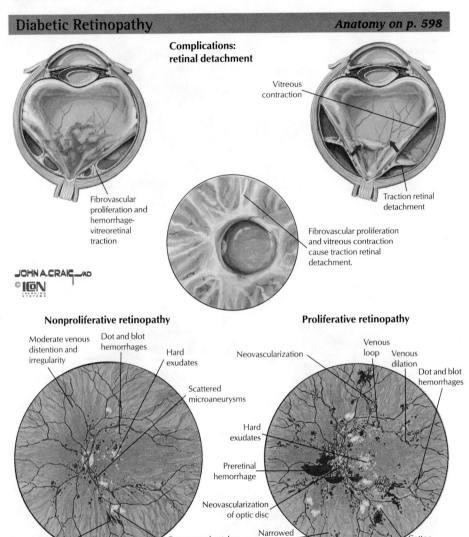

Complications: retinal detachment

Vitreous contraction

Fibrovascular proliferation and hemorrhage-vitreoretinal traction

Traction retinal detachment

Fibrovascular proliferation and vitreous contraction cause traction retinal detachment.

JOHN A.CRAIG—AD
©ICN
LEARNING SYSTEMS

Nonproliferative retinopathy

Moderate venous distention and irregularity

Dot and blot hemorrhages

Hard exudates

Scattered microaneurysms

Hard exudates

Flame-shaped hemorrhages

Cotton wool patches (retinal infarcts)

Proliferative retinopathy

Neovascularization

Venous loop

Venous dilation

Dot and blot hemorrhages

Preretinal hemorrhage

Neovascularization of optic disc

Narrowed arteriole

Cotton wool patches

Diabetic retinopathy develops in nearly all patients with type 1 DM and 50-80% of those with type 2 DM of 20 years' duration or more. It can rapidly progress in pregnant women with type 1 DM. It is the number one cause of blindness in middle-aged individuals and the fourth leading cause overall in the United States.

CHARACTERISTIC	DESCRIPTION
Etiology	Hyperglycemia through an interaction of hemodynamic, biochemical, and hormonal mechanisms leading to capillary endothelial cell damage (retinal hemorrhages, venous distention, microaneurysms, edema, and microangiopathy)
Types	Nonproliferative and proliferative (abnormal neovascularization and fibrosis)
Complications	Vitreous hemorrhage, retinal edema, retinal detachment

Clinical Correlation

Glaucoma

Anatomy on p. 598

Open angle

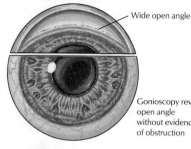

Wide open angle

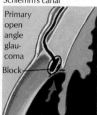

Primary impedance at Schlemm's canal

Primary open angle glaucoma

Block

Gonioscopy reveals open angle without evidence of obstruction

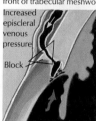

Obstruction or distortion of trabecular meshwork

Block

Secondary impedance at or in front of trabecular meshwork

Increased episcleral venous pressure

Block

Secondary impedance due to venous back pressure

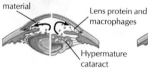

Pseudoexfoliation material

Lens protein and macrophages

Hypermature cataract

Pigment particles

Lens-induced glaucoma

Pigment-induced glaucoma

Primary closed angle

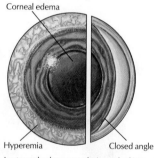

Corneal edema

Hyperemia

Closed angle

Pupillary block

Secondary block in angle

Primary block at pupil

Central anterior chamber shallow

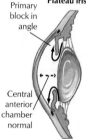

Primary block in angle

Central anterior chamber normal

Plateau iris

JOHN A.CRAIG—AD
© ICON LEARNING SYSTEMS

Acute angle closure results in marked increase in intraocular pressure with conjunctival hyperemia, corneal edema, and fixed middilated pupil.

Angle closure may result from primary pupillary block with bulging iris or from less common plateau iris (primary occlusion at periphery of iris).

Glaucoma is an optic neuropathy that can lead to visual field deficits and is often associated with increased intraocular pressure (IOP).

CHARACTERISTIC	DESCRIPTION
Etiology	Usually increased resistance to outflow of aqueous humor, which leads to increased IOP (reference range, 10-21 mm Hg)
Types	Primary open angle (POAG) most common; closed angle (iris blocks trabecular meshwork)
Risk factors	African-American, family history, age, increased IOP
POAG pathogenesis	Blocked canal of Schlemm (angle is normal) or from obstruction or malfunction of anterior segment angle
Closed-angle pathogenesis	Age-related anatomical changes that block angle or secondary to diseases that pull iris over angle

Clinical Correlation

Cataract

Anatomy on p. 598

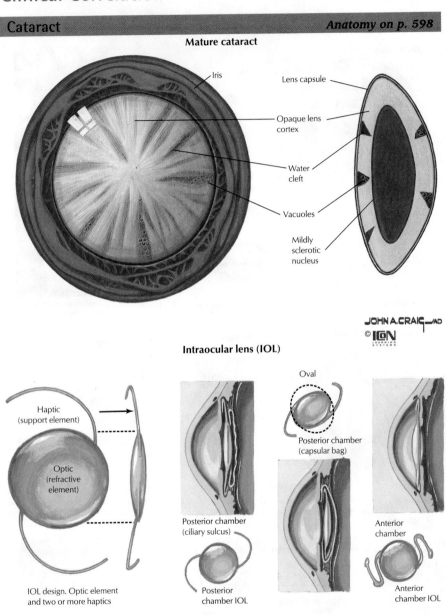

Mature cataract

Iris

Lens capsule

Opaque lens cortex

Water cleft

Vacuoles

Mildly sclerotic nucleus

JOHN A. CRAIG—MD
© ICON
LEARNING SYSTEMS

Intraocular lens (IOL)

Haptic (support element)

Optic (refractive element)

IOL design. Optic element and two or more haptics

Posterior chamber (ciliary sulcus)

Posterior chamber IOL

Oval

Posterior chamber (capsular bag)

Anterior chamber

Anterior chamber IOL

IOLs placed in either posterior or anterior chamber to replace focusing power lost in cataract removal

A cataract is an opacity, or cloudy area, in the crystalline lens. Risk factors for cataracts include age, smoking, alcohol use, sun exposure, low education status, diabetes, and systemic steroid use. Treatment is most often surgical, involving lens removal (patient becomes markedly farsighted), with vision corrected with glasses, contact lenses, or an implanted plastic lens (intraocular lens).

Clinical Correlation

Orbital Blow-out Fracture *Anatomy on pp. 545, 598, 628*

Clinical findings in orbital blow-out fractures

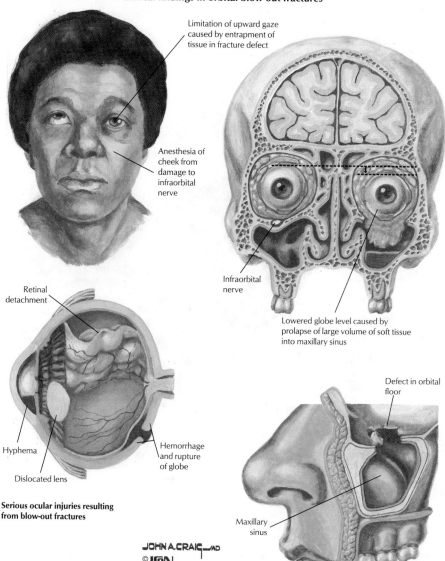

Limitation of upward gaze caused by entrapment of tissue in fracture defect

Anesthesia of cheek from damage to infraorbital nerve

Infraorbital nerve

Lowered globe level caused by prolapse of large volume of soft tissue into maxillary sinus

Retinal detachment

Defect in orbital floor

Hyphema

Hemorrhage and rupture of globe

Dislocated lens

Serious ocular injuries resulting from blow-out fractures

Maxillary sinus

JOHN A. CRAIG—AD
© ICON
LEARNING
SYSTEMS

A massive zygomaticomaxillary complex fracture or direct blow to the front of the orbit (e.g., by a baseball or fist) may cause a rapid increase in intraorbital pressure and a resulting blow-out fracture of the thin orbital floor. In severe comminuted fractures of the orbital floor, the orbital soft tissues may herniate into the underlying maxillary sinus. Clinical signs include diplopia, infraorbital nerve paresthesia, enophthalmos, edema, and ecchymosis.

Temporal Region: Infratemporal Fossa

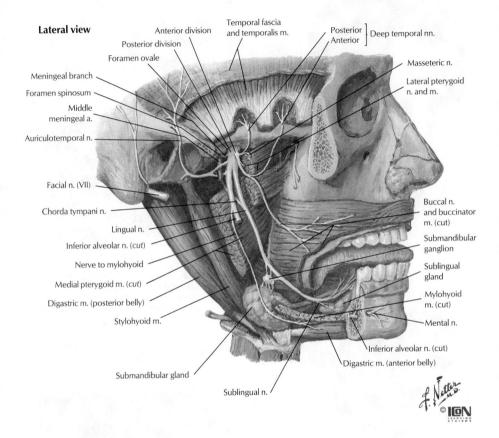

Lateral view

Anterior division
Posterior division
Foramen ovale
Temporal fascia and temporalis m.
Posterior ⎱ Deep temporal nn.
Anterior ⎰
Masseteric n.
Lateral pterygoid n. and m.

Meningeal branch
Foramen spinosum
Middle meningeal a.
Auriculotemporal n.

Facial n. (VII)
Chorda tympani n.
Lingual n.
Inferior alveolar n. (*cut*)
Nerve to mylohyoid
Medial pterygoid m. (*cut*)
Digastric m. (posterior belly)
Stylohyoid m.

Buccal n. and buccinator m. (cut)
Submandibular ganglion
Sublingual gland
Mylohyoid m. (cut)
Mental n.
Inferior alveolar n. (cut)
Digastric m. (anterior belly)

Submandibular gland
Sublingual n.

The infratemporal fossa is the space inferior to the zygomatic arch, medial to the mandibular ramus, and posterior to the maxilla. CN V$_3$ exits the foramen ovale, and several of its larger branches pass through this region:

Auriculotemporal: sensory to auricle and temple
Buccal: sensory to cheek
Lingual: sensory to tongue
Inferior alveolar: sensory to mandibular teeth, gums, and chin (via mylohyoid nerve)
Motor branches: to muscles of mastication, tensor veli palatini, mylohyoid, anterior belly of the digastric, and tensor tympani (in middle ear)

Temporal Region: Muscles of Mastication

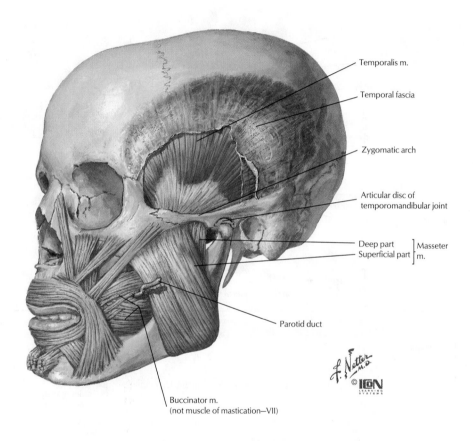

Temporalis m.

Temporal fascia

Zygomatic arch

Articular disc of
temporomandibular joint

Deep part] Masseter
Superficial part [m.

Parotid duct

Buccinator m.
(not muscle of mastication—VII)

Temporal Region: Muscles of Mastication (continued)

The muscles of mastication provide a coordinated set of movements that facilitate biting and chewing (grinding action of the jaws). These muscles participate in movements of elevation, retrusion (retraction), and protrusion of the mandible; are derivatives of the first pharyngeal (branchial) arch; and all are innervated by the mandibular division of the trigeminal nerve. Opening the jaw (depression) is performed largely by the digastric and geniohyoid muscles.

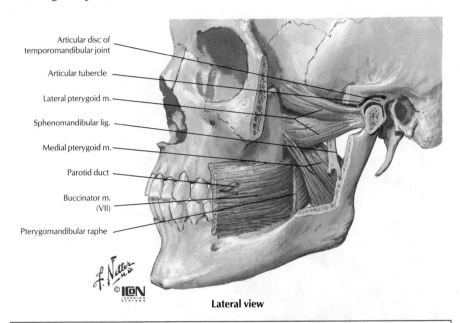

Articular disc of temporomandibular joint

Articular tubercle

Lateral pterygoid m.

Sphenomandibular lig.

Medial pterygoid m.

Parotid duct

Buccinator m. (VII)

Pterygomandibular raphe

Lateral view

MUSCLE	ORIGIN	INSERTION	INNERVATION	MAIN ACTIONS
Temporalis	Floor of temporal fossa and deep temporal fascia	Coronoid process and anterior ramus of mandible	Mandibular nerve (V_3)	Elevates mandible; posterior fibers retrude mandible
Masseter	Zygomatic arch	Ramus of mandible and coronoid process	Mandibular nerve	Elevates and protrudes mandible; deep fibers retrude it
Lateral pterygoid	*Superior head*: infratemporal surface of greater wing of sphenoid *Inferior head*: lateral pterygoid plate	Neck of mandible, articular disc, and capsule of TMJ	Mandibular nerve	Acting together, protrude mandible and depress chin; acting alone and alternately, produce side-to-side movements
Medial pterygoid	*Deep head*: medial surface of lateral pterygoid plate and palatine bone *Superficial head*: tuberosity of maxilla	Ramus of mandible, inferior to mandibular foramen	Mandibular nerve	Elevates mandible; acting together, protrude mandible; acting alone, protrude side of jaw; acting alternately, produce grinding motion

Temporal Region: Maxillary Artery

The blood supply of the infratemporal region and nasal cavities is via the maxillary artery. It is divided for descriptive purposes into three parts:

Retromandibular: arteries enter foramina and supply dura, mandibular teeth and gums, ear, and chin
Pterygoid: branches supply muscles of mastication and buccinator
Pterygopalatine: branches enter foramina and supply maxillary teeth and gums, orbital floor, nose, paranasal sinuses, palate, auditory tube, and superior pharynx

Major branches of the maxillary include the inferior alveolar and middle meningeal (from first part), branches to the muscles of mastication (from second part), and the superior alveolar, infraorbital, greater palatine, and sphenopalatine (from third part).

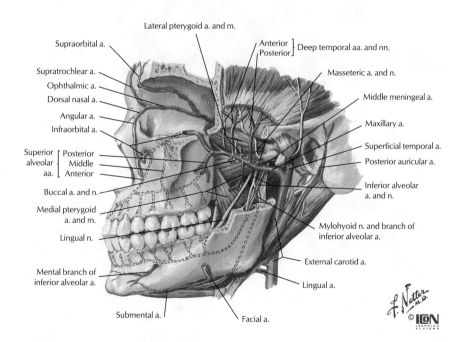

Ear: General Anatomy

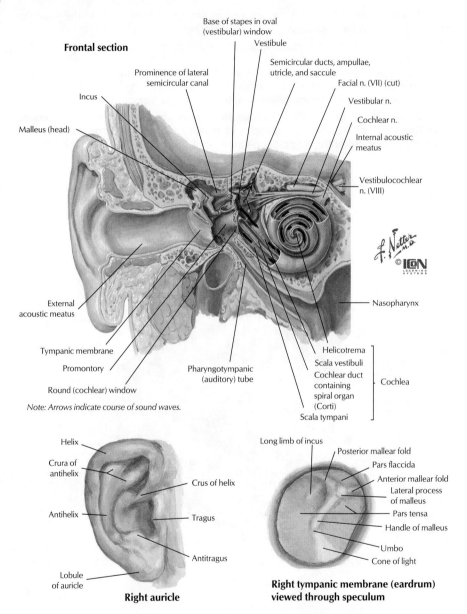

Frontal section

Base of stapes in oval (vestibular) window

Vestibule

Prominence of lateral semicircular canal

Semicircular ducts, ampullae, utricle, and saccule

Facial n. (VII) (cut)

Incus

Vestibular n.

Malleus (head)

Cochlear n.

Internal acoustic meatus

Vestibulocochlear n. (VIII)

Nasopharynx

External acoustic meatus

Tympanic membrane

Promontory

Round (cochlear) window

Note: Arrows indicate course of sound waves.

Pharyngotympanic (auditory) tube

Helicotrema

Scala vestibuli

Cochlear duct containing spiral organ (Corti)

Scala tympani

Cochlea

Helix

Crura of antihelix

Crus of helix

Antihelix

Tragus

Antitragus

Lobule of auricle

Right auricle

Long limb of incus

Posterior mallear fold

Pars flaccida

Anterior mallear fold

Lateral process of malleus

Pars tensa

Handle of malleus

Umbo

Cone of light

Right tympanic membrane (eardrum) viewed through speculum

The ear consists of three parts:

External: auricle (pinna), external acoustic meatus, and tympanic membrane (eardrum)

Middle: tympanic cavity (between eardrum and labyrinthine wall) that contains ossicles (malleus, incus, stapes) and stapedius and tensor tympani muscles and communicates with the mastoid antrum posteriorly and auditory (eustachian) tube anteriorly

Internal: acoustic apparatus (cochlea) and vestibular apparatus (vestibule with utricle and saccule, and the semicircular canals)

Clinical Correlation

Acute Otitis Externa
Anatomy on p. 610

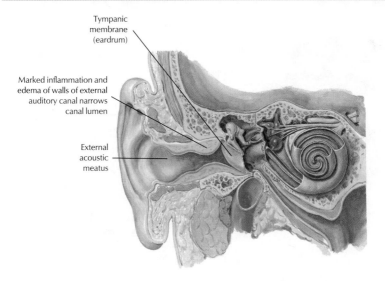

Tympanic membrane (eardrum)

Marked inflammation and edema of walls of external auditory canal narrows canal lumen

External acoustic meatus

In otitis externa, inflammation, edema, and discharge are limited to external auditory canal and its walls.

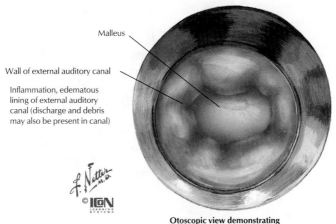

Malleus

Wall of external auditory canal

Inflammation, edematous lining of external auditory canal (discharge and debris may also be present in canal)

Otoscopic view demonstrating clinical appearance of otitis externa

Acute otitis externa, better known as swimmer's ear, involves inflammation or infection of the external ear (external acoustic meatus).

CHARACTERISTIC	DESCRIPTION
Etiology	Compromised protective effects of cerumen (earwax) by bacterial infection, commonly with *Pseudomonas aeruginosa* or *Staphylococcus aureus*
Presentation	Pruritus, sensation of ear fullness, pain especially with mastication
Signs and symptoms	Erythema, edema, discharge, and pain when tragus or auricle is moved; fever if advanced infection

Clinical Correlation

Acute Otitis Media   *Anatomy on p. 610*

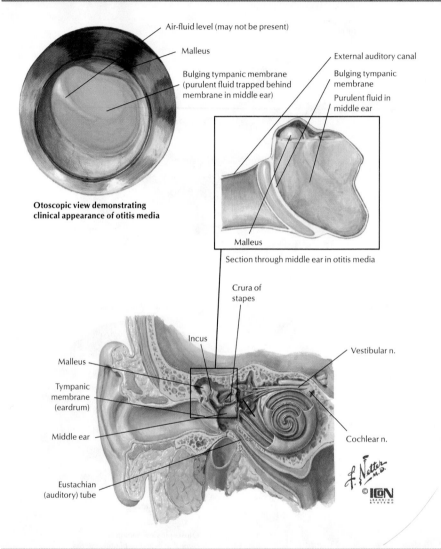

Air-fluid level (may not be present)

Malleus

Bulging tympanic membrane
(purulent fluid trapped behind
membrane in middle ear)

External auditory canal

Bulging tympanic
membrane

Purulent fluid in
middle ear

**Otoscopic view demonstrating
clinical appearance of otitis media**

Malleus

Section through middle ear in otitis media

Crura of
stapes

Incus

Malleus

Tympanic
membrane
(eardrum)

Middle ear

Eustachian
(auditory) tube

Vestibular n.

Cochlear n.

Acute otitis media—inflammation of the middle ear—is common in children younger than 15 years because the auditory tube is short and relatively more horizontal, which limits drainage by gravity and provides a route for infection from the nasopharynx.

CHARACTERISTIC	DESCRIPTION
Etiology	*Streptococcus pneumoniae* (40%), nontypeable *Haemophilus influenzae* (20%), *Moraxella catarrhalis* (10%), and group A streptococcus; also viral etiologies (30-40%)
Presentation	Pain, decreased hearing, fever, preceding upper respiratory infection
Signs and symptoms	Loss of normal translucent appearance of tympanic membrane, which may be erythematous and bulging; absent cone of light

Clinical Correlation

Weber and Rinne Tests
Anatomy on p. 610

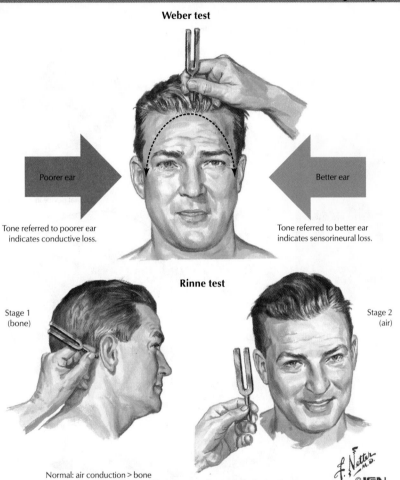

Weber test

Poorer ear

Better ear

Tone referred to poorer ear
indicates conductive loss.

Tone referred to better ear
indicates sensorineural loss.

Rinne test

Stage 1
(bone)

Stage 2
(air)

Normal: air conduction > bone
In ear with decreased hearing, if bone > air, evidence of conduction loss
In ear with decreased hearing, if air > bone, evidence of sensineural loss

Sensineural hearing loss suggests a disorder of the inner ear or cochlear division of CN VIII; conductive hearing loss suggests a disorder of the external or middle ear (eardrum, ossicles, or both).

TEST	SITE	FINDINGS
Weber	Fork placed on forehead	Sound heard in middle if normal hearing or equal deafness exists; lateralization to one side indicates a conductive loss on that side or a sensineural loss on the opposite side
Rinne	Handle placed on mastoid process	Reveals bone conduction hearing loss
	Tines of fork held beside ear	Reveals air conduction hearing loss

Clinical Correlation

Cochlear Implantation
Anatomy on pp. 610

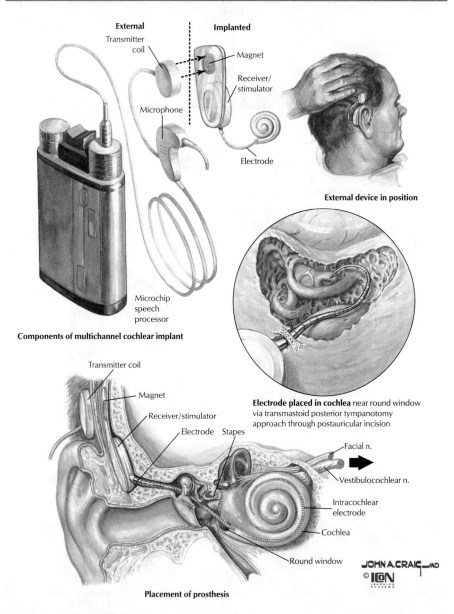

External
Transmitter coil
Microphone

Implanted
Magnet
Receiver/stimulator
Electrode

Microchip speech processor

Components of multichannel cochlear implant

External device in position

Electrode placed in cochlea near round window via transmastoid posterior tympanotomy approach through postauricular incision

Transmitter coil
Magnet
Receiver/stimulator
Electrode   Stapes
Facial n.
Vestibulocochlear n.
Intracochlear electrode
Cochlea
Round window

JOHN A. CRAIG—AD
© ICON

Placement of prosthesis

Approximately 2 million Americans have profound bilateral deafness. One option available to them is a cochlear implant, which consists of a speech processor and implanted electrodes. An external microphone detects sound, which is converted by the processor into electrical signals transmitted to the cochlear implant and vestibulocochlear nerve.

Clinical Correlation

Vertigo

Anatomy on pp. 573, 610

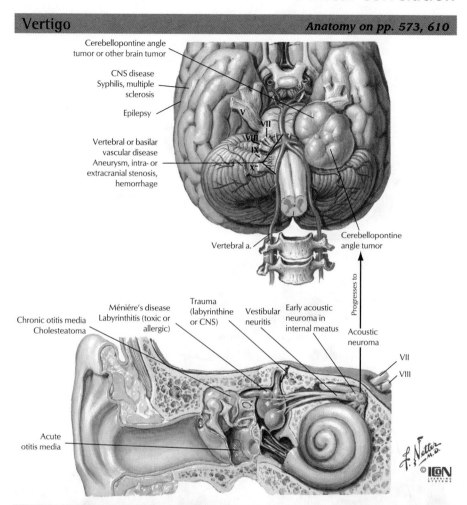

Cerebellopontine angle tumor or other brain tumor

CNS disease Syphilis, multiple sclerosis

Epilepsy

Vertebral or basilar vascular disease Aneurysm, intra- or extracranial stenosis, hemorrhage

Vertebral a.

Cerebellopontine angle tumor

Progresses to

Chronic otitis media Cholesteatoma

Ménière's disease Labyrinthitis (toxic or allergic)

Trauma (labyrinthine or CNS)

Vestibular neuritis

Early acoustic neuroma in internal meatus

Acoustic neuroma

VII

VIII

Acute otitis media

A symptom involving the peripheral vestibular system or its CNS connections and characterized by the illusion or perception of motion is called vertigo.

PERIPHERAL TYPE	CAUSE
Acute vestibulopathy	Viral infection
Endolymphatic hydrops (Ménière's disease)	Excess endolymph secondary to impaired resorption
Benign paroxysmal positional vertigo	Accumulation of otoconial debris in semicircular canals
Vestibular schwannoma (acoustic neuroma)	Benign tumor of vestibulocochlear nerve
Chronic otitis media	Infection or cholesteatoma

Central types of vertigo may be caused by multiple sclerosis (MS), migraine, vascular disease (vestibulobasilar region), or brainstem tumors (cerebellopontine angle).

Clinical Correlation

Removal of Acoustic Neuroma

Anatomy on pp. 545, 610

Superior semicircular canal

Lateral semicircular canal

Facial n.

Sigmoid venous sinus

Posterior semicircular canal

f. Netter
©ICN LEARNING SYSTEMS

Portion of bony capsule of semicircular canals removed

Prominence of facial n. canal

Posterior semicircular canal opened

Prominence of sigmoid venous sinus

Facial n.

Dura mater

Vertical crest

Facial n.

Superior vestibular n.

Inferior vestibular n.

Internal acoustic meatus

Pons

Tumor

Cerebellum

Dura opened, exposing cerebellopontine angle and acoustic neuroma. Vestibular nerve cut and tumor separated from facial nerve

Labyrinth removed and internal acoustic meatus opened. Vertical crest separates facial nerve from superior vestibular nerve

The translabyrinthine approach to acoustic neuroma removal takes advantage of the anatomy of CN VIII. The tumor is first encapsulated within the vestibular division of CN VIII in the internal acoustic meatus. The approach is via the mastoid air cells, with removal of semicircular canals and resection of the tumor. Early treatment can spare the cochlear division of CN VIII, and thus hearing, and the facial nerve.

Oral Cavity: Mouth and Palate

The mouth consists of an oral vestibule (space between the lips and/or cheeks, and the teeth-gums), and the oral cavity proper. Features of the oral cavity proper include the palate (hard and soft), teeth, gums (gingivae), tongue, and salivary glands.

The mucosa of the hard palate, cheeks, tongue, and lips contain numerous minor salivary glands that secrete directly into the oral cavity. Note the position of the palatine tonsils (lymphoid tissue) between the palatoglossal and palatopharyngeal folds (muscles).

Anterior view

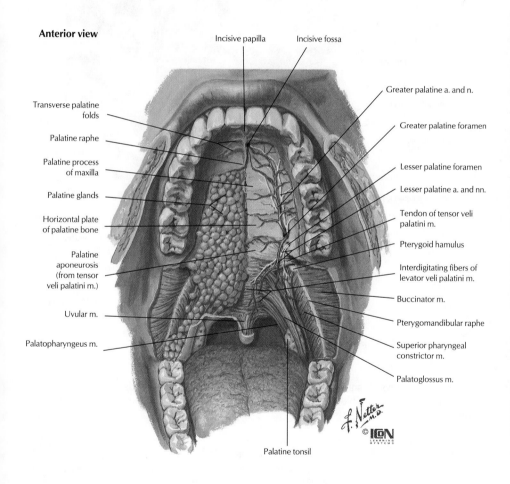

Incisive papilla

Incisive fossa

Transverse palatine folds

Palatine raphe

Palatine process of maxilla

Palatine glands

Horizontal plate of palatine bone

Palatine aponeurosis (from tensor veli palatini m.)

Uvular m.

Palatopharyngeus m.

Greater palatine a. and n.

Greater palatine foramen

Lesser palatine foramen

Lesser palatine a. and nn.

Tendon of tensor veli palatini m.

Pterygoid hamulus

Interdigitating fibers of levator veli palatini m.

Buccinator m.

Pterygomandibular raphe

Superior pharyngeal constrictor m.

Palatoglossus m.

Palatine tonsil

Oral Cavity: Salivary Glands

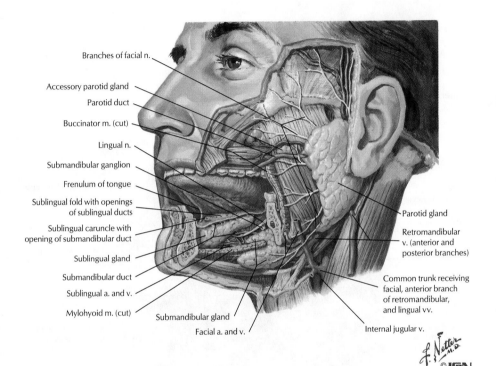

Branches of facial n.

Accessory parotid gland

Parotid duct

Buccinator m. (cut)

Lingual n.

Submandibular ganglion

Frenulum of tongue

Sublingual fold with openings
of sublingual ducts

Sublingual caruncle with
opening of submandibular duct

Sublingual gland

Submandibular duct

Sublingual a. and v.

Mylohyoid m. (cut)

Submandibular gland

Facial a. and v.

Parotid gland

Retromandibular
v. (anterior and
posterior branches)

Common trunk receiving
facial, anterior branch
of retromandibular,
and lingual vv.

Internal jugular v.

The paired parotid, submandibular, and sublingual salivary glands are primary salivary glands. Minor salivary glands exist in the mucosa of the hard palate, cheeks, tongue, and lips.

GLAND	GLAND TYPE AND INNERVATION
Parotid	Serous gland innervated by CN IX parasympathetics that course to gland via auriculotemporal nerve (branch of CN V_3)
Submandibular	Serous and mucous gland innervated by CN VII parasympathetics that course to gland via lingual nerve (branch of CN V_3)
Sublingual	Largely mucous gland innervated by CN VII parasympathetics that course to gland via lingual nerve (branch of CN V_3)

Oral Cavity: Tongue

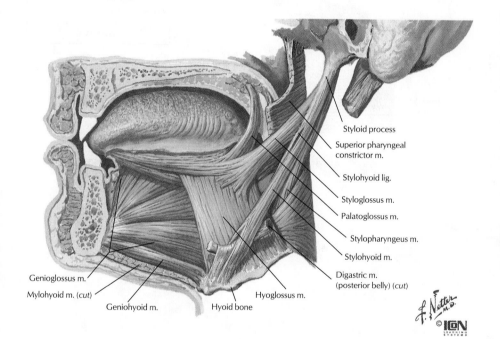

Styloid process

Superior pharyngeal constrictor m.

Stylohyoid lig.

Styloglossus m.

Palatoglossus m.

Stylopharyngeus m.

Stylohyoid m.

Digastric m. (posterior belly) (cut)

Genioglossus m.

Mylohyoid m. (cut)

Geniohyoid m.

Hyoid bone

Hyoglossus m.

Oral Cavity: Tongue (continued)

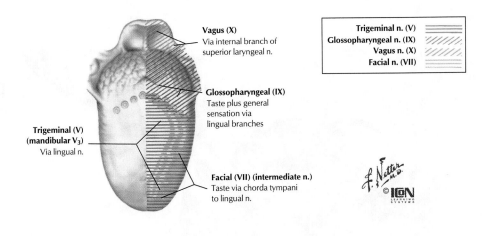

Vagus (X)
Via internal branch of
superior laryngeal n.

Trigeminal n. (V)	≡
Glossopharyngeal n. (IX)	/////
Vagus n. (X)	/////
Facial n. (VII)	≡

Glossopharyngeal (IX)
Taste plus general
sensation via
lingual branches

**Trigeminal (V)
(mandibular V₃)**
Via lingual n.

Facial (VII) (intermediate n.)
Taste via chorda tympani
to lingual n.

The tongue is a strong muscular (genioglossus) organ that has several extrinsic muscles to assist with movement. Sensory (pain and taste) innervation is via multiple cranial nerves.

MUSCLE	ORIGIN	INSERTION	INNERVATION	MAIN ACTIONS
Genioglossus	Mental spine of mandible	Dorsum of tongue and hyoid bone	Hypoglossal nerve (XII)	Depresses tongue; posterior part protrudes tongue
Hyoglossus	Body and greater horn of hyoid bone	Side and inferior aspect of tongue	Hypoglossal nerve	Depresses and retracts tongue
Styloglossus	Styloid process and stylohyoid ligament	Side and inferior aspect of tongue	Hypoglossal nerve	Retracts tongue and draws it up for swallowing
Palatoglossus	Palatine aponeurosis of soft palate	Side of tongue	Vagus nerve and pharyngeal plexus	Elevates posterior tongue

Oral Cavity: Palate

Pharyngeal mucosa removed

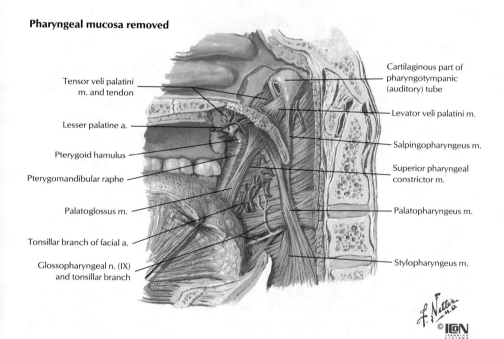

Tensor veli palatini m. and tendon

Lesser palatine a.

Pterygoid hamulus

Pterygomandibular raphe

Palatoglossus m.

Tonsillar branch of facial a.

Glossopharyngeal n. (IX) and tonsillar branch

Cartilaginous part of pharyngotympanic (auditory) tube

Levator veli palatini m.

Salpingopharyngeus m.

Superior pharyngeal constrictor m.

Palatopharyngeus m.

Stylopharyngeus m.

Oral Cavity: Palate (continued)

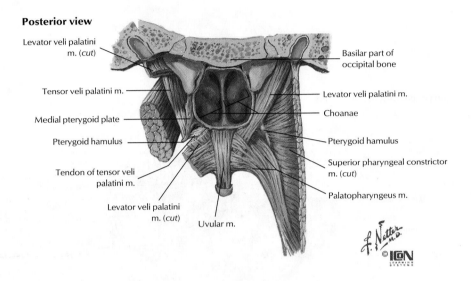

Posterior view

Levator veli palatini m. (*cut*)

Basilar part of occipital bone

Tensor veli palatini m.

Levator veli palatini m.

Medial pterygoid plate

Choanae

Pterygoid hamulus

Pterygoid hamulus

Tendon of tensor veli palatini m.

Superior pharyngeal constrictor m. (*cut*)

Levator veli palatini m. (*cut*)

Palatopharyngeus m.

Uvular m.

The hard palate makes up the anterior four fifths of the palate; the soft palate is a fibromuscular extension demarcated by the palatoglossal and palatopharyngeal folds (mucosa covers underlying muscles of the same names).

MUSCLE	SUPERIOR ATTACHMENT (ORIGIN)	INFERIOR ATTACHMENT (INSERTION)	INNERVATION	MAIN ACTIONS
Levator veli palatini	Auditory tube and temporal bone	Palatine aponeurosis	Vagus nerve via pharyngeal plexus	Elevates soft palate during swallowing
Tensor veli palatini	Scaphoid fossa of medial pterygoid plate, spine of sphenoid, and auditory tube	Palatine aponeurosis	Mandibular nerve	Tenses soft palate and opens auditory tube during swallowing and yawning
Palatopharyngeus	Hard palate and palatine aponeurosis	Lateral wall of pharynx	Vagus nerve via pharyngeal plexus	Tenses soft palate; pulls walls of pharynx superiorly, anteriorly, and medially during swallowing
Musculus uvulae	Nasal spine and palatine aponeurosis	Mucosa of uvula	Vagus nerve via pharyngeal plexus	Shortens and elevates uvula

Clinical Correlation

Common Oral Lesions   *Anatomy on pp. 617, 619*

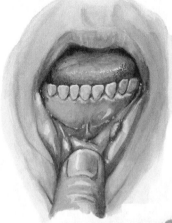

Recurrent aphthous ulcer

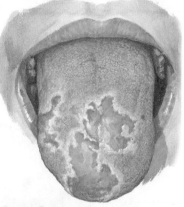

Geographic tongue

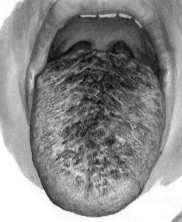

Hairy tongue

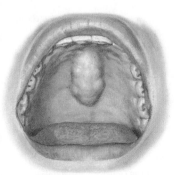

Torus palatinus

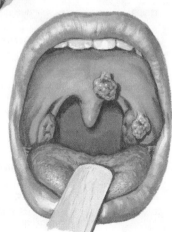

Papillomas of soft palate and anterior pillar

Clinical Correlation

Common Oral Lesions (continued)   *Anatomy on pp. 617, 619*

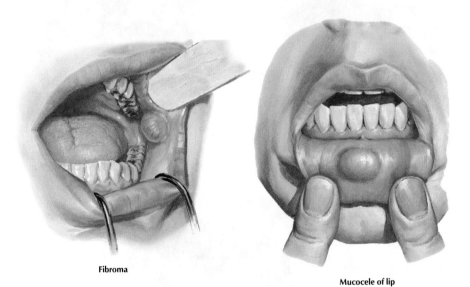

Fibroma

Mucocele of lip

LESION	DESCRIPTION
Recurrent aphthous ulcer (canker sore)	Common; etiology uncertain (nutrition, hormonal, bacterial or viral infection, genetic, Crohn's disease)
Viral stomatitis	Herpes simplex; occurs on lip, gums, tongue, and hard palate; heals spontaneously in 10-14 days
Oral candidiasis (oral thrush)	Most common fungal infection (30-60% of healthy adults); white, plaquelike lesions with hemorrhagic underlying mucosa
Hairy tongue	Benign condition caused by accumulation of keratin and bacteria on filiform papillae of tongue
Geographic tongue	Benign condition; etiology unknown; area of atrophied filiform papillae; sensitivity to some foods and liquids
Torus palatinus	Benign smooth, hard lesions on midline hard palate
Oral papilloma	Infection with strains of human papillomavirus; pedunculated, cauliflowerlike squamous epithelial masses that can be excised
Fibroma	Soft lesions at sites of chronic trauma that lead to inflammation and fibrous hyperplasia
Mucocele	Salivary extrusion from a minor salivary gland into surrounding tissue, usually lower lip; may burst and recur

Clinical Correlation

Cancer of the Oral Cavity and Oropharynx

Anatomy on pp. 617-619, 635

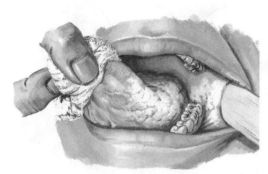

Moderately advanced leukoplakia of tongue and cheek

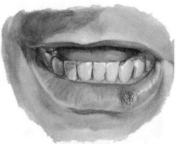

Carcinoma of lip

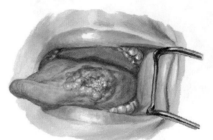

Squamous cell carcinoma (SCC) of tongue

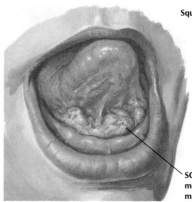

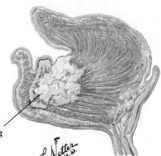

SCC of floor of mouth invading mandible

Clinical Correlation

Cancer of the Oral Cavity and Oropharynx (continued)

Anatomy on pp. 617-619, 635

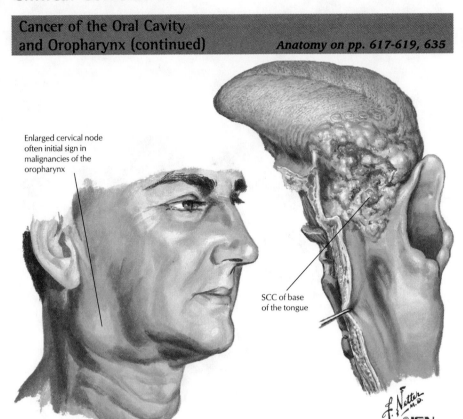

Enlarged cervical node often initial sign in malignancies of the oropharynx

SCC of base of the tongue

Squamous cell carcinoma (SCC) accounts for more than 90% of cancers in this region, so the information here is limited to SCC. All of these lesions may present with palpable submental, submandibular, and upper deep cervical lymph nodes.

TYPE AND SITE OF LESION	PRESENTATION	RISK FACTORS
Premalignant		
Erythroplasia	Red, raised lesion or a smooth, atrophic red lesion	Alcohol, tobacco use (synergistic effect)
Leukoplakia	White patchy mucosa	Alcohol, tobacco use
Malignant		
Lip SCC (90% lower lip)	Nonhealing, crusting ulcerative lesion or scaly, hyperkeratotic lesion at vermilion border of lip	Ultraviolet (sun) exposure
Tongue SCC	Anterolateral tongue; nonhealing ulcer; exophytic lesion	Alcohol, tobacco use
Floor of mouth	Anterior tongue; may infiltrate mandible; trismus if muscles of mastication involved	Alcohol, tobacco use
Oropharynx SCC	Ulcerative or infiltrating mucosal lesions; pain; dysphagia	Alcohol, tobacco use

Nose: Walls of the Nasal Cavity

The lateral nasal wall features three conchae covered with sensitive and highly vascular mucosa. The vascular supply is via branches of the sphenopalatine artery (from the maxillary artery); the nerves are from the maxillary nerve (CN V$_2$) (general sensation), CN I (olfaction), and CN VII (secretomotor to mucous glands via the pterygopalatine ganglion).

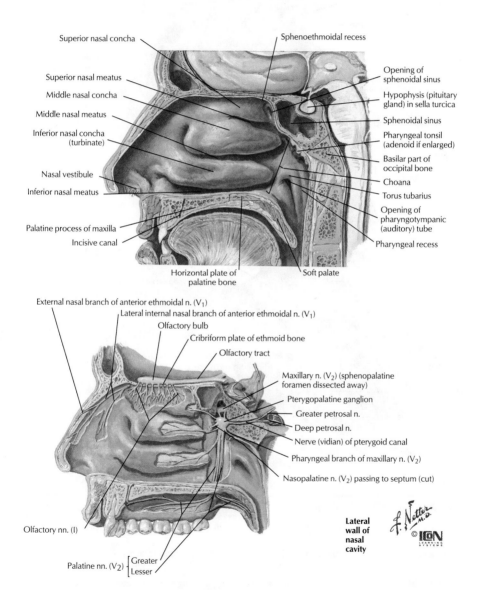

Superior nasal concha

Superior nasal meatus

Middle nasal concha

Middle nasal meatus

Inferior nasal concha (turbinate)

Nasal vestibule

Inferior nasal meatus

Palatine process of maxilla

Incisive canal

Horizontal plate of palatine bone

Sphenoethmoidal recess

Opening of sphenoidal sinus

Hypophysis (pituitary gland) in sella turcica

Sphenoidal sinus

Pharyngeal tonsil (adenoid if enlarged)

Basilar part of occipital bone

Choana

Torus tubarius

Opening of pharyngotympanic (auditory) tube

Pharyngeal recess

Soft palate

External nasal branch of anterior ethmoidal n. (V$_1$)

Lateral internal nasal branch of anterior ethmoidal n. (V$_1$)

Olfactory bulb

Cribriform plate of ethmoid bone

Olfactory tract

Maxillary n. (V$_2$) (sphenopalatine foramen dissected away)

Pterygopalatine ganglion

Greater petrosal n.

Deep petrosal n.

Nerve (vidian) of pterygoid canal

Pharyngeal branch of maxillary n. (V$_2$)

Nasopalatine n. (V$_2$) passing to septum (cut)

Olfactory nn. (I)

Palatine nn. (V$_2$) {Greater / Lesser

Lateral wall of nasal cavity

Nose: Paranasal Sinuses

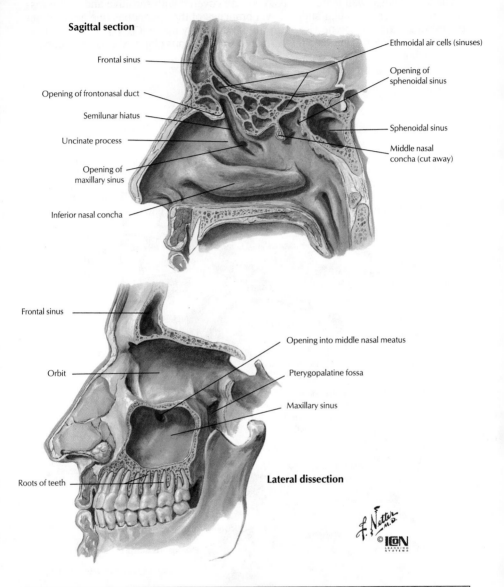

Sagittal section

Frontal sinus

Opening of frontonasal duct

Semilunar hiatus

Uncinate process

Opening of maxillary sinus

Inferior nasal concha

Ethmoidal air cells (sinuses)

Opening of sphenoidal sinus

Sphenoidal sinus

Middle nasal concha (cut away)

Frontal sinus

Orbit

Roots of teeth

Opening into middle nasal meatus

Pterygopalatine fossa

Maxillary sinus

Lateral dissection

SINUS	DESCRIPTION
Frontal	Paired sinuses, lying anteriorly in frontal bone and draining into semilunar hiatus of middle meatus
Ethmoid	Paired anterior and middle draining into middle meatus (hiatus semilunaris and ethmoid bulla, respectively) and posterior draining into superior nasal meatus
Sphenoidal	Paired sinuses, in sphenoid bone, draining into sphenoethmoidal recess
Maxillary	Paired sinuses, in maxilla, draining into middle meatus (semilunar hiatus); largest sinus (20-30 ml)

Clinical Correlation

Rhinosinusitis   *Anatomy on p. 628*

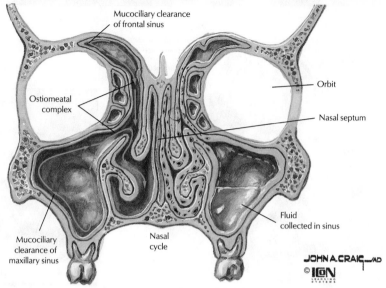

Mucociliary clearance of frontal sinus

Orbit

Ostiomeatal complex

Nasal septum

Mucociliary clearance of maxillary sinus

Nasal cycle

Fluid collected in sinus

JOHN A. CRAIG—AD
© ICON

Cilia drain sinuses by propelling mucus toward natural ostia (mucociliary clearance)

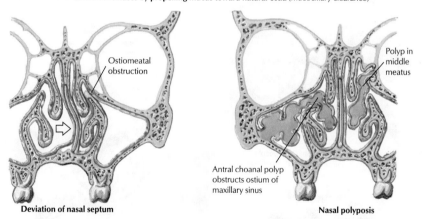

Ostiomeatal obstruction

Polyp in middle meatus

Antral choanal polyp obstructs ostium of maxillary sinus

Deviation of nasal septum

Nasal polyposis

Rhinosinusitis is an inflammation of the paranasal sinuses (usually ethmoid and maxillary sinuses) and nasal cavity.

CHARACTERISTIC	DESCRIPTION
Etiology	Respiratory viral infection or bacterial infection (often secondary); deviation of nasal septum
Pathogenesis	Obstruction of discharge of normal sinus secretions compromises normal sterility of sinuses
Signs and symptoms	Nasal congestion, facial pain and/or pressure, purulent discharge, fever, headache, painful maxillary teeth, halitosis

Clinical Correlation

Physical Examination of the Paranasal Sinuses
Anatomy on pp. 617, 628

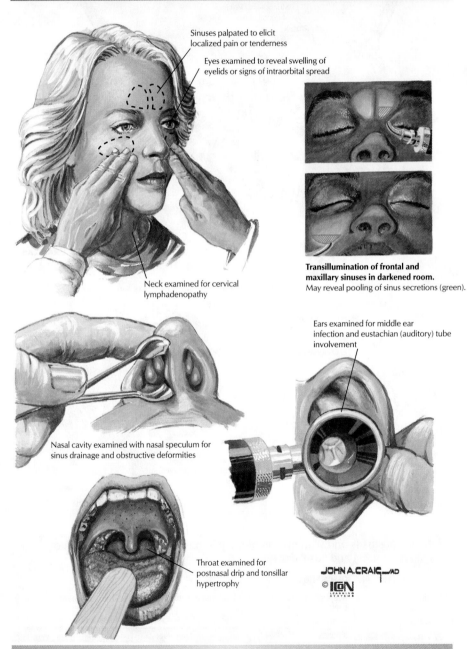

Sinuses palpated to elicit localized pain or tenderness

Eyes examined to reveal swelling of eyelids or signs of intraorbital spread

Neck examined for cervical lymphadenopathy

Transillumination of frontal and maxillary sinuses in darkened room.
May reveal pooling of sinus secretions (green).

Ears examined for middle ear infection and eustachian (auditory) tube involvement

Nasal cavity examined with nasal speculum for sinus drainage and obstructive deformities

Throat examined for postnasal drip and tonsillar hypertrophy

JOHN A. CRAIG—AD
© ICN

The physical examination is usually sufficient to make the diagnosis, although computed tomography of the sinus may help in difficult cases.

Pharynx: Subdivisions

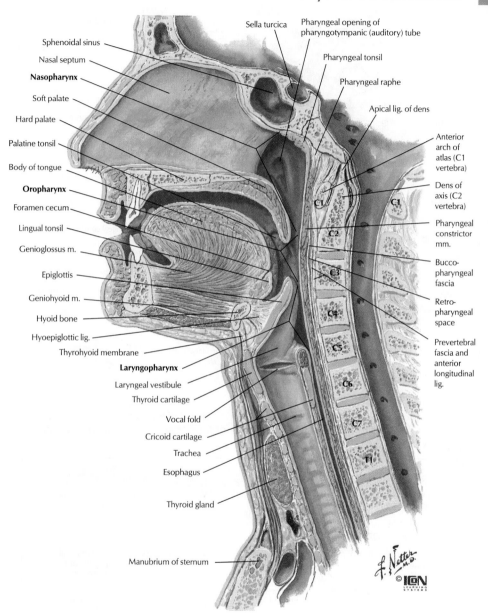

Sella turcica

Pharyngeal opening of pharyngotympanic (auditory) tube

Sphenoidal sinus

Nasal septum

Pharyngeal tonsil

Nasopharynx

Pharyngeal raphe

Soft palate

Hard palate

Apical lig. of dens

Palatine tonsil

Anterior arch of atlas (C1 vertebra)

Body of tongue

Oropharynx

Dens of axis (C2 vertebra)

Foramen cecum

Lingual tonsil

Pharyngeal constrictor mm.

Genioglossus m.

Bucco-pharyngeal fascia

Epiglottis

Retro-pharyngeal space

Geniohyoid m.

Hyoid bone

Hyoepiglottic lig.

Prevertebral fascia and anterior longitudinal lig.

Thyrohyoid membrane

Laryngopharynx

Laryngeal vestibule

Thyroid cartilage

Vocal fold

Cricoid cartilage

Trachea

Esophagus

Thyroid gland

Manubrium of sternum

C1

C1

C2

C3

C4

C5

C6

C7

T1

The pharynx (throat) is subdivided into the

Nasopharynx: lies posterior to the nasal cavity above the soft palate

Oropharynx: extends from the soft palate to the superior tip of the epiglottis and lies posterior to the oral cavity

Laryngopharynx: extends from the tip of the epiglottis to the inferior aspect of the cricoid cartilage; also known by clinicians as the hypopharynx

The palatine, lingual, pharyngeal, and tubal tonsils comprise Waldeyer's tonsillar ring of lymphoid tissues, which guard the entry to the digestive and respiratory tracts.

Pharynx: Muscles

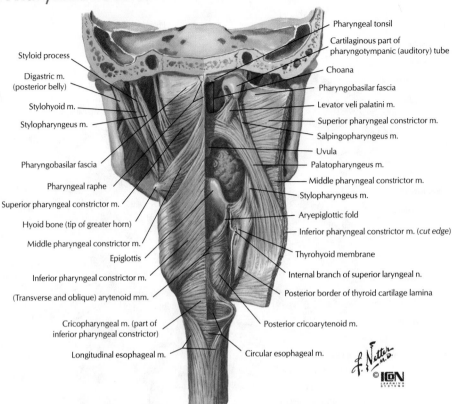

The muscles of the pharynx participate in swallowing (deglutition) and contract serially from superior to inferior to move a bolus of food from the oropharynx and laryngopharynx into the proximal esophagus.

MUSCLE	ORIGIN	INSERTION	INNERVATION	MAIN ACTIONS
Superior pharyngeal constrictor	Hamulus, pterygomandibular raphe, mylohyoid line of mandible, and side of tongue	Median raphe of pharynx and pharyngeal tubercle	Vagus via pharyngeal plexus	Constricts wall of pharynx during swallowing
Middle pharyngeal constrictor	Stylohyoid ligament and horns of hyoid bone	Median raphe of pharynx	Vagus via pharyngeal plexus	Constricts wall of pharynx during swallowing
Inferior pharyngeal constrictor	Oblique line of thyroid cartilage, and cricoid cartilage	Median raphe of pharynx	Vagus via pharyngeal plexus	Constricts wall of pharynx during swallowing
Salpingo-pharyngeus	Auditory tube	Side of pharynx	Vagus via pharyngeal plexus	Elevates pharynx and larynx during swallowing and speaking
Stylo-pharyngeus	Styloid process	Posterior and superior borders of thyroid cartilage	Glossopharyngeal nerve	Elevates pharynx and larynx during swallowing and speaking

Vascular Summary: Arteries

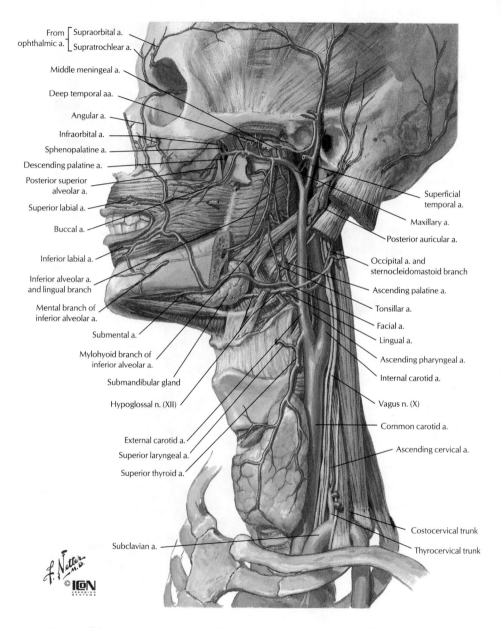

From ophthalmic a. [Supraorbital a.
Supratrochlear a.

Middle meningeal a.

Deep temporal aa.

Angular a.

Infraorbital a.

Sphenopalatine a.

Descending palatine a.

Posterior superior alveolar a.

Superior labial a.

Buccal a.

Inferior labial a.

Inferior alveolar a. and lingual branch

Mental branch of inferior alveolar a.

Submental a.

Mylohyoid branch of inferior alveolar a.

Submandibular gland

Hypoglossal n. (XII)

External carotid a.

Superior laryngeal a.

Superior thyroid a.

Subclavian a.

Superficial temporal a.

Maxillary a.

Posterior auricular a.

Occipital a. and sternocleidomastoid branch

Ascending palatine a.

Tonsillar a.

Facial a.

Lingual a.

Ascending pharyngeal a.

Internal carotid a.

Vagus n. (X)

Common carotid a.

Ascending cervical a.

Costocervical trunk

Thyrocervical trunk

Arteries of the head and neck include branches derived from the following:

Subclavian: supply lower neck, thoracic wall, shoulder, upper back, and brain (vertebrals)

External carotid: supply thyroid, larynx, pharynx, neck, oral cavity, face, nasal cavity, meninges, and temporal and infratemporal regions

Internal carotid: supply brain, orbit, eyeball, lacrimal glands, forehead, and ethmoid sinuses

Vascular Summary: Veins

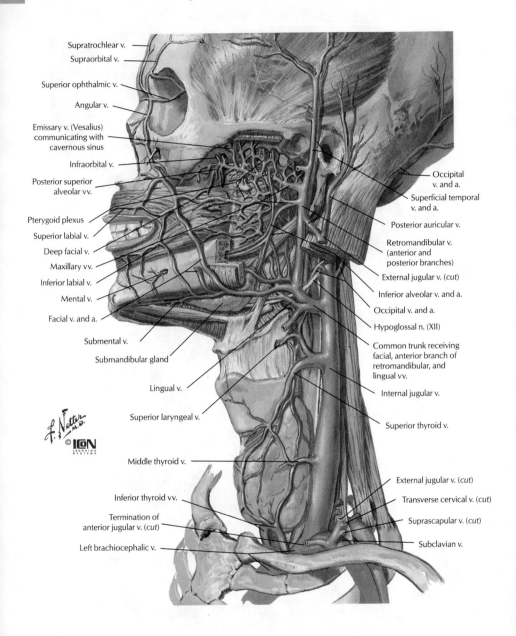

Supratrochlear v.
Supraorbital v.
Superior ophthalmic v.
Angular v.
Emissary v. (Vesalius) communicating with cavernous sinus
Infraorbital v.
Posterior superior alveolar vv.
Pterygoid plexus
Superior labial v.
Deep facial v.
Maxillary vv.
Inferior labial v.
Mental v.
Facial v. and a.
Submental v.
Submandibular gland
Lingual v.
Superior laryngeal v.
Middle thyroid v.
Inferior thyroid vv.
Termination of anterior jugular v. (cut)
Left brachiocephalic v.

Occipital v. and a.
Superficial temporal v. and a.
Posterior auricular v.
Retromandibular v. (anterior and posterior branches)
External jugular v. (cut)
Inferior alveolar v. and a.
Occipital v. and a.
Hypoglossal n. (XII)
Common trunk receiving facial, anterior branch of retromandibular, and lingual vv.
Internal jugular v.
Superior thyroid v.
External jugular v. (cut)
Transverse cervical v. (cut)
Suprascapular v. (cut)
Subclavian v.

Venous drainage of the head and neck ultimately collects blood into these major veins (numerous anastomoses exist between these veins):

Retromandibular: receives tributaries from temporal and infratemporal regions (pterygoid plexus), nasal cavity, pharynx, and oral cavity
Internal jugular: drains brain, face, thyroid gland, and neck
External jugular: drains superficial neck, lower neck and shoulder, and upper back (often communicates with retromandibular vein)

Vascular Summary: Lymphatics

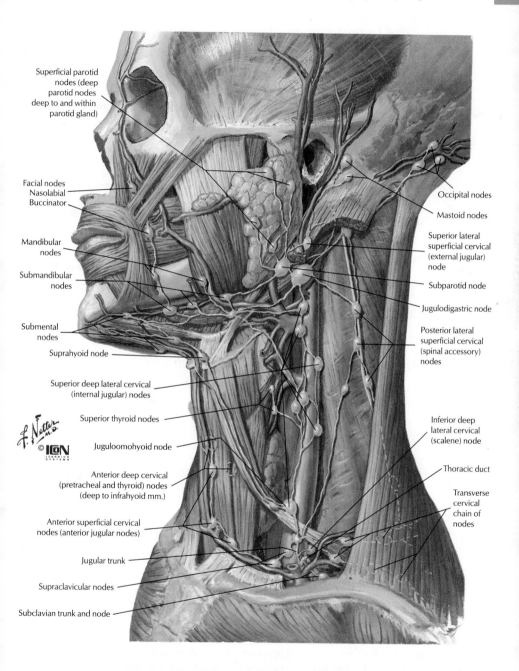

Superficial parotid nodes (deep parotid nodes deep to and within parotid gland)

Facial nodes
Nasolabial
Buccinator

Mandibular nodes

Submandibular nodes

Submental nodes

Suprahyoid node

Superior deep lateral cervical (internal jugular) nodes

Superior thyroid nodes

Juguloomohyoid node

Anterior deep cervical (pretracheal and thyroid) nodes (deep to infrahyoid mm.)

Anterior superficial cervical nodes (anterior jugular nodes)

Jugular trunk

Supraclavicular nodes

Subclavian trunk and node

Occipital nodes

Mastoid nodes

Superior lateral superficial cervical (external jugular) node

Subparotid node

Jugulodigastric node

Posterior lateral superficial cervical (spinal accessory) nodes

Inferior deep lateral cervical (scalene) node

Thoracic duct

Transverse cervical chain of nodes

Lymph nodes and vessels of the head and neck tend to follow the vascular supply draining back to the deep cervical nodes (jugulodigastric and juguloomohyoid nodes) that course along the internal jugular vein. Superficial cervical nodes drain more superficial structures of the neck along vessels that parallel the external jugular vein.

Nerve Summary: Autonomic Innervation

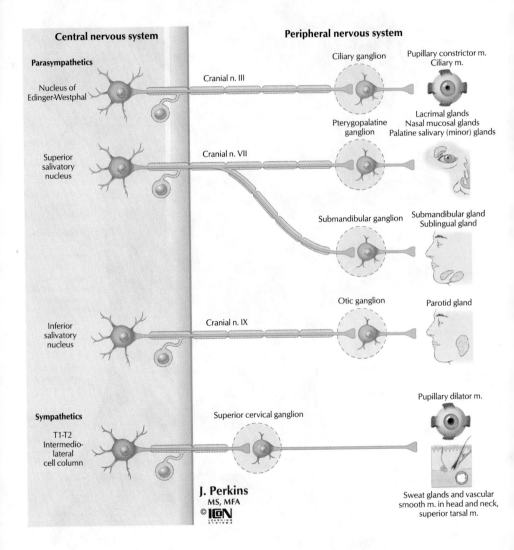

Autonomic distribution to the head involves preganglionic axons that arise from neurons in the CNS and synapse in peripheral ganglia. Postganglionic axons arise from neurons in these ganglia and course to their respective targets (smooth muscle and glands). Postganglionic sympathetics from the superior cervical ganglion (SCG) follow vessels, existing nerves, or both to their targets (largely vasomotor, sweat glands and some smooth muscle).

Nerve Summary: Oculomotor, Trochlear, and Abducent Nerve Distribution

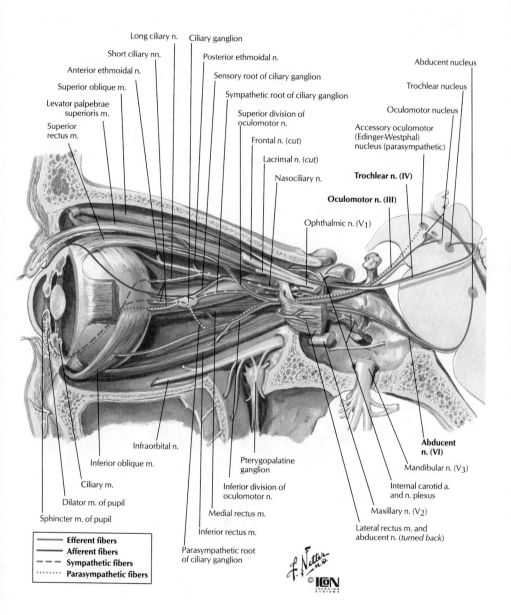

Long ciliary n.
Ciliary ganglion
Short ciliary nn.
Posterior ethmoidal n.
Anterior ethmoidal n.
Abducent nucleus
Superior oblique m.
Sensory root of ciliary ganglion
Trochlear nucleus
Levator palpebrae superioris m.
Sympathetic root of ciliary ganglion
Oculomotor nucleus
Superior rectus m.
Superior division of oculomotor n.
Accessory oculomotor (Edinger-Westphal) nucleus (parasympathetic)
Frontal n. (cut)
Lacrimal n. (cut)
Trochlear n. (IV)
Nasociliary n.
Oculomotor n. (III)
Ophthalmic n. (V₁)
Infraorbital n.
Abducent n. (VI)
Inferior oblique m.
Pterygopalatine ganglion
Mandibular n. (V₃)
Ciliary m.
Inferior division of oculomotor n.
Internal carotid a. and n. plexus
Dilator m. of pupil
Maxillary n. (V₂)
Sphincter m. of pupil
Medial rectus m.
Lateral rectus m. and abducent n. (turned back)
Inferior rectus m.
Parasympathetic root of ciliary ganglion

——— Efferent fibers
——— Afferent fibers
- - - Sympathetic fibers
········· Parasympathetic fibers

The oculomotor nerve (CN III) innervates five muscles in the orbit (general somatic efferents) and conveys parasympathetic preganglionics to the ciliary ganglion (postganglionics mediate pupillary constriction and accommodation). The trochlear nerve (CN IV) innervates the SO muscle, and the abducent nerve (CN VI) innervates the lateral rectus muscle.

Nerve Summary: Trigeminal Nerve Distribution

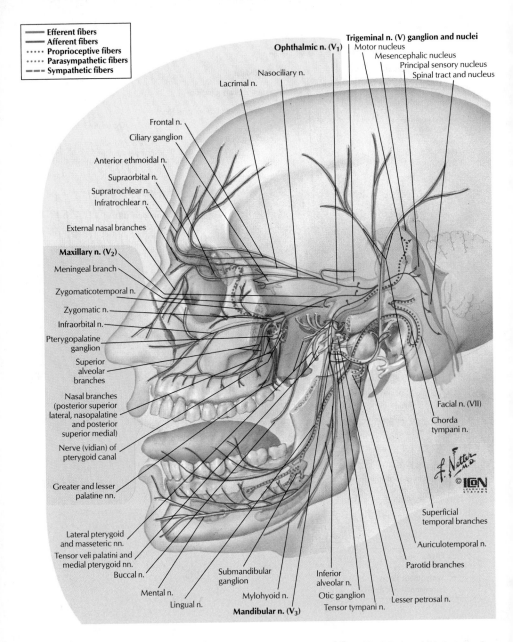

Efferent fibers
Afferent fibers
Proprioceptive fibers
Parasympathetic fibers
Sympathetic fibers

Ophthalmic n. (V₁)

Trigeminal n. (V) ganglion and nuclei
Motor nucleus
Mesencephalic nucleus
Principal sensory nucleus
Spinal tract and nucleus

Nasociliary n.
Lacrimal n.
Frontal n.
Ciliary ganglion
Anterior ethmoidal n.
Supraorbital n.
Supratrochlear n.
Infratrochlear n.
External nasal branches
Maxillary n. (V₂)
Meningeal branch
Zygomaticotemporal n.
Zygomatic n.
Infraorbital n.
Pterygopalatine ganglion
Superior alveolar branches
Nasal branches (posterior superior lateral, nasopalatine and posterior superior medial)
Nerve (vidian) of pterygoid canal
Greater and lesser palatine nn.
Lateral pterygoid and masseteric nn.
Tensor veli palatini and medial pterygoid nn.
Buccal n.
Mental n.
Lingual n.
Submandibular ganglion
Mylohyoid n.
Mandibular n. (V₃)
Inferior alveolar n.
Otic ganglion
Tensor tympani n.
Lesser petrosal n.
Facial n. (VII)
Chorda tympani n.
Superficial temporal branches
Auriculotemporal n.
Parotid branches

The trigeminal nerve (CN V), the major sensory nerve of the head, provides general somatic afferents via its ophthalmic, maxillary, and mandibular divisions. Its mandibular division innervates muscles derived from the first branchial arch. Because of this nerve's extensive distribution, many parasympathetic fibers from CNs III, VII, and IX course with branches of CN V to reach their targets (smooth muscle and glands).

Nerve Summary: Facial Nerve Distribution

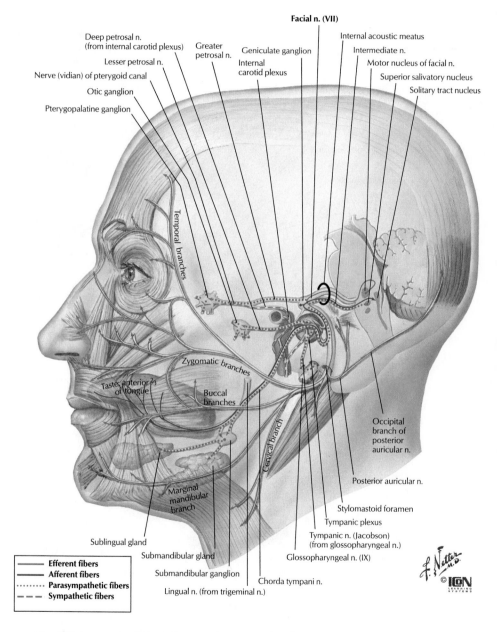

Facial n. (VII)

Deep petrosal n. (from internal carotid plexus)
Greater petrosal n.
Geniculate ganglion
Internal acoustic meatus
Intermediate n.
Lesser petrosal n.
Internal carotid plexus
Motor nucleus of facial n.
Nerve (vidian) of pterygoid canal
Superior salivatory nucleus
Otic ganglion
Solitary tract nucleus
Pterygopalatine ganglion

Temporal branches

Zygomatic branches

Taste, anterior ⅔ of tongue

Buccal branches

Cervical branch

Occipital branch of posterior auricular n.

Marginal mandibular branch

Posterior auricular n.

Sublingual gland

Stylomastoid foramen
Tympanic plexus

Submandibular gland

Tympanic n. (Jacobson) (from glossopharyngeal n.)

Submandibular ganglion

Glossopharyngeal n. (IX)

Chorda tympani n.

Lingual n. (from trigeminal n.)

—— Efferent fibers
—— Afferent fibers
········· Parasympathetic fibers
– – – Sympathetic fibers

The facial nerve (CN VII), the major motor nerve of the head, provides general somatic efferents to muscles derived from the second branchial arch and parasympathetics to the pterygopalatine and submandibular ganglia. It also conveys special visceral afferents from taste receptors on the anterior two thirds of the tongue.

Nerve Summary: Glossopharyngeal Nerve Distribution

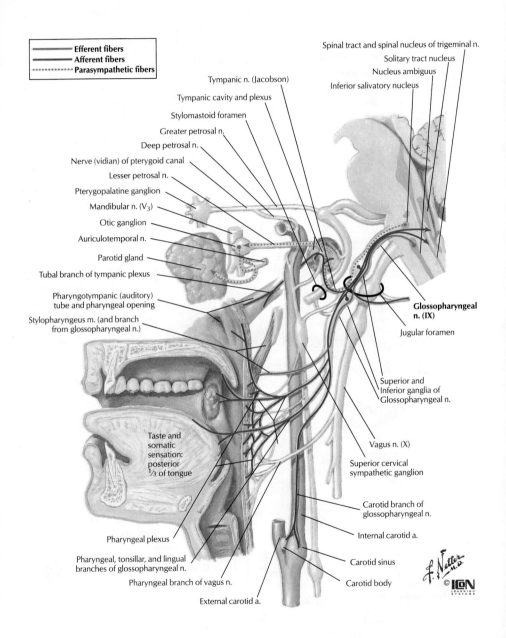

	Efferent fibers
	Afferent fibers
	Parasympathetic fibers

Spinal tract and spinal nucleus of trigeminal n.

Solitary tract nucleus

Nucleus ambiguus

Inferior salivatory nucleus

Tympanic n. (Jacobson)

Tympanic cavity and plexus

Stylomastoid foramen

Greater petrosal n.

Deep petrosal n.

Nerve (vidian) of pterygoid canal

Lesser petrosal n.

Pterygopalatine ganglion

Mandibular n. (V₃)

Otic ganglion

Auriculotemporal n.

Parotid gland

Tubal branch of tympanic plexus

Pharyngotympanic (auditory) tube and pharyngeal opening

Stylopharyngeus m. (and branch from glossopharyngeal n.)

Glossopharyngeal n. (IX)

Jugular foramen

Taste and somatic sensation: posterior ⅓ of tongue

Superior and Inferior ganglia of Glossopharyngeal n.

Vagus n. (X)

Superior cervical sympathetic ganglion

Carotid branch of glossopharyngeal n.

Internal carotid a.

Pharyngeal plexus

Pharyngeal, tonsillar, and lingual branches of glossopharyngeal n.

Pharyngeal branch of vagus n.

Carotid sinus

Carotid body

External carotid a.

The glossopharyngeal nerve (CN IX) innervates the stylopharyngeus muscle, sends parasympathetics to the otic ganglion (parotid gland), and conveys special visceral afferents from taste receptors on the posterior third of the tongue. General visceral afferents also return from the carotid sinus and body, tongue, pharynx, and middle ear.

Nerve Summary: Sympathetic Ganglia and Nerves

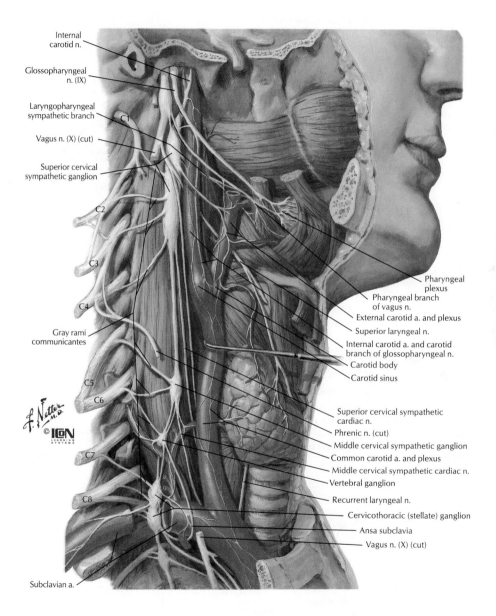

Internal carotid n.

Glossopharyngeal n. (IX)

Laryngopharyngeal sympathetic branch

C1

Vagus n. (X) (cut)

Superior cervical sympathetic ganglion

C2

C3

C4

Gray rami communicantes

C5

C6

C7

C8

Subclavian a.

Pharyngeal plexus
Pharyngeal branch of vagus n.
External carotid a. and plexus
Superior laryngeal n.
Internal carotid a. and carotid branch of glossopharyngeal n.
Carotid body
Carotid sinus

Superior cervical sympathetic cardiac n.
Phrenic n. (cut)
Middle cervical sympathetic ganglion
Common carotid a. and plexus
Middle cervical sympathetic cardiac n.
Vertebral ganglion
Recurrent laryngeal n.
Cervicothoracic (stellate) ganglion
Ansa subclavia
Vagus n. (X) (cut)

Preganglionic sympathetics from the upper thoracic spinal cord levels (T1-T2) ascend via the sympathetic trunk and synapse in the SCG. Postganglionic axons from the SCG then course along blood vessels or existing nerves to reach their targets (smooth muscle and glands).

Embryology: Brain Development

Folding of the neural tube (ectoderm) forms the CNS (brain and spinal cord). Cranially, the neural tube expands to form a forebrain, midbrain, and hindbrain.

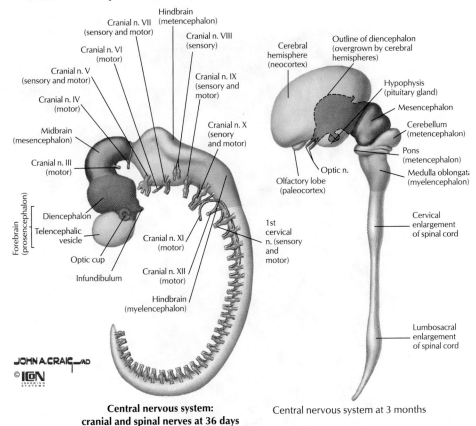

Cranial n. VII (sensory and motor)
Hindbrain (metencephalon)
Cranial n. VIII (sensory)
Cranial n. VI (motor)
Cranial n. V (sensory and motor)
Cranial n. IX (sensory and motor)
Cranial n. IV (motor)
Midbrain (mesencephalon)
Cranial n. X (senory and motor)
Cranial n. III (motor)
Diencephalon
Telencephalic vesicle
Optic cup
Infundibulum
Cranial n. XI (motor)
Cranial n. XII (motor)
1st cervical n. (sensory and motor)
Hindbrain (myelencephalon)
Forebrain (prosencephalon)

Cerebral hemisphere (neocortex)
Outline of diencephalon (overgrown by cerebral hemispheres)
Hypophysis (pituitary gland)
Mesencephalon
Cerebellum (metencephalon)
Pons (metencephalon)
Optic n.
Medulla oblongata (myelencephalon)
Olfactory lobe (paleocortex)
Cervical enlargement of spinal cord
Lumbosacral enlargement of spinal cord

JOHN A.CRAIG—AD
©ICN

Central nervous system: cranial and spinal nerves at 36 days

Central nervous system at 3 months

ADULT DERIVATIVES OF THE FOREBRAIN, MIDBRAIN, AND HINDBRAIN			
Forebrain	Telencephalon	Cerebral hemispheres Olfactory cortex Hippocampus Basal ganglia/corpus striatum Lateral and 3rd ventricles	Nerves: Olfactory (I)
	Diencephalon	Optic cup/nerves Thalamus Hypothalamus Mammillary bodies Part of 3rd ventricle	Optic (II)
Midbrain	Mesencephalon	Tectum Cerebral aqueduct Red nucleus Substantia nigra Crus cerebelli	Oculomotor (III) Trochlear (IV)
Hindbrain	Metencephalon	Pons Cerebellum	Trigeminal (V) Abducens (VI) Facial (VII) Vestibulocochlear (VIII) Glossopharyngeal (IX) Vagus (X) Hypoglossal (XI)
	Myelencephalon	Medulla oblongata	

Clinical Correlation

Craniosynostosis   *Anatomy on pp. 545, 546, 642*

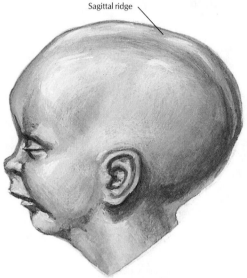

Sagittal ridge

Scaphocephaly due to sagittal craniosynostosis

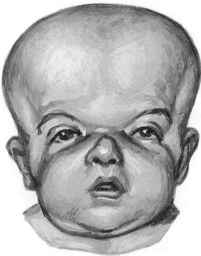

Limitation of growth of sagittal suture

Brachycephaly due to coronal craniosynostosis

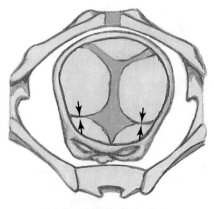

Limitation of growth of coronal sutures

JOHN A. CRAIG—MD
© ICON
LEARNING SYSTEMS

As the brain grows, so does the neurocranium, by bone deposition along suture lines. If this process is interrupted (because of unknown reasons or genetic factors), the cranium may compensate by depositing more bone along other sutures. If the sagittal suture closes prematurely, growth in width is altered, so growth occurs lengthwise and leads to a long, narrow cranium; coronal and lambdoid suture closure results in a short, wide cranium. The disorder occurs in approximately 1 in 2000 births and is more common in males than in females.

Embryology: Pharyngeal Arch Development

Pharyngeal arches develop from the vertebrate ancestral gill (branchial) arch system as an evolutionary adaptation to terrestrial life. The original six pairs of arches develop into four pairs, with a cranial nerve, the muscles it innervates, a cartilage/bone element, and an aortic arch associated with each arch.

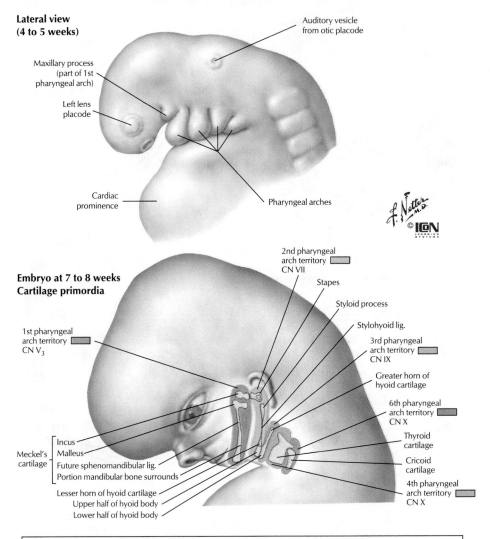

Lateral view (4 to 5 weeks)

Auditory vesicle from otic placode

Maxillary process (part of 1st pharyngeal arch)

Left lens placode

Cardiac prominence

Pharyngeal arches

Embryo at 7 to 8 weeks Cartilage primordia

2nd pharyngeal arch territory CN VII

Stapes

Styloid process

Stylohyoid lig.

1st pharyngeal arch territory CN V₃

3rd pharyngeal arch territory CN IX

Greater horn of hyoid cartilage

6th pharyngeal arch territory CN X

Thyroid cartilage

Meckel's cartilage
- Incus
- Malleus
- Future sphenomandibular lig.
- Portion mandibular bone surrounds

Cricoid cartilage

4th pharyngeal arch territory CN X

Lesser horn of hyoid cartilage
Upper half of hyoid body
Lower half of hyoid body

PHARYNGEAL ARCH BONES AND CARTILAGE	
Arch No.	Derivatives of Arch Cartilages
1	Malleus, incus, sphenomandibular ligament
2	Stapes, styloid process, stylohyoid ligament, upper half of hyoid
3	Lower half and greater horns of hyoid
4	Thyroid and epiglottic cartligages
6	Cricoid, arytenoid, and corniculate cartilages

Embryology: Pharyngeal Pouch Derivatives

Sagittal section

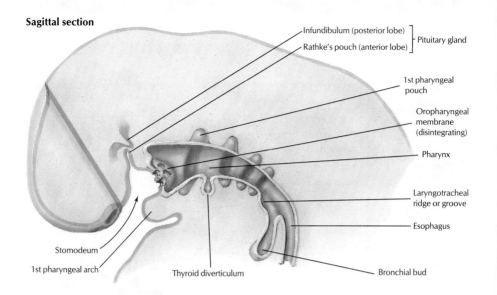

Infundibulum (posterior lobe)
Rathke's pouch (anterior lobe)
Pituitary gland

1st pharyngeal pouch

Oropharyngeal membrane (disintegrating)

Pharynx

Laryngotracheal ridge or groove

Esophagus

Stomodeum

1st pharyngeal arch

Thyroid diverticulum

Bronchial bud

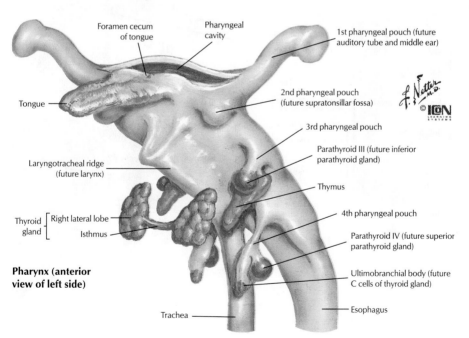

Foramen cecum of tongue

Pharyngeal cavity

1st pharyngeal pouch (future auditory tube and middle ear)

Tongue

2nd pharyngeal pouch (future supratonsillar fossa)

3rd pharyngeal pouch

Parathyroid III (future inferior parathyroid gland)

Thymus

Laryngotracheal ridge (future larynx)

4th pharyngeal pouch

Thyroid gland

Right lateral lobe

Isthmus

Parathyroid IV (future superior parathyroid gland)

Pharynx (anterior view of left side)

Ultimobranchial body (future C cells of thyroid gland)

Esophagus

Trachea

Internally, each arch is also associated with an endoderm-derived pharyngeal pouch, an outpocketing of the foregut in the head and neck. The four pharyngeal pouches give rise to various important structures, but the thyroid gland develops as its own diverticulum from the tongue and migrates to its final position anterior to the trachea.

Clinical Correlation

Pharyngeal Arch and Pouch Anomalies   *Anatomy on pp. 644, 645*

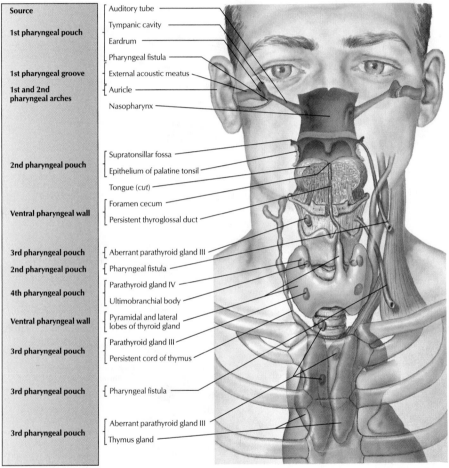

Source

1st pharyngeal pouch
- Auditory tube
- Tympanic cavity
- Eardrum
- Pharyngeal fistula

1st pharyngeal groove
- External acoustic meatus

1st and 2nd pharyngeal arches
- Auricle
- Nasopharynx

2nd pharyngeal pouch
- Supratonsillar fossa
- Epithelium of palatine tonsil
- Tongue (*cut*)

Ventral pharyngeal wall
- Foramen cecum
- Persistent thyroglossal duct

3rd pharyngeal pouch
- Aberrant parathyroid gland III

2nd pharyngeal pouch
- Pharyngeal fistula

4th pharyngeal pouch
- Parathyroid gland IV
- Ultimobranchial body

Ventral pharyngeal wall
- Pyramidal and lateral lobes of thyroid gland

3rd pharyngeal pouch
- Parathyroid gland III
- Persistent cord of thymus

3rd pharyngeal pouch
- Pharyngeal fistula

3rd pharyngeal pouch
- Aberrant parathyroid gland III
- Thymus gland

Most anomalies of the pharyngeal apparatus involve fistulas, cysts, or ectopic glandular tissue. Some common anomalies and their sources—the associated pharyngeal pouch or wall—are shown here.

Embryology: Facial Development

The face develops by fusion of an unpaired frontonasal prominence with bilateral maxillary, nasal, and mandibular prominences that meet in the midline. Fusion along the midline by portions of the maxilla and palatine bone gives rise to the hard palate.

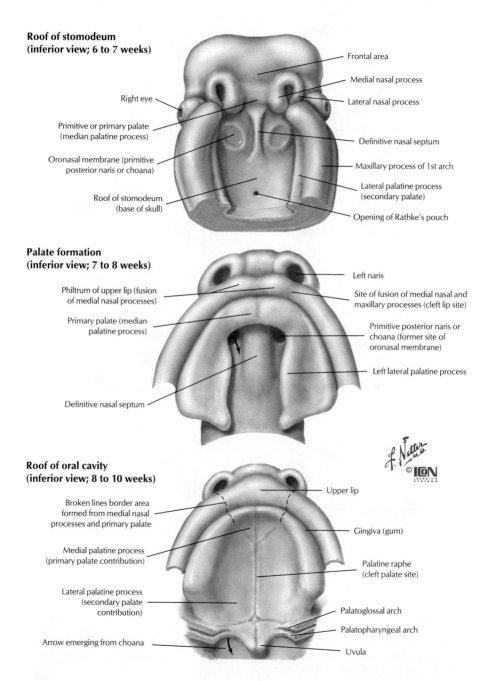

Roof of stomodeum (inferior view; 6 to 7 weeks)

- Frontal area
- Medial nasal process
- Right eye
- Lateral nasal process
- Primitive or primary palate (median palatine process)
- Definitive nasal septum
- Oronasal membrane (primitive posterior naris or choana)
- Maxillary process of 1st arch
- Roof of stomodeum (base of skull)
- Lateral palatine process (secondary palate)
- Opening of Rathke's pouch

Palate formation (inferior view; 7 to 8 weeks)

- Left naris
- Philtrum of upper lip (fusion of medial nasal processes)
- Site of fusion of medial nasal and maxillary processes (cleft lip site)
- Primary palate (median palatine process)
- Primitive posterior naris or choana (former site of oronasal membrane)
- Left lateral palatine process
- Definitive nasal septum

Roof of oral cavity (inferior view; 8 to 10 weeks)

- Upper lip
- Broken lines border area formed from medial nasal processes and primary palate
- Gingiva (gum)
- Medial palatine process (primary palate contribution)
- Palatine raphe (cleft palate site)
- Lateral palatine process (secondary palate contribution)
- Palatoglossal arch
- Palatopharyngeal arch
- Arrow emerging from choana
- Uvula

Clinical Correlation

Congenital Anomalies of the Oral Cavity   *Anatomy on pp. 647*

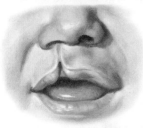

Unilateral cleft lip—partial

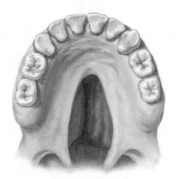

Partial cleft of palate

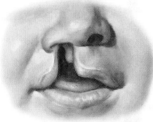

Unilateral cleft of primary palate—
complete, involving lip and alveolar ridge

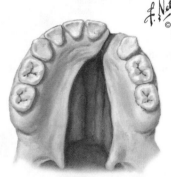

**Complete cleft of secondary palate
and unilateral cleft of primary palate**

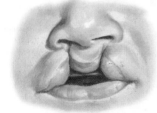

Bilateral cleft lip

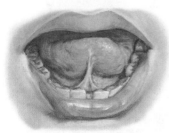

Ankyloglossia—restricted tongue movement
from a short lingual frenulum

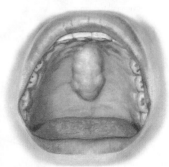

Torus palatinus—bone deposition on palate

Because the face and oral cavity develop largely by midline fusion of various prominences, incomplete or failed fusion can lead to cleft formation (lips and palate) or
anomalous features (ankyloglossia, torus formations). The etiology is multifactorial,
but genetics seems to play some role.

Review Questions

What are the boundaries of the posterior cervical triangle, and what nerve innervates the muscles that define this region?	Trapezius, SCM, and middle third of the clavicle bound this triangle, and both muscles are innervated by CN XI (spinal accessory), which courses through the triangle.
What nerve(s) innervate the infrahyoid muscles (strap muscles) of the neck?	Ansa cervicalis (C1-C3) of the cervical plexus.
Where can one find the phrenic nerve in the neck, and what does it innervate?	The phrenic nerve (C3-C5) appears on the anterior surface of the anterior scalene muscle and innervates the diaphragm.
What is the relationship of the subclavian vessels to the scalene muscles?	The subclavian artery passes between the anterior and middle scalenes; the vein passes anterior to the anterior scalene muscle.
What are the arterial branches of the thyrocervical trunk?	Inferior thyroid, transverse cervical, and suprascapular.
What are the two terminal branches of the external carotid artery?	Maxillary and superficial temporal.
What is the retropharyngeal space, and why is it important?	A potential space between the alar and prevertebral fascial layers. An infection in this space can spread superiorly to the base of the skull or inferiorly into the posterior mediastinum.
Identify several signs of Graves' disease (hyperthyroidism).	Thyrotoxicosis, lid lag, exophthalmos, pretibial myxedema, and goiter.
During thyroid surgery, what nerve must be identified and preserved?	Recurrent laryngeal nerve, which innervates the muscles of the larynx.
Clinically, why are the posterior cricoarytenoid muscles important?	They are the only laryngeal muscles that abduct the vocal folds, keeping the rima glottidis open for respiration.
What is the principal function of the prevertebral neck muscles?	Flexion of the neck.
For each foramen below, identify the nerve(s) that pass through that foramen. Superior orbital fissure: Rotundum: Ovale: Internal acoustic meatus: Jugular:	Oculomotor, trochlear, abducent, and V_1 V_2 V_3, lesser petrosal (occasionally) Facial and vestibulocochlear Glossopharyngeal, vagus, and spinal accessory
What are the four types of skull fractures?	Linear, comminuted, diastasis, and basilar.
What is a Le Fort I fracture of the face?	Horizontal detachment of the maxilla at the level of the nasal floor, resulting in a free-floating maxillary segment.
What type of joint is the TMJ?	Modified hinge joint that also has some gliding action.
Why do mandibular fractures often present with multiple fracture lines?	The U shape of the mandible offers two potentially vulnerable sites for fracture, which include the canine and third molar areas.

Review Questions

In Bell's palsy, if the facial nerve is lesioned unilaterally in the facial canal, what symptoms result?	Facial paralysis, loss of taste in the anterior portion of the tongue, hyperacusis, and decreased salivation. All of these symptoms occur ipsilaterally.
In trigeminal neuralgia, one of the trigger points is the lower eyelid. What cutaneous branch is stimulated?	Infraorbital branch of V2.
Shingles (herpes zoster) commonly affects one or several contiguous unilateral dermatomes. What sensory sites are most often involved?	Generally, T5 to L2 dermatomes and CNs V and VII.
Approximately how much CSF is produced a day, and where is it reabsorbed into the venous system?	Approximately 500 ml/day is produced; CSF is reabsorbed by the arachnoid granulations (most significant site) and small capillaries along the brainstem and spinal cord.
Trace venous blood in the superior petrosal sinus to the right atrium.	Superior petrosal sinus to sigmoid sinus to internal jugular vein to brachiocephalic vein (right or left) to superior vena cava to right atrium.
If a pituitary adenoma expands into the cavernous sinus, which nerves may be vulnerable to compression?	CNs III, IV, VI, and/or V1 and V2.
The central sulcus of the brain divides what two functional regions?	The anterior primary motor cortex from the posterior primary somatosensory cortex.
What is the distribution of the posterior cerebral artery?	It arises from the basilar artery and supplies the inferior cerebrum and occipital lobe.
What artery demonstrates the highest predilection for cerebral aneurysm?	Anterior communicating, followed by the posterior communicating artery of the circle of Willis.

For each intracranial hematoma, suggest the most likely vascular source.
    Epidural:
    Subdural:
    Subarachnoid:
	
	Arterial, usually the middle meningeal or its branches
	Venous, often the cortical bridging veins
	Arterial, often from saccular (berry) aneurysms

Why might one hear an orbital bruit after a cavernous sinus fistula?	Bleeding into the sinus results in an increase in venous pressure draining the blood from the sinus, in this case via the ophthalmic veins, which communicates directly with the sinus and with veins of the pterygoid plexus and face.
How are strokes classified, and which type is most common?	Ischemic (80% of strokes) and hemorrhagic.
If the IC artery becomes occluded in the carotid canal, how might blood reach the brain and orbit?	Via branches of the external carotid artery (facial and maxillary and their branches), which will supply the ophthalmic and fill the IC by reversal of blood flow, and by the circle of Willis (vertebrals and contralateral IC arteries).
What are the two most common types of brain tumors?	Gliomas (50% in adults and higher in children) and meningiomas (20%).

Review Questions

How does herpes simplex virus gain access to the brain?	The virus can gain access from cutaneous or mucosal infection and be transported in a retrograde fashion to the sensory nerve ganglia, where the virus replicates and becomes latent, before reactivating and infecting the brain by spreading in an antero-grade fashion along meningeal branches of the nerve (often CN V, or spinal meningeal branches).
Trace the pathway of tears from the lacrimal gland to the nasal cavity.	Lacrimal gland (CN VII secretomotor fibers) to lacrimal ducts to bulbar conjunctival and corneal surfaces, then to lacrimal lake, to lacrimal punctum (superior and inferior) to lacrimal canaliculi to lacrimal sac, down the nasolacrimal duct, and into the inferior meatus of the inferior nasal concha.
During clinical testing of the extraocular muscles, which two muscles elevate the eye and, what nerves innervate them?	SR (CN III) and IO (CN III), in abduction and adduction, respectively.
What clinical signs would be present if the oculomotor nerve was unilaterally damaged?	Ptosis (levator palpebrae superioris muscle), abduction and depression of the globe (lateral rectus and superior oblique muscles unopposed), and a dilated pupil (mydriasis) (loss of parasympathetics) ipsilaterally. The patient would probably have diplopia and might lose accommodation ability.
What site on the retina is responsible for the most acute vision?	Fovea centralis in the macula lutea.
What causes bloodshot eyes?	Irritants that cause local dilation of conjunctival vessels (conjunctival hyperemia).

Define these refractive disorders.
  Myopia:
 	
  Hyperopia:
 	
  Presbyopia:
	Nearsightedness; difficulty seeing distant objects clearly
	Farsightedness; difficulty seeing close objects clearly
	Progressive loss of ability to accommodate the lens and focus on close objects clearly

What is glaucoma, and which type is most common?	Resistance to the outflow of aqueous humor, usually primary open angle, resulting from impedance at the canal of Schlemm or of the trabecular meshwork, or from venous back-pressure.
In a blow-out fracture of the orbit, what nerve is particularly vulnerable to injury?	Blow-out fractures involve the orbital floor, placing the infraorbital nerve (V_2) at risk.
Account for each clinical sign of Horner's syndrome.	Ptosis: loss of innervation of the superior tarsal (smooth) muscle (distal part of levator palpebrae muscle of upper eyelid) Miosis: loss of innervation of the dilator muscle of the pupil Anhydrosis: loss of innervation of sweat glands Flushed face: unopposed vasodilation of cutaneous vessels (each sign represents loss of sympathetic innervation)
What is the action of the medial pterygoid muscles?	Elevate the mandible; acting together, they protrude the mandible, and acting alternately, they produce a grinding motion.

Review Questions

Which branches of the maxillary artery supply the teeth and gums?	Superior alveolar (posterior, middle, and anterior) to maxillary teeth and inferior alveolar to the mandibular teeth.
Pain in the ear from acute otitis media is conveyed by which cranial nerve?	Tympanic branch of the glossopharyngeal.
In the Rinne test, where is the tuning fork placed to assess bone conduction hearing?	The fork's handle is placed on the mastoid process.
What are some primary causes of peripheral vertigo?	Infection, impaired resorption of endolymph, accumulation of otoconial debris in the semicircular canals, and tumors of the vestibulocochlear nerve.
What deficits might be expected if the chorda tympani nerve is damaged?	Loss of salivary secretion in the submandibular and sublingual salivary glands and loss of taste from the anterior two thirds of the tongue.
During swallowing, which muscle pulls the tongue back and upward?	Styloglossus.
Identify the five nerves innervating the tongue.	Motor: CN XII; sensory: CN V_3 (anterior), CN IX (posterior), and CN X (epiglottis); taste: CN VII (anterior) and CN IX (posterior).
What is the innervation of the lateral nasal wall?	Sensory: CN V_2; olfaction: CN I; secretomotor to glands: CN VII.
Which paranasal sinuses drain into the middle meatus beneath the middle nasal concha?	Frontal, maxillary, and anterior and middle ethmoid sinuses.
What nerve is formed by the union of the deep and greater petrosal nerves?	Nerve of the pterygoid canal (vidian), composed of postganglionic sympathetics (from SCG) and preganglionic parasympathetics (from CN VII).
What are the three subdivisions of the pharynx?	Nasopharynx, oropharynx, and laryngopharynx (called hypopharynx by most clinicians).
Which of the pharyngeal constrictor muscles lies posterior to the hyoid bone, and what is its innervation?	Middle constrictor, innervated by pharyngeal plexus (motor via the vagus) and sensory by the glossopharyngeal to the pharyngeal plexus.
What is an adenoid?	Swollen, inflamed nasopharyngeal tonsil caused by acute or chronic infection.
What is Waldeyer's tonsillar ring?	A ring of lymphoid tissues around the oropharynx, including the palatine, lingual, and nasopharyngeal tonsils.
Why might pain in the throat be referred to the ear?	Both receive sensory innervation from CN IX.
Lymph from the head drains ultimately into what group of lymph nodes?	Deep cervical lymph nodes; on the left side, these nodes drain into the thoracic duct, and on the right side, they drain into the subclavian duct.
Which portion of the trigeminal nerve conveys efferent, afferent, and proprioceptive fibers?	Mandibular division.
Where are the neurons located that give rise to all postganglionic sympathetic fibers innervating the head?	Superior cervical ganglion.

Review Questions

The facial nerve is associated with which pharyngeal arch?	Second arch.
Developmentally, the hindbrain gives rise to what CNS regions?	Metencephalon (pons and cerebellum) and myelencephalon (medulla oblongata).
Which pharyngeal pouch gives rise to the inferior parathyroid glands?	Third pouch. They actually migrate further than the superior pair of glands and can be found inferior to the thyroid lobes (and vary in number).
What connection may remain between the thyroid gland and the tongue?	Persistent thyroglossal duct between the pyramidal lobe and the foramen cecum.

How would you clinically test each CN?

NERVE	EXAMINATION	FINDINGS/DEFICITS
I	Test smell in each nostril	Trauma, infection leading to Hyposmia (partial loss) Anosmia (total loss) Hyperosmia (exaggerated) Dysosmia (distorted sense)
II	Test acuity, fields, optic disc	Altered acuity or blindness, hemianopsia, papilledema, optic atrophy
II, III	Pupillary reflex to light	Horner's syndrome, tonic pupil, Argyll Robertson pupil, gaze paresis
III, IV, IV	Test ocular movements	Diplopia, strabismus, nystagmus, ophthalmoplegia, nerve palsies
V	Test sensory over its three divisions, motor to jaw muscles, corneal reflex	Lesion to higher centers or nerve Corneal reflex tests integrity ofV1 (and VII for blink)
VII	Test muscles of facial expression, taste anterior two thirds tongue	Lesion centrally or to nerve as in Bell's palsy, parotid tumor, MS
VIII	Weber test (lateralization) and Rinne test (air-bone conduction)	Perceptive or conductive deafness, tinnitus, vertigo
IX, X	Gag reflex, swallowing, soft palate elevation with "ahhh"	Usually central lesions, stroke, malignancy, motor neuron disease
XI	Rotate head against resistance, elevate shoulders	SCM/trapezius weakness/ atrophy, tumor, spasmodic torticollis
XII	Inspect and protrude tongue, listen to patient's articulation	Unilateral nerve lesion: tongue protrudes to affected side, atrophy

Frank H. Netter, MD

Frank H. Netter was born in 1906 in New York City. He studied art at the Art Student's League and the National Academy of Design before entering medical school at New York University, where he received his MD degree in 1931. During his student years, Dr. Netter's notebook sketches attracted the attention of the medical faculty and other physicians, allowing him to augment his income by illustrating articles and textbooks. He continued illustrating as a sideline after establishing a surgical practice in 1933, but he ultimately opted to give up his practice in favor of a full-time commitment to art. After service in the United States Army during World War II, Dr. Netter began his long collaboration with the CIBA Pharmaceutical Company (now Novartis Phamaceuticals). This 45-year partnership resulted in the production of the extraordinary collection of medical art so familiar to physicians and other medical professionals worldwide.

Icon Learning Systems acquired the Netter Collection in July 2000 and continues to update Dr. Netter's original paintings and to add newly commissioned paintings by artists trained in the style of Dr. Netter.

Dr. Netter's works are among the finest examples of the use of illustration in the teaching of medical concepts. The 13-book *Netter Collection of Medical Illustrations*, which includes the greater part of the more than 20,000 paintings created by Dr. Netter, became and remains one of the most famous medical works ever published. *The Netter Atlas of Human Anatomy*, first published in 1989, presents the anatomical paintings from the Netter Collection. Now translated into 11 languages, it is the anatomy atlas of choice among medical and health professions students the world over.

The Netter illustrations are appreciated not only for their aesthetic qualities, but more importantly, for their intellectual content. As Dr. Netter wrote in 1949 "...clarification of a subject is the aim and goal of illustration. No matter how beautifully painted, how delicately and subtly rendered a subject may be, it is of little value as a *medical illustration* if it does not serve to make clear some medical point." Dr. Netter's planning, conception, point of view, and approach are what inform his paintings and what makes them so intellectually valuable.

Frank H. Netter, MD, physician and artist, died in 1991.

Contributing Illustrators

In addition to the art done by Dr. Frank Netter, the following medical artists were involved in either the conceptualization or painting of the art on the following pages:

KIP CARTER
378, 381

JOHN CRAIG, MD
24, 30, 32, 34, 49, 55, 56, 57, 58, 83, 85, 86, 87, 96, 113, 174, 181, 186, 188, 190, 191, 193, 195, 206, 225, 228, 244, 245, 266, 282, 283, 285, 302, 303, 304, 305, 306, 307, 331, 345, 346, 361, 362, 380, 440, 442, 477, 491, 492, 493, 499, 502, 506, 510, 517, 563, 584, 585, 590, 592, 611, 612

DRAGONFLY MEDIA GROUP
14, 15, 17

ENID HATTON
601, 611, 612

CRAIG LUCE
162, 165

CARLOS A. MACHADO, MD
2, 3, 4, 5, 6, 7, 8, 9, 13, 19, 21, 22, 23, 27, 28, 30, 31, 32, 34, 45, 46, 47, 51, 54, 55, 56, 57, 66, 83, 85, 87, 88, 89, 96, 106, 124, 141, 170, 172, 174, 175, 182, 204, 211, 212, 244, 245, 278, 282, 284, 285, 300, 323, 331, 344, 345, 346, 350, 354, 362, 363, 364, 366, 373, 376, 379, 440, 442, 466, 467, 470, 471, 477, 495, 498, 511, 611, 612

DAVID MASCARO
24, 282, 283, 361, 362, 411, 491, 563, 590, 614

JAMES PERKINS
10, 18, 20, 33, 38, 40, 42, 44, 99, 100

STEVE MOON
357

FRANK NETTER
411, 591